The

HUMAN
BRAIN

An Introduction to Its
Functional Anatomy

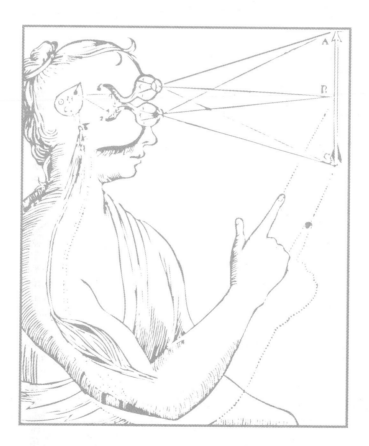

Reproduction of a woodcut in *De Homine,* 1662, by René Descartes, who thought that the pineal gland was the seat of the soul, monitoring the movement of "animal spirits" in sensory nerves and controlling the movement of animal spirits through motor nerves.

The brain, and the brain alone, is the source of our pleasures, joys, laughter, and amusement, as well as our sorrow, pain, grief, and tears. It is especially the organ we use to think and learn, see and hear, to distinguish the ugly from the beautiful, the bad from the good, and the pleasant from the unpleasant. The brain is also the seat of madness and delirium, of the fears and terrors that assail by night or by day, of sleeplessness, awkward mistakes, and thoughts that will not come, of pointless anxieties, forgetfulness, and eccentricities.

Hippocrates, ca. 400 BC

The human mind can be described as a slow-clockrate modified-digital machine with multiple distinguishable parallel processing, all working in salt water.

Philip Morrison: The mind of the machine, **Technology Review 75:17, 1973**

One of the difficulties in understanding the brain is that it is like nothing so much as a lump of porridge.

R.L. Gregory: **Eye and brain: the psychology of seeing,** *New York, 1966, McGraw-Hill*

Were I to await perfection,
My book would never be finished.

Tai T'ung, 13th century Chinese scholar: The six scripts: principles of chinese writing.
Quoted in Edmunds LN Jr: **Cellular and molecular bases of biological clocks,**
New York, 1988, Springer-Verlag

The
HUMAN
BRAIN

An Introduction to Its Functional Anatomy

John Nolte, PhD
Professor of Cell Biology and Anatomy
Director, Division of Academic Resources
The University of Arizona College of Medicine
Tucson, Arizona

THREE-DIMENSIONAL BRAIN RECONSTRUCTIONS
by John Sundsten, PhD
University of Washington
School of Medicine
Seattle, Washington

Fourth Edition

with 567 illustrations

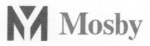

St. Louis Baltimore Boston Carlsbad Chicago Minneapolis New York Philadelphia Portland
London Milan Sydney Tokyo Toronto

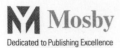

Mosby
Dedicated to Publishing Excellence

A Times Mirror
Company

Publisher: Richard Furn
Editor: Beverly Copland
Senior Developmental Editor: Linda Caldwell
Project Manager: Carol Sullivan Weis
Production Editor: Karen M. Rehwinkel
Designer: Jen Marmarinos
Manufacturing Manager: David Graybill

Fourth Edition
Copyright © 1999 by Mosby, Inc.

Printed in the United States of America
Composition and Lithography/color film by Graphic World, Inc.
Printing/binding by Von Hoffmann Press, Inc.

Mosby-Year Book, Inc.
11830 Westline Industrial Drive
St. Louis, Missouri 63146

Library of Congress Cataloging-in-Publication Data
Nolte, John.
   The human brain : an introduction to its functional anatomy / John
Nolte ; three-dimensional brain reconstructions by John Sundsten. --
4th ed.
      p.   cm.
   Includes bibliographical references and index.
   ISBN 0-8151-8911-7
   1. Neuroanatomy.   2. Brain—Anatomy.   I. Title.
   [DNLM: 1. Nervous System—anatomy & histology.   2. Brain—anatomy
& histology.   WL 101 N789h 1998]
QM451.N64   1998
611.8—dc21
DNLM/DLC
for Library of Congress   98-17069
                                                              CIP

98 99 00 01 02/9 8 7 6 5 4 3 2 1

PREFACE

As the Decade of the Brain draws to a close, growth in our knowledge of neurobiology continues unabated. New techniques allow the exploration of the nervous system at virtually all levels, ranging from watching the behavior of individual ion channels in neuronal membranes to watching the areal changes in blood flow in the brains of subjects as they perform various mental tasks. These changes provided the incentive for a new edition. In addition, back in what seems like a former life I started out as a photoreceptor physiologist, and the sparse consideration of neurophysiology in earlier editions has always represented to me an uncomfortable omission. The Human Neuroscience course at The University of Arizona has become a wonderful, long-sought melding of neural structure and function, and it motivated me to add a substantial amount of neurophysiology to this edition.

As a result, many major changes have been incorporated into this new edition.

- **Two chapters are brand new:** Chapter 7, Electrical Signaling by Neurons, and Chapter 8, Synaptic Transmission Between Neurons.
- Other topics were expanded to include additional coverage of neurophysiological and clinical topics and are presented as separate chapters: Chapter 2, Development of the Nervous System; Chapter 13, The Chemical Senses of Taste and Smell; Chapter 14, Hearing and Balance: The Eighth Cranial Nerve; and Chapter 21, Control of Eye Movements.
- Illustrations, images, and design are in **full color.** Vivid color illustrations and brain images present the complexity of neuroanatomical structures and physiological processes clearly and graphically. A full-color design enhances textual presentation and highlights important content.
- **Expanded coverage of neurophysiology** has been woven throughout the book, providing an integrated presentation of neurological mechanisms.
- **New clinical content** has been added, including many images depicting neurological disorders, providing real-life application of neuroanatomy and neurophysiological concepts.
- A new layout and design highlights and emphasizes important information. **Summary statement headings** describe and summarize key section concepts and are also provided as an **outline that introduces each chapter.** Many more tables set off significant data and content. Boxes highlight ancillary topics. Key terms are boldface.
- Chapters have been reorganized and streamlined, so that there are more chapters (24) with fewer pages in most. Information in each chapter is more accessible and manageable.
- There are **nearly 600 illustrations:** Those carried over from the last edition have been reworked and many new ones added.

I tried to follow the same principles used since the inception of this book. Although the book has grown in length, a minimum of detail has been added. In writing or updating various sections, I tried not to include facts simply for their own sake. Rather, new observations and concepts were added where they help to illuminate function. Because much of our new knowledge has been made possible by new techniques, illustrations of these techniques have been maintained, updated, and to some extent distributed throughout the book: anatomical labeling and tract-tracing methods, magnetic resonance imaging, positron emission tomography, and electrophysiological techniques are presented in abundance. The Suggested Readings have been updated, but the same philosophy was retained: the intent in choosing references was not only to document recent findings but also to provide access through those references to the vast neuroscientific literature. For these reasons, the emphasis is on recent reviews and research papers. Many classic and scientifically more important papers have been omitted, although some older or peripherally-related articles that make interesting reading are listed.

The challenge of writing a clear, accurate, up-to-date survey of human neurobiology is a formidable one, and it is inevitable that I have committed errors of hyperbole, obfuscation, and ignorance. I welcome the comments and suggestions of students and colleagues who use this book. They will improve my knowledge and my teaching, and make the next edition that much better. A comment card is included in the back of the book for this purpose.

John Nolte
Tucson, Arizona

ACKNOWLEDGMENTS

As in the case of the first three editions, this revision was far from a solitary accomplishment, and I am indebted to many. Friends and colleagues from around the world kindly provided illustrations. The sources are acknowledged, with my gratitude, in the figure legends, but I would especially like to thank Jay Angevine for giving me access to the wonderful Weigert-stained brain sections and for being a mainstay for me here in Arizona in discussing things neuroanatomical; John Sundsten, for the stunning three-dimensional reconstructions that appear throughout the book and for the fun we had making them; Pam Eller, for preparing the brainstem sections used in Chapters 11 through 15 and elsewhere and for being my buddy all these years; Ray Carmody for his unstinting help with clinical images over the last 7 years; Nate McMullen and Allen Bell, for the light micrographs in Chapter 1 and elsewhere; Drs. Ennio Pannese and Alan Peters for the beautiful electron micrographs; Grant Dahmer and Norm Koelling for the brain dissections; and Ken Catania for the mole stories and pictures. Thanks also to Jay Angevine, Dave Asher, Pam Eller, Tom Finger, Ted Glattke, Jill Keller, Norm Koelling, Gail Koshland, Chris Leadem, Nate McMullen, Erwin Montgomery, Frank Porreca, Carol Swanson, Lyn Turkstra, Gary Wenk, and Steve Wright for their helpful and valued comments on various parts of the manuscript. Drs. Allen Siegel, J.F. Rodriquez-Sierra, Susan Billings-Gagliardi, and Frank Willard reviewed the third edition and made suggestions for this new edition. Thanks to my teaching colleagues in Arizona for their enthusiasm and good humor and for new ways of looking at things; and to the students of The University of Arizona College of Medicine, who use the book and offer many helpful comments and suggestions, and who by their curiosity and caring continue to make teaching fun. Thanks also to the ever-evolving cast of characters at Mosby for their patience and support. Finally, my love and thanks to Carol for sharing me with The Book for the last couple of years.

John Nolte
Tucson, Arizona
February, 1998

CONTENTS

The

HUMAN
BRAIN

An Introduction to Its
Functional Anatomy

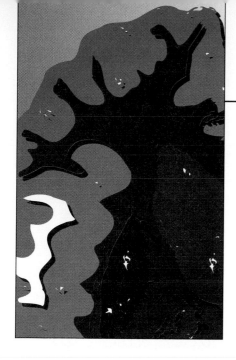

CHAPTER 1

INTRODUCTION TO THE NERVOUS SYSTEM

The object of this book is to present and explain some basic anatomical facts about how the brain is put together and to discuss a few aspects of how it works. This introductory chapter describes in a very general way the subdivisions of the nervous system, then focuses on the cellular elements found within it and some anatomical specializations that adapt these cellular elements to their respective functions.

THE NERVOUS SYSTEM HAS CENTRAL AND PERIPHERAL PARTS

The nervous system is broadly subdivided into the **peripheral nervous system** and the **central nervous system** (Figure 1-1). The peripheral nervous system (PNS) is the collection of spinal and cranial nerves whose branches infiltrate virtually all parts of the body, conveying messages

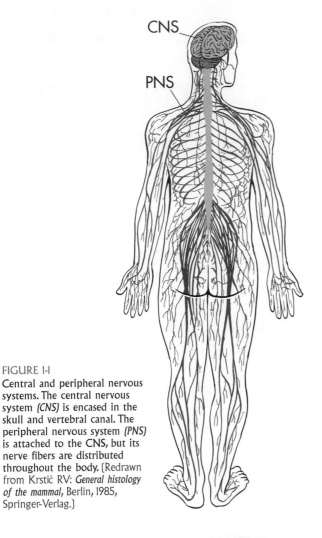

FIGURE I-I
Central and peripheral nervous
systems. The central nervous
system *(CNS)* is encased in the
skull and vertebral canal. The
peripheral nervous system *(PNS)*
is attached to the CNS, but its
nerve fibers are distributed
throughout the body. (Redrawn
from Krstić RV: *General histology
of the mammal,* Berlin, 1985,
Springer-Verlag.)

to and from the central nervous system. The central nervous system (CNS) is composed of the **brain** and the **spinal cord** (Figure 1-2). The brain itself has multiple subdivisions and is composed of the **cerebrum,** the **cerebellum,** and the **brainstem.** The cerebrum, in turn, is composed of the two massive **cerebral hemispheres** (separated from one another by the **longitudinal fissure**) and the **diencephalon★;** in an intact human brain most of the diencephalon is hidden from view by the massive cerebral hemispheres. The brainstem is that part of the CNS, exclusive of the cerebellum, that lies between the cerebrum and the spinal cord.

THE PRINCIPAL CELLULAR ELEMENTS OF THE NERVOUS SYSTEM ARE NEURONS AND GLIAL CELLS

Despite the large size and widespread distribution of the nervous system, it contains only two principal categories of cells—**nerve cells,** or **neurons,** which are the information-processing and signaling elements, and **glial cells,** which play a variety of supporting roles. Both neurons and glial cells are present in enormous numbers. There are around 100 billion neurons in the

★ Much seemingly arcane neuroanatomical terminology has a Latin or Greek derivation that actually makes sense. In this case, *encephalon* is Greek for "in the head" (i.e., "brain"). *Diencephalon* means "in-between-brain," signifying that this part of the CNS is interposed between the cerebral hemispheres and the brainstem.

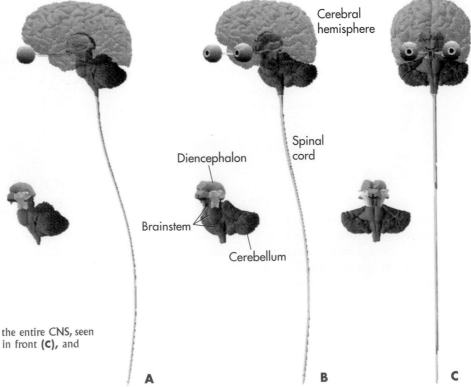

FIGURE I-2
Three-dimensional reconstruction of the entire CNS, seen from the left side **(A),** from directly in front **(C),** and from halfway between **(B).**

human nervous system and several times that many glial cells.

Neurons Come in a Variety of Sizes and Shapes, But All Are Variations on the Same Theme

Neurons are in the business of conveying information. They do so by a combination of electrical and chemical signaling mechanisms: electrical signals are used to convey signals rapidly from one part of a neuron to another, whereas chemical messengers are typically used to carry signals between neurons. Hence there are anatomically specialized zones for receiving, transmitting, and passing on information (Figure 1-3, Table 1-1). All neurons have a cell body (or **soma,** or **perikaryon★**) that supports the metabolic and synthetic needs of the rest of the neuron. Most neurons have a series of branching, tapering processes called **dendrites** that receive information from other neurons via **synaptic contacts** (or **synapses**) and one long, cylindrical process called an **axon** that conducts information away from the cell body. The axon gives rise

---

★*Karyon* is Greek for "nucleus," and, strictly speaking, the perikaryon is the cytoplasm surrounding the nucleus of a neuron. However, the term is commonly used to refer to the entire cell body.

Table I-I   Parts of a Typical Neuron

Part	Description	Major organelles	Primary function(s)
Dendrites	Tapered extensions of cell body	Cytoskeleton, mitochondria	Receive information from other neurons
Soma (cell body)	May have one, two, or many processes; typically one axon, many dendrites	Nucleus, Golgi apparatus, Nissl substance, cytoskeleton, mitochondria	Synthesize macromolecules
Axon	Single, cylindrical; may be many cm long; may be myelinated or unmyelinated	Cytoskeleton, mitochondria, transport vesicles	Conduct information to other neurons
Synaptic endings	Vesicle-filled apposition to part of another neuron; most are axodendritic or axosomatic, but other configurations occur	Synaptic vesicles, mitochondria	Transmit information to other neurons

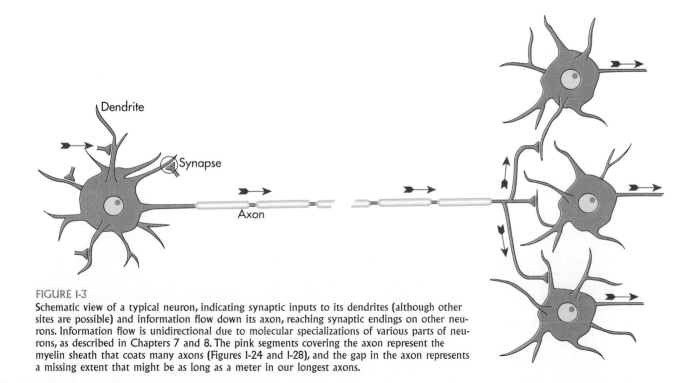

FIGURE I-3
Schematic view of a typical neuron, indicating synaptic inputs to its dendrites (although other sites are possible) and information flow down its axon, reaching synaptic endings on other neurons. Information flow is unidirectional due to molecular specializations of various parts of neurons, as described in Chapters 7 and 8. The pink segments covering the axon represent the myelin sheath that coats many axons (Figures 1-24 and 1-28), and the gap in the axon represents a missing extent that might be as long as a meter in our longest axons.

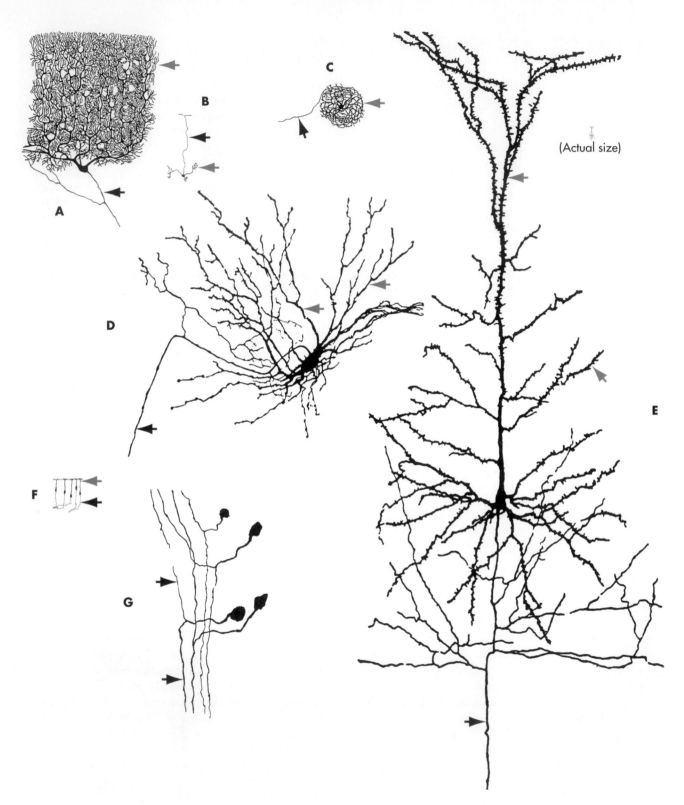

(Actual size)

FIGURE 1-4

Examples of multipolar (**A-E**), bipolar (**F**), and unipolar (**G**) neurons, all drawn to about the same scale to demonstrate the range of neuronal sizes and shapes. All were stained by the Golgi method (Figure 1-14); dendrites are indicated by green arrows, axons by blue arrows. **A,** Purkinje cell from the cerebellar cortex; **B,** granule cell from the cerebellar cortex; **C,** projection neuron from the inferior olivary nucleus; **D,** spinal cord motor neuron; **E,** large pyramidal neuron from the cerebral cortex; **F,** olfactory receptor neurons; **G,** dorsal root ganglion cells (whose processes have axonal properties along almost their entire course). The tiny inset at the upper right shows the actual size of the pyramidal neuron. [Modified from Ramón y Cajal S: *Histologie du système nerveux de l'homme et des vertébrés*, Paris, 1909, 1911, Maloine.]

Box 1-1 Making the Morphology of Individual Neurons Visible

One drawback of Golgi staining is that it stains a subset of neurons indiscriminately (Figure 1-14, *A*), revealing relatively little about the function of an individual cell. The last few decades have seen the development of increasingly sophisticated techniques for demonstrating the morphology of functionally identified neurons.

A mainstay in the study of the electrophysiological properties of individual neurons has been the use of micropipette electrodes that either impale single neurons or attach to their surfaces (see Chapter 7). The same electrodes can be used as tiny hypodermic needles to inject a dye or marker substance, allowing study of the anatomy of the same neuron (Figure 1-5). Such injections can reveal morphological detail comparable to that shown by Golgi staining (Figures 1-5 and 1-6).

Different classes of neurons also have chemically different interiors, and it is possible to make labeled antibodies that demonstrate some of these differences (Figure 1-6, *D*). Correlations of neuronal morphology and location with neurotransmitter content have been particularly instructive. For example, neurons that use norepinephrine as the chemical transmitter at their synapses contain this substance throughout their axons and cell bodies. Appropriate fixation and processing causes these neurons to be fluorescent. Alternatively, it is possible to make a labeled antibody to an enzyme involved in the formation of a neurotransmitter or a labeled antibody to a receptor for a given transmitter. Such methods have made it possible to map out "chemically coded" neural pathways in recent years (see Chapter 11). Methods for studying neurotransmitter content and electrophysiological properties can be combined to produce particularly elegant structure-function correlations (Figure 1-6).

to a series of terminal branches that form synapses on other neurons. Hence neurons are anatomically and functionally polarized, with electrical signals traveling in only one direction under ordinary physiological circumstances. (The molecular underpinnings of this anatomical and functional polarization are discussed in Chapters 7-9.)

Despite the basic similarity of neurons to one another, there is wide variability in the details of their shapes and sizes (Figure 1-4). Certain aspects of somatic, dendritic, and axonal morphology give rise to a descriptive terminology for neurons. The vast majority of vertebrate neurons are **multipolar,** meaning that there are multiple dendritic projections from the cell body and almost always an axon as well (Figure 1-4, *A-E*); in many cases the pattern of the dendritic processes is characteristic of that type of neuron. Some neurons are **bipolar** (Figure 1-4, *F*) or **unipolar**★ (Figure 1-4, *G*), having two processes or only one, respectively. There is a wide spectrum not only of neuronal shapes but also of neuronal sizes. Cell bodies range from about 5 to 100 μm in diameter. Many axons are short, only a millimeter or so in length; but some, like those that extend from the cerebral cortex to the sacral spinal cord, measure a meter or more.†

★ Although true unipolar neurons are common in invertebrate nervous systems, vertebrate neurons with a unipolar appearance are actually **pseudounipolar.** They start out as bipolar neurons, and the two processes swing around to one side of the cell and fuse during development.
† Diagrams and drawings such as those in Figures 1-3 and 1-4 do not convey a sense of the relative sizes of neurons and their parts. If you envision the spinal motor neuron shown in Figure 1-4, *D* as being the size of a tennis ball, then its dendrites would spread out through a room-size volume and its axon would correspond to a half-inch garden hose nearly half a mile long. Using the same scale, the small interneuron shown in Figure 1-4, *B* would be little larger than the head of a pin; its axon would be a hair-thin process only 1 or 2 feet long.

For many years, the major technique available for studying the shapes and sizes of neurons was Golgi staining, a method that infiltrates all the processes of a small percentage of neurons with heavy metals, causing them to stand out from an unstained or counterstained background (Figures 1-4 and 1-14, *A*). More recently, however, a variety of methods relying on microinjection or immunocytochemical techniques have become available (Box 1-1). These now make it possible to correlate the structure of an individual neuron with aspects of its function.

Neurons may also be classified according to their connections. **Sensory neurons** are either directly sensitive to various stimuli (such as touch or temperature changes) or they receive direct connections from non-neuronal **receptor cells. Motor neurons** end directly on muscles or glands. Most sensory and motor neurons live partly in the PNS and partly in the CNS (Figure 1-8), whereas almost all other neurons reside in the CNS and interconnect other neurons. Some are local **interneurons** and have all their projections confined to a single small area of the CNS. Others are **projection neurons,** with long axons connecting different areas, as in a neuron in the cerebral cortex whose axon reaches the spinal cord. In a strict sense, the human nervous system is composed almost entirely of interneurons and projection neurons: there are at most 20 million sensory fibers in all of the spinal and cranial nerves combined and no more than a few million motor neurons. Even taking into account the autonomic neurons that innervate muscles and glands (see Chapter 10), more than 99% of our neurons are interneurons or projection neurons. However, the words "sensory" and "motor" are often used in a much broader sense to refer to cells and axons that carry information related to sensory stimuli and to the generation of responses, respectively.

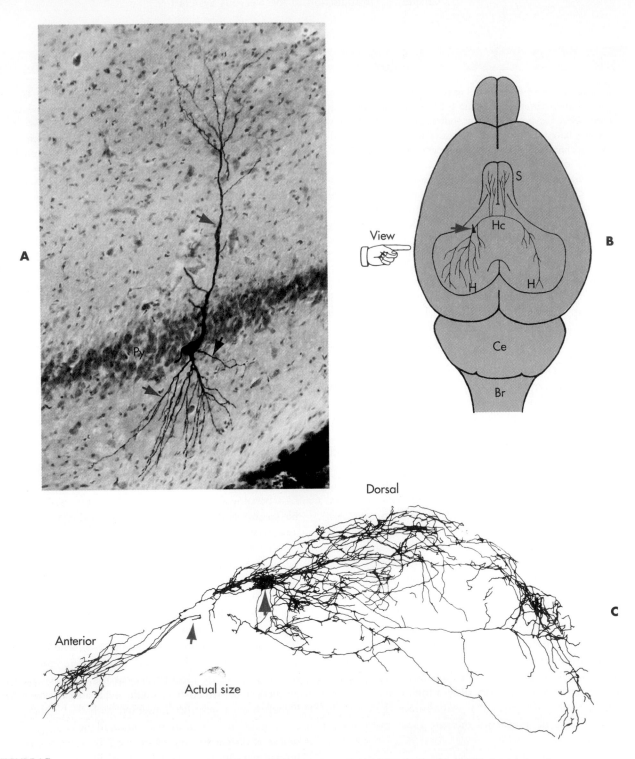

FIGURE 1-5

Morphology of individual neurons revealed by injection of marker substances from intracellular recording electrodes. This study not only shows the striking degree of anatomical detail that can be demonstrated using this technique but also shows that, although we tend to draw neurons as fairly simple cells with a single axon going from one place to another, they are in reality far more complicated. **A,** A pyramidal neuron from the hippocampus of a rat, injected with horseradish peroxidase. The marker was subsequently visualized using an immunocytochemical technique, and the cell body *(blue arrow)* of the injected neuron stands out from the neighboring neurons in the pyramidal cell layer *(Py)*; dendrites *(red arrows)* and a single axon *(black arrow)* emerge from the cell body. Examining stained processes of this neuron in many adjacent sections led to the conclusion that the axon had a long, complex set of branches, shown schematically in **B.** This is a view of the dorsal surface of a rat's brain. The hippocampus *(H)* is a specialized area of cerebral cortex buried within the cerebral hemisphere (see Chapter 23). The labeled hippocampal pyramidal neuron *(blue arrow)* sent axonal branches to the septal nuclei *(S)* bilaterally, to the hippocampus in which the neuron resided, and to the opposite hippocampus by way of the hippocampal commissure *(Hc)*. *Ce,* Cerebellum; *Br,* brainstem. **C,** Drawing of a reconstruction of the neuron and its branches in the injected hemisphere, compiled from numerous adjacent parasagittal sections. The view is from the side, as indicated by the hand in **B.** At this magnification the cell body is a small structure *(large blue arrow)* surrounded by dendrites. The axon branches extensively and sends projections both anteriorly and posteriorly. In this reconstruction, it ends at the point *(small blue arrow)* where one of its branches prepares to cross the midline and project to the contralateral hemisphere. (Modified from Tamamaki N, Watanabe K, Nojyo Y: A whole image of the hippocampal pyramidal neuron revealed by intracellular pressure-injection of horseradish peroxidase, *Brain Res* 307:336, 1984.)

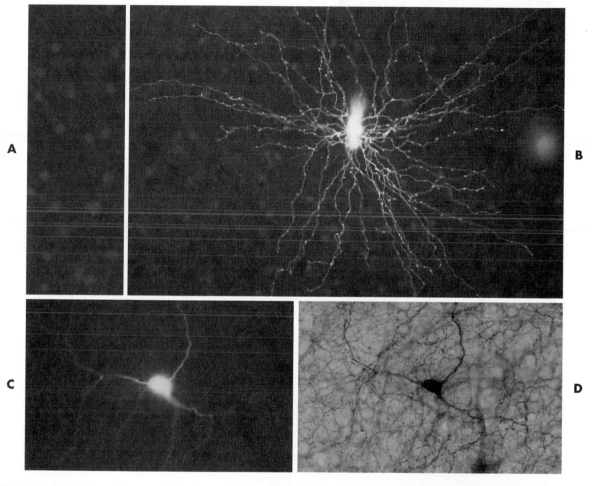

FIGURE 1-6

Combined use of a neurotransmitter identification technique and intracellular injection of dye. A subset of retinal amacrine cells (see Chapter 17) uses serotonin as a neurotransmitter. These neurons accumulate serotonin from the surrounding medium and also accumulate certain analogs of serotonin. **A,** A fluorescent analog (5,7-dihydroxytryptamine) was applied to a living, flat-mounted rabbit retina, which was then viewed using ultraviolet illumination. Serotonin-accumulating amacrine cells fluoresce blue under these conditions, allowing chemically identified neurons to be impaled by dye-filled micropipette electrodes. **B,** A serotonin-containing amacrine cell injected with a fluorescent dye (Lucifer Yellow). Details of the long, mostly unbranched dendrites of this neuron are readily apparent. **C** and **D,** An additional example of combined use of a neurotransmitter identification technique and intracellular injection of dye. Another subset of retinal amacrine cells uses dopamine as a neurotransmitter. One such amacrine cell was first injected with a fluorescent dye (Lucifer Yellow, **C**). The same area of retina was then stained with an antibody to tyrosine hydroxylase (an enzyme involved in the synthesis of dopamine) as shown in **D.** The obvious correspondence between the two images indicates that the injected amacrine cell manufactures dopamine. (**A** and **B** courtesy Dr. David I. Vaney, National Vision Research Institute of Australia. **C** and **D** courtesy Dr. Dennis M. Dacey, University of Washington School of Medicine.)

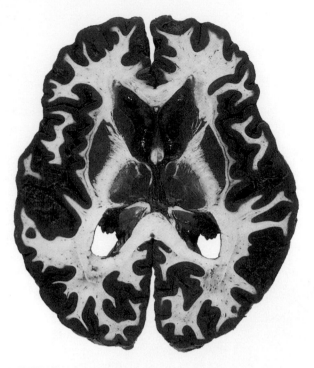

Horizontal slice of a whole human brain, approximately 6 mm thick, stained by a method that differentiates between gray and white matter. Pretreatment with phenol makes the white matter resistant to the blue copper sulfate stain, so white matter appears white and gray matter appears bright blue. (Prepared by Pam Eller, Rocky Mountain Taste and Smell Center, University of Colorado Medical School.)

Neuronal Cell Bodies and Axons Are Largely Segregated Within the Nervous System

For the most part, the CNS is easily divisible into **gray matter** and **white matter** (Figures 1-7 and 1-8). *Gray matter* refers to areas where there is a preponderance of cell bodies and dendrites; however, it is actually a pinkish–gray color because of its abundant blood supply. *White matter* refers to areas where there is a preponderance of axons; many axons have a **myelin** sheath (described later in this chapter) that is mostly lipid and therefore has a fatty, white appearance.

Specific areas of gray matter are often called **nuclei★**, particularly if the contained cell bodies are functionally related to one another. An area where gray matter forms a layered surface covering on some part of the CNS is referred to as a **cortex.** The cerebral and cerebellar cortices are two prominent examples. Occasionally, descriptive names are used for particular areas of gray matter (e.g., the putamen, a nucleus in the cerebral hemisphere named for its shape and location), but these are relatively infrequent.

In contrast, subdivisions of white matter (i.e., collections of axons) go by a bewildering variety of names, such

★Thus the term *nucleus* has two meanings in the CNS—it can mean either the nucleus of an individual neuron or a collection of neuronal cell bodies.

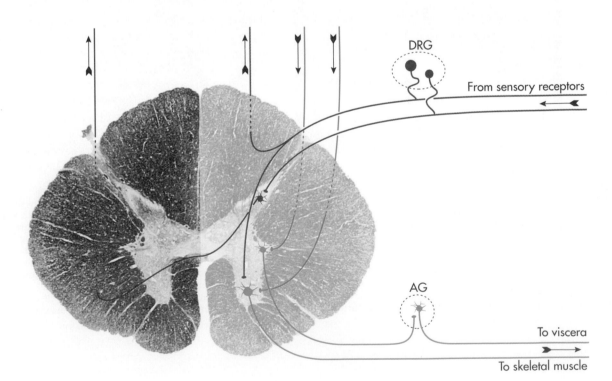

Division of the CNS into gray matter and white matter, as typified by the spinal cord in cross section. Gray matter contains interneurons, projection neurons, motor neurons, and endings of sensory fibers and fibers arriving from other parts of the CNS. White matter contains ascending and descending pathways. Neurons in the peripheral nervous system are clustered in ganglia, some containing sensory neurons (*DRG,* dorsal root ganglia) and some containing autonomic neurons (*AG,* autonomic ganglia).

as **fasciculus, funiculus, lemniscus, peduncle,** and, most commonly, **tract.** Many tracts have two-part names that provide some free information about the nature of the tract; the first part of the name refers to the location of the neuronal cell bodies from which these axons originate, and the second part refers to the site where they terminate. Thus a spinocerebellar tract is one that starts in the spinal cord and ends in the cerebellum.

The spinal cord provides a reasonably clear example of the separation of neural tissue into gray matter and white matter (Figure 1-8). Sensory axons, whose unipolar cell bodies are located in the dorsal root ganglia of spinal nerves, enter the spinal cord and divide into a large number of branches, most of which terminate on neuronal processes in the spinal gray matter. Motor axons, whose multipolar cell bodies are located in the spinal gray matter, leave the spinal cord and enter spinal nerves. The white matter contains **long descending tracts** (from the brainstem and cerebrum), **long ascending tracts** (to the brainstem, cerebellum, and cerebrum), and local axons interconnecting different spinal levels. The gray matter, on the other hand, contains motor neurons, the endings of incoming sensory axons and long descending tracts, local interneurons, and projection neurons whose axons enter long ascending tracts. This division into white and gray matter is not absolute anywhere in the CNS; for example, axons in long descending tracts obviously must pass through some gray matter before reaching their targets.

Peripheral nerves are, for most of their courses, collections of axons on their way to or from places such as skin, muscle, or internal organs, accompanied by glial and connective tissue sheaths (see Figure 9-18). Many of these axons have cell bodies that also reside in the PNS, and these somata are typically clustered in **ganglia** at predictable sites along the nerve (Figure 1-8).

Neuronal Organelles Are Distributed in a Pattern That Supports Neuronal Function

Neurons need mechanisms to deal not only with their electrical and chemical signaling functions, but also with other consequences of their extended anatomy. A large neuron with a long axon (e.g., one of the neurons shown in Figure 1-4 *A, D,* and *E*) may have 99% of its cytoplasm in the axon, much of it many centimeters away from the cell body; hence its single nucleus and associated synthetic apparatus must have efficient mechanisms for communicating with distant parts of its appendages. In addition, brains have no bones, but neurons have long, delicate processes, so there is a need for mechanical stabilization that can be met only partially by the external suspension mechanisms described in Chapters 4 and 5. To address these issues, neurons, like other cells, contain a nucleus and an assortment of organelles—mitochondria, endoplasmic reticulum, Golgi apparatus, and cytoskeletal

elements—but their abundance and configuration in different parts of a neuron reflect the function of each of these parts.

Neuronal cell bodies synthesize macromolecules

The neuronal cell body is the site of synthesis of nearly all of the neuron's enzymes, structural proteins, membrane components, and organelles, as well as some of its chemical messengers. Its structure (Figure 1-9) reflects this function. The nucleus is large and pale-staining, with most of its chromatin dispersed and available for transcription; it contains one or more prominent nucleoli, which are actively involved in the transcription of ribosomal RNA. The cytoplasm contains abundant rough endoplasmic reticulum and free ribosomes for protein synthesis, together with stacks of Golgi cisternae for further processing and packaging of synthesized proteins. Many mitochondria are also present, to meet the energy requirements of continuous, very active protein synthesis.

Ribosomes, whether studding the surface of the rough endoplasmic reticulum or free in the cytoplasm between the cisternae, are stained intensely by basic dyes, appearing light microscopically as clumps called **Nissl bodies** or **Nissl substance** (Figure 1-10). Nissl bodies are particularly prominent in large neurons, a consequence of the large total volume of cytoplasm contained in their processes, and appear in characteristic configurations in different neuronal types (Figure 1-11).

The organelles just described are embedded in a network of three kinds of filamentous protein polymers that extend throughout the neuron and its processes, collectively comprising the neuronal cytoskeleton. **Microtubules** are cylindrical assemblies, about 25 nm in diameter, of 13 strands (protofilaments) of protein arranged around a hollow core. Each protofilament is a polymer of the protein **tubulin;** an assortment of additional proteins associated with the microtubules link them to each other, to other cytoskeletal elements, and to various organelles as they travel toward or away from the cell body. **Neurofilaments,** the neuron's version of the intermediate filaments found in most cells, are multiply twisted, ropelike assemblies of strands that are polymers involving at least three different proteins from the cytokeratin family. Neurofilaments are about 10 nm in diameter, much too small to be seen under the light microscope, but they aggregate in response to certain chemical fixatives. When silver stains are applied, such aggregates can be visualized as **neurofibrils** (Figure 1-12). Finally, **microfilaments,** the thinnest cytoskeletal element (7 nm), are twisted pairs of actin filaments. All three kinds of cytoskeletal elements contribute to maintaining the shape of the neuron. Microtubules also serve as the substrate along which organelles are transported through neuronal processes (as described in more detail later in the chapter), and microfilaments are im-

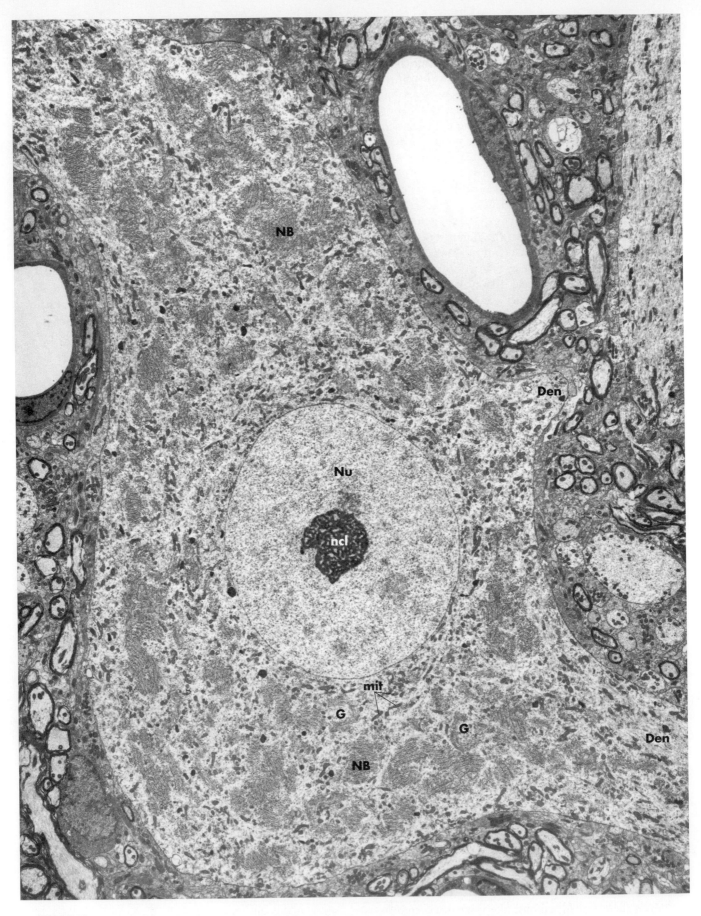

FIGURE 1-9
Cell body and some of the proximal dendrites (Den) of a spinal cord motor neuron. The nucleus (Nu) and prominent nucleolus (ncl) are apparent, as are other organelles typical of neuronal cell bodies—Nissl bodies (NB), Golgi cisternae (G), and mitochondria (mit). Cytoskeletal elements, although present, are difficult to resolve at this low magnification. The actual size of the area shown in this micrograph is about 55 μm × 70 μm. (From Peters A, Palay SL, Webster H deF: *The fine structure of the nervous system: neurons and their supporting cells*, ed 3, New York, 1991, Oxford University Press.)

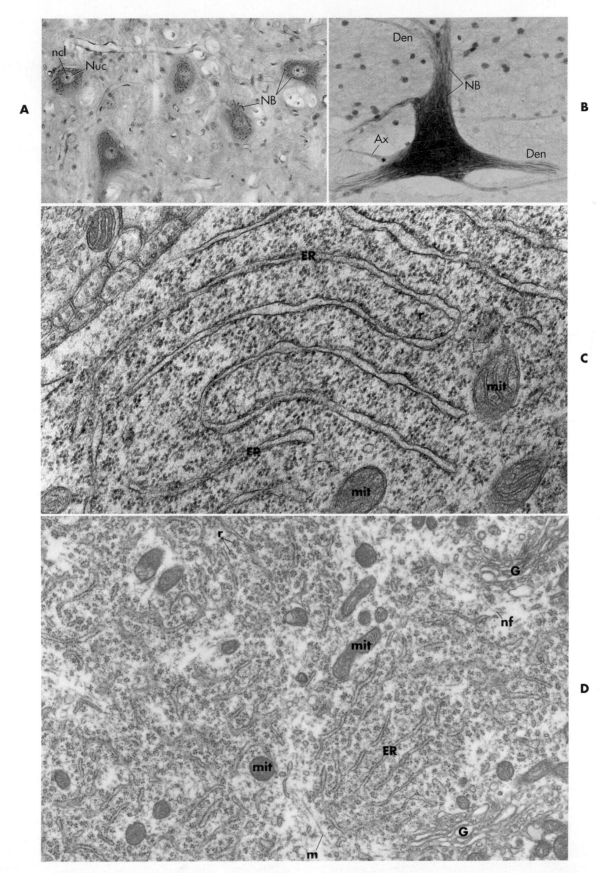

FIGURE 1-10

Nissl bodies in spinal cord motor neurons. At the light microscopic level (**A** and **B**) Nissl bodies *(NB)* appear as clumps of basophilic material distributed throughout the cell body and extending into dendrites *(Den)* but not axons *(Ax)* or their point of origin (the axon hillock, *[*]*). Electron microscopy (**C** and **D**) reveals that Nissl bodies are stacks of rough endoplasmic reticulum *(ER)* with interspersed clusters of free ribosomes *(r)*, embedded in neuronal cytoplasm containing Golgi cisternae *(G)*, mitochondria *(mit)*, microtubules *(m)*, and neurofilaments *(nf)*. The actual size of the Nissl body in **C** is about 3 μm × 2 μm. *Nuc,* Nucleus; *ncl,* nucleolus. (**A** courtesy Dr. Nathaniel T. McMullen, Department of Cell Biology and Anatomy, The University of Arizona College of Medicine. **B** courtesy Dr. Allen L. Bell, Anatomy Department, University of New England College of Osteopathic Medicine. **C** from Pannese E: *Neurocytology: fine structure of neurons, nerve processes, and neuroglial cells*, New York, 1994, Thieme Medical Publishers, Inc. **D** from Peters A, Palay SL, Webster H deF: *The fine structure of the nervous system: neurons and their supporting cells*, ed 3, New York, 1991, Oxford University Press.)

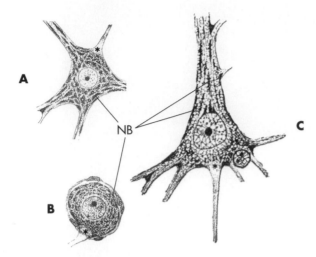

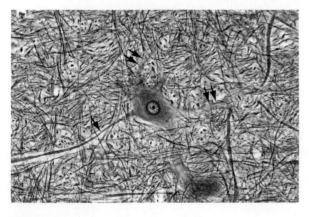

portant for anchoring membrane molecules in place (e.g., receptor molecules at synapses) and for movement of the advancing tip of growing axons.

Dendrites receive synaptic inputs

Dendrites are tapering extensions of the neuronal cell body. Although the total array of dendrites—a neuron's **dendritic tree**—can have an elaborate structure (Figure 1-4), each individual dendrite has a cytoplasmic construction similar to that of the cell body. Hence microtubules, neurofilaments, and microfilaments extend into

the dendrites (Figure 1-13). Nissl bodies may extend into the proximal parts of dendrites (Figures 1-10 and 1-11), as may parts of the Golgi apparatus. Mitochondria are abundant, particularly near synaptic endings where they meet the energetic requirements of the synaptic electrical signaling processes described in Chapter 8. As the principal input structures of neurons, dendrites are surrounded by a dense meshwork of synaptic terminals and processes of glial cells (Figures 1-13 and 1-21, *A*). The dendrites of many neurons are studded with small protuberances called **dendritic spines** (Figure 1-14), which are the preferred sites for some kinds of synaptic contacts.

Axons convey electrical signals over long distances

The single axon of each neuron looks different from the dendrites. Rather than being a tapered extension of the neuronal cell body, the axon is a cylindrical process that arises abruptly from an **axon hillock** on one side of the neuronal cell body or one of its proximal dendrites. Bundles of microtubules, accompanied by neurofilaments and mitochondria, funnel through the axon hillock into the **initial segment** of the axon (Figure 1-15). Nissl substance stays behind (Figures 1-10 and 1-11), so the relatively vast volume of axonal cytoplasm depends on the soma for virtually all the macromolecules needed by it and its synaptic terminals. The initial segment is typically the most electrically excitable part of the neuron; as described in more detail in Chapters 7 and 8, all the synaptic inputs to the dendrites, cell body, and initial segment itself are summed up here to determine the electrical response that will be propagated along the axon.

Beyond the initial segment, many axons are encased in a spiral wrapping of glial membranes called **myelin** (Figure 1-16). As discussed in Chapter 7, myelin is a mammalian invention that greatly increases the speed of propagation of electrical signals along axons.

Organelles and macromolecules are transported in both directions along axons

Axons are much too long to depend on diffusion for the delivery of macromolecules and organelles synthesized in the soma, and an active process of **axonal transport** is used instead. Similarly, a variety of substances ranging from "used" organelles to intracellular chemical messengers need to be transported from synaptic endings back to the soma. Transport away from the soma is termed **anterograde,** and transport toward the soma is termed **retrograde.** There are two general categories of axonal transport in terms of speed, appropriately enough called **slow** and **fast.** Slow axonal transport moves soluble pro-

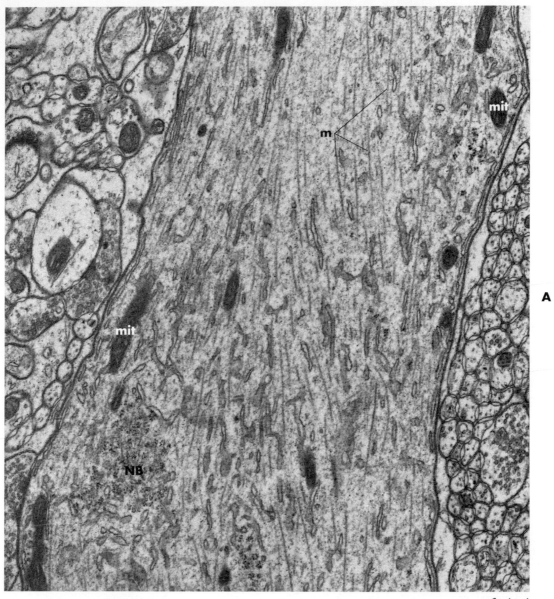

Continued

FIGURE I-13

Cytoskeletal elements and other organelles of dendrites, seen in a longitudinal section of a cerebellar Purkinje cell dendrite **(A)** and a transverse section of a spinal cord motor neuron dendrite **(B).** Microtubules *(m)* and neurofilaments *(nf)* extend longitudinally through the dendrites, accompanied by mitochondria *(mit)* and, in parts close to the soma, Nissl bodies *(NB)*. As the principal input site of neurons, dendrites are typically surrounded by axon terminals *(At)*, forming synaptic endings either directly on the shaft of the dendrite *(arrows)* or on small spines *(sp)* protruding from the dendrite. The actual diameters of these two dendrites are about 4 µm and 7 µm, respectively. [**A** from Pannese E: *Neurocytology: fine structure of neurons, nerve processes, and neuroglial cells*, New York, 1994, Thieme Medical Publishers, Inc. **B** from Peters A, Palay SL, Webster H deF: *The fine structure of the nervous system: neurons and their supporting cells*, ed 3, New York, 1991, Oxford University Press.]

teins—such as cytoskeletal proteins and cytoplasmic enzymes—in the anterograde direction at rates of a few millimeters a day; the mechanism of this movement is still not understood. Fast axonal transport moves membrane-associated substances—mitochondria, lysosomes, vesicles of neurotransmitter precursors, and membrane components—at rates up to 400 mm a day. Microtubules serve as the "railroad tracks" for fast transport. Some

things move preferentially in the anterograde direction, others in the retrograde direction. This is made possible by the longitudinal polarity of microtubules: tubulin is a structurally polarized molecule and can only be added in one orientation to one end (called the *plus end*) of an existing microtubule. Axonal microtubules are oriented with their plus ends pointing away from the soma. Two ATPases associated with microtubules serve as the mo-

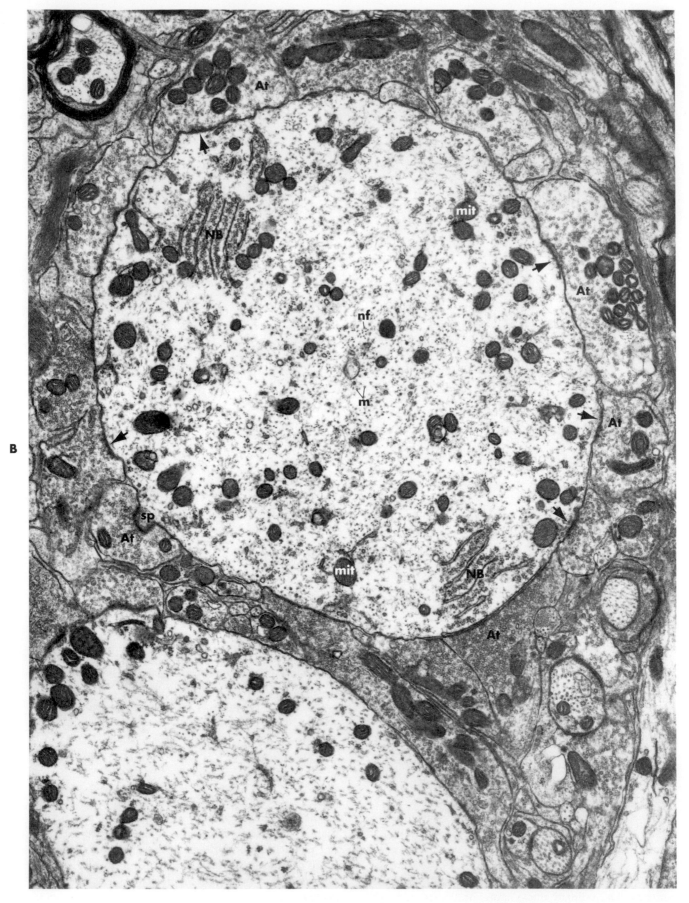

FIGURE 1-13, cont'd
For legend see page 13.

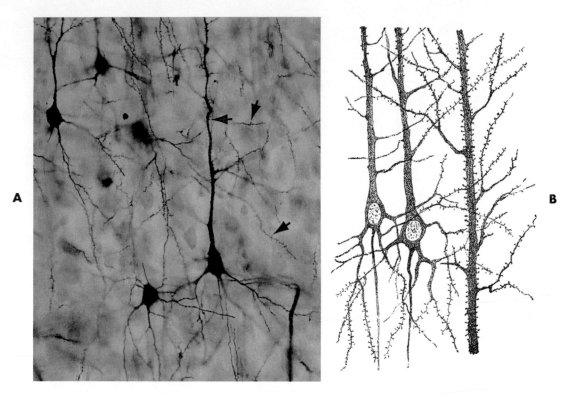

FIGURE 1-14
Dendritic spines on pyramidal neurons of the cerebral cortex, visible as tiny protuberances *(arrows)* from the dendrites of neurons stained by a Golgi/Nissl method **(A)** or with methylene blue **(B)**. (**A** courtesy Dr. Nathaniel T. McMullen, Department of Cell Biology and Anatomy, The University of Arizona College of Medicine. **B** from Ramón y Cajal S: *Histologie du système nerveux de l'homme et des vertébrés*, Paris, 1909, 1911, Maloine.)

tors for fast transport. **Kinesin** bridges between microtubules and some membrane-associated cell components and moves them toward the plus end of the microtubule (i.e., in the anterograde direction). **Dynein** moves some components in the retrograde direction (Figure 1-17).

Modern neuroanatomical techniques take advantage of axonal transport to map out the connections between neurons (Box 1-2 and Figure 1-18). Appropriate tracer substances injected into or near known neuronal cell bodies are transported anterogradely, revealing the locations of the neurons' synaptic terminals. Conversely, tracers injected near synaptic endings are taken up by the endings and transported retrogradely to the cell bodies (a method used covertly by some viruses, such as herpes, to gain access to the nervous system).

Synaptic contacts mediate information transfer between neurons

Information is collected and integrated by a neuron's cell body and dendrites, transmitted along its axon, and finally conveyed to other neurons at synapses (Figure 1-3). The vast majority of vertebrate synapses are variations on a common theme. An enlargement (the **presynaptic** ele-

ment) of a distal axonal branch abuts part of another neuron (the **postsynaptic** element), separated from it by a **synaptic cleft** 10 to 20 nm across. The presynaptic ending contains membrane-bound packets **(synaptic vesicles)** of neurotransmitter molecules (Figure 1-19), some of which are released into the synaptic cleft in response to electrical activity. The neurotransmitter diffuses across the synaptic cleft, binds to receptor molecules in the postsynaptic membrane, and causes an electrical signal in the postsynaptic neuron. At first telling, this seems like an inordinately labor-intensive way to transfer a message from one neuron to another. However, there are major computational advantages to this strategy, as discussed further in Chapter 8.

Most synapses have an axonal ending as the presynaptic element and part of a dendrite as the postsynaptic element, but in fact any part of a neuron can be presynaptic to any part of another neuron (or sometimes even to itself). This gives rise to names for categories of synapses based on the identities of the presynaptic and postsynaptic elements (Figure 1-20).

The total number of synapses in a human CNS is almost unimaginably huge (Figure 1-21) and ultimately makes possible our complex mental abilities. The number of synapses on a given neuron is roughly

Text continued on p. 23

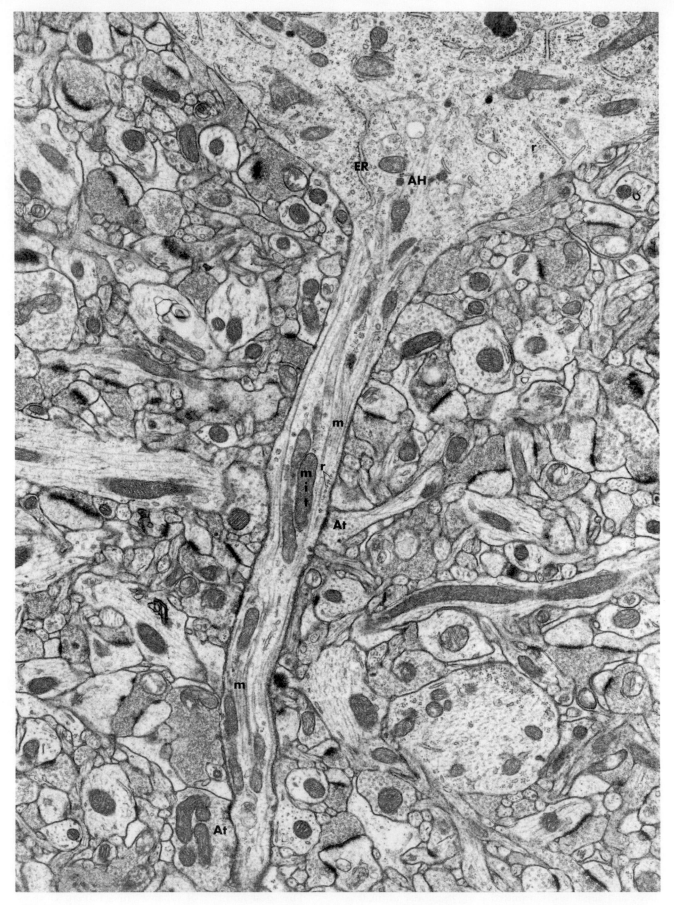

FIGURE 1-15

The initial segment of the axon of a pyramidal neuron from the cerebral cortex. Many microtubules *(m)* funnel into the axon from the axon hillock *(AH)*. The axon also contains mitochondria *(mit)* and clusters of ribosomes *(r)*, but no Nissl bodies *(ER)*. Axon terminals *(At)* also reach the initial segment, but not more distal portions of the axon (except for the axon terminals, which can receive synaptic contacts). The actual diameter of this axon is about 1 μm. (From Peters A, Palay SL, Webster H deF: *The fine structure of the nervous system: neurons and their supporting cells*, ed 3, New York, 1991, Oxford University Press.)

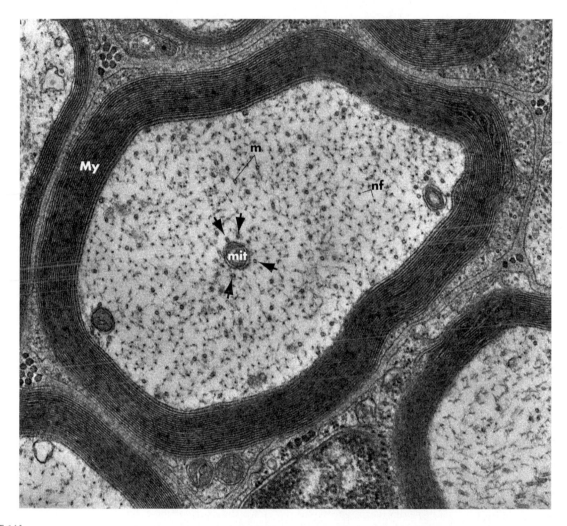

FIGURE I-I6
Cross section of a myelinated axon in the peripheral nervous system. Beyond the initial segment, many axons of the CNS and PNS acquire a myelin sheath *(My)* provided by glial cells (Figures I-24 and I-28) in addition to the usual complement of mitochondria *(mit)*, microtubules *(m)*, and neurofilaments *(nf)*. Microtubules are involved in the transport of organelles along axons (Figure I-I7) and are often found closely associated with mitochondria *(arrows)*. The actual diameter of this axon is about I.5 μm, and the thickness of the myelin sheath is about 0.25 μm. [From Pannese E: *Neurocytology: fine structure of neurons, nerve processes, and neuroglial cells*, New York, 1994, Thieme Medical Publishers, Inc.]

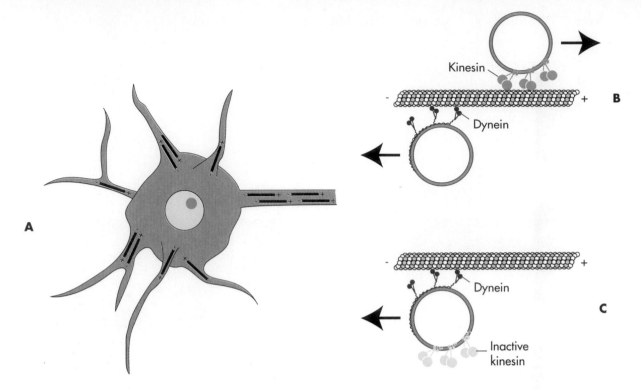

FIGURE 1-17

Mechanism of fast axonal transport. **A,** Schematic neuron with microtubules arranged longitudinally in its axon and dendrites. Axonal microtubules are arranged with plus ends directed away from the cell body and toward the axon's terminals. In contrast, dendritic microtubules can be oriented in either direction. Part of a single microtubule is shown enlarged in **B** and **C,** with tubulin molecules shown as small spheres. The two slightly different forms of tubulin (shaded and white in the figure) are arranged in strands, like beads on a string, with 13 longitudinally oriented strands forming the walls of each microtubule. Tubulin "beads" can only be added at the plus end. Kinesin and dynein bind to membranous organelles (e.g., mitochondria, vesicles) and form temporary cross-bridges with microtubules, allowing the organelles to "walk" along the microtubule toward its plus (kinesin) or minus (dynein) end. Because all the plus ends of axonal microtubules point in the same direction, kinesin mediates anterograde transport and dynein mediates retrograde transport. Some types of organelles may bind just one of these motor molecules preferentially **(A).** Alternatively, organelles may bind both but only have one of the two in an active state at any given time **(B).** (**A** based on an illustration in Pannese E: *Neurocytology: fine structure of neurons, nerve processes, and neuroglial cells,* New York, 1994, Thieme Medical Publishers, Inc. **B** and **C,** redrawn from Vallee RB, Bloom GS: Mechanisms of fast and slow axonal transport, *Annu Rev Neurosci* 14:59, 1991, © 1991 by Annual Reviews, Inc.)

Box 1-2 Using Axonal Transport to Study Neuronal Connections

Neurons are embedded in a seemingly impenetrable thicket of processes of other neurons (Figures 1-12 and 1-15), but are nevertheless interconnected in systematic ways. Mapping these interconnections has been a formidable challenge. **Degeneration techniques** have been used since the 19th century and are based on the reactions of neurons to injury. If an axon is severed, its formerly attached cell body undergoes a characteristic series of cytological changes **(chromatolysis).** Therefore examining brain sections for chromatolytic cells can reveal the locations of the cell bodies of origin of the severed axons. While the cell body undergoes chromatolysis, the portion of the axon distal to the cut degenerates **(wallerian degeneration).** The same distal changes occur if the damage is inflicted at the ultimate proximal location (that is, if the cell body is destroyed). Special staining methods can be used to selectively stain degenerating axons or their synaptic terminals. Therefore if a particular nucleus is destroyed, the path of axons originating there and the sites of their termination can be determined.

Although a great deal of information has been gained over the years with the aid of degeneration techniques, their use is not without pitfalls. It is technically difficult, and sometimes impossible, to completely destroy a particular structure without also damaging nearby structures. In addition, because the segregation of gray and white matter is not absolute, axons passing through a given nucleus can be destroyed along with the cell bodies forming the nucleus. For these and other reasons, techniques that take advantage of axonal transport have proven to be a great advance. Early methods of this type used radioactive substances (usually tritiated amino acids) introduced into an area of gray matter, taken up by the resident neurons, incorporated into macromolecules, and transported down the axons of these neurons. Eventually, the synaptic terminals of these axons become radioactive. Subsequent methods have used the introduction of a marker substance (often a protein) into selected areas of gray matter, where it encounters synaptic terminals. The terminals take up the protein and transport it back to the parent neurons. A protein commonly used in such experiments is an enzyme called **horseradish peroxidase,** which can be detected with great sensitivity and resolution by appropriate histochemical procedures (Figure 1-5). Although this technique is typically used for retrograde transport studies, it can be used simultaneously for anterograde transport studies, labeling not only the neurons that project to a given area of gray matter but also the targets of axons that leave it (Figure 1-18). Certain fluorescent dyes can also be used in retrograde transport studies. By injecting two different dyes at two different sites in the nervous system, it is possible to determine whether any neurons have branching axons that project to both sites.

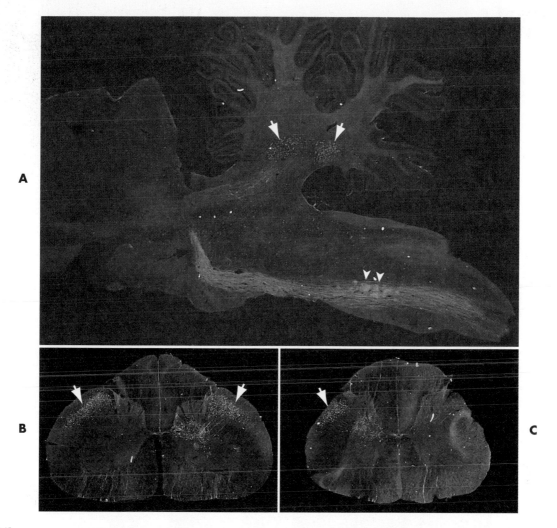

FIGURE 1-18

Use of bidirectional transport to demonstrate projections to and from the red nucleus, an area of gray matter in the rostral brainstem. Inputs to the red nucleus include projections from the cerebellum; outputs include projections to the spinal cord. Both inputs and outputs are organized topographically so that a given part of the red nucleus receives inputs from a specific part of the contralateral half of the cerebellum and sends outputs to specific parts of the contralateral half of the brainstem and spinal cord. These connections were traced in the CNS of a cat by injecting a marker substance (horseradish peroxidase conjugated with wheat germ agglutinin [WGA-HRP] for increased sensitivity and specificity), localizing it histochemically, and viewing labeled CNS sections with polarized darkfield microscopy. **A,** Parasagittal section through one side of a cat's brainstem after injection of WGA-HRP into the contralateral red nucleus; rostral is to the left. The red nucleus itself cannot be seen in this plane of section, but retrogradely labeled neurons can be seen in two deep cerebellar nuclei (anterior and posterior interposed nuclei; *white arrows*), and anterogradely labeled fibers of the rubrospinal tract *(red arrows)* can be seen traversing the brainstem. Along the course of the rubrospinal tract, some fibers terminate in the lateral reticular nucleus of the brainstem *(arrowheads)*. **B,** Section through the cervical spinal cord of a cat after injection of WGA-HRP into the forelimb area of the left red nucleus and the hindlimb area of the right red nucleus. Because both red nuclei were injected, both rubrospinal tracts are labeled *(white arrows)*, but only fibers contralateral to the forelimb area injection terminate in the spinal gray matter at this level *(red arrow)*. **C,** Section through the lumbar spinal cord of the same cat as in **B.** No labeled rubrospinal fibers remain on the right side, contralateral to the forelimb area injection, because they all terminated rostral to this level. However, labeled fibers can be seen in the left rubrospinal tract *(white arrow)* and ending in the spinal gray matter on the left side *(red arrow)*, contralateral to the hindlimb area injection. [From Robinson FR, Houk JC, Gibson AR: Limb specific connections of the cat magnocellular red nucleus, *J Comp Neurol* 257:553, 1987.]

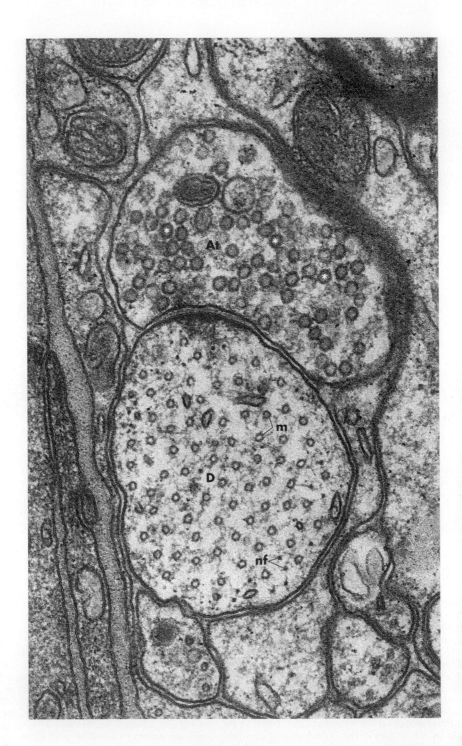

FIGURE 1-19

A synapse in the gray matter of a rat's spinal cord. The presynaptic element is an axon terminal *(At)*, filled with synaptic vesicles (*) and abutting the postsynaptic element, which is a dendrite *(D)* of another neuron. The two elements are separated by a synaptic cleft, and the postsynaptic membrane is thickened, an indication of the presence of specialized molecules in and near the membrane at this site. The dendrite is cut transversely in this image, and microtubules *(m)* and neurofilaments *(nf)* can be seen cut in cross section. The actual diameter of the postsynaptic dendrite is about 0.75 μm. (From Pannese E: *Neurocytology: fine structure of neurons, nerve processes, and neuroglial cells*, New York, 1994, Thieme Medical Publishers, Inc.)

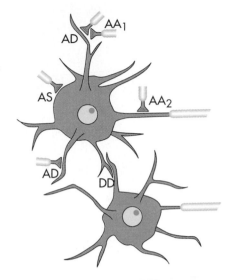

FIGURE I-20
Potential sites of synaptic contacts. Most synapses consist of an axon terminal contacting a dendrite, and so are called *axodendritic synapses (AD)*. However, all other possible
combinations occur at least occasionally, giving rise to two-part names for the synapse
type, with the first part indicating the presynaptic element and the second part indicating the postsynaptic element. These include axosomatic *(AS)* and dendrodendritic
(DD) synapses and axoaxonic synapses with the postsynaptic element being another
axon terminal *(AAI)* or the initial segment of an axon *(AA$_2$)*. [Based on an illustration in
Pannese E: *Neurocytology: fine structure of neurons, nerve processes, and neuroglial cells*, New
York, 1994, Thieme Medical Publishers, Inc.]

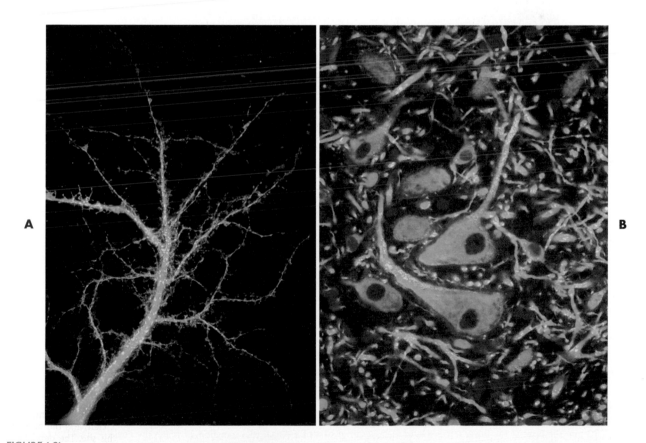

FIGURE I-21
Synapses densely distributed over the surface of CNS neurons. **A,** Double immunofluorescence micrograph of a dendrite of a hippocampal
neuron developing in tissue culture. The cell body (not seen in this field of view) and dendrites were stained with a fluorescent antibody directed against MAP2, a microtubule-associated protein restricted to the perikaryal-dendritic region of neurons (green fluorescence). Axon terminal projections originating from other neurons not visible in this field form a dense network of synaptic contact sites and were stained with
a fluorescent antibody directed against synaptotagmin, an integral membrane protein of synaptic vesicles. (Overlapping red and green fluorescence, from sites where an axon terminal is superimposed on part of the dendrite, appears yellow.) **B,** Triple fluorescence micrograph of
CNS gray matter (deep cerebellar nuclei of a rat). MAP2 was stained as in **A,** showing neuronal cell bodies and dendrites (green fluorescence).
Axon terminals, which almost completely cover the cell bodies and dendrites, were stained with a fluorescent antibody directed against synap-
tojanin, another protein concentrated in presynaptic terminals (red fluorescence). A third dye (DAPI) was used to stain the nuclei of neurons
and glial cells (blue fluorescence). [**A** courtesy Drs. Olaf Mundigl and Pietro De Camilli, Yale University School of Medicine. **B** from the cover
photograph accompanying McPherson PS et al: A presynaptic inositol-5-phosphatase, *Nature* 379:353, 1996.]

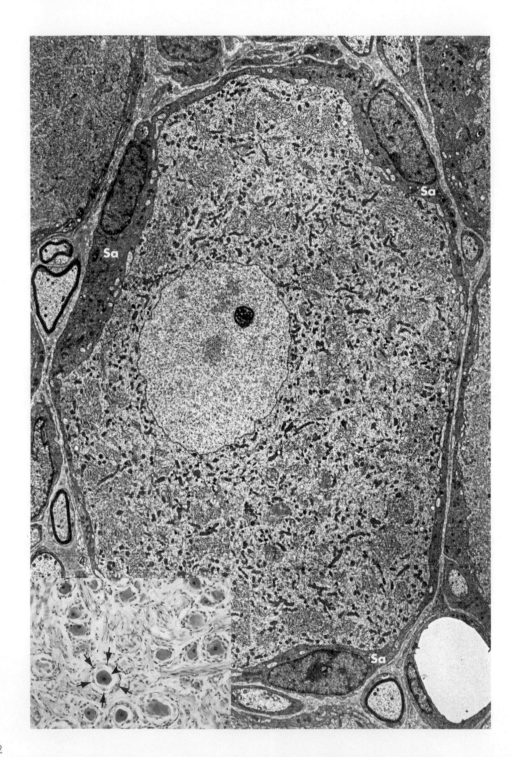

FIGURE 1-22

Schwann cells flattened out as satellite cells *(Sa)* surrounding a single dorsal root ganglion cell from a rat. The actual size of the cell is about 20 μm × 30 μm. The inset at the lower left is a light micrograph of part of a dorsal root ganglion, in which the nuclei *(arrows)* can be seen in flattened satellite cells surrounding individual, much larger, dorsal root ganglion cells *(arrowhead).* [Electron micrograph from Pannese E: *Neuro-cytology: fine structure of neurons, nerve processes, and neuroglial cells,* New York, 1994, Thieme Medical Publishers, Inc. Inset courtesy Dr. Nathaniel T. Mc-Mullen, Department of Cell Biology and Anatomy, The University of Arizona College of Medicine.]

related to the extent of its dendrites and ranges from a few dozen on a small neuron such as a cerebellar granule cell (Figure 1-4, *B*) to hundreds of thousands on the elaborate dendritic tree of a cerebellar Purkinje cell (Figure 1-4, *A*).

Schwann Cells Are the Principal PNS Glial Cells

Neurons in the PNS (Table 1-2) and their parts, with few exceptions, are almost completely enveloped by processes of glial cells. The general roles of these glial processes are to provide metabolic support and electrical insulation; PNS neurons and processes, unlike those in the CNS, are mechanically supported by connective tissue sheaths (described in Chapter 9). All PNS glial cells are variants of one cell type, the **Schwann cell.** Some Schwann cells are flattened out as **satellite cells** that surround the neuronal cell bodies in PNS ganglia (Figure 1-22). Most, however, envelop axons as they travel through peripheral nerves.

PNS axons can be myelinated or unmyelinated

Many peripheral nerve fibers are **myelinated,** vaguely resembling a string of sausages. Each link of sausage corresponds to a length of axon wrapped in myelin, with adjacent links separated by a gap in the myelin. The gaps are **nodes of Ranvier,** sites about 1 μm long where the axon is separated from extracellular space only by fingerlike projections from Schwann cells (Figure 1-23). The myelin between two nodes is an **internode** and is formed by a single Schwann cell (Figure 1-24); adjacent internodes form the projections that cover the node between them. Internodes range in length from about 0.2 to 2 mm, with larger-diameter axons having longer internodes and thicker myelin sheaths. As explained in Chapter 7, this arrangement is part of what allows larger axons to conduct electrical signals more rapidly.

Most of the smaller axons in peripheral nerves do not acquire myelin sheaths. Rather, groups of up to a dozen or so **unmyelinated** axons are simply embedded in individual Schwann cells (Figure 1-25). This lack of myelin, together with their small diameter, leads to relatively slow conduction of electrical signals by unmyelinated axons (see Chapter 7).

Although the enhancing of axonal conduction velocity by myelin is their best-understood function, Schwann cells have been implicated in several other functions, including facilitating the regrowth of axons after peripheral nerve injury, helping to regulate extracellular ionic concentrations around neurons and their processes, and collaborating with neurons in some metabolic processes.

Table 1-2	Components of the PNS	
Cells/ parts of cells	Types	Locations/forms
Neuronal cell bodies	Sensory neurons	Spinal and cranial nerve ganglia, some sensory epithelia
	Autonomic ganglion cells	Sympathetic, parasympathetic, enteric ganglia
Parts of neurons	Axons of motor neurons, axons of autonomic neurons, peripheral processes of sensory neurons	Spinal and cranial nerves
Glial cells	Schwann cells	Myelin sheaths, sheaths of unmyelinated axons, satellite cells

CNS Glial Cells Include Oligodendrocytes, Astrocytes, Ependymal Cells, and Microglial Cells

Glia is Greek for "glue." Historically, glia were so named because they fill up most of the spaces between neurons and appear to hold them in place. Although some glial cells do provide structural support, it is now clear that CNS glial cells play a wide variety of additional roles. In contrast to the PNS, there are multiple kinds of glial cells in the CNS (Figure 1-26, Table 1-3).

Some CNS axons are myelinated by oligodendrocytes; others are unmyelinated

Many CNS axons are wrapped in myelin sheaths (Figure 1-27) that are fundamentally similar to those of PNS axons, except that in the CNS the sheaths are formed by a different population of glial cells called **oligodendrocytes.** As in the periphery, larger axons have thicker myelin and longer internodes. However, as the name implies (*oligodendro-* is Greek for "tree with few branches"), individual oligodendrocytes produce multiple internodes on multiple axons (compare Figures 1-24 and 1-28). A single oligodendrocyte may have dozens of branches, each ending as an internode (Figures 1-29 and 1-30). Unlike Schwann cells, oligodendrocyte processes do not envelop unmyelinated CNS axons, which can be directly exposed to the extracellular environment (Figure 1-31). Given their role as myelin-producing cells, oligodendrocytes are

Text continued on p. 31

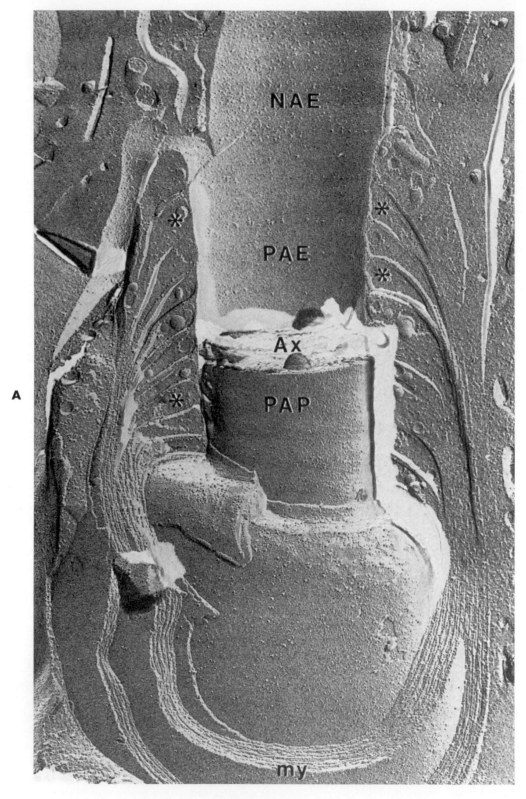

FIGURE 1-23

Myelin sheaths and nodes of Ranvier in peripheral nerves. **A,** Freeze-fracture study of a node of Ranvier from a cat peripheral nerve. This technique involves freezing and splitting a tissue sample, then coating the exposed surfaces with a heavy metal, such as gold or platinum, and examining them with a scanning electron microscope. Sometimes the fracture cuts across cell membranes, but it often splits membranes in two, revealing their interiors. In the latter case, the part of the membrane whose other side faces the extracellular space is called the *E* (for external) face and the part whose other side faces the cell's interior is called the *P* (for protoplasmic) face. (If you imagine a cell membrane as a peanut butter and jelly sandwich oriented so that the peanut butter is closer to the cell interior, then freeze-fracturing would involve prying the sandwich apart; the P face would correspond to the peanut butter, and the E face would correspond to the jelly.) In part of the picture, the fracture cuts through the myelin *(my)* near the node, through pockets of Schwann cell cytoplasm (*) adjacent to the node, or through the axon itself *(Ax)* near the node. On either side of the transection of the axon, its membrane is split, revealing the P face *(PAP)* and the E face *(PAE)* of the paranodal axonal membrane. The split through the membrane continues into the node, revealing the E face of the axonal membrane there *(NAE)*. The numerous particles exposed on the E face of the nodal membrane are thought to correspond to specialized ion channels that are concentrated in this region (see Chapter 7). (**A** from Pannese E: *Neurocytology: fine structure of neurons, nerve processes, and neuroglial cells*, New York, 1994, Thieme Medical Publishers, Inc.)

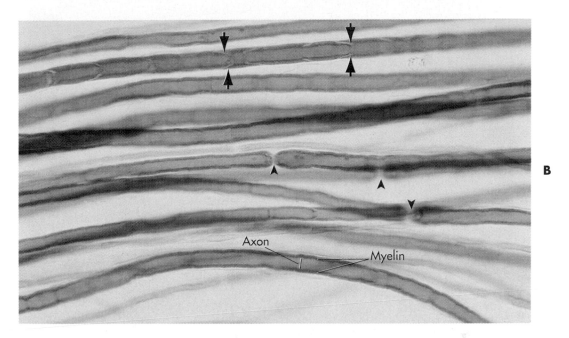

FIGURE I-23, cont'd

B, A fixed peripheral nerve was teased apart so that individual nerve fibers were visible and stained with osmium (a lipophilic stain for membranes). The axon is the central pale area in each fiber, and the myelin sheath stands out on both sides of each axon as a more densely stained area; a few nodes of Ranvier *(arrowheads)* are visible. The occasional diagonal clefts *(arrows)* that appear to cross the myelin sheaths are known as *Schmidt–Lanterman incisures;* they correspond to thin extensions of Schwann cell cytoplasm that spiral around with the myelinating membranes (Figure I-24). (**B** courtesy Dr. Nathaniel T. McMullen, Department of Cell Biology and Anatomy, The University of Arizona College of Medicine.)

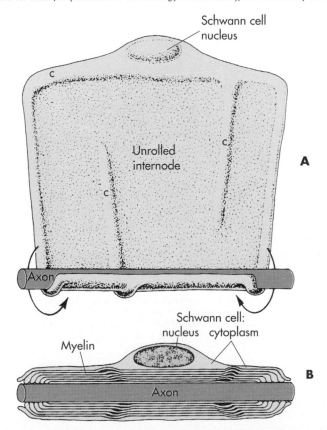

FIGURE I-24

Schematic diagram of the formation of myelin in the PNS. **A,** The single Schwann cell that forms an internode, unrolled from the axon it would normally be wrapped around. The cell is flattened into a two-membrane-thick sheet, with cytoplasm *(c)* remaining only as a thin rim around the periphery and as a few thin fingers extending between the membranes. **B,** A longitudinal section through the internode resulting from the Schwann cell in A spiraling around the axon. Most of the internode consists simply of tightly wrapped Schwann cell membranes. Some cytoplasm remains on the surface of the internode near the nucleus, as small pockets near the node, and as Schmidt-Lanterman incisures. (Redrawn from Krstić RV: *Illustrated encyclopedia of human histology,* Berlin, 1984, Springer-Verlag.)

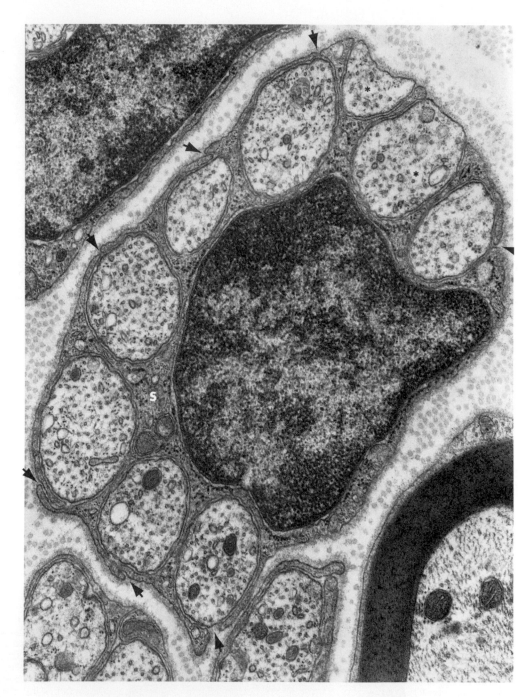

FIGURE 1-25
Unmyelinated nerve fibers in a dorsal root of a rat. Nine axons, each with the usual complement of microtubules, neurofilaments, and mito-chondria, are embedded in a single Schwann cell *(S)*. Even though no myelin is present, seven of the axons are almost completely ensheathed, communicating with the adjacent extracellular spaces only through small clefts *(arrows)* in the Schwann cell wrapping. The other two axons (*)
are partially exposed at the surface of the Schwann cell. [From Pannese E: *Neurocytology: fine structure of neurons, nerve processes, and neuroglial cells,*
New York, 1994, Thieme Medical Publishers, Inc.]

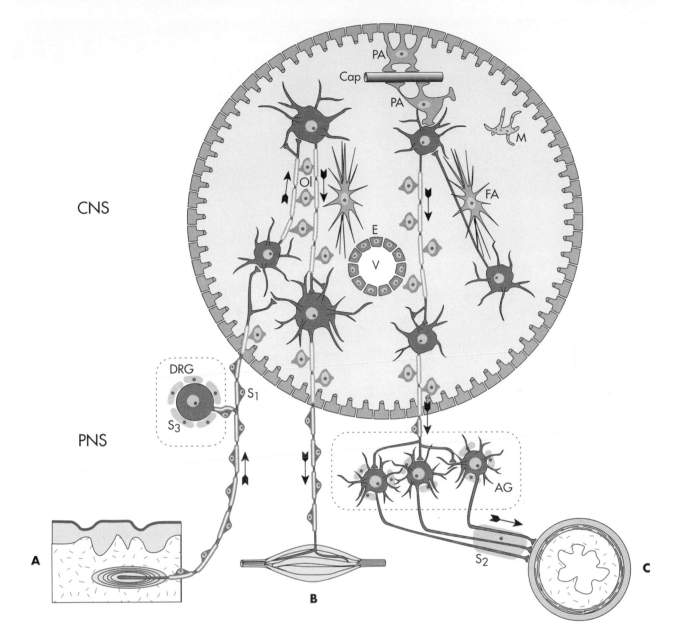

FIGURE 1-26

Summary diagram of cell types in the nervous system, showing the distribution of glial cell types in the CNS and PNS. A layer of end-feet of protoplasmic astrocytes *(PA)* forms a leaky membrane that covers the surface of the CNS, separating it from the PNS. Other end-feet of protoplasmic astrocytes are distributed in the gray matter, abutting either neurons or capillaries *(Cap)*. Fibrous astrocytes *(FA)* are interspersed among nerve fibers in the white matter, many of which are myelinated by oligodendrocytes *(Ol)*. Small microglial cells *(M)* act as scavengers in response to injury, and ependymal cells *(E)* line the ventricular cavities *(V)* of the CNS. Schwann cells and their variants are the principal glial cells of the PNS, forming the myelin of peripheral nerve fibers *(S₁)*, enveloping unmyelinated axons *(S₂)*, and forming satellite cells *(S₃)* surrounding sensory neurons in peripheral ganglia such as dorsal root and autonomic ganglia *(DRG, AG)*. The direction of information flow in various neurons is indicated by arrows. Processes of sensory neurons convey information to the CNS (**A**, in this case from skin). Information leaves the CNS to reach skeletal muscle directly (**B**) or to reach smooth muscle and glands (**C**) after a synapse in an autonomic ganglion *(AG)*. (Based on a drawing in Krstić RV: *General histology of the mammal*, Berlin, 1985, Springer-Verlag.)

Table 1-3   Cell Types in the Central Nervous System

Cells / parts of cells	Principal location(s)	Principal function(s)
Neurons, dendrites, synapses	Gray matter	Receive and integrate information, synthesize macromolecules
Axons	White matter	Transmit information
Oligodendrocytes	White matter	CNS myelin sheaths
Protoplasmic astrocytes	Gray matter	Mechanical and metabolic support, response to injury
Fibrous astrocytes	White matter	Mechanical and metabolic support, response to injury
Microglia	Gray (and white) matter	Phagocytosis
Ependymal cells	Walls of ventricles	Line ventricles and choroid plexus, secrete cerebrospinal fluid

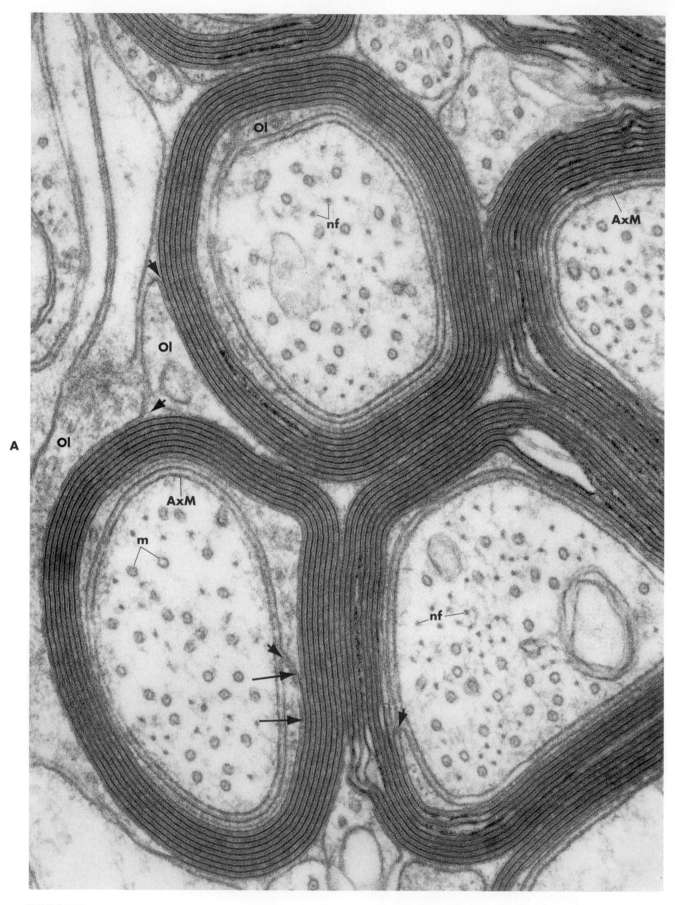

FIGURE 1-27

CNS myelin sheaths. **A,** Transverse section of myelinated fibers in a rat's optic nerve. Each axon contains microtubules *(m)* and neurofilaments *(nf)* and is bounded by a cell membrane *(AxM)*. Processes of oligodendrocytes *(Ol)* wrap around each axon to form its myelin sheath. Tongues of oligodendrocyte cytoplasm at the inside and outside of the myelin sheath narrow until the inner surfaces of their membranes fuse, forming the dense line that spirals through the myelin *(long arrows)*. The clefts between adjoining oligodendrocyte processes *(short arrows)* lead to the fainter zones between the dense lines. The actual diameter of each axon is about 0.5 μm.

Continued

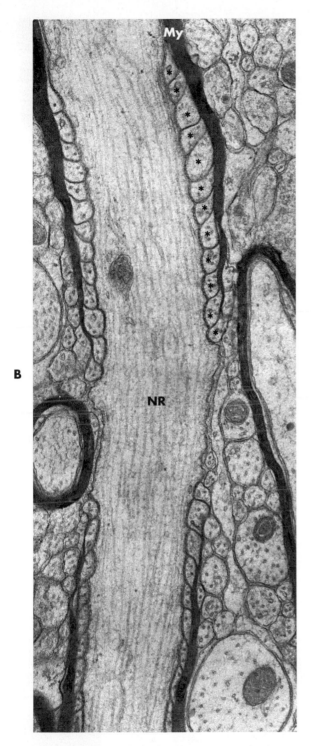

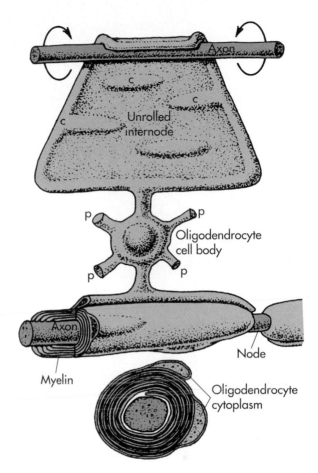

FIGURE 1-28

Schematic diagram of the formation of myelin in the CNS. A series of processes *(p)* emanate from an oligodendrocyte, each one giving rise to a flattened expansion that wraps around an axon to form an internode. As in the case of PNS myelin (Figure 1-24), most of the internode consists of tightly wrapped membranes, but small rims and fingers of oligodendrocyte cytoplasm *(c)* are also carried along. (Redrawn from Krstić RV: *Illustrated encyclopedia of human histology*, Berlin, 1984, Springer-Verlag.)

FIGURE 1-27, cont'd

B, Longitudinal section of a myelinated axon and node of Ranvier in a rat spinal cord. Numerous microtubules run longitudinally through the axon. At the node *(NR)* the myelin *(My)* ends as a series of pockets of oligodendrocyte cytoplasm *(*)*, leaving the axon bare. The actual diameter of this axon is about 1 μm. (**A** from Peters A, Palay SL, Webster H deF: *The fine structure of the nervous system: neurons and their supporting cells*, ed 3, New York, 1991, Oxford University Press. **B** from Pannese E: *Neurocytology: fine structure of neurons, nerve processes, and neuroglial cells*, New York, 1994, Thieme Medical Publishers, Inc.)

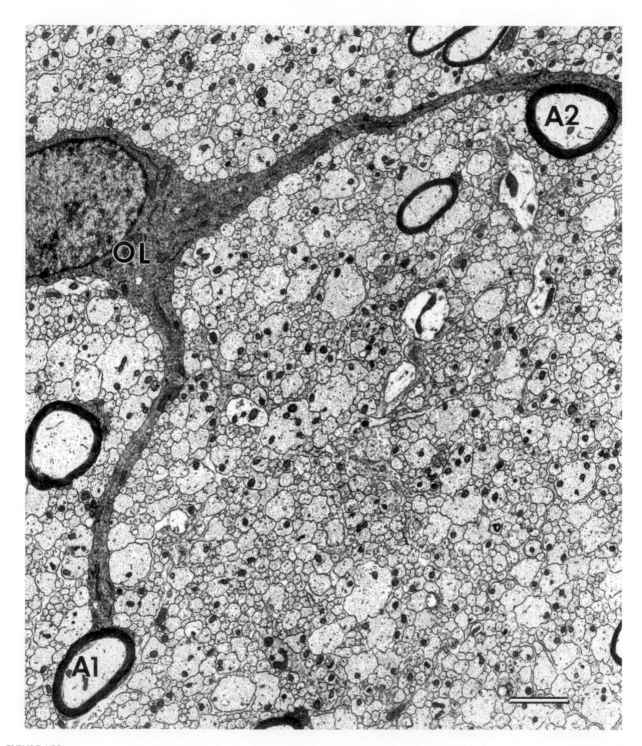

FIGURE 1-29

A single oligodendrocyte *(OL)* in the spinal cord white matter of a young rat, myelinating two different axons *(A1, A2)*. This cell and its processes stand out because in young rats, like many other young mammals, myelin has not yet developed around many axons. Note that the oligodendrocyte is connected to its myelin sheaths via thin processes; this tenuous connection has been cited as a possible reason for the paucity of remyelination after injury to myelin sheaths in the brain and spinal cord. Scale mark equals 2 μm. [From Waxman SG, Sims TJ: Specificity in central myelination: evidence for local regulation of myelin thickness, *Brain Res* 292:179, 1984.]

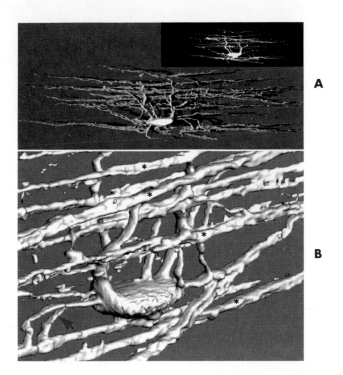

FIGURE 1-30
Three views of a single oligodendrocyte from the cerebellar white matter of a rat. Individual cells in fixed brain tissue were injected with Lucifer Yellow using a dye-filled micropipette and reconstructed with a confocal laser scanning microscope. Further processing of images such as that in the inset in **A** yielded the three-dimensional reconstruction seen in **A** and, at higher magnification and from a different viewpoint, in **B**. Numerous processes emerge from the cell body (*arrow*; the same one is indicated in both parts of the figure). Each process ends as an internode (***). The actual size of the area shown in the inset in **A** is about 330 μm × 100 μm, and the actual longest diameter of the oligodendrocyte's cell body is about 25 μm. (Courtesy Dr. Peter S. Eggli, Institute of Anatomy, University of Bern. Inset from Weruaga-Prieto E, Eggli P, Celio MR: Topographic variations in rat brain oligodendrocyte morphology elucidated by injection of Lucifer Yellow in fixed tissue slices, *J Neurocytol* 25:19, 1996.)

most prominent in white matter, but they are also found in the gray matter. Here they provide myelin sheaths for axons traversing gray matter and also participate (along with other glial cell types) in surrounding neurons and their processes in a manner analogous to satellite cells in the PNS.

Astrocytes provide structural and metabolic support to neurons

Astrocytes, named for their typical star shapes, form the second major category of CNS glial cells. Adult astrocytes fall into two broad classes—**protoplasmic** astrocytes (Figure 1-32), found in gray matter, and **fibrous** astrocytes (Figure 1-33), found in white matter. (Astrocytes of a third category, called **radial glia,** are present during development and form a scaffolding that helps guide growing axons.) Despite their somewhat different appearances, protoplasmic and fibrous astrocytes have basically similar characteristics. Astrocytes have a well-developed cytoskeleton (Figure 1-34) that is dominated by intermediate filaments but also includes microtubules and actin filaments, consistent with a role as structural support elements

in the CNS. In addition, some astrocyte processes have enlarged end-feet that are applied either to the surface of CNS capillaries or to the surface of the CNS itself (Figure 1-32); other processes abut neurons, dendrites, synaptic endings, and nodes of Ranvier. This carpeting of otherwise exposed surfaces with astrocyte processes suggests that these cells have a role in CNS metabolism and the regulation of extracellular ionic concentrations. Finally, astrocytes are a major part of the limited armamentarium available to the CNS in responding to injury; they multiply, increase their production of intermediate filaments, and form dense, gliotic scars.

Ependymal cells line the ventricles

The CNS, as described in Chapter 2, develops embryologically from a neuroepithelial tube. The cavity of the tube persists in the adult CNS as a system of ventricles (see Chapter 5) with an epithelial lining of **ependymal cells.** In some locations the ependymal cells are specialized as a secretory epithelium that produces the cerebrospinal fluid (CSF) that fills the ventricles and bathes the CNS (see Figure 5-5).

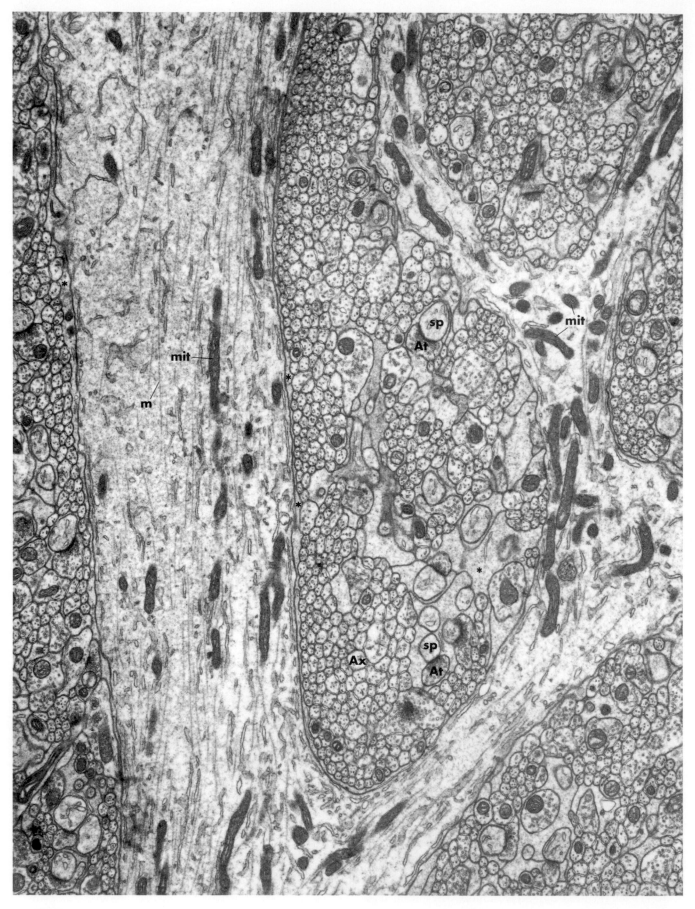

FIGURE 1-31
Unmyelinated axons in the CNS. Hundreds of tiny axons (*Ax*, actual diameter about 0.25 μm) are cut transversely as they pass between large branches of a Purkinje cell dendrite in the cerebellar cortex. The dendrite contains longitudinally oriented microtubules *(m)* and mitochondria *(mit)* and is almost completely covered by thin processes of astrocytes (*), except where dendritic spines *(sp)* are contacted by the terminals of the un-myelinated axons *(At)*. In contrast to the glial covering of unmyelinated PNS axons, unmyelinated axons in the CNS are typically bare. (From Peters A, Palay SL, Webster H deF: *The fine structure of the nervous system: neurons and their supporting cells,* ed 3, New York, 1991, Oxford University Press.)

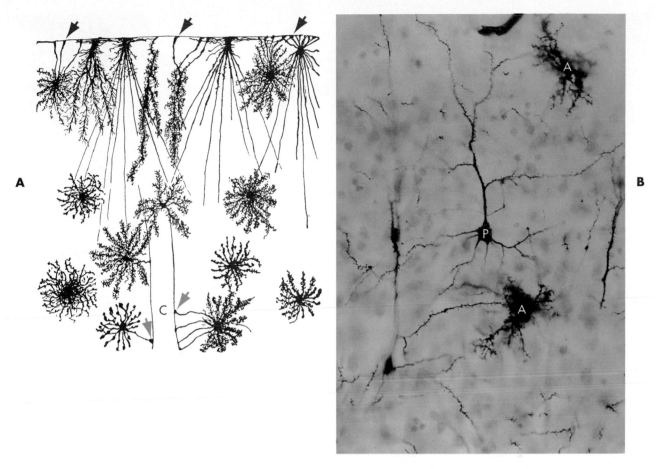

FIGURE 1-32
Protoplasmic astrocytes in the cerebral cortex, stained by the Golgi method. **A,** Astrocytes have enlarged end-feet, covering the surface of the CNS *(blue arrows)*, contacting capillaries *(C, green arrows)* and contacting neurons (not shown). **B,** Golgi-stained astrocytes *(A)* and pyramidal neurons *(P).* (**A** from Ramón y Cajal S: *Histologie du système nerveux de l'homme et des vertébrés*, Paris, 1909, 1911, Maloine. **B** courtesy Dr. Nathaniel T. Mc-Mullen, Department of Cell Biology and Anatomy, The University of Arizona College of Medicine.)

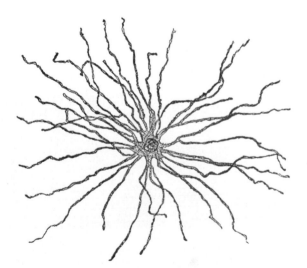

FIGURE 1-33
A fibrous astrocyte isolated from spinal cord white matter. (From Ramón y Cajal S: *Histologie du système nerveux de l'homme et des vertébrés*, Paris, 1909, 1911, Maloine.)

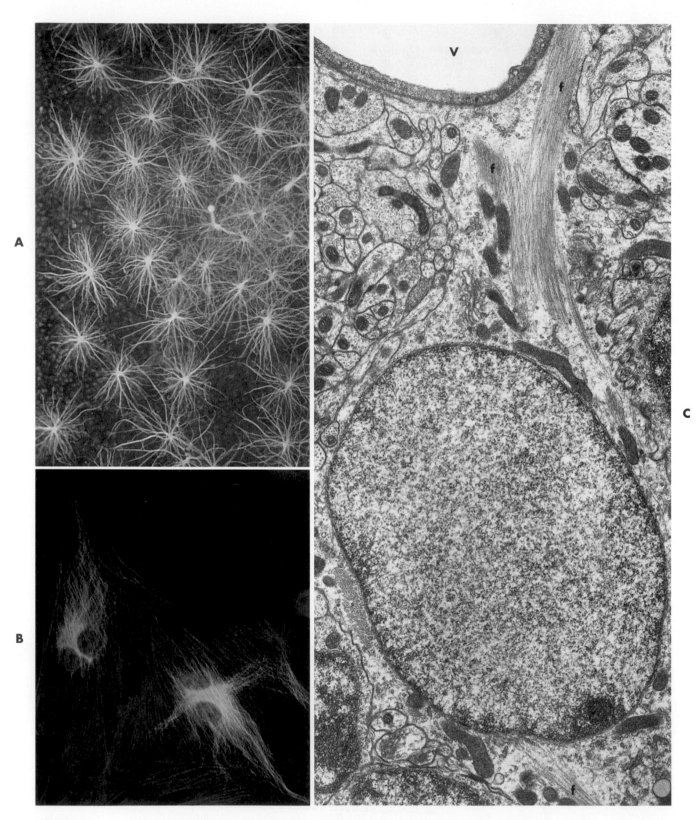

FIGURE I-34

Cytoskeletal elements of astrocytes. **A,** Retinal astrocytes stained with a fluorescent antibody directed against a specific protein in astrocyte intermediate filaments (glial fibrillary acidic protein, or GFAP). This spectacular image illustrates why astrocytes (Greek for "star cell") got their name. **B,** Triple fluorescence micrograph of astrocytes isolated from rat cerebral cortex and developing in tissue culture. Actin filaments were stained with fluorescent phalloidin (red fluorescence), microtubules with a fluorescent antibody directed against tubulin (green fluorescence), and cell nuclei with DAPI (blue fluorescence). **C,** Electron micrograph of a fibrous astrocyte in the cerebellar cortex of a rat. Prominent bundles of intermediate filaments *(f)* are apparent, one of them leading into an expanded end-foot that partly surrounds a blood vessel *(V)*. (**A** courtesy Dr. Andreas Karschin, Max-Planck-Institut für Biophysikalische Chemie. **B** courtesy Drs. Olaf Mundigl and Pietro De Camilli, Yale University School of Medicine. **C** from Pannese E: *Neurocytology: fine structure of neurons, nerve processes, and neuroglial cells*, New York, 1994, Thieme Medical Publishers, Inc.)

Microglial cells respond to CNS injury

Microglial cells, as their name implies, are smaller than oligodendrocytes and astrocytes (which together are sometimes called **macroglia**). Microglia seem not to be involved in the minute-to-minute metabolism and electrical signaling of the nervous system, and their role in the normal, healthy nervous system is not clear. However, they play the other major role in the nervous system's response to injury. When microglia detect neuronal damage, they proliferate, migrate to the site of damage or disease, transform into macrophages,* and devour pathogens and neuronal debris.

SUGGESTED READINGS

Abbott NJ, editor: Glial-neuronal interaction, *Ann NY Acad Sci* vol 633, 1991.

Angevine JB: The nervous tissue. In Fawcett DW: *Bloom and Fawcett: a textbook of histology*, New York, 1994, Chapman and Hall.

Burgoyne RD, editor: *The neuronal cytoskeleton*, New York, 1991, Wiley-Liss, Inc.

Cherniak C: The bounded brain: toward quantitative neuroanatomy, *J Cog Neurosci* 2:1, 1990. *An interesting account of the widely varying estimates of a number of aspects of the human brain.*

Federoff S, Zhai R, Novak JP: Microglia and astroglia have a common progenitor cell, *J Neurosci Res* 50:477, 1997.

Gehrmann J, Matsumoto Y, Kreutzberg GW: Microglia: intrinsic immunoeffector cell of the brain, *Brain Res Rev* 20:269, 1995.

Heimer L, Robards MJ: *Neuroanatomical tract-tracing methods*, New York, 1981, Plenum Press.

Heimer L, Záborszky L: *Neuroanatomical tract-tracing methods 2. Recent progress*, New York, 1989, Plenum Press.

Ibrahim M, Butt AM, Berry M: Relationship between myelin sheath diameter and internodal length in axons of the anterior medullary velum of the adult rat, *J Neurol Sci* 133:119, 1995.

Kettenmann H, Ransom BR: *Neuroglia*, New York, 1995, Oxford University Press.

Kimelberg HK, Norenberg MD: Astrocytes, *Sci Am* 260(4):66, 1989.

Mesulam M-M: Tracing neural connections of human brain with selective silver impregnation: observations on geniculocalcarine, spinothalamic, and entorhinal pathways, *Arch Neurol* 36:814, 1979.

Miklossy J, Clarke S, Van der Loos H: The long distance effects of brain lesions: visualization of axonal pathways and their terminations in the human brain by the Nauta method, *J Neuropath Exp Neurol* 50:595, 1991.

Palay SL et al: The axon hillock and initial segment, *J Cell Biol* 38:193, 1968.

Pannese E: *Neurocytology: fine structure of neurons, nerve processes, and neuroglial cells*, New York, 1994, Thieme Medical Publishers, Inc. *A succinct yet thorough review, and the source of a number of beautiful micrographs in this book.*

Paxinos G, editor: *The human nervous system*, San Diego, 1990, Academic Press. *A detailed, extensive review of human neuroanatomy.*

Peters A, Palay SL, Webster H deF: *The fine structure of the nervous system: the neurons and their supporting cells,* ed 3, New York, 1991, Oxford University Press. *A classic reference work on electron microscopy of neural tissues and also the source of a number of beautiful micrographs in this book.*

Streit WJ, Kincaid-Colton CA: The brain's immune system, *Sci Am* 273(5), 1995. *A recent review of the role of microglia in responding to disease and possibly sometimes contributing to it.*

Vallee RB, Bloom GS: Mechanisms of fast and slow axonal transport, *Annu Rev Neurosci* 14:59, 1991.

Waxman SG, Kocsis JD, Stys PK, editors: *The axon: structure, function, and pathophysiology*, New York, 1995, Oxford University Press. *A terrific compendium of work on all aspects of axonal structure and function—central and peripheral, myelinated and unmyelinated.*

Weruaga-Prieto E, Eggli P, Celio MR: Topographic variations in rat brain oligodendrocyte morphology elucidated by injection of Lucifer Yellow in fixed tissue slices, *J Neurocytol* 25:19, 1996.

---

*The origin of microglia has long been controversial. Their resemblance to white blood cells after neuronal injury has been taken as evidence that microglia are derived from monocyte-related stem cells that invade the nervous system early in embryogenesis. Other evidence, however, suggests that they may be derived from the same neural epithelium as macroglia.

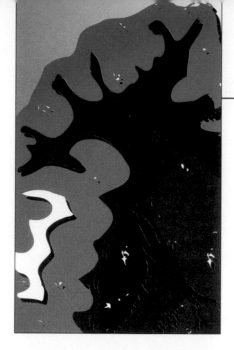

DEVELOPMENT OF THE NERVOUS SYSTEM

THE NEURAL TUBE AND NEURAL CREST GIVE RISE TO THE CENTRAL AND PERIPHERAL NERVOUS SYSTEMS
    The Sulcus Limitans Separates Sensory and Motor Areas of the Spinal Cord and Brainstem
    The Neural Tube Has a Series of Bulges and Flexures
        There are three primary vesicles
        There are five secondary vesicles
    Growth of the Telencephalon Overshadows Other Parts of the Nervous System
    The Cavity of the Neural Tube Persists as a System of Ventricles
ADVERSE EVENTS DURING DEVELOPMENT CAN CAUSE CONGENITAL MALFORMATIONS OF THE NERVOUS SYSTEM
    Defective Closure of the Neural Tube Can Cause Spina Bifida or Anencephaly
    Defective Secondary Neurulation Can Cause a Distinctive Set of Abnormalities
    The Prosencephalon Can Develop Abnormally Even if Neural Tube Closure Is Complete

As complex as the human nervous system is, its embryonic origin is as a simple, tubular, ectodermal structure. An understanding of the development of the nervous system helps make sense of its adult configuration and organization. Similarly, the relatively frequent congenital malformations of the CNS are more easily understood in light of its embryological development; such malformations also provide clues that aid in the understanding of normal development.

The focus in this chapter is on the events that lead to the shape of the CNS and the configuration of its major components. There is clearly much more to building a nervous system than this—neurons must proliferate in enormous numbers, migrate from their places of birth to their final destinations, and establish appropriate connections with other neurons. Consideration of these events is beyond the scope of this chapter.

THE NEURAL TUBE AND NEURAL CREST GIVE RISE TO THE CENTRAL AND PERIPHERAL NERVOUS SYSTEMS

During the third week of embryonic development a longitudinal band of ectoderm thickens to form the **neural plate.** Shortly thereafter, the neural plate begins to fold inward, forming a longitudinal **neural groove** in the midline flanked by a parallel **neural fold** on each side (Figures 2-1 and 2-2). The neural groove deepens, and the neural folds approach each other in the dorsal midline. At the end of the third week the two folds begin to fuse midway along the neural groove at a level corresponding to the future cervical spinal cord, forming the **neural tube** (Figure 2-3). This process is referred to as **primary neurulation.** As the neural tube closes, it separates from the ectodermal (i.e., skin) surface and becomes enclosed

36

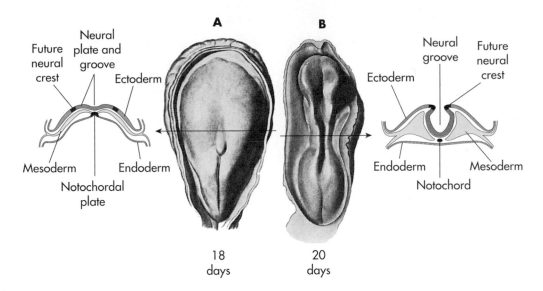

FIGURE 2-1

The neural plate and beginning neural groove at about 18 days of development (A), and the neural groove 2 days later (B), shortly before the neural tube begins to close. The schematic cross sections to the left and right are at the levels indicated by arrows in A and B, respectively. (A and B from Arey LB: *Developmental anatomy*, ed 4, Philadelphia, 1941, WB Saunders.)

within the body. As this fusion occurs, groups of cells from the crest of each neural fold dissociate from the neural tube (Figure 2-4). These **neural crest cells** develop into a variety of cell types (Figure 2-5), including the sensory neurons of the ganglia of spinal nerves and some cranial nerves,★ the postganglionic neurons of the autonomic nervous system, and the Schwann cells and satellite cells of the PNS. The neural tube, on the other hand, develops into virtually the entire CNS; its cavity becomes the ventricular system of the brain. (The sacral spinal cord forms by a slightly different mechanism. After the neural tube closes, a secondary cavity extends into the mass of cells at its caudal end, in a process of **secondary neurulation**.)

The Sulcus Limitans Separates Sensory and Motor Areas of the Spinal Cord and Brainstem

During the fourth week a longitudinal groove appears in the lateral wall of the neural tube. This groove, called the **sulcus limitans,** extends throughout the future spinal cord and brainstem and subdivides the gray matter in the walls of the neural tube into a more dorsal **alar plate** and a more ventral **basal plate** (Figures 2-2 and 2-6). This is a distinction of some functional importance because alar plate derivatives are primarily concerned with sensory processing, whereas motor neurons are located in basal plate derivatives. In the adult spinal cord, even though the

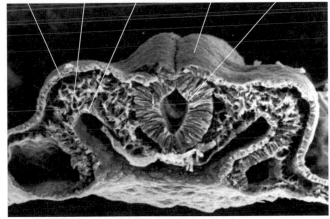

FIGURE 2-2

Scanning electron micrograph of the just-closing neural tube of a chick embryo, fractured at about the level of the future midbrain. (From the cover photograph accompanying Schoenwolf GC, Smith JL: Mechanisms of neurulation: traditional viewpoint and recent advances, *Devel* 109:243, 1990.)

sulcus limitans can no longer be found, the central gray matter can be divided into a **posterior horn** and an **anterior horn** on each side (Figure 2-6, C). The central processes of sensory neurons (derived from neural crest cells) end mainly in the posterior horn, which contains most of the cells whose axons form ascending sensory pathways. In contrast, the anterior horn contains the cell bodies of motor neurons, whose axons leave the spinal cord and innervate skeletal muscles. The same distinction between sensory alar plate derivatives and motor basal plate derivatives holds true in the brainstem, as discussed briefly in this chapter and in more detail in Chapter 12. (The sulcus limitans is thought not to extend beyond the

★ Thickenings of the cranial epithelium, called **placodes**, are induced by the underlying neural tube and give rise to additional neural crest-like cells. Placodal derivatives include the olfactory epithelium, the lens of the eye, hair cells of the inner ear, and parts or all of the ganglia of cranial nerves V, VII, VIII, IX, and X.

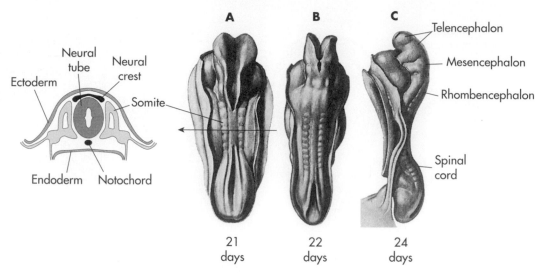

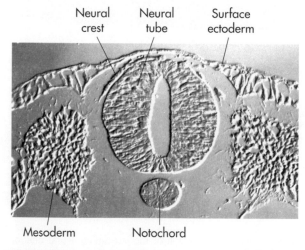

FIGURE 2-3

Neural tube closure during the fourth week. Neural folds begin to fuse at the cervical level of the future spinal cord at about day 21 **(A)**; total length of neural tube at this time is about 2.5 mm. The area of fusion expands rapidly in both rostral and caudal directions **(B).** By about day 24 **(C)** the rostral end of the neural tube has closed; the caudal end will close about 2 days later. Even before the neural tube has finished closing, local enlargements (the primary vesicles) and bends begin to appear **(C)**. The notochord is the forerunner of the skeletal axis, helping to form the vertebral column. The mesodermally derived somites, adjacent to the neural tube, go on to form most of the vertebral column, as well as segmental structures such as skeletal muscle and dermis corresponding to spinal cord segments (see Chapter 10). **(A-C** from Arey LB: *Developmental anatomy,* ed 4, Philadelphia, 1941, WB Saunders.)

FIGURE 2-4

Section through the just-closed neural tube of a chick embryo at the level of the future spinal cord. Neural crest cells have been pinched off as the neural tube closed. (From Schoenwolf GC, Smith JL: Mechanisms of neurulation: traditional viewpoint and advances, *Devel* 109:243, 1990.)

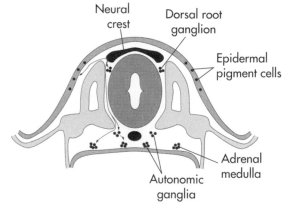

FIGURE 2-5

Migratory paths and some fates of neural crest cells. Neural crest cells give rise to an extraordinary variety of tissues and structures, only some of which are indicated here.

brainstem, so the alar/basal plate distinction is not useful for cerebral structures, even though some deal primarily with sensory processes and others with motor processes.)

The Neural Tube Has a Series of Bulges and Flexures

The neural tube is never a simple, straight cylinder. Even before the rostral and caudal neuropores close, bulges begin to appear in the rostral end of the neural tube in the region of the future brain, and bends begin to appear as well (Figure 2-3, *C*).

There are three primary vesicles

During the fourth week, three bulges, or vesicles, are apparent and are referred to as the **primary vesicles** (Figure 2-7). From rostral to caudal, these are the **prosencephalon** (forebrain), the **mesencephalon** (midbrain), and the **rhombencephalon** (hindbrain), which merges smoothly with the spinal portion of the neural tube. The prosencephalon develops into the cerebrum. The mesencephalon becomes the midbrain of the adult brainstem, and the rhombencephalon becomes the rest of the brainstem and the cerebellum (Table 2-1).

The three primary vesicles are not arranged in a straight line, but rather are associated with two bends or flexures in the neural tube (Figure 2-7, *A*). One of these,

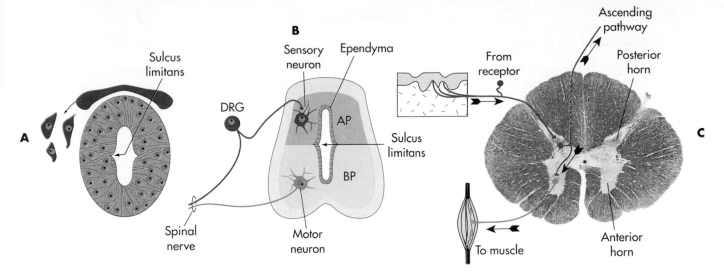

FIGURE 2-6
Sulcus limitans and alar and basal plates. **A,** Neural tube during the fourth week. **B,** Embryonic spinal cord during the sixth week; dorsal root ganglion (*DRG*) cells, derived from the neural crest, send their central processes into the spinal cord to terminate mainly on alar plate (*AP*) cells; basal plate (*BP*) cells become motor neurons, whose axons exit in the ventral roots. **C,** Adult spinal cord.

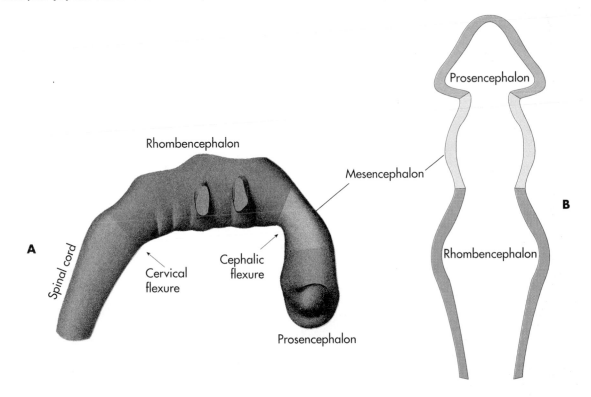

FIGURE 2-7
Primary vesicles at the end of the fourth week. **A,** Lateral view of the neural tube, showing vesicles and flexures. **B,** Schematic longitudinal section, as though the flexures had been straightened out. (**A** modified from Hochstetter F: *Beiträge zur Entwicklungsgeschichte des menschlichen Gehirns.* I. Teil, Vienna, 1919, Franz Deuticke.)

Table 2-1 Derivatives of Vesicles of the Neural Tube			
Primary vesicle	Secondary vesicle	Neural derivatives	Cavity
Prosencephalon	Telencephalon	Cerebral hemispheres★	Lateral ventricles
	Diencephalon	Thalamus, hypothalamus, other structures	Third ventricle
Mesencephalon	Mesencephalon	Midbrain	Cerebral aqueduct
Rhombencephalon	Metencephalon	Pons, cerebellum	Part of fourth ventricle
	Myelencephalon	Medulla	Part of fourth ventricle
			Part of central canal

★A few structures that appear in sections to be part of the cerebral hemisphere, most notably the globus pallidus (part of the basal ganglia), are actually diencephalic derivatives.

the **cervical flexure,** occurs between the rhomben-cephalon and spinal cord but does not persist in the adult CNS. The second, the **cephalic** (or **mesencephalic) flexure,** occurs at the level of the future midbrain; it persists in the adult as the bend between the axes of the brainstem and the forebrain (see Figure 3-1).

There are five secondary vesicles

As the brain continues to develop, two of the primary vesicles become subdivided. During the fifth week, five **secondary vesicles** can be distinguished (Figure 2-8). The prosencephalon gives rise to the **telencephalon** (Greek for "end-brain") and the **diencephalon** (Greek for "in-between-brain"); the mesencephalon remains undivided; the rhombencephalon gives rise to the **metencephalon** and the **myelencephalon.** The telencephalon becomes the cerebral hemispheres of the adult brain. The diencephalon gives rise to the **thalamus** (a large mass of gray matter interposed between the cerebral cortex and other structures), the **hypothalamus** (an autonomic control center), the neural part of the eye, and several other structures.

The metencephalon becomes the **pons** (part of the brainstem) and the cerebellum. The myelencephalon becomes the **medulla** (the part of the brainstem that merges with the spinal cord).

In addition, a **pontine flexure** appears in the dorsal surface of the brainstem between the metencephalon and the myelencephalon (Figure 2-8, *A*). This flexure does not persist as a bend in the axis of the brainstem, but it does have important consequences for the configuration of the caudal brainstem. As the flexure develops, the walls of the neural tube spread apart to form a diamond-shaped cavity (hence the name *rhombencephalon*) so that only a thin membranous roof remains over what will become the **fourth ventricle** (Figure 2-9). Thus the alar and basal plates, still separated by the sulcus limitans, come to lie in the floor of the fourth ventricle. The result is that in the corresponding part of the adult brainstem (rostral medulla and caudal pons), sensory nuclei are located lateral, rather than posterior, to motor nuclei. As discussed further in Chapter 12, this is of some utility in making sense of the arrangement of cranial nerve nuclei.

Lateral portions of the alar plate in the rostral metencephalon thicken considerably and form the **rhombic lips.** These continue to enlarge, finally fusing in the midline to form a transverse ridge that will eventually become the cerebellum★ (Figure 2-10).

★ Although the cerebellum develops from the alar plate, it is involved in motor functions in the sense that cerebellar lesions cause impairments of posture and movement but not of sensation (see Chapter 20).

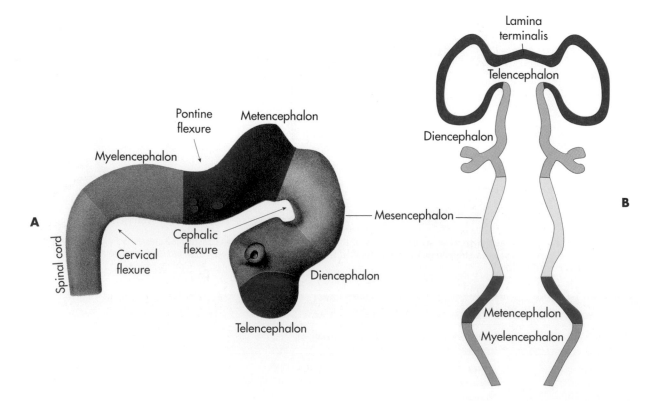

FIGURE 2-8
Secondary vesicles during the sixth week. **A,** Lateral view of the neural tube, showing vesicles and flexures. **B,** Schematic longitudinal section, as though the flexures had been straightened out. (**A** modified from Hochstetter F: *Beiträge zur Entwicklungsgeschichte des menschlichen Gehirns.* I. Teil, Vienna, 1919, Franz Deuticke.)

Growth of the Telencephalon Overshadows Other Parts of the Nervous System

Subsequent events are dominated by the tremendous growth of the telencephalon. This portion of the neural tube begins as two swellings connected across the midline by a thin membrane, the **lamina terminalis*** (Figure 2-8, *B*). The basal part of the wall of the telencephalon, adjacent to the diencephalon, thickens to form the primordia of gray masses called the **basal ganglia** or **basal nuclei.** At the same time, the walls of the diencephalon thicken to form the thalamus and hypothalamus, separated by the **hypothalamic sulcus.** With continued growth, the telencephalon folds down alongside the diencephalon until eventually the two fuse (Figure 2-11). The telencephalic surface overlying the area of fusion develops into a portion of the cerebral cortex called the **insula.** The cortex adjoining the insula expands greatly during the ensuing months (Figure 2-12) until the insula itself is completely hidden from view (Figure 2-11, *C*). Each cerebral hemisphere ultimately assumes the shape of a great arc encircling the insular cortex, and parts of the hemisphere that started out dorsal to the insula get pushed around into the temporal lobe (Figure 2-12). As discussed and demonstrated in the next chapter, knowledge of this growth of each cerebral hemisphere in a great **C** shape is of considerable

importance for understanding the anatomical organization of the forebrain (see Figure 3-16).

The expansion of cortical area that begins as an evagination of two telencephalic vesicles, and continues as the growth of each hemisphere into a **C** shape, concludes with development of extensive folds in the surface of the hemisphere. Thus each cerebral hemisphere starts out with a smooth surface (Figure 2-13) and becomes progressively more convoluted (Figures 2-14 and 2-15). A critical part of this growth of the cerebral cortex (and of the cerebellum [Figure 2-10] and other parts of the CNS) is massive proliferation and migration of neurons and glial cells. Most neuronal production and migration occurs during the third through fifth months of development, and the formation of neuronal connections and production of myelin sheaths continue well after birth (Figure 2-16).

The Cavity of the Neural Tube Persists as a System of Ventricles

The cavity of the neural tube persists as the ventricular system of the adult brain (Figure 2-17; see also Figures 5-1 and 5-2). Except for the rudimentary central canal of the spinal cord and caudal medulla, the ventricles comprise a continuous, fluid-filled series of spaces extending through all the major divisions of the CNS. The cavity of the pons and rostral medulla is the fourth ventricle; that of the diencephalon is the **third ventricle.** A large **C**-shaped **lateral ventricle** occupies each cerebral hemisphere. Each lateral ventricle communicates with the third ventricle through an **interventricular foramen** (Figure 2-18), and the third ventricle communicates with the fourth ventricle through the **cerebral aqueduct** of the midbrain.

---

* The lamina terminalis thus starts out as a bridge between the two cerebral hemispheres and as such is the site where bundles of fibers interconnecting the hemispheres begin to grow. In the adult brain the two most prominent of these commissures, or crossing bundles—the anterior commissure and the corpus callosum—are still attached to the thin lamina terminalis (see Figures 3-2 and 3-13).

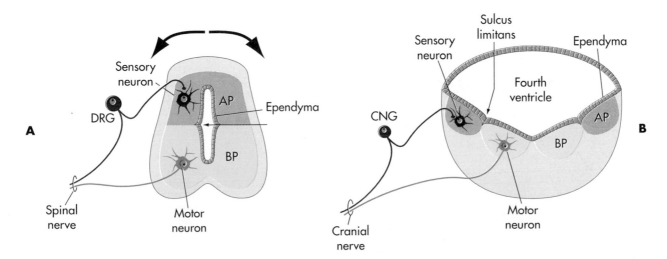

FIGURE 2-9

Formation of the floor of the fourth ventricle. Walls of the neural tube are spread apart by the pontine flexure so that they and the sulcus limitans become the floor of the ventricle and the roof becomes a thin membrane. The dorsal-ventral arrangement of sensory and motor areas in the spinal cord **(A)** becomes a lateral-medial arrangement in the brainstem **(B)**. *CNG,* Cranial nerve ganglion cell; *DRG,* dorsal root ganglion; *AP,* alar plate; *BP,* basal plate.

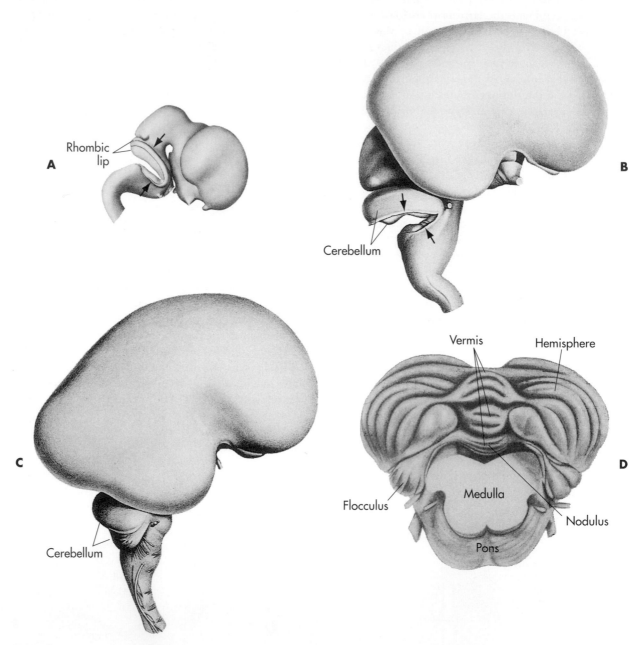

FIGURE 2-10

Development of the cerebellum. During the second month of development lateral parts of the alar plate in the rostral metencephalon thicken to form rhombic lips **(A).** These continue to enlarge during the third and fourth month **(B** and **C),** forming the cerebellum. By about five months **(D)** a series of deep fissures develops in the cerebellar surface, and both midline (vermis) and lateral (hemisphere) zones are apparent. (The nodulus is a special part of the vermis, continuous laterally with the flocculus; see Chapter 20 for additional details.) Arrows indicate the cut edge of the thin roof of the fourth ventricle in **A** and **B.** (From Hochstetter F: *Beiträge zur Entwicklungsgeschichte des menschlichen Gehirns.* I. Teil **(A-C)** and II. Teil **(D),** Vienna, 1919 and 1929, Franz Deuticke.)

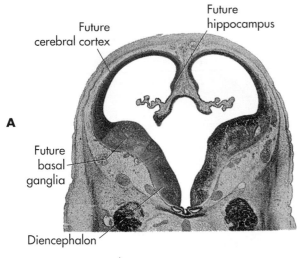

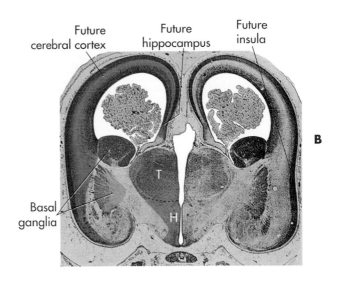

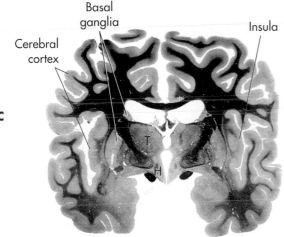

FIGURE 2-11

Fusion between diencephalon and telencephalon as the cerebral hemispheres enlarge. **A,** During the second month the telencephalon, including zones that will become the cerebral cortex and basal ganglia, is a separate vesicle connected to the diencephalon. As a result of subsequent rapid telencephalic growth, the basal ganglia portion folds down toward the diencephalon. At the end of the third month **(B)** the telencephalon and diencephalon have fused. After further rapid growth the insula, overlying the point of fusion, becomes overgrown by other cerebral cortex in the adult brain **(C).** The hippocampus is one example of a telencephalic structure that starts out in a dorsal position and is pushed around into the temporal lobe (slightly posterior to the plane of section in **C;** see Figures 3-20 to 3-22). *H,* Hypothalamus; *T,* thalamus. (**A** and **B** from Hochstetter F: *Beiträge zur Entwicklungsgeschichte des menschlichen Gehirns.* I. Teil, Vienna, 1919, Franz Deuticke.)

Where the walls of the rhombencephalon spread apart to form the fourth ventricle, the roof of the ventricle becomes extremely thin (Figure 2-9). An area covering the roof of the third ventricle and extending onto the surface of the telencephalon becomes similarly thin (Figure 2-18). At each of these locations, tufts of small blood vessels invaginate the ventricular roof to form the **choroid plexus,** which is responsible for the production of most of the **cerebrospinal fluid** that fills the ventricles. As each cerebral hemisphere grows around in a **C** shape, so too does the choroid plexus, which protrudes into its lateral ventricle.

ADVERSE EVENTS DURING DEVELOPMENT CAN CAUSE CONGENITAL MALFORMATIONS OF THE NERVOUS SYSTEM

A large number of intricate events need to happen in a precisely coordinated fashion for the nervous system to develop properly. Sometimes a flaw in the process causes a congenital malformation of the nervous system, and the nature of the malformation frequently provides clues

about the timing of the defect (Table 2-2). Although the nature of the insult or event responsible for a given malformation is usually unknown, malformations sometimes are seen in chromosomal disorders or after viral infections or exposure to various environmental agents at particular times during gestation.

Defective Closure of the Neural Tube Can Cause Spina Bifida or Anencephaly

Defective closure of the neural tube is a frequent cause of congenital malformations of the nervous system (about one per thousand live births). Because the neural tube forms and closes under the influence of certain dorsal portions of the embryo situated just beneath the neural ectoderm, defects related to these events are referred to as **defects of dorsal induction.** Complete failure of the neural tube to close results in a fatal deformity called **craniorachischisis** (from Greek words meaning "cleft skull and spine"), in which the CNS appears as an open furrow on the dorsal surface of the head and body. Failure of the caudal neuropore to close can result in a severe form of **spina bifida** called **myelomeningocele** (from

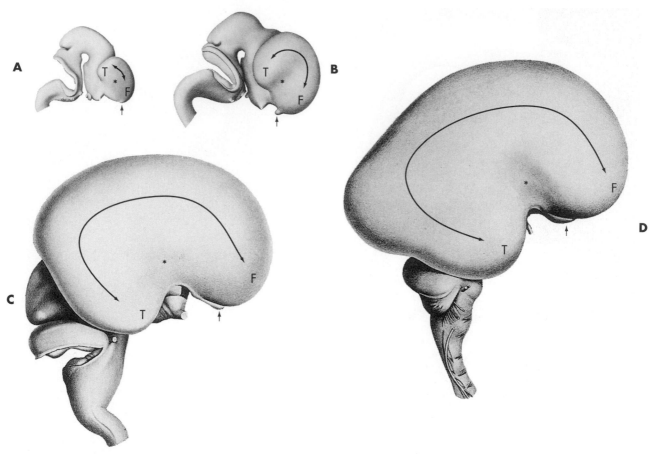

FIGURE 2-12
"Rotation" of the cerebral hemispheres into a C shape. Although commonly described as a rotation, the change in shape is actually caused by disproportionate growth of cortex (neocortex, described in Chapter 22) above the location of the future insula (*). The frontal (*F*) and temporal (*T*) poles actually move little, but expansion of the cortex between them causes development of the C shape during the second (**A** and **B**), third (**C**), and fourth (**D**) months. The olfactory bulb is indicated by arrows. (From Hochstetter F: *Beiträge zur Entwicklungsgeschichte des menschlichen Gehirns.* I. Teil, Vienna, 1919, Franz Deuticke.)

FIGURE 2-13
Magnetic resonance image of a 23-week-old fetus in utero. Fluid-filled spaces are dark in this T1-weighted image (see Chapter 5), and the anterior (*A*) and posterior (*P*) horns of the lateral ventricles, the midline third ventricle (*3*), and abundant subarachnoid space (*) surrounding the brain can all be seen. The surface of the cerebral hemispheres is still smooth at this stage, except for a depression (*arrow*) at the site of the insula. (From Girard N, Raybaud C, Poncet M: In vivo study of brain maturation in normal fetuses, *AJNR Am J Neuroradiol* 16:407, 1995.)

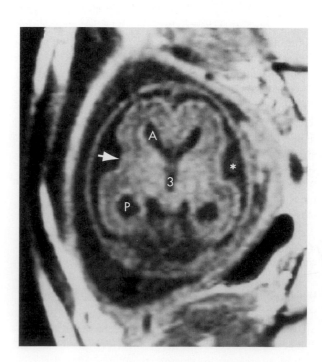

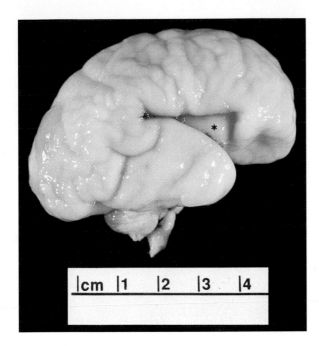

FIGURE 2-14
The brain of a 26-week-old who died shortly after birth as the result of an intraventricular hemorrhage. Sulci are still few and shallow, and the insula (*) is still exposed. (Courtesy Dr. Naomi Rance, The University of Arizona College of Medicine.)

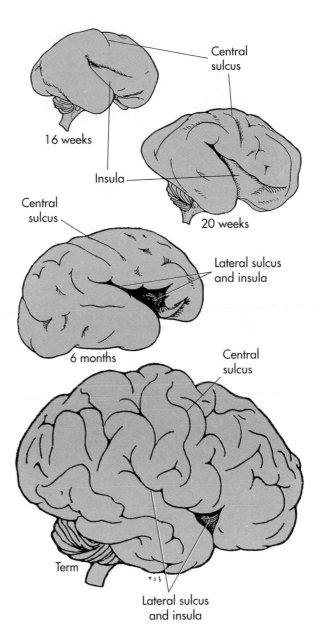

FIGURE 2-15
Progressive development of cortical convolutions. (From Mettler FA: *Neuroanatomy*, ed 2, St. Louis, 1948, Mosby.)

Greek words meaning "herniated spinal cord and meninges"). In myelomeningocele the alar and basal plates on both sides are visible as four distinct bands on the exposed neural plate. The sulcus limitans on each side and the midline ventral groove between the basal plates also are visible on the body surface (Figure 2-19). Vertebrae fail to form over the defect, the caudal walls of the neural tube are still continuous with the skin of the back, and the cord and meninges are displaced into a saclike cavity on the back. Myelomeningocele is accompanied by an **Arnold-Chiari malformation** in which the cerebellum and caudal brainstem are elongated and pushed down into the foramen magnum. Frequently there is obstruction to the flow of cerebrospinal fluid and hydrocephalus results. The reason these two deformities accompany one another is not known with certainty, but it has been proposed that both arise from a single misalignment at the site where the neural tube first begins to close.

If the rostral neuropore fails to close, **anencephaly,** in which much of each cerebral hemisphere is absent, can result. As in spina bifida, the walls of the neural tube then may be continuous with the skin of the head, and the central cavity of the neural tube may be open to the outside.

Neural tube defects can be detected by ultrasound examination or indicated by elevated levels of **alpha-feto-**

protein. This protein is a major component of fetal serum, and an open neural tube allows some to leak out into amniotic fluid (and ultimately to reach the maternal circulation, where it can also be detected). Although the causes of many cases of neural tube defect remain unknown, the majority can be prevented if the maternal diet contains sufficient levels of **folate** at the time of neural tube closure. Because closure occurs at the end of the first month of gestation, when a woman may be unaware of the pregnancy, routine folate supplementation has been recommended for potentially child-bearing women or as part of the general food supply.

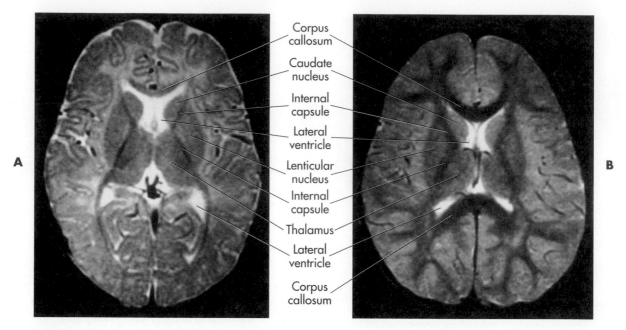

Corpus
callosum

Caudate
nucleus

Internal
capsule

Lateral
ventricle

Lenticular
nucleus

Internal
capsule

Thalamus

Lateral
ventricle

Corpus
callosum

FIGURE 2-16

Magnetic resonance images from 5-month-old (**A**) and 2-year-old (**B**) children. Fluid-filled spaces are bright and white matter is dark in this T2-weighted image (see Chapter 5). Little myelin has developed yet in the 5-month-old in areas that will contain many myelinated fibers at 2 years of age (e.g., internal capsule, corpus callosum, deep cerebral white matter). (Courtesy Dr. Roger Bird, St. Joseph's Hospital and Medical Center, Phoenix, Arizona.)

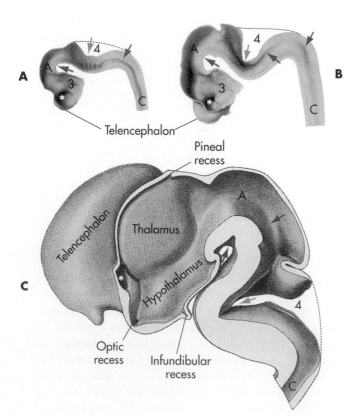

Telencephalon

Pineal
recess

Thalamus

Telencephalon

Hypothalamus

Optic
recess

Infundibular
recess

FIGURE 2-17

Development of the ventricular system at 37 days (**A**), 41 days (**B**), and 50 days (**C**). By 50 days the thalamus and hypothalamus form the walls of the slit-shaped midline third ventricle; several small recesses, described further in Chapter 5, protrude from this ventricle. As each cerebral hemisphere grows around in a C shape (Figure 2-12), so too does its lateral ventricle; the adult configuration is shown in Figures 5-1 and 5-2. The location of the thin, membranous roof of the fourth ventricle is indicated by dotted lines. *Blue arrows*, cephalic flexure; *green arrows*, pontine flexure; *red arrows*, sulcus limitans; *, interventricular foramen; *3*, third ventricle; *4*, fourth ventricle; *A*, aqueduct; *C*, central canal of the spinal cord and caudal medulla. (**A** and **B** from Hines M: Studies in the growth and differentiation of the telencephalon in man: the fissura hippocampi, *J Comp Neurol* 34:73, 1922. **C** from Hochstetter F: *Beiträge zur Entwicklungsgeschichte des menschlichen Gehirns.* II. Teil, Vienna, 1929, Franz Deuticke.)

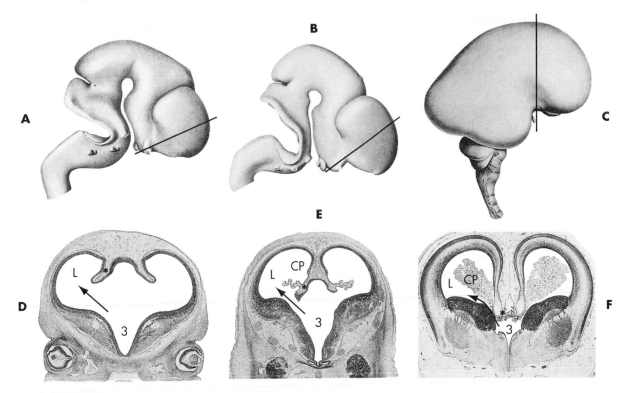

FIGURE 2-18

Formation of choroid plexus. **A-C** are nervous systems at about 6, 7, and 15 weeks; **D-F** are sections in the indicated planes. At 6 weeks (**A** and **D**) the third (*3*) and lateral (*L*) ventricles are in open continuity through the interventricular foramen (*arrow*); the thinned-out roof of the neural tube begins to invaginate into the lateral ventricle at the choroid fissure (*). At 7 weeks (**B** and **E**) fronds of choroid plexus (*CP*) begin to form at the site of invagination. By 15 weeks (**C** and **F**) the choroid plexus is a vascular, convoluted mass occupying much of the lateral ventricle; both the choroid fissure and choroid plexus curve around in a C shape with the cerebral hemisphere. Similar but less extensive choroid plexus forms in the roof of the third ventricle (**F**) and in the roof of the fourth ventricle (not shown). [From Hochstetter F: *Beiträge zur Entwicklungsgeschichte des menschlichen Gehirns.* I. Teil, Vienna, 1919, Franz Deuticke.]

Defective Secondary Neurulation Can Cause a Distinctive Set of Abnormalities

The cell mass at the caudal end of the neural tube gives rise not only to the sacral spinal cord, but also to some adjacent tissues. Hence defective secondary neurulation can be associated with a unique spectrum of abnormalities, including traction injuries to the spinal cord as a result of tethering of its caudal end, and a variety of cysts and tumors. Dimpling, hairiness, or discoloration of the overlying skin may provide an indication of an otherwise hidden defect.

The Prosencephalon Can Develop Abnormally Even if Neural Tube Closure Is Complete

The complex changes and subdivisions in the forebrain develop under the influence of more ventrally situated

portions of the embryo. Hence malformations in this region are referred to as **defects of ventral induction;** they are typically associated with marked facial abnormalities as well. A spectrum of malformations known as **holoprosencephaly** (from Greek words meaning "affecting the entire forebrain") results from partial or complete failure of the prosencephalon to separate into the diencephalon and the paired telencephalic vesicles during the second month of development. Malformations such as holoprosencephaly are rare and usually fatal. However, a variety of other influences during development, such as environmental insults, can cause less profound structural abnormalities that may still have major neurological consequences (Figure 2-20, *A*).

Disruptions occurring later in development may affect neuronal proliferation or migration. This can lead to abnormal gyral patterns, even though all the basic elements of the CNS may be present (Figure 2-20, *B*).

Table 2-2   Timing of Developmental Events

Week	Major developments	Appearance*	Malformations
3	Neural groove and folds Three primary vesicles visible Cervical and cephalic flexures Motor neurons appear		Neural tube defects
4	Neural tube starts to close (day 22) Rostral neuropore closes (day 24) Caudal neuropore closes (day 26) Neural crest cells begin to migrate Secondary neurulation starts Motor nerves emerge		Neural tube defects
5	Optic vesicle, pontine flexure Five secondary vesicles visible Sulcus limitans, sensory ganglia Sensory nerves grow into CNS Rhombic lips Basal ganglia begin Thalamus, hypothalamus begin Autonomic ganglia, lens, cochlea start		Holoprosencephaly, sacral cord abnormalities
6–7	Telencephalon enlarged Basal ganglia prominent Secondary neurulation complete Cerebellum and optic nerve begin Choroid plexus Insula		
8–12	Neuronal proliferation and migration Cerebral and cerebellar cortex begin First cortical sulci Anterior commissure, optic chiasm Internal capsule Reflexes appear		Migration/proliferation problems (e.g., abnormal cortex or gyri)
12–16	Neuronal proliferation and migration Glial differentiation Corpus callosum More cortical sulci; lobes apparent		Migration/proliferation problems (e.g., abnormal cortex or gyri)
16–40	Neuronal migration Glial proliferation, some myelination Synapse formation		Hemorrhage, other destructive events

*Top two figures from Arey LB: *Developmental anatomy,* ed 4, Philadelphia, 1941, WB Saunders; Bottom figure courtesy Dr. Naomi Rance, The University of Arizona College of Medicine; all others from Hochstetter F: *Beiträge zur Entwicklungsgeschichte des menschlichen Gehirns.* I. Teil, Vienna, 1919, Franz Deuticke.

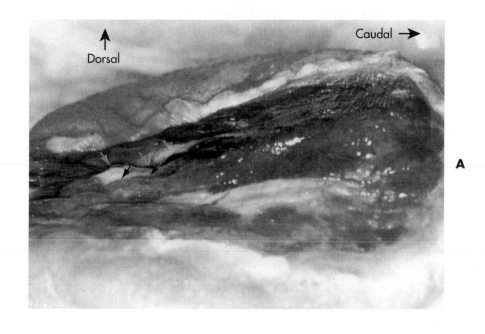

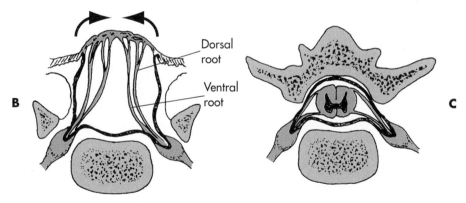

FIGURE 2-19

Myelomeningocele, an embryologic remnant. **A,** Photograph of cystic spina bifida, or myelomeningocele. The patient is in his first day of life, and the spinal defect is about to be closed surgically. The neural placode, representing the unfused spinal part of the embryonic neural tube, is the central element in the myelomeningocele. The midline ventral groove (*green arrows*) and the sulcus limitans on each side (*red arrows*) can be seen clearly on the left side of the photograph. More rostrally (to the left and out of the photograph), the spinal cord is normal; more caudally (right side of photograph), the neural placode is more primitive and heavily vascularized. **B,** Within the defect, the open spinal cord is exposed at the body surface and is continuous with the skin. Spinal rootlets are attached to the ventral surface of the neural placode. **C,** Rostral to the defect, the neural tube has closed, and the spinal cord has a normal appearance in cross section. (**A** courtesy Dr. Theodore J. Tarby. **B** and **C** modified from an illustration in Mori K: *Anomalies of the central nervous system,* New York, 1985, Thieme-Stratton.)

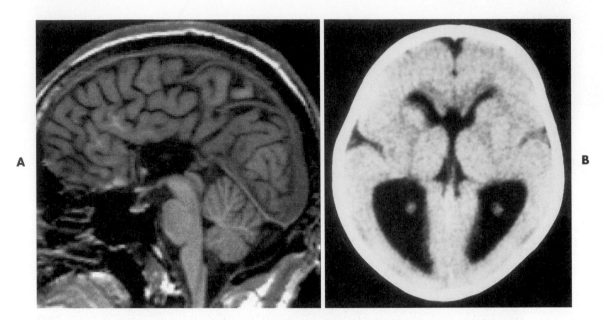

FIGURE 2-20

Malformations not related to defective neural tube closure. **A,** Magnetic resonance image of a 26-year-old man with fetal alcohol syndrome, a common cause of congenital malformations of the face and CNS. The major structural abnormality visible in the MRI is complete absence of the corpus callosum (compare to Figures 3-2 and 5-16), but this individual also had mild facial abnormalities and an IQ of 77. **B,** CT image of a 5-month-old male with a seizure disorder and developmental delay. Although all the major elements of the CNS appear to be present, cortical folding is almost completely absent. This condition, called *lissencephaly* (Greek for "smooth brain") is thought to be due to defective migration of neurons during the third and fourth month of development. (**A** from Swayze VW et al: Magnetic resonance imaging of brain anomalies in fetal alcohol syndrome, *Pediatrics* 99:232, 1997. **B** courtesy Dr. Raymond F. Carmody, Department of Radiology, The University of Arizona College of Medicine.)

SUGGESTED READINGS

Chi JG, Dooling EC, Gilles FH: Gyral development of the human brain, *Ann Neurol* 1:86, 1977.

Copp AJ et al: The embryonic development of mammalian neural tube defects, *Prog Neurobiol* 35:363, 1990.

Crelin ES: Development of the nervous system, *CIBA Clin Symp* 26(2), 1974.

Dobyns WB, Truwit CL: Lissencephaly and other malformations of cortical development: 1995 update, *Neuroped* 26:132, 1995.

Drews U: *Color atlas of embryology*, Stuttgart, 1995, Georg Thieme Verlag. *A compact, well-illustrated review.*

Gordon N: Folate metabolism and neural tube defects, *Brain and Devel* 17:307, 1995.

Huttenlocher PR: Morphometric study of human cerebral cortex development, *Neuropsychologia* 28:517, 1990. *A look at developmental changes in numbers of neurons and numbers of synapses, with some consideration of how these might relate to the development of cognitive abilities.*

Jennings MT et al: Neuroanatomic examination of spina bifida aperta and the Arnold-Chiari malformation in a 130-day human fetus, *J Neurol Sci* 54:325, 1982.

Kier EL, Fulbright RK, Bronen RA: Limbic lobe embryology and anatomy: dissection and MR of the medial surface of the fetal cerebral hemisphere, *AJNR Am J Neuroradiol* 16:1847, 1995.

Le Douarin NM, Fontaine-Pérus J, Couly G: Cephalic ectodermal placodes and neurogenesis, *Trends Neurosci* 9:175, 1986.

Le Douarin NM, Smith J: Development of the peripheral nervous system, *Ann Rev Cell Biol* 4:375, 1988.

Lemire RJ et al: *Normal and abnormal development of the human nervous system*, New York, 1975, Harper & Row.

Miller RH: Oligodendrocyte origins, *Trends Neurosci* 19:92, 1996.

Moore KL: *The developing human*, ed 5, Philadelphia, 1993, WB Saunders.

Norman MC et al: *Congenital malformations of the brain: pathological, embryological, clinical, radiological and genetic aspects*, New York, 1995, Oxford University Press.

O'Rahilly R, Müller F: *The embryonic human brain: an atlas of developmental stages*, New York, 1994, Wiley-Liss, Inc.

Roessler E et al: Mutations in the human *Sonic hedgehog* gene cause holoprosencephaly, *Nature Gen* 14:357, 1996.

Schoenwolf GC, Smith JL: Mechanisms of neurulation: traditional viewpoint and recent advances, *Devel* 109:243, 1990. *A recent review of the sources of the forces that cause the neural plate to indent and form the neural groove and tube.*

Schole H et al: Transcription factor AP-2 essential for cranial closure and craniofacial development, *Nature* 381:235, 1996. *Zeroing in on the molecular bases of neural tube and other developmental defects.*

Swayze VW et al: Magnetic resonance imaging of brain anomalies in fetal alcohol syndrome, *Pediatrics* 99:232, 1997.

Tuchmann-Duplessis H, Auroux M, Haegel P: *Illustrated human embryology, vol 3, Nervous system and endocrine glands*, New York, 1974, Springer-Verlag.

Van Allen MI et al: Evidence for multi-site closure of the neural tube in humans, *Am J Med Genet* 47:723, 1993. *Although the primary site of neural tube closure described in this chapter is the longitudinally most extensive closure, there are probably several other sites that start shortly thereafter; failure of any one of these closures can cause a neural tube defect in a distinctive pattern.*

Volpe JJ: *Neurology of the newborn*, ed 3, Philadelphia, 1995, WB Saunders.

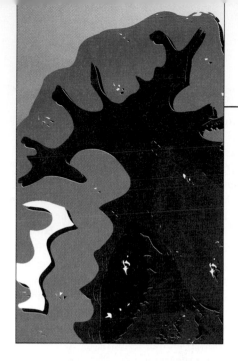

GROSS ANATOMY AND GENERAL ORGANIZATION OF THE CENTRAL NERVOUS SYSTEM

The human central nervous system (CNS) is composed of the brain and spinal cord. This chapter briefly discusses the major surface and internal structures of the brain (summarized in Figure 3-23) and, together with the following six chapters, lays the groundwork for the more detailed discussion of the functional anatomy of the CNS in ensuing chapters.

THE LONG AXIS OF THE CNS BENDS AT THE CEPHALIC FLEXURE

Before considering the parts of the brain in more detail, it is helpful to discuss some terms used for planes and directions in the nervous system. The **sagittal** plane divides the brain into two symmetrical halves. **Parasagittal** planes are those parallel to the sagittal plane. **Frontal** planes (also called **coronal** planes) are parallel to the long axis of the body and perpendicular to the sagittal plane (e.g., a vertical plane passing through both of your ears). These terms are fairly straightforward and have the same meaning with respect to any part of the nervous system. However, directional terms such as **anterior, dorsal,** and **rostral** change their meanings relative to each other in different parts of the nervous system. The reason for this, as indicated in Figure 3-1, is the bend of about 80° in going from the long axis of the brainstem to the long axis of the cerebrum. This bend is a consequence of the

cephalic flexure, which appears early in the embryological development of the nervous system (see Figure 2-7) and persists in the mature brain. Dorsal/ventral terminology ignores this bend, as though we had a linear CNS and walked around on all fours, so that the directional meaning of "dorsal" changes by 80° at the midbrain-diencephalon junction. The terms *anterior* and *superior,* in contrast, retain a constant meaning relative to the normal upright orientation of the body as a whole. This means, for example, that the ventral surface of the spinal cord is also its *anterior* surface, but the ventral surface of the diencephalon is its *inferior* surface. Rostral/caudal terminology may cause additional confusion because it has a functional connotation for many (implying "toward the telencephalon"), so that the posterior end of the cerebral hemispheres could be considered rostral to all parts of the diencephalon. Use of anterior/posterior and superior/inferior (or dorsal/ventral) terminology in reference to the cerebrum avoids any ambiguity.

HEMISECTING A BRAIN REVEALS PARTS OF THE DIENCEPHALON, BRAINSTEM, AND VENTRICULAR SYSTEM

The cerebral hemispheres conceal most of the rest of an intact brain (Figure 3-2, *A*). Hemisection reveals many parts of the diencephalon, brainstem, and cerebellum, and addi-

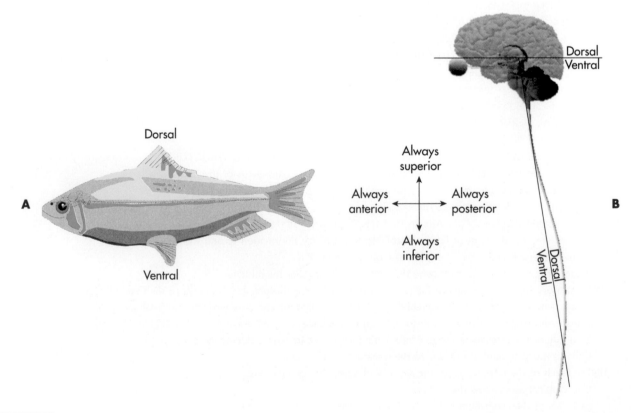

FIGURE 3-1
Various directional terms used when referring to different parts of the CNS. For animals that move through the world horizontally (**A**), dorsal/ventral is always equivalent to superior/inferior. As a result of our upright posture and the cephalic flexure (**B**), dorsal/ventral is equivalent to superior/inferior in the forebrain, but to posterior/anterior in the spinal cord and brainstem.

tional features of the cerebral hemispheres as well (Figure 3-2, *B*). The cephalic flexure is visible at the junction between the brainstem and the diencephalon. The brainstem itself is subdivided into (1) the **midbrain,** which is continuous with the diencephalon, (2) the **pons,** and (3) the **medulla,** which is continuous with the spinal cord. The two cerebral hemispheres are joined by a huge fiber bundle, the **corpus callosum,** which has an enlarged and rounded posterior **splenium,** a **body,** and an anterior, curved **genu,** which tapers gently into a ventrally directed **rostrum** that merges into the lamina terminalis (where development of the corpus callosum started).

The nervous system develops embryologically from a neuroectodermal tube; the cavity of the tube persists in the adult as a system of ventricles (see Figure 5-1), part of which is apparent in the sagittal plane (Figure 3-2, *B*). Portions of the medial surfaces of the diencephalon form the walls of the narrow, slitlike **third ventricle,** which opens into the large **lateral ventricle** of each cerebral hemi-sphere through an **interventricular foramen** (or **foramen of Monro**). Posteriorly, the third ventricle is continuous with a narrow channel through the midbrain, the **cerebral aqueduct** (or **aqueduct of Sylvius**). The aqueduct in turn is continuous with the **fourth ventricle** of the pons and medulla, and the fourth ventricle is continuous with the microscopically tiny **central canal** of the caudal medulla and the spinal cord.

HUMANS, RELATIVE TO OTHER ANIMALS, HAVE LARGE BRAINS

One impressive feature of the human brain is its size, and our distinctively human mental capacities are commonly attributed to this. Our brains weigh about 400 g at birth, and this weight triples during the first 3 years of life (resulting from addition of myelin and growth of neuronal processes, rather than the addition of more neurons). The

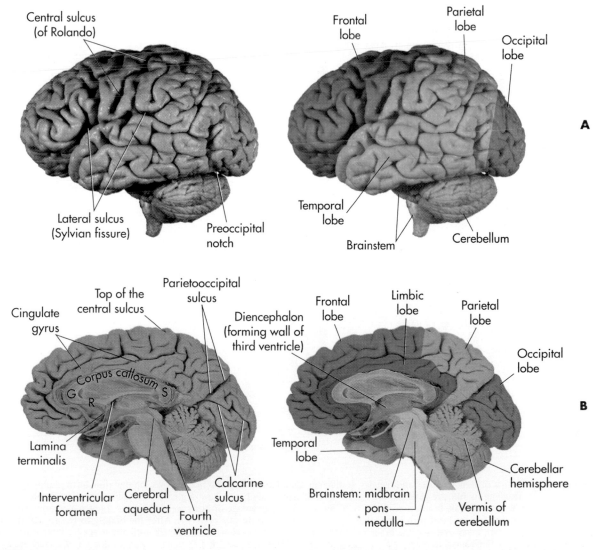

FIGURE 3-2

Major regions of the adult brain as seen in lateral (**A**) and medial (**B**) views. *R, G,* and *S* indicate the rostrum, genu, and splenium, respectively, of the corpus callosum.

rate of growth then slows, and the maximum brain weight of around 1400 g is reached by age 18. This weight holds steady until about the age of 50, when a slow decline sets in (Figure 3-3). The weight of 1400 g is only an average figure; brain weights for normal individuals range from 1100 g (or less) to around 1700 g. This large range of sizes is surprising, and its significance is not well understood. However, we do know that within this range larger brains do not work better in any obvious way than smaller brains.

Part of the large brain size is simply a reflection of our body size: big animals tend to have big brains. Elephants, for example, have 5000 g brains. Similarly, the size difference between the bodies of human males and females explains, at least to a great extent, the fact that male brains are slightly larger than female brains (Figure 3-3). However, this is not the whole story; many animals that are larger than we nevertheless have smaller brains (Figure 3-4). Overall, then, relative to our body size, humans have larger brains than most other animals. It is tempting to attribute our mental abilities to our relatively large brains, but this is an oversimplification. Relative to body size, dolphins, some small primates and rodents, and even some

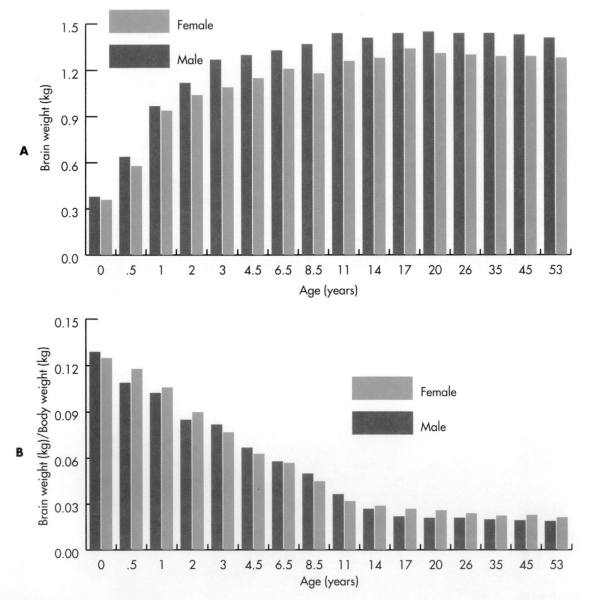

FIGURE 3-3

A, Average brain weights of human males and females at different ages. Notice how the brain grows rapidly after birth, doubling in the first year of life, before reaching its full size at about the age of 11. At all ages, male brains have a greater average weight than female brains. However, as indicated in **B,** adult female brains actually account for a greater percentage of body weight than do adult male brains. Brain growth is substantial in utero, and we are born with brains that are very large relative to our body size. After the brain growth spurt of the first 1 to 3 years of life, body growth takes over and the brain weight/body weight ratio declines progressively until about age 17. (Plotted from the data in Dekaban AS, Sadowsky D: Changes in brain weights during the span of human life: relation of brain weights to body heights and body weights, *Ann Neurol* 4:345, 1978.)

fish have larger brains than we do. The key differences in our brains appear to lie in an increased complexity of neuronal interconnections and in a selective increase in the size of certain areas of the cerebral cortex thought to be involved in higher functions (see Figure 22-13).

NAMED SULCI AND GYRI COVER THE CEREBRAL SURFACE

A striking aspect of human cerebral hemispheres is the degree to which their surface is folded and convoluted. Each ridge is called a **gyrus,** and each groove between ridges is called a **sulcus;** particularly deep sulci are often called **fissures.** This folding into gyri and sulci is a mechanism for increasing the total cortical area; each of us has about 2.5 ft² of cortex, two thirds of which is hidden from view in the walls of sulci. The appearance of various gyri and sulci varies considerably from one brain to another, to the point where they may not even be continuous structures (e.g., a particular gyrus may be transected by one or more sulci). Major features, however, are reasonably constant.

In the discussion that follows, the principal surface features of the hemispheres are described, with some broad generalizations regarding the function of various cortical areas. These functional descriptions are highly oversimpli-

fied and are offered primarily for purposes of initial orientation. Cortical function is discussed in more detail in Chapter 22.

Each Cerebral Hemisphere Includes a Frontal, Parietal, Occipital, Temporal, and Limbic Lobe

Four prominent sulci—the **central sulcus,** the **lateral sulcus,** the **parietooccipital sulcus,** the **cingulate sulcus**—together with the **preoccipital notch** and parts of a few other sulci are used to divide each cerebral hemisphere into five lobes (Figures 3-2 and 3-5):

1. The **frontal lobe** extends from the anterior tip of the brain (the **frontal pole**) to the central sulcus (or **sulcus of Rolando**). Inferiorly it ends at the lateral sulcus **(fissure of Sylvius).** On the medial surface of the brain, it extends posteriorly to an imaginary line from the top of the central sulcus to the cingulate sulcus.

2. The **parietal lobe** extends from the central sulcus to an imaginary line connecting the top of the parietooccipital sulcus and the preoccipital notch. Inferiorly it is bounded by the lateral sulcus and the imaginary continuation of this sulcus to the posterior boundary of the parietal lobe. On the medial

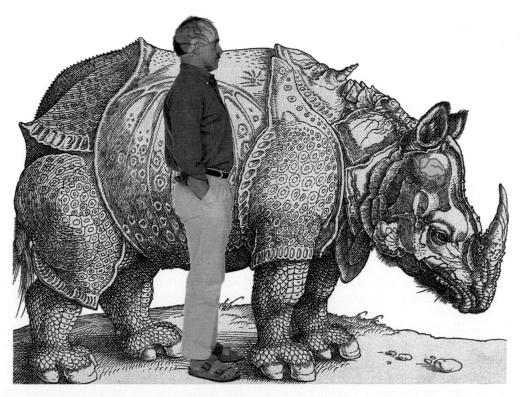

FIGURE 3-4
The relative sizes of the brain of a rhinoceros and the alleged brain of the author. Although the rhino's body weight is about 30 times greater, its brain weight is likely to be only half as great. (Drawing of rhino courtesy of Albrecht Dürer; author courtesy of Mr. and Mrs. Nolte; suggested by an illustration in Cobb S: Brain size, *Arch Neurol* 12:555, 1965.)

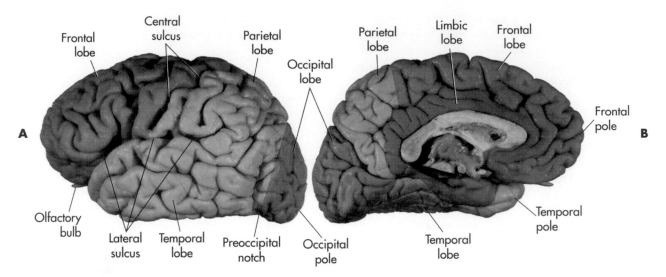

FIGURE 3-5
Lobes of the cerebral hemisphere. **A,** The boundaries of the frontal, parietal, occipital, and temporal lobes on the lateral surface of the hemisphere. **B,** The boundaries of the frontal, parietal, occipital, temporal, and limbic lobes on the medial surface of the hemisphere.

surface of the brain, it is bounded inferiorly by the cingulate and calcarine sulci, anteriorly by the frontal lobe, and posteriorly by the parietooccipital sulcus.

3. The **temporal lobe** extends superiorly to the lateral sulcus and the line forming the inferior boundary of the parietal lobe; posteriorly it extends to the line connecting the top of the parietooccipital sulcus and the preoccipital notch. On the medial surface its posterior boundary is an imaginary line extending from the preoccipital notch toward the splenium of the corpus callosum, and part of its superior boundary is the **collateral sulcus.**

4. The **occipital lobe** is bounded anteriorly by the parietal and temporal lobes on both the lateral and medial surfaces of the hemisphere.

5. The **limbic lobe** is a strip of cortex that appears to more or less encircle the telencephalon-diencephalon junction. It is interposed between the corpus callosum and the frontal, parietal, and occipital lobes, and curves around to occupy part of the medial surface of what would otherwise be called the *temporal lobe.*

These separations correspond only approximately to functional subdivisions, but they do provide a meaningful basis for discussion and reference.

An additional area of cerebral cortex not usually included in any of the five lobes discussed above lies buried in the depths of the lateral sulcus, concealed from view by portions of the frontal, parietal, and temporal lobes. This cortex, called the **insula,** overlies the site where the telencephalon and diencephalon fused during embryological development (see Chapter 2). It can be revealed by prying open the lateral sulcus or by removing the overly-

ing portions of other lobes (Figure 3-6). The portion of a given lobe overlying the insula is called an **operculum** (Latin for "lid"); there are frontal, parietal, and temporal opercula. The **circular sulcus** outlines the insula and marks its borders with the opercular areas of cortex.

The frontal lobe contains motor areas

Four gyri make up the lateral surface of the frontal lobe (Figure 3-7). The **precentral gyrus** is anterior to the central sulcus and parallel to it, extending to the **precentral sulcus.** The **superior, middle,** and **inferior frontal gyri** are oriented parallel to one another and roughly perpendicular to the precentral gyrus. The superior frontal gyrus continues onto the medial surface of the hemisphere as far as the cingulate sulcus. The inferior frontal gyrus is visibly divided into three parts: (1) the **orbital part,** which is most anterior and is continuous with the inferior **(orbital)** surface of the frontal lobe; (2) the **opercular part,** which is most posterior and forms a portion of the frontal operculum; and (3) the wedge-shaped **triangular part,** which lies between the other two. The inferior, or orbital, surface of the frontal lobe is mostly occupied by a group of gyri of variable appearance that are collectively called **orbital gyri** or **orbitofrontal cortex.** The only named gyrus on this surface is the **gyrus rectus** (Greek for "straight gyrus"), which is most medial and extends onto the medial surface of the hemisphere. Between the gyrus rectus and the orbital gyri is the **olfactory sulcus,** which contains the olfactory bulb and tract. The medial surface of the lobe contains extensions of the superior frontal gyrus, precentral gyrus, and gyrus rectus; certain small cortical areas near the rostrum of the corpus callosum are part of the limbic lobe.

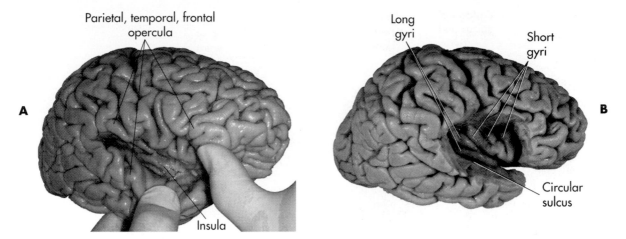

FIGURE 3-6
Location of the insula, demonstrated by prying open the lateral sulcus (**A**) and then cutting away the frontal, parietal, and temporal opercula (**B**). The surface of the insula is convoluted like other cortical areas, typically into about three short gyri and two long gyri.

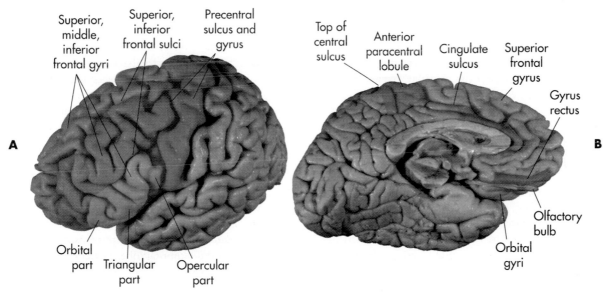

FIGURE 3-7
Lateral, medial, and inferior surfaces of the frontal lobe, seen from above and in front (**A**) and from medially and below (**B**).

The frontal lobe contains four general functional areas:
1. The **primary motor cortex** occupies much of the precentral gyrus. It contains many of the cells of origin of descending motor pathways and is involved in the initiation of voluntary movements.
2. The **premotor area** is made up of the remainder of the precentral gyrus together with adjacent portions of the superior and middle frontal gyri; it is also functionally related to the initiation of voluntary movements.
3. **Broca's area**, the opercular and triangular parts of the inferior frontal gyrus of one hemisphere (usually the left), is important in the production of written and spoken language.

4. The **prefrontal cortex,** a very large and somewhat confusingly named area comprising the remainder of the frontal lobe, is involved with what may very generally be described as personality, insight, and foresight.

The parietal lobe contains somatosensory areas

The lateral surface of the parietal lobe is divided into three areas: the **postcentral gyrus** and the **superior** and **inferior parietal lobules** (Figure 3-8). The postcentral gyrus is posterior to the central sulcus and parallel to it, extending to the **postcentral sulcus.** The **intraparietal sulcus** runs posteriorly from the postcentral sulcus toward the

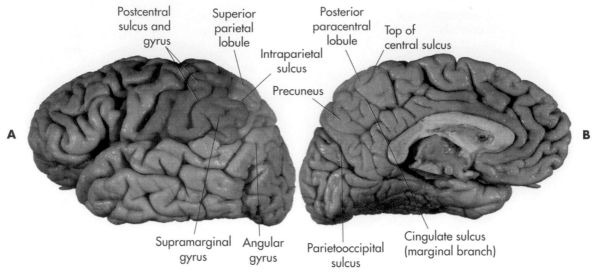

FIGURE 3-8
Lateral **(A)** and medial **(B)** surfaces of the parietal lobe.

occipital lobe, separating the superior and inferior parietal lobules. The inferior parietal lobule in turn is composed of the **supramarginal gyrus,** which caps the upturned end of the lateral sulcus, and the **angular gyrus,** which similarly caps the **superior temporal sulcus.** The angular gyrus is typically broken up by small sulci and may overlap the supramarginal gyrus. The medial surface of the parietal lobe contains the medial extension of the postcentral gyrus and is completed by an area called the **precuneus,** which is bounded by the cingulate sulcus, the parietooccipital sulcus, and the **marginal branch** of the cingulate sulcus. The extensions of the precentral and postcentral gyri onto the medial surface of the hemisphere are sometimes referred to together as the **paracentral lobule,** which is partly in the frontal lobe and partly in the parietal lobe.

The parietal lobe is associated, in a very general sense, with three functions:

1. The postcentral gyrus corresponds to **primary somatosensory cortex;** that is, it is concerned with the initial cortical processing of tactile and proprioceptive (sense of position) information.
2. Much of the inferior parietal lobule of one hemisphere (usually the left), together with portions of the temporal lobe, is involved in the comprehension of language.
3. The remainder of the parietal cortex subserves complex aspects of spatial orientation and perception.

The temporal lobe contains auditory areas

The lateral surface of the temporal lobe is composed of the **superior, middle,** and **inferior temporal gyri** (Figure 3-9). The superior surface of the temporal lobe continues into the lateral sulcus, where it forms the temporal operculum. The inferior temporal gyrus continues

onto the inferior surface of the lobe. The rest of the inferior surface is made up of the broad and often discontinuous **occipitotemporal (fusiform)** gyrus, which is separated from the limbic lobe by the collateral sulcus. The occipitotemporal gyrus, as its name implies, is partly in the occipital lobe and partly in the temporal lobe.

The temporal lobe is associated in a general way with four functions:

1. Part of the superior surface of the temporal lobe, continuing as a small area of the superior temporal gyrus, is the **primary auditory cortex.**
2. **Wernicke's area,** the posterior portion of the superior temporal gyrus of one hemisphere (usually the left), is important in the comprehension of language.
3. Much of the temporal lobe, particularly the inferior surface, is involved in higher order processing of visual information.
4. The most medial part of the temporal lobe* is involved in complex aspects of learning and memory.

The occipital lobe contains visual areas

The lateral surface of the occipital lobe is of variable configuration, and its gyri are usually referred to simply as **lateral occipital gyri.** On the medial surface, the wedge-shaped area between the parietooccipital and calcarine sulci is called the **cuneus** (Latin for "wedge") (Figure 3-10). The gyrus inferior to the calcarine sulcus is the **lingual gyrus.** The lingual gyrus is adjacent to the posterior portion of the occipitotemporal gyrus, separated from it

---

*The structures important in learning and memory (discussed in Chapter 23) are actually parts of the limbic lobe and underlying limbic-related structures, and are not part of the temporal lobe as defined in this chapter. However, because of their gross anatomical location, these structures critical for memory are commonly referred to as "medial temporal."

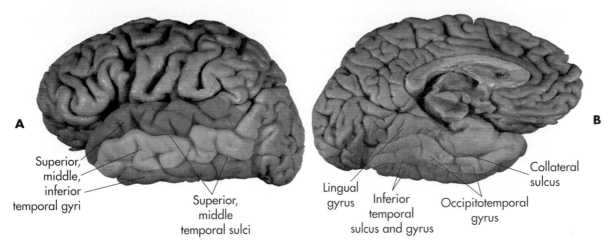

FIGURE 3-9
Lateral, medial, and inferior surfaces of the temporal lobe, seen from the side **(A)** and from medially and below **(B).**

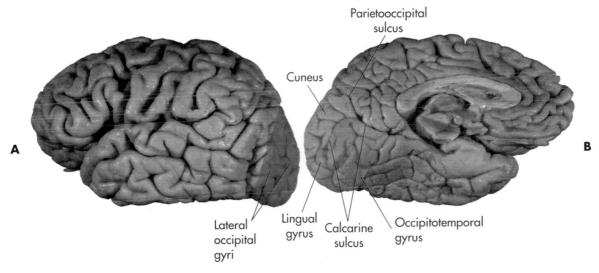

FIGURE 3-10
Lateral, medial, and inferior surfaces of the occipital lobe, seen from the side **(A)** and from medially and below **(B).**

by the collateral sulcus, and usually continuous anteriorly with the **parahippocampal gyrus.** The transition from lingual to parahippocampal gyrus occurs at the **isthmus** of the cingulate gyrus (Figure 3–11).

The occipital lobe is more or less exclusively concerned with visual functions. **Primary visual cortex** is contained in the walls of the calcarine sulcus and a bit of the surrounding cortex. The remainder of the lobe is referred to as **visual association cortex** and is involved in higher order processing of visual information; visual association cortex extends into the temporal lobe as well, reflecting the importance of vision for primates like us.

The limbic lobe is interconnected with other limbic structures buried in the temporal lobe

The **limbic lobe** (Figure 3–11) is mostly composed of the **cingulate** and **parahippocampal gyri.** The cingulate gyrus, immediately superior to the corpus callosum, can

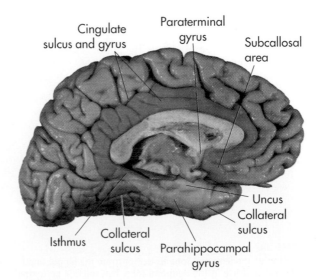

FIGURE 3-11
Limbic lobe as seen on the medial surface of a hemisected brain from which the brainstem and cerebellum were removed.

be followed posteriorly to the splenium of the corpus callosum, where it turns inferiorly as the narrow **isthmus** of the cingulate gyrus and continues as the parahippocampal gyrus of the temporal lobe. These two gyri give the appearance of encircling the diencephalon and they, together with certain other small cortical areas near the lamina terminalis (paraterminal gyrus) and inferior to the genu of the corpus callosum (subcallosal area), comprise the limbic lobe (from the Latin word *limbus,* meaning "border"). The anterior end of the parahippocampal gyrus hooks backward on itself, forming a medially directed bump called the **uncus.** The superior border of the parahippocampal gyrus is the **hippocampal sulcus.** Folded into the temporal lobe at the hippocampal sulcus is a limbic-related area of cortex called the **hippocampus** (Figure 3-12). The limbic lobe and many of the structures with which it is interconnected (such as the hippocampus) make up the **limbic system,** which is important in emotional responses, drive-related behavior, and memory.

THE DIENCEPHALON INCLUDES THE THALAMUS AND HYPOTHALAMUS

The diencephalon accounts for less than 2% of the weight of the brain, but nevertheless is extremely important. It has four divisions: **thalamus, hypothalamus, epithalamus,** and **subthalamus.** Portions of three of these divisions can be seen on a hemisected brain (Figure 3-13); the subthalamus is an internal structure that can be seen only in sections through the brain.

The Thalamus Conveys Information to the Cerebral Cortex

The thalamus is an ovoid nuclear mass, part of which borders on the third ventricle. The line of attachment of the roof of this ventricle is marked by a horizontally oriented ridge, the **stria medullaris thalami.** Parts of the medial surfaces of the two thalami fuse in many brains in an area called the **interthalamic adhesion** or **massa interme-**

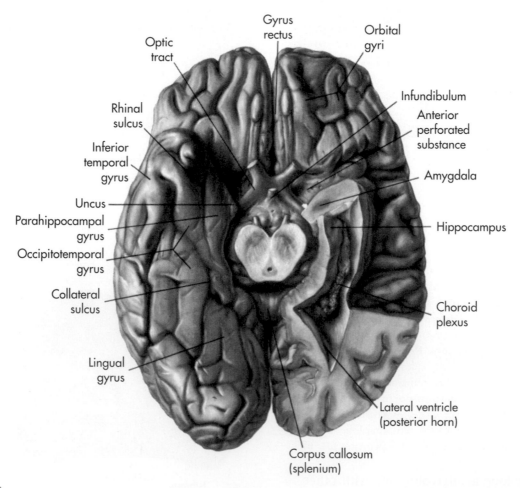

FIGURE 3-12

Dissection of the temporal lobe to demonstrate the hippocampus. The hippocampus is a cortical area that has folded into the inferior horn of the lateral ventricle in the temporal lobe. The anterior perforated substance is an area of the base of the brain where many small blood vessels enter the cerebrum. The rhinal sulcus looks like an anterior continuation of the collateral sulcus, but is actually a separate landmark. [From Mettler FA: *Neuroanatomy,* ed 2, St. Louis, 1948, Mosby.]

dia. (Because the massa intermedia is absent in many normal brains, it apparently performs no unique function.) Posteriorly, the thalamus protrudes over the most rostral portion of the brainstem. Anteriorly, it abuts the interventricular foramen. The thalamus is a nuclear mass of major importance in most functional systems. No sensory information, with the exception of olfactory information, reaches the cerebral cortex without prior processing in thalamic nuclei. In addition, the anatomical loops characteristic of motor systems, which involve pathways between the cerebellum and cerebral cortex and between basal ganglia and cerebral cortex, typically involve thalamic nuclei as well. Finally, limbic projections to the cerebral cortex also traverse the thalamus.

The Hypothalamus Controls the Autonomic Nervous System

The hypothalamus is inferior to the thalamus, separated from it by the **hypothalamic sulcus** in the wall of the third ventricle. It also forms the floor of this ventricle, and its inferior surface is one of the few parts of the diencephalon visible on an intact brain. This inferior surface (Figures 3-14 and 3-15) includes the **infundibular stalk** and two rounded protuberances called the **mammillary bodies.** The hypothalamus is the major visceral control center of the brain and is involved in limbic system functions as well.

The epithalamus comprises the midline **pineal gland** and several small nearby neural structures visible in sections.

MOST CRANIAL NERVES ARE ATTACHED TO THE BRAINSTEM

The brainstem plays major roles in cranial nerve functions, in conveying information to and from the cerebrum, and in some special functions of its own. It is divided into the midbrain, the pons, and the medulla (Figure 3-2, *B*). The **tectum** (Latin for "roof") of the midbrain, that portion dorsal to the cerebral aqueduct, consists of paired bumps called the **superior** and **inferior colliculi** (Latin for "little hills"). The paired **cerebral peduncles** make up most of the remainder of the midbrain (see Figures 3-20 and 3-21). The pons consists of a protruding **basal pons,** oval in sagittal section, and the overlying **pontine tegmentum,** which forms part of the floor of the fourth ventricle. The medulla consists of a rostral **open** portion, containing part of the fourth ventricle, and a caudal **closed** portion, continuous with the spinal cord (Figure 3-13).

The points of attachment of most cranial nerves, as well as additional brainstem structures, can be seen in an inferior view of the brain (Figures 3-14 and 3-15). The **olfactory tract** is located in the olfactory sulcus, lateral to the gyrus rectus, and is attached directly to the cerebral

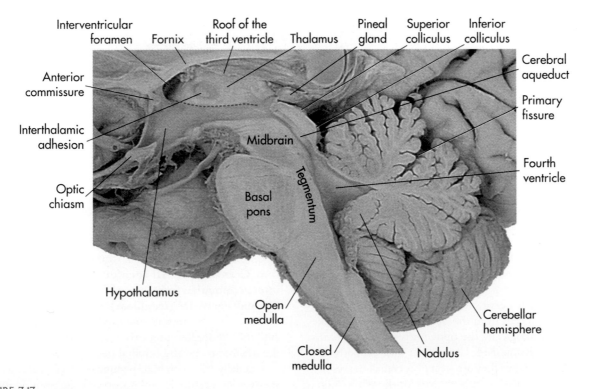

FIGURE 3-13
Major features of the diencephalon, brainstem, and cerebellum as seen in a hemisected brain, shown actual size. The dotted line in the wall of the third ventricle indicates the location of the hypothalamic sulcus.

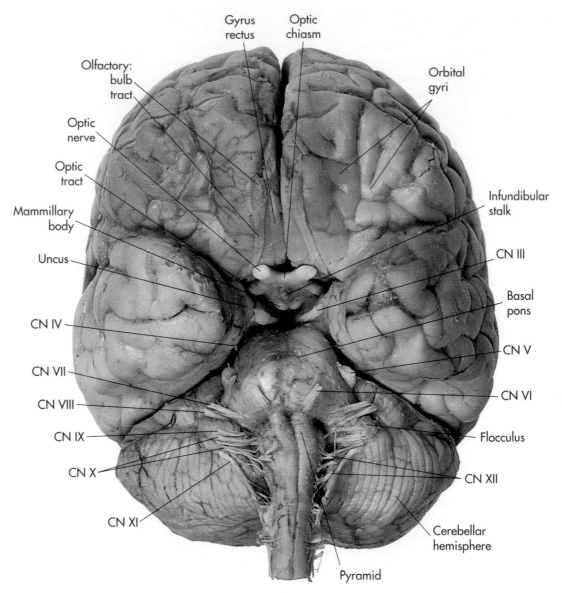

Gyrus rectus

Optic chiasm

Olfactory: bulb tract

Optic nerve

Optic tract

Mammillary body

Uncus

CN IV

CN VII

CN VIII

CN IX

CN X

CN XI

Orbital gyri

Infundibular stalk

CN III

Basal pons

CN V

CN VI

Flocculus

CN XII

Cerebellar hemisphere

Pyramid

FIGURE 3-14
Inferior surface of a brain, showing the locations of the cranial nerves. (Dissection by Dr. Norman Koelling, The University of Arizona College of Medicine.)

hemisphere. **Cranial nerve I (olfactory)** is actually a collection of bundles of very fine axons called **olfactory fila** that terminate in the **olfactory bulb** at the anterior end of the tract. Slightly posterior to the attachment points of the olfactory tracts, the **optic nerves (cranial nerve II)** join to form the **optic chiasm,** in which half the fibers of each nerve cross to the opposite side. The **optic tract** proceeds from the optic chiasm to a thalamic nucleus. Embryologically, the optic nerves are outgrowths of the diencephalon (see Chapter 2) and properly are tracts of the CNS, but they are treated as cranial nerves because of their course outside the rest of the brain. Considered in this way, cranial nerve II is the only one that projects directly to the diencephalon.

Located farther posteriorly are the cerebral peduncles of the midbrain, each of which contains a massive fiber bundle that carries a great deal of the descending projection from the cerebral cortex to the brainstem and spinal cord. **Cranial nerve III (oculomotor)** emerges into the **interpeduncular fossa** between the cerebral peduncles. **Cranial nerve IV (trochlear)** emerges from the dorsal surface of the brainstem just caudal to the inferior colliculi, then proceeds anteriorly through the space between the brainstem and the cerebral hemisphere.

Caudally, the cerebral peduncles disappear into the transversely oriented basal portion of the pons. Dorsolaterally, this part of the pons narrows into a large fiber bundle that enters the cerebellum. This is the **middle cere-**

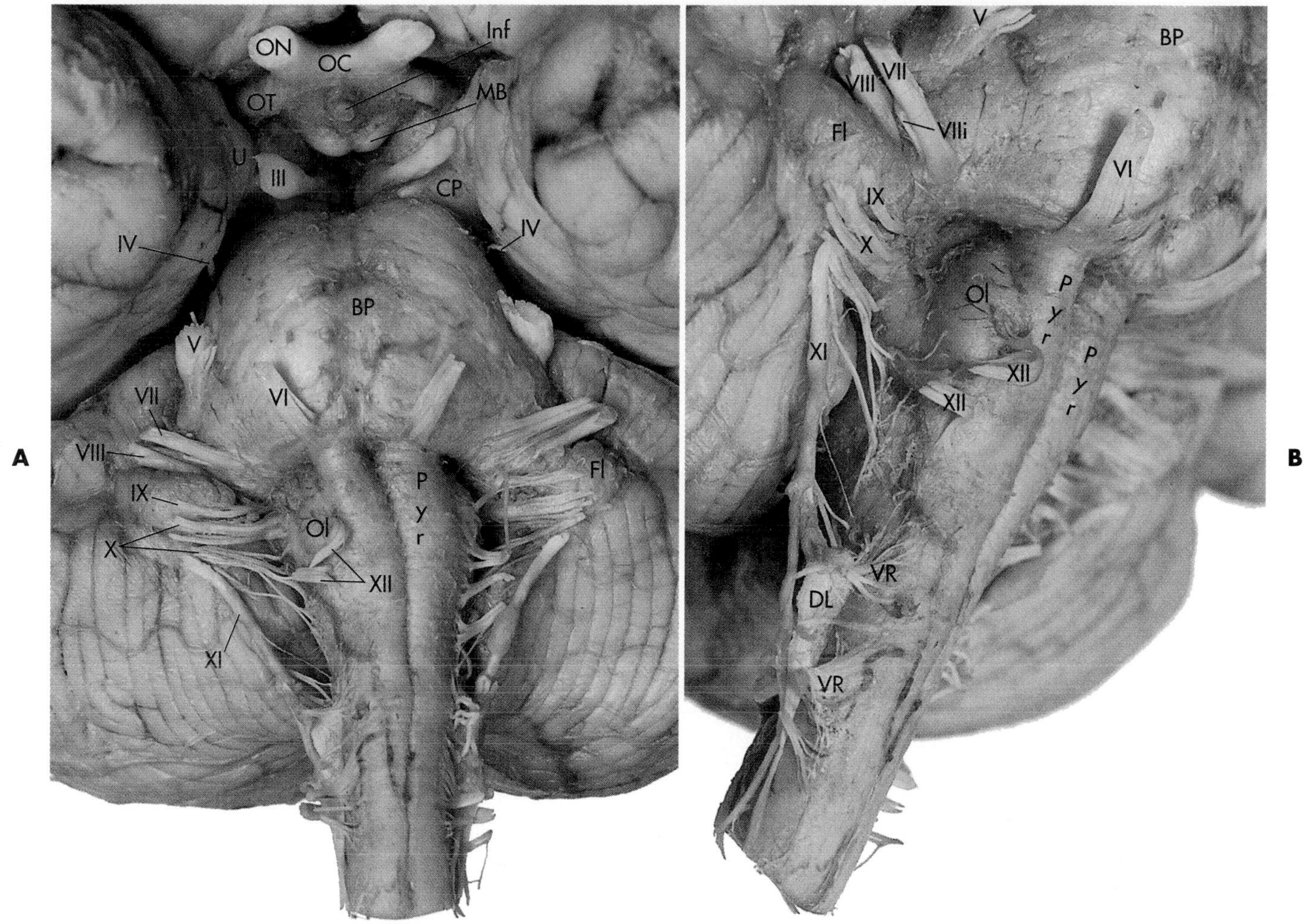

FIGURE 3-15
Closeups of the anterior (**A**) and lateral (**B**) surfaces of the same brain shown in Figure 3-14. Cranial nerves III-XII indicated by Roman numerals; *VIIi*, intermediate nerve (part of the facial nerve). *BP*, Basal pons; *CP*, cerebral peduncle; *DL*, denticulate ligament (suspensory ligament of the spinal cord); *Fl*, flocculus; *Inf*, infundibular stalk (former attachment of the pituitary gland); *MB*, mammillary body; *Ol*, olive; *OC*, optic chiasm; *ON*, optic nerve (cranial nerve II); *OT*, optic tract; *Pyr*, pyramid; *U*, uncus; *VR*, cervical ventral root. (Dissection by Dr. Norman Koelling, The University of Arizona College of Medicine.)

bellar peduncle (brachium pontis), which carries the major input from the cerebral hemispheres to the cerebellum by way of relays in nuclei of the basal pons (see Figure 3-31). **Cranial nerve V (trigeminal)** emerges from the lateral aspect of the basal pons. **Cranial nerve VI (abducens)** emerges near the midline at the caudal edge of the pons. **Cranial nerves VII (facial)** and **VIII (vestibulocochlear)** emerge more laterally near the cerebellum, at the caudal edge of the pons. The area of attachment of cranial nerves VII and VIII is called the **cerebellopontine angle** and is a common site of development of tumors, such as tumors of the Schwann cells of cranial nerve VIII.

Caudal to the pons are two thick fiber bundles that resemble the cerebral peduncles but are considerably smaller. These are the **pyramids** of the medulla, which carry those fibers of the cerebral peduncles that are di-

rected to the spinal cord. The two pyramids decussate* in the area of transition from brainstem to spinal cord. Dorsolateral to each pyramid is an ovoid protuberance called the **olive**. **Cranial nerve XII (hypoglossal)** emerges from the sulcus between the pyramid and the olive. The more or less continuous series of filaments that will form **cranial nerves IX (glossopharyngeal)** and **X (vagus)** emerge from the sulcus dorsal to the olive. (The most caudal of these filaments are sometimes considered separately as a **cranial part of nerve XI [accessory nerve].**)

---

* A *decussation* is a site where nerve fibers joining unlike areas of the CNS cross, such as where fibers cross on their way from one side of the cerebrum to the opposite side of the spinal cord. In contrast, a *commissure* is a crossing site for fibers connecting similar areas.

THE CEREBELLUM INCLUDES A VERMIS AND TWO HEMISPHERES

The cerebellum can be subdivided in several different ways, two of which are briefly considered here. In one sense the cerebellum comprises a midline **vermis,** which is hemisected in a hemisected brain (Figure 3-2, *B*), and a much larger, lateral **hemisphere** on each side (Figure 3-2). Using any other method of subdividing the cerebellum, a given division has both a vermal and a hemispheral component.

Lobes of the cerebellum, which roughly correspond to separate functional areas, are also recognized. The **anterior lobe** is that portion anterior to the **primary fissure** (Figure 3-13). This lobe receives a large proportion of its afferent inputs from the spinal cord and plays a prominent role in coordinating leg movements. The **flocculonodular lobe** consists of three small components: the **nodulus,** which is the vermal portion of the lobe (Figure 3-13), and a small **flocculus** on each side near the vestibulocochlear nerve (Figure 3-14). The nodulus is actually continuous with the flocculus of each side, but this continuity is difficult to see without dissecting the cerebellum. The flocculonodular lobe receives afferent inputs from the vestibular system and is involved in controlling eye movements and postural adjustments to gravity. All of the cerebellum posterior to the primary fissure, exclusive of the flocculonodular lobe, constitutes the **posterior lobe,** which is the largest of the three. The posterior lobe receives the majority of the afferent input from the cerebral cortex by way of relays in **pontine nuclei** and transmission through the middle cerebellar peduncle. This lobe plays a prominent role in the coordination of voluntary movements. In reality, cerebellar function is not quite so neatly parceled out among the anatomical subdivisions; the details of cerebellar function are discussed in Chapter 20.

SECTIONS OF THE CEREBRUM REVEAL THE BASAL GANGLIA AND LIMBIC STRUCTURES

Before consideration of the internal structures of the brain, it is useful to discuss certain consequences of the shape of the cerebral hemispheres. As a result of the embryological development of the hemispheres (see Figure 2-12), the cortical lobes are arranged in a C shape from the frontal lobe, through the parietal and occipital lobes, and into the temporal lobe. A number of other structures, such as the lateral ventricles (Figure 3-16, *D*), are similarly C shaped, with the result that sections through the brain may cut these structures in two different places. The hippocampus, together with its efferent fiber bundle (the **fornix**), is another example (Figure 3-16, *C*). The hippocampus is folded into the temporal lobe, forming part of the wall of the lateral ventricle there (Figure 3-12). It

becomes smaller as the temporal lobe curves into the parietal lobe, and it ends near the splenium of the corpus callosum. The fornix continues this curved course, arching anteriorly under the corpus callosum, then turning inferiorly and posteriorly toward the hypothalamus, where many of its fibers end in the mammillary bodies.

The Caudate Nucleus, Putamen, and Globus Pallidus Are Major Components of the Basal Ganglia

The basal ganglia are a group of nuclei that form part of each cerebral hemisphere. They are internal structures of the hemisphere, visible only in sections. The major basal ganglia are the **caudate** and **lenticular nuclei** (together with some brainstem structures with which they are interconnected). The caudate nucleus, another example of a C-shaped structure, has an enlarged **head** deep in the frontal lobe, and its increasingly attenuated **body** and **tail** follow the lateral ventricle around into the temporal lobe (Figure 3-16, *A*). The lenticular nucleus, which is subdivided into the **putamen** and the **globus pallidus,** lies lateral and partially anterior to the thalamus. It is separated from the thalamus and from much of the head of the caudate nucleus by a thick sheet of fibers called the **internal capsule.** The internal capsule contains most of the fibers interconnecting the cerebral cortex and deep structures such as the thalamus and basal ganglia.

The Amygdala and Hippocampus Are Major Limbic Structures

The **amygdala,** another nucleus contained within each cerebral hemisphere, was historically considered to be one of the basal ganglia. However, it is now known that the amygdala and the hippocampus are major components of the limbic system. The amygdala lies beneath the uncus of the temporal lobe (Figure 3-19). The hippocampus extends posteriorly from the level of the amygdala, underlying the medial temporal lobe.

Cerebral Structures Are Arranged Systematically

Figures 3-17 to 3-22 are intended as an introduction to the configuration of internal structures of the brain. Each section is in a coronal plane and has been stained for myelin,★ thus differentiating gray matter from white matter. Only major structures are labeled, but the same sections are presented in more detail elsewhere in this book and in a companion atlas (Nolte J, Angevine JB Jr: *The human brain in photographs and diagrams*, St Louis, 1995, Mosby). Figure 3-23 diagrams the interrelationships (and some of the functions) of the major structures that make up the CNS.

★ Weigert's hematoxylin (Loyez method).

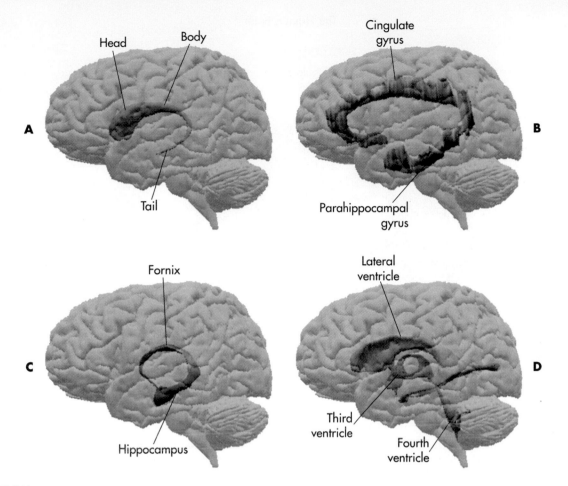

FIGURE 3-16

Four examples of C-shaped telencephalic structures: the caudate nucleus **(A)**, limbic lobe **(B)**, hippocampus/fornix system **(C)**, and lateral ventricle **(D)**.

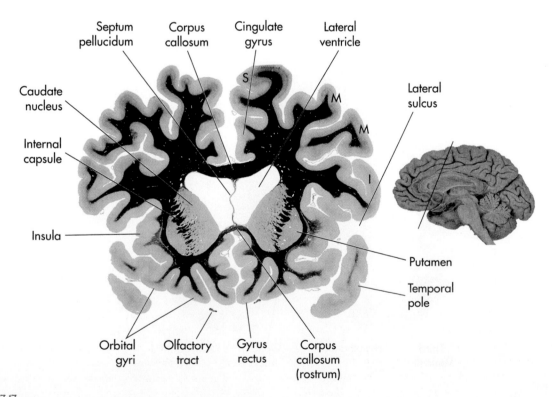

FIGURE 3-17

Section through the frontal lobes, slightly posterior to the genu of the corpus callosum. Inferior to the body of the corpus callosum is the septum pellucidum, a thin, paired membrane that intervenes between the corpus callosum and the fornix and separates portions of the two lateral ventricles. At this level, which is anterior to the diencephalon, the basal ganglia are represented by the putamen and the head of the caudate nucleus, with part of the internal capsule between them. Inferiorly, note the continuity between these nuclei. *I*, Inferior frontal gyrus; *M*, middle frontal gyrus; *S*, superior frontal gyrus.

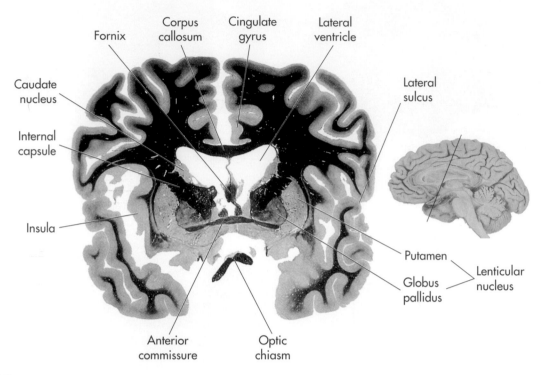

FIGURE 3-18
Section through the anterior commissure, which interconnects portions of the temporal lobes, as well as certain olfactory structures. At this level both parts of the lenticular nucleus (the putamen and the globus pallidus) are present. The section is at the anterior end of both the interventricular foramen and the thalamus, and cuts through the fornix tangentially as it curves down toward the hypothalamus.

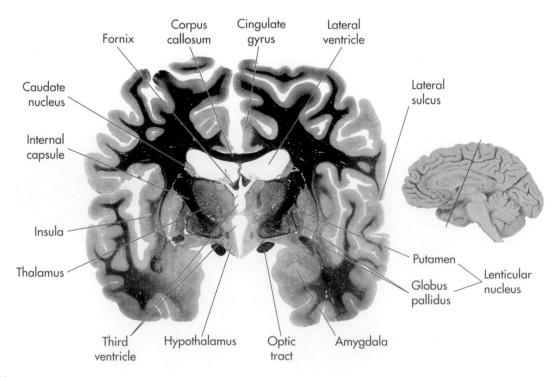

FIGURE 3-19
Section through the anterior part of the diencephalon. Parts of both the thalamus and the hypothalamus can be seen. At this level and at more posterior levels, the internal capsule is found between the lenticular nucleus and the thalamus. The third ventricle can be seen in the midline, above and below the interthalamic adhesion. The section passes through the anterior part of the uncus, revealing the amygdala.

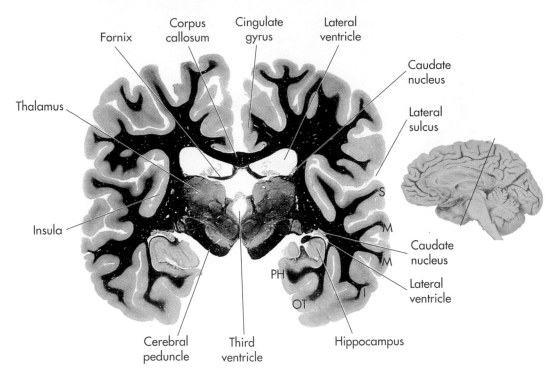

FIGURE 3-20
Section through the posterior thalamus and the brainstem. The thalamus is partially posterior to the lenticular nucleus, accounting for the presence of one but not the other at this level. The section is also posterior to the uncus, and the amygdala has been replaced by the hippocampus. Note that the caudate nucleus and lateral ventricle can now be seen in two places; because of their C shapes, they were transected twice in this and the next section. *I*, Inferior temporal gyrus; *M*, middle temporal gyrus; *OT*, occipitotemporal gyrus; *PH*, parahippocampal gyrus; *S*, superior temporal gyrus.

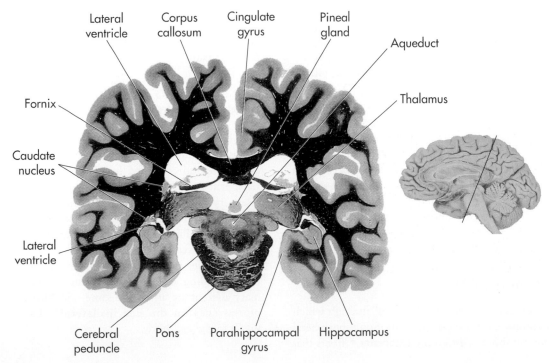

FIGURE 3-21
Section through the brainstem and the most posterior part of the thalamus. The two portions of the lateral ventricle on each side are closer together than in previous sections because the posterior edge of their C shape is being approached. The thalamus protrudes posteriorly and is superior and lateral to part of the midbrain.

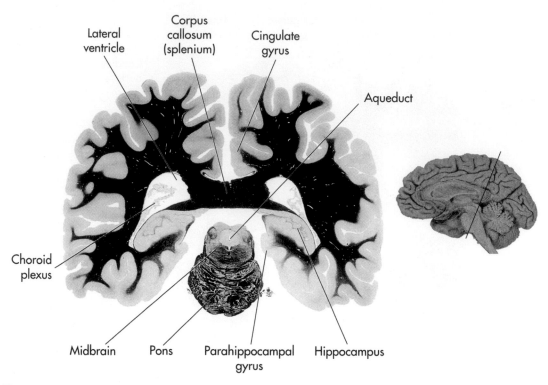

Lateral ventricle · Corpus callosum (splenium) · Cingulate gyrus · Aqueduct · Choroid plexus · Midbrain · Pons · Parahippocampal gyrus · Hippocampus

FIGURE 3-22
Section through the splenium of the corpus callosum. The lateral ventricle is no longer cut in two places because this section is tangential to the posterior edge of its C shape. The final portion of the hippocampus can be seen as it ends near the splenium.

PARTS OF THE NERVOUS SYSTEM ARE INTERCONNECTED IN SYSTEMATIC WAYS

The functional subdivisions of the CNS discussed thus far (Figure 3-23) interact with one another as the substrate for perception, motivation, and behavior. Despite the seemingly impenetrable thicket of interconnections among neurons in the nervous system (see Figure 1-15), there are in fact some "wiring principles" that govern many of these interconnections. This section is an overview of such principles, primarily using somatic sensation and body movement as examples. None of these wiring principles is an absolute rule; rather, much like the "rules" of English grammar and spelling, they are guidelines rife with exceptions. Nevertheless, such general guidelines may be helpful in navigating subsequent chapters.

Primary Afferents and Axons of Lower Motor Neurons Convey Information to and From the CNS

Peripheral nerves are the electrical "cables" through which the CNS communicates with the body. Some peripheral nerve axons are those of **primary afferents,** ★ fibers that convey information into the CNS from the periphery. Others are axons of **lower motor neurons,** fibers that convey messages to skeletal muscles directing them to contract. (Peripheral nerves also contain autonomic fibers, contacting visceral structures, but these are not included in this discussion.)

Primary afferents enter the CNS without crossing the midline

The only way the CNS can receive information about things touching the skin, or about the position of limbs, is as information conveyed by axons in peripheral nerves. Each primary afferent neuron involved has its cell body in a sensory ganglion, a peripherally directed process ending in skin, a muscle, or a joint, and a central process ending in the CNS (Figure 3-24). Primary afferents terminate in the CNS on second-order neurons, which in turn project to third-order neurons, etc. With few exceptions, the receptive ending, cell body, and central terminals of a primary afferent are all on the same side. That is, the central process ends on the side **ipsilateral**★ (Latin for "same side") to the cell body.

★ *Afferent* and *efferent* refer to the direction of information flow in an axon, relative to some structure. Hence axons that convey information from structure A to structure B are both efferent from structure A and afferent to structure B.

★ *Ipsilateral* and *contralateral* are relative terms, just like *afferent* and *efferent*. Any site in the nervous system is ipsilateral to some structures and contralateral to others.

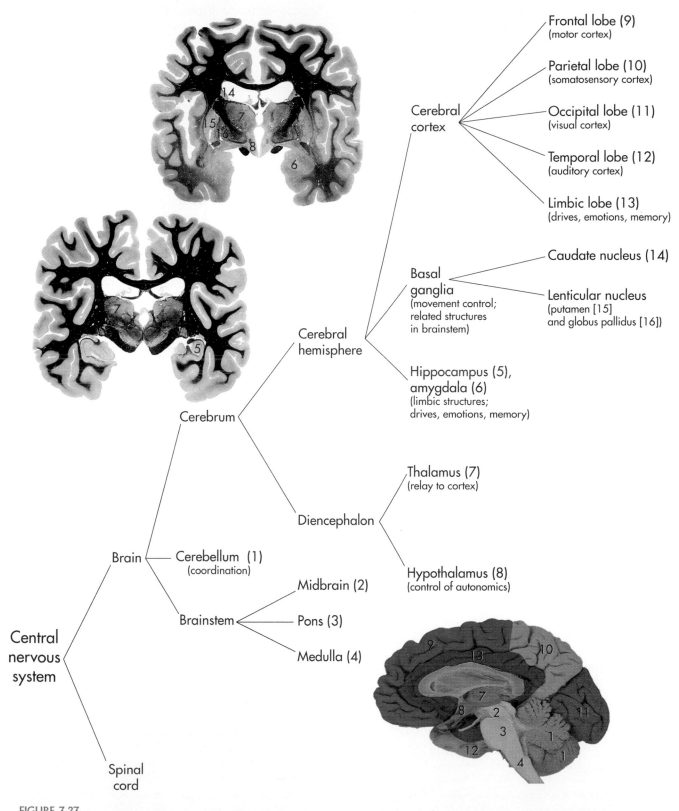

FIGURE 3-23
Overview of the subdivisions of the CNS. The major structures listed here, as well as many related structures, are the subjects of subsequent chapters.

Axons of lower motor neurons leave the CNS without crossing the midline

Similarly, the only way the CNS can induce muscles to contract in response to a stimulus is by way of messages conveyed by axons of lower motor neurons. Lower motor neurons have their cell bodies within the CNS, and axons that travel through peripheral nerves to end (again, with few exceptions) on ipsilateral muscle fibers (Figure 3-24).

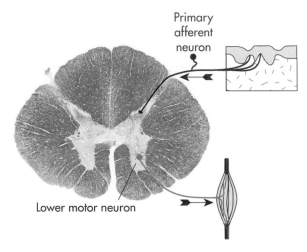

FIGURE 3-24
Wiring pattern of primary afferents and lower motor neurons.

Somatosensory Inputs Participate in Reflexes, Pathways to the Cerebellum, and Pathways to the Cerebral Cortex

Most types of sensory information do at least three different things. They feed into local functions such as reflexes, and they distribute to both the cerebral cortex (via the thalamus) and the cerebellum. An individual primary afferent, together with the interneurons with which it is connected, commonly does all three (Figure 3-25).

The somatosensory system provides a nice example of this distribution in three different spheres. *Somatosensory* literally means "body sense," and encompasses several different types of sensation, including pain, temperature, simple touch, proprioception (perception of position), kinesthesia (perception of movement), and stereognosis (perception of the size and shape of objects by touch). In addition to sending their information to the thalamus and cerebellum, somatosensory afferents feed into things like stretch reflexes (e.g., the familiar knee-jerk reflex) and withdrawal reflexes (e.g., blinking in response to something touching a cornea).

Somatosensory pathways to the cerebral cortex cross the midline and pass through the thalamus

Somatosensory *pathways* (not necessarily individual *fibers*) typically cross the midline someplace between their origin and their destination so that, for example, information

FIGURE 3-25
Typical distribution pattern of somatosensory information (and other types of sensory information) to reflex arcs, the cerebellum, and the cerebral cortex (via the thalamus).

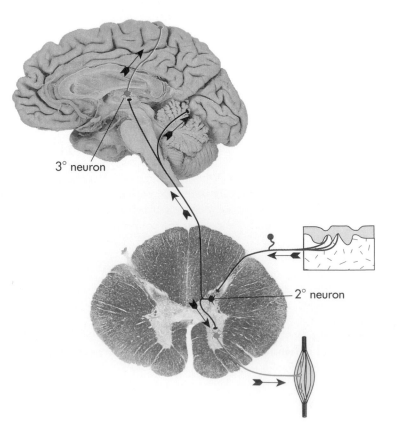

about one hand reaches the **contralateral** (Latin for "opposite side") postcentral gyrus. This crossing of sensory pathways is a curious and unexplained fact of vertebrate evolution. It applies not only to those pathways representing spinal nerves but often to those representing cranial nerves as well (except for taste and olfaction; see Chapter 13). A number of hypotheses have been advanced to explain this phenomenon, including the notion that it is an early evolutionary mistake still awaiting correction.★ Whatever its explanation, it would be even more peculiar if information from the *right* hand reached the left cerebral hemisphere, which in turn controlled the *left* hand. This is not the case, however, because descending pathways also cross the midline at some point between their origins and their terminations (Figure 3-30).

The thalamus and cerebral cortex of each side reside in the same half of the cerebrum, and thalamocortical fibers are uncrossed. Because primary afferents are also uncrossed, this implies that the shortest path to the cerebral cortex is three neurons long: a primary afferent, a neuron that crosses the midline, and a thalamic neuron (Figure 3-26). (This is the shortest possible path; many pathways are more than three neurons long.)

The location in the CNS where the midline-crossing takes place is different for different pathways, and knowledge of these crossover points can be crucial in deciding where a lesion is. In the case of the somatosensory system, for example, the pain and temperature pathway crosses at a different point than the main pathway for touch (Figure 3-27). Note that one-sided damage affecting these two pathways at level *A* would have the curious result of diminution of touch on the side ipsilateral to the lesion and diminution of pain on the side contralateral to the lesion. Reflexes would be unaffected because they are mediated by local connections near the level of entry of the primary afferents.

Somatosensory cortex contains a distorted map of the body

Somatosensory information from different parts of the body enters the spinal cord at different levels (see Figures 10-3 and 10-17). Representations of different parts within a pathway thereafter remain contiguous but separate (e.g., Figure 10-20). The end result is that the contralateral half of the body is mapped out systematically in each postcentral gyrus in a little humanoid **somatotopic** map called a **homunculus** (Latin for "little human"). The map is spatially distorted, however, emphasizing areas such as the fingertips and lips, for which somatosensory acuity is most important (Figure 3-28, *A*). Systematic, distorted maps are a repeated theme in the CNS; many cases in which they have not been found are probably simply reflections of our not knowing which parameter to map.

★ Zill, Sasha N: Personal communication, 1977.

Each side of the cerebellum receives information about the ipsilateral side of the body

The cerebellum receives large amounts of sensory information and uses it not in perceptual processes, but rather in helping with the coordination of movement; somatosensory information is particularly germane. The cerebellum is also a major exception to the generalization about pathways crossing the midline: a given side of the cerebellum is related to the ipsilateral side of the body. One of the anatomical bases for this uncrossed relationship is that somatosensory pathways from the periphery to the cerebellum are typically uncrossed. Somatosensory pathways from the periphery to the cerebellum do not pass through the thalamus and can involve as few as two neurons (Figure 3-29).

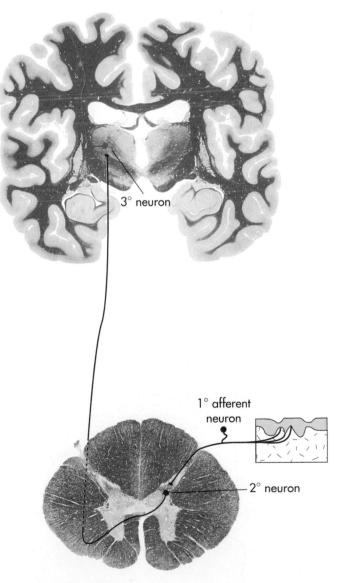

FIGURE 3-26
The minimum sensory pathway from the periphery to the cerebral cortex.

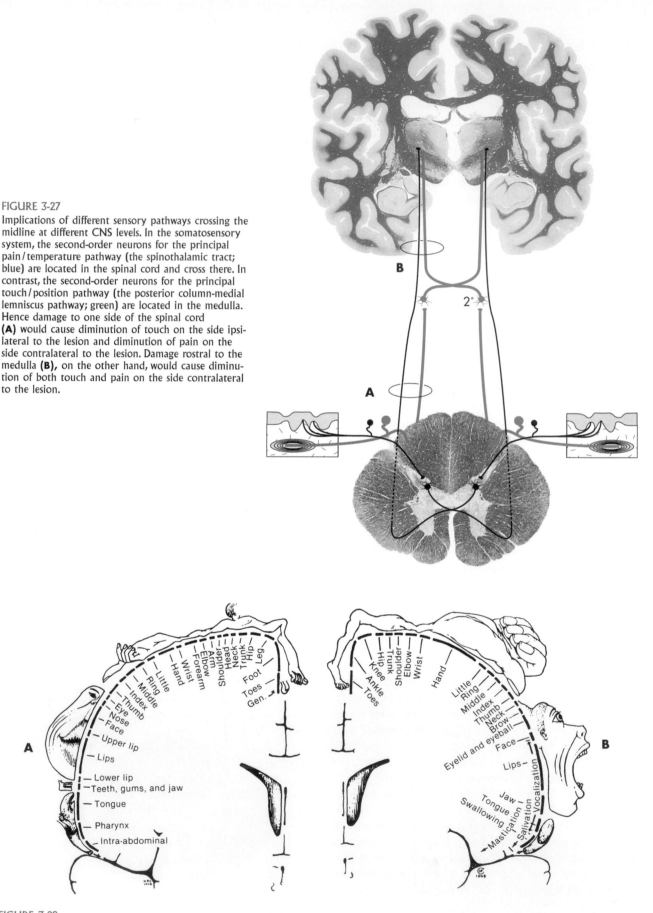

FIGURE 3-27

Implications of different sensory pathways crossing the midline at different CNS levels. In the somatosensory system, the second-order neurons for the principal pain/temperature pathway (the spinothalamic tract; blue) are located in the spinal cord and cross there. In contrast, the second-order neurons for the principal touch/position pathway (the posterior column-medial lemniscus pathway; green) are located in the medulla. Hence damage to one side of the spinal cord **(A)** would cause diminution of touch on the side ipsilateral to the lesion and diminution of pain on the side contralateral to the lesion. Damage rostral to the medulla **(B)**, on the other hand, would cause diminution of both touch and pain on the side contralateral to the lesion.

FIGURE 3-28

Somatotopic mapping in human somatosensory **(A)** and motor **(B)** cortex obtained by electrical stimulation of the surface of the brains of conscious patients during neurosurgery. The size of a given part of the homunculus is roughly proportional to the size of the cortical area devoted to that body part. (From Penfield W, Rasmussen T: *The cerebral cortex of man.* © 1950 by Macmillan Publishing Co., Inc., renewed 1978 by T. Rasmussen.)

Other sensory systems are similar to the somatosensory system

The somatosensory system is one of the better understood sensory systems, but others are organized according to similar anatomical principles—primary afferents that terminate without crossing, participation in reflexes, pathways to the cerebral cortex that involve at least three neurons and a relay in the thalamus, distorted maps, and projections to the cerebellum. One area of variability is the pattern of crossing the midline. Some systems project bilaterally to the thalamus. For example, we need to compare the inputs from both ears to localize sound; this comparison begins to take place in the brainstem, and each ear is represented bilaterally in the brainstem, thalamus, and cerebral cortex. The olfactory,* taste, and some visceral pathways are uncrossed, for reasons as unclear as those for the crossing of other pathways. Most or all kinds of sensory information reach the cerebellum, but many of the connections involved are not as well understood as the somatosensory connections.

Higher Levels of the CNS Influence the Activity of Lower Motor Neurons

Lower motor neurons are subject to a variety of influences, such as reflex circuitry and descending impulses from the

---

*The olfactory pathway is also unusual in bypassing the thalamus, at least initially. The olfactory bulb is an outgrowth of the telencephalon, and the olfactory nerve projects directly to it, and from there to certain cortical areas.

brainstem (e.g., the automatic posture-adjustment signals from the vestibular nuclei). Most important in terms of voluntary movement is the **corticospinal tract,** a collection of fibers that, as the name implies, descend from cell bodies in motor areas of the cerebral cortex and terminate in the spinal cord. These are often referred to clinically as **upper motor neurons.*** Systematic maps are found in motor cortex just as in somatosensory cortex, and the cell bodies of corticospinal neurons are distributed in the precentral gyrus in a pattern parallel to the somatosensory homunculus (Figure 3-28, *B*). Damage to the corticospinal tract causes weakness of half of the body, even though reflexes may still be functional (or even exaggerated).

The cerebellum and basal ganglia also influence movement, but have few or no outputs of their own that reach the spinal cord. Rather, they act indirectly by affecting the activity of motor areas of the cerebral cortex. Damage to the cerebellum or basal ganglia leaves motor cortex and lower motor neurons intact, so movements are defective—they may, for example, be slow or uncoordinated—but weakness is not prominent.

Corticospinal axons cross the midline

Just as somatosensory pathways cross the midline between the periphery and the cerebral cortex, so too does the corticospinal tract (Figure 3-30). Hence damage to one cerebral hemisphere can result in both somatosensory deficits and weakness in the contralateral arm and leg.

Each side of the cerebellum indirectly affects movements of the ipsilateral side of the body

The cerebellum (discussed further in Chapter 20), in a very general sense, helps to plan the details of movements and to correct them while they are still in progress. For example, to lift a glass to your lips you need to contract your biceps and relax your triceps, both by just the right amount at just the right time; as the glass approaches your lips, you need to make fine adjustments in its trajectory. The cerebellum plays a role in both processes. To do so, it needs to know not only what you intend to do (i.e., input from the cerebral cortex), but also the moment-to-moment position of your arm (i.e., somatosensory inputs). Cerebellar outputs return to motor cortex, affecting corticospinal activity; this requires a trip through the thalamus. The final element in the general pattern of cerebellar connectivity is dictated by the fact that one side of the cerebellum is related to the ipsilateral side of the body. Because one side of the cerebrum is related to the contralateral side of the body, this means that pathways interconnecting the cerebellum and cerebrum must cross the midline (Figure 3-31). Because cerebellar outputs are di-

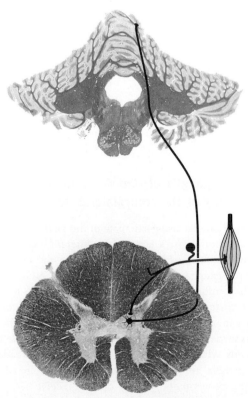

FIGURE 3-29
The minimum sensory pathway from the periphery to the cerebellum.

---

* For the purposes of this discussion, *corticospinal neurons* are synonymous with *upper motor neurons.* As will be discussed further in subsequent chapters, however, the two terms are often used variably and inconsistently.

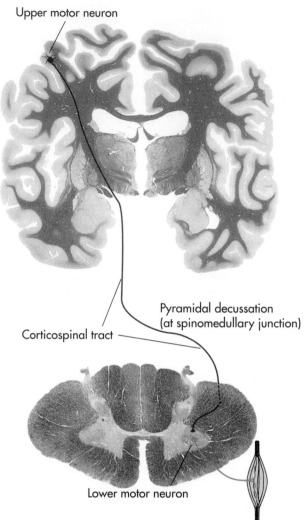

Upper motor neuron

Pyramidal decussation
(at spinomedullary junction)

Corticospinal tract

Lower motor neuron

FIGURE 3-30
Overview of the corticospinal tract. Corticospinal neurons project directly to the spinal cord, bypassing the thalamus.

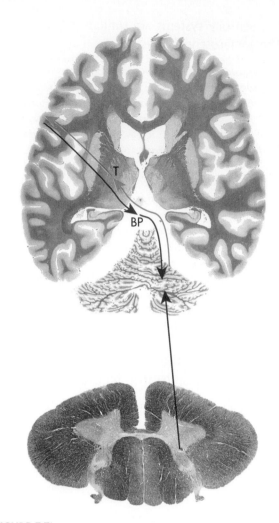

FIGURE 3-31
Overview of cerebellar connections, explained in more detail in Chapter 20. (The spinal cord section is inverted relative to its appearance in most other sections in this book, so that anterior is up in both parts of the figure.) *BP,* Basal pons; *T,* thalamus.

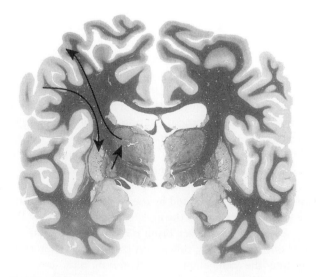

FIGURE 3-32
Overview of the major circuit involved in basal ganglia functions, explained in more detail in Chapter 19. Because the basal ganglia of one hemisphere influence motor cortex of the ipsilateral hemisphere, damage to the basal ganglia on one side can cause a contralateral movement disorder.

rected toward motor cortex (via the thalamus), cerebellar damage causes problems with movement but not with sensation.

The basal ganglia of one side indirectly affect movements of the contralateral side of the body

The basal ganglia also participate in the planning of movements, although in a somewhat different way than the cerebellum does (see Chapter 19). Like the cerebellum, the basal ganglia receive input from the cerebral cortex and then influence movement by affecting the output of motor cortex (Figure 3-32). One set of this cortex-basal ganglia-thalamus circuitry resides in each half of the cerebrum, so damage to the basal ganglia on one side causes problems with movement on the contralateral side. The basal ganglia are not prominently involved in adjusting ongoing movements, so they do not receive sensory information as directly as the cerebellum does (compare Figures 3-31 and 3-32).

SUGGESTED READINGS

Armstrong E: Brains, bodies and metabolism, *Brain Behav Evol* 36:166, 1990.

Blinkov SM, Glezer II: *The human brain in figures and tables*, New York, 1968, Plenum Press and Basic Books.

DeArmond SJ, Fusco MM, Dewey MM: *Structure of the human brain: a photographic atlas,* ed 3, New York, 1989, Oxford University Press.

Dekaban AS, Sadowsky D: Changes in brain weights during the span of human life: relation of brain weights to body heights and body weights, *Ann Neurol* 4:345, 1978.

Duvernoy HM: *The human brain: surface, three-dimensional sectional anatomy and MRI,* Vienna, 1991, Springer-Verlag.

Filipek PA et al: The young adult human brain: an MRI-based morphometric analysis, *Cer Cortex* 4:344, 1994. *Relative volumes of different brain parts.*

Gluhbegovic N, Williams TH: *The human brain: a photographic guide,* New York, 1980, Harper & Row. *Includes a series of beautiful dissections.*

Haines DE: *Neuroanatomy: an atlas of structures, sections, and systems,* ed 4, Baltimore, 1995, Williams & Wilkins.

Igarashi S, Kamiya T: *Atlas of the vertebrate brain: morphological evolution from cyclostomes to mammals,* Baltimore, 1972, University Park Press. *Ever wonder what an anteater's brain looks like?*

Ludwig E, Klingler J: *Atlas cerebri humani,* Boston, 1956, Little, Brown & Co. *A series of technically spectacular dissections of human brains.*

Nieuwenhuys R, Voogd J, van Hurjzen C: *The human central nervous system: a synopsis and atlas,* ed 3, New York, 1988, Springer-Verlag. *Includes many beautiful drawings of the brain and various subsystems of the CNS, as well as a brief but thorough text portion.*

Nolte J, Angevine JB Jr: *The human brain in photographs and diagrams,* St Louis, 1995, Mosby.

Ono M, Kubik S, Abernathey CD: *Atlas of the cerebral sulci,* New York, 1990, Thieme Medical Publishers. *A good place to get a sense of the variability of the cortical surface from one brain to another.*

Roberts M, Hanaway J, Morest DK: *Atlas of the human brain in section,* ed 2, Philadelphia, 1987, Lea & Febiger.

Schnitzlein HN, Murtagh FR: *Imaging anatomy of the head and spine: a photographic color atlas of MRI, CT, gross, and microscopic anatomy in axial, coronal, and sagittal planes,* ed 2, Baltimore, 1990, Urban and Schwarzenberg.

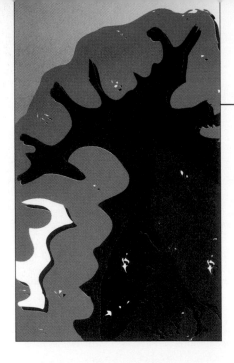

MENINGEAL COVERINGS OF THE BRAIN AND SPINAL CORD

Living brain is on the soft and mushy side, despite the network of cytoskeletal proteins contained in neurons and glial cells. Without support of some kind, the CNS would be unable to maintain its shape, particularly as we walk and run around and occasionally bump our heads. The brain and spinal cord are protected from outside forces by their encasement in the skull and vertebral column, respectively. In addition, the CNS is suspended within a series of three membranous coverings, the **meninges** (from the Greek word *meninx,* meaning "membrane"), that stabilize the shape and position of nerve tissue in two different ways during head and body movements. First, the brain is

mechanically suspended within the meninges, which in turn are anchored to the skull so that the brain is constrained to move with the head. Second, there is a layer of **cerebrospinal fluid (CSF)** within the meninges; the buoyant effect of this fluid environment greatly decreases the tendency of various forces (such as gravity) to distort the brain. Thus a brain weighing 1500 g in air effectively weighs less than 50 g in its normal CSF environment, where it is easily able to maintain its shape. In contrast, an isolated fresh brain, unsupported by its usual surroundings, becomes seriously distorted and may even tear under the influence of gravity (Figure 4-1).

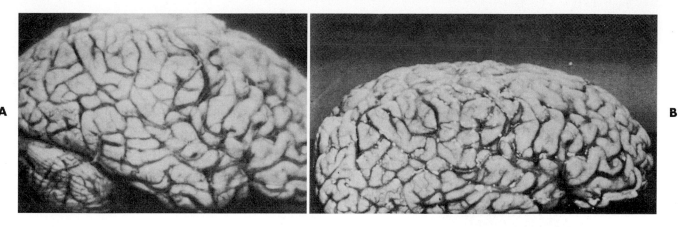

FIGURE 4-1
Effects of gravity and of partial flotation on brain. **A,** An unfixed human brain in a vat of isotonic saline; normal shape is maintained. **B,** The same brain in air, obviously distorted by its own weight. (From Oldendorf W: *The quest for an image of brain*, New York, 1980, Raven Press.)

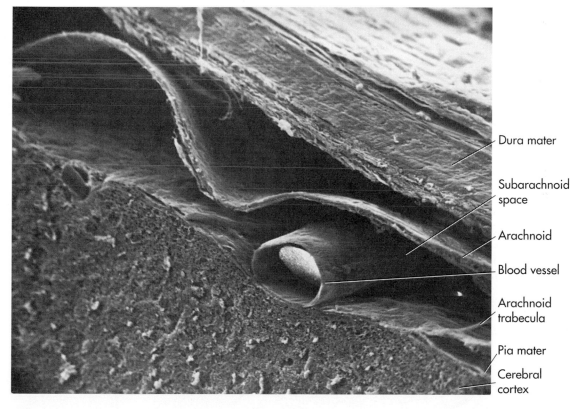

Dura mater

Subarachnoid
space

Arachnoid

Blood vessel

Arachnoid
trabecula

Pia mater

Cerebral
cortex

FIGURE 4-2
Scanning electron micrograph of the cranial meninges of a young dog. The apparent space between the dura mater and the arachnoid is an artifact of processing and would not normally be present. (Courtesy Dr. Delmas J. Allen, Medical College of Ohio.)

THERE ARE THREE MENINGEAL LAYERS: THE DURA MATER, ARACHNOID, AND PIA MATER

The three meninges, from the outermost layer inward, are the **dura mater,** the **arachnoid,** and the **pia mater** (Figure 4-2). In common usage the dura mater and pia mater are often referred to simply as the *dura*

and *pia.* The dura mater is by far the most substantial of the three meninges, and for this reason is also called the **pachymeninx** (from the Greek word *pachy* meaning "thick," as in thick-skinned pachyderms). The arachnoid and pia mater, in contrast, are thin and delicate. They are similar to and continuous with each other and so are sometimes referred to together as the *pia-arachnoid* or the **leptomeninges** (from the Greek word *lepto,* meaning "thin" or "fine"). The dura mater is attached to the inner surface of the skull, and the arachnoid adheres to the inner surface of the dura mater. The pia mater is attached to the brain, following all its contours, and the space between the arachnoid and pia mater is filled with CSF.

Because of the differences between cranial and spinal meninges, those of the spinal cord are described separately at the end of this chapter.

THE DURA MATER PROVIDES MECHANICAL STRENGTH

The cranial dura is a thick, tough, collagenous membrane that adheres firmly to the inner surface of the skull (*dura* is the Latin word for "hard," as in durable). It is often described as consisting of two layers: an outer layer that serves as the periosteum of the inner surface of the skull and an inner layer, the meningeal dura. Because these two layers are tightly fused, with no sharp histological bound-

ary between them, the entire complex is ordinarily referred to as *dura mater.*

No space exists on either side of the dura under normal circumstances because one side is attached to the skull and the other side adheres to the arachnoid. However, two **potential spaces,** the **epidural** and **subdural** spaces, are associated with the dura (Table 4-1, Figure 4-14). Epidural space refers to the potential space between the cranium

Table 4-1	Spaces in the Cranial Meninges
Space	**Location**
Epidural	Potential space between dura and calvaria
Subdural	Potential space in the innermost dural layer
Subarachnoid	Normally present, CSF-filled space; enlarged in cisterns

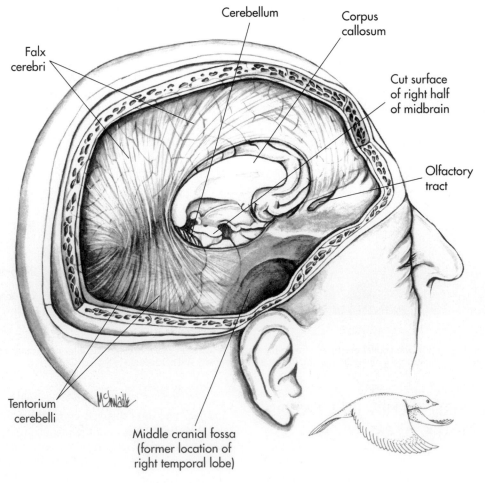

FIGURE 4-3

Shape and spatial relationships of the dural reflections. The cerebellum and part of the left cerebral hemisphere are drawn in on the other side of the falx cerebri and tentorium cerebelli. The small bird in the corner reminds certain individuals of the shape of the tentorium cerebelli. (Drawn from a dissection by Gary Jenison, University of Colorado Health Sciences Center.)

and the periosteal layer. Subdural space is commonly described as the potential space between dura and arachnoid and is sometimes said to contain a thin film of fluid. However, electron microscopic evidence indicates that the dura and arachnoid are normally attached to each other, and when they appear to separate the splitting actually occurs within the innermost cellular layers of the dura. Parts of these potential spaces can become actual fluid-filled cavities in certain pathological conditions, most often as a result of hemorrhage.

Dural Septa Partially Separate Different Intracranial Compartments

There are several places where the inner dural layer folds in on itself as a sheetlike protrusion, each called a **dural reflection** or **dural septum,** into the cranial cavity. The principal dural reflections are the **falx cerebri,** which intervenes between the two cerebral hemispheres, and the **tentorium cerebelli,** which intervenes between the cerebral hemispheres and the cerebellum (Figure 4-3). The **falx cerebelli** is a small reflection that partially separates the two cerebellar hemispheres. The **diaphragma sellae,** another small reflection, covers the pituitary fossa, admitting the infundibulum through a small perforation.

The falx cerebri (from the Latin word *falx,* meaning "sickle") is a long, arched, vertical dural sheet (Figures 4-3 and 4-4, *A*) that occupies the longitudinal fissure and separates the two cerebral hemispheres. Anteriorly it is at-

tached to the crista galli of the ethmoid bone. The falx curves posteriorly and fuses with the middle of the tentorium cerebelli at the internal occipital protuberance. The inferior, free edge of the falx generally parallels the corpus callosum, but the falx is somewhat broader posteriorly than it is anteriorly, so the free edge comes closer to the splenium of the corpus callosum than to the genu. The anterior portion of the falx is frequently incomplete, containing a number of perforations.

The tentorium cerebelli separates the superior surface of the cerebellum from the occipital lobes, defining **supratentorial** and **infratentorial** compartments. The supratentorial compartment contains the cerebrum, and the infratentorial compartment (or **posterior fossa**) contains the brainstem and cerebellum. Because the interval between the cerebrum and cerebellum is not horizontal or flat, neither is the tentorium. Rather, it is roughly the shape of a bird with its wings extended in front of it; the bird's body would correspond to the midline region where the falx joins the tentorium, and its wings would correspond to the rest of the tentorium, which is prolonged anteriorly (Figure 4-3). Posteriorly the tentorium is attached mainly to the occipital bone. This line of attachment continues anteriorly and inferiorly along the petrous temporal bone. The free edge of the tentorium also curves anteriorly on each side, almost encircling the midbrain (Figure 4-5). This space in the tentorium through which the brainstem passes is called the **tentorial notch** (or **tentorial incisure**) and is of great clinical significance, as discussed later in this chapter.

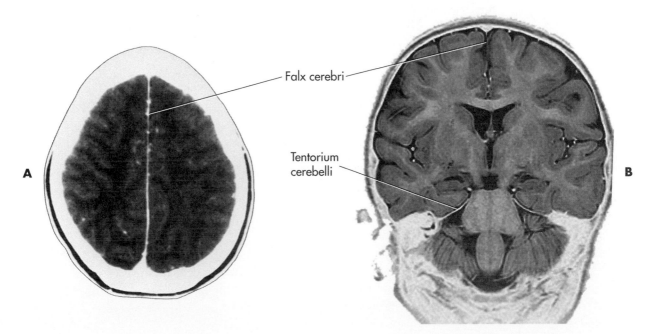

A   **B**

Falx cerebri

Tentorium cerebelli

FIGURE 4-4
Major dural septa as seen in clinical images. **A,** A contrast-enhanced CT scan (see Chapter 6) showing the falx cerebri between the two cerebral hemispheres. **B,** A coronal MRI (see Chapter 5) showing the falx cerebri and tentorium cerebelli. (From Nolte J, Angevine JB Jr: *The human brain in photographs and diagrams,* St. Louis, 1995, Mosby.)

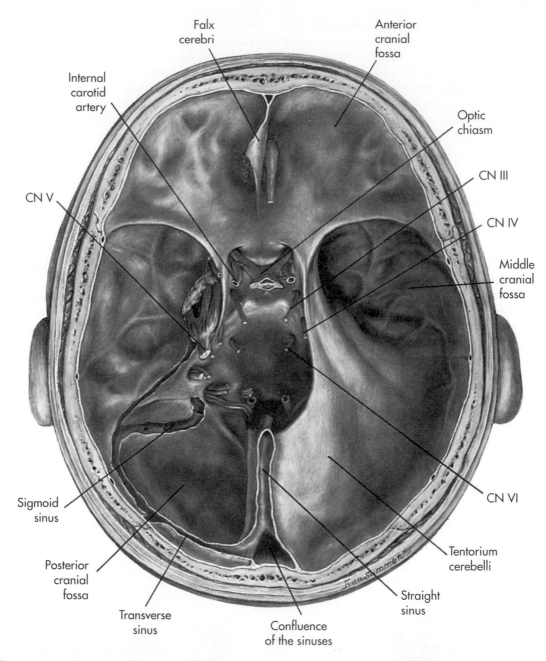

Falx
cerebri

Anterior
cranial
fossa

Internal
carotid
artery

Optic
chiasm

CN V

CN III

CN IV

Middle
cranial
fossa

Sigmoid
sinus

CN VI

Posterior
cranial
fossa

Tentorium
cerebelli

Transverse
sinus

Confluence
of the sinuses

Straight
sinus

FIGURE 4-5
Dural lining of the base of the skull. The falx has been removed except for a small anterior portion. The left half of the tentorium has also been removed, exposing the posterior fossa (where the cerebellum was). [From Mettler FA: *Neuroanatomy*, ed 2, St. Louis, 1948, Mosby.]

The Dura Mater Contains Venous Sinuses That Drain the Brain

As noted previously, the two layers of the cranial dura are tightly fused, and there are no pathological conditions in which an intradural space (i.e., a space between the two layers) develops. However, at some edges of dural reflections (most often attached edges), the two layers are normally separated to form channels, called **dural venous sinuses,** into which the cerebral veins empty. These sinuses are roughly triangular in cross section and are lined with endothelium (Figure 4-6). The locations of the major sinuses can be inferred by considering the lines of attachment of the falx and the tentorium. The **superior sagittal sinus** is found along the attached edge of the falx, the left and right **transverse sinuses** along the posterior line of attachment of the tentorium, and the **straight sinus** along the line of attachment of the falx and tentorium (Figures 4-5 and 4-7). All four of these sinuses meet in the **confluence of the sinuses** (also called the **torcular,** or **torcular Herophili**—"the winepress of Herophilus") near the internal occipital protuberance. Venous blood flows posteriorly in the superior sagittal and straight sinuses into the confluence, and from there through the transverse sinuses. Each transverse sinus continues, from the point where it leaves the tentorium, as the **sigmoid sinus,** which proceeds anteriorly and inferiorly through an S-shaped course and empties into the internal jugular vein (Figures 4-5 and 4-7; see also Figure 6-29).

The confluence of the sinuses is generally not a symmetrical structure. Usually most of the blood from the superior sagittal sinus flows into the right transverse sinus, whereas blood from the straight sinus flows into the left transverse sinus (Figures 4-5 and 4-7). Not uncommonly, the two transverse sinuses are not interconnected at all.

In addition to receiving cerebral veins, the major dural sinuses are connected with several smaller sinuses (see Figure 6-28). The **inferior sagittal sinus,** in the free edge of the falx cerebri, empties into the straight sinus. The small **occipital sinus,** in the attached edge of the falx cerebelli, empties into the confluence of the sinuses (Figure 4-7). The **superior petrosal sinus,** in the edge of the tentorium attached to the petrous temporal bone, carries blood from the cavernous sinus to the transverse sinus at the point where the latter leaves the tentorium to become the sigmoid sinus. The **inferior petrosal sinus** follows a groove between the temporal and occipital bones, carrying blood from the cavernous sinus to the internal jugular vein.

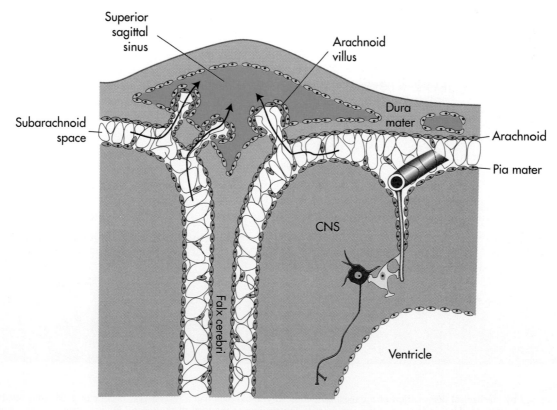

FIGURE 4-6
Section through the superior sagittal sinus showing the movement of CSF from subarachnoid space, through the arachnoid villi, and into the sinus. (Modified from Hamilton WJ: *Textbook of human anatomy,* ed 2, St. Louis, 1976, Mosby.)

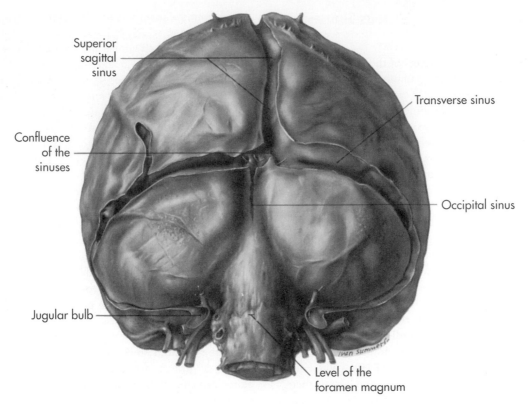

Superior
sagittal
sinus

Confluence
of the
sinuses

Transverse sinus

Occipital sinus

Jugular bulb

Level of the
foramen magnum

FIGURE 4-7
The brain, still encased in dura, viewed from behind. Note the asymmetry of the confluence of the sinuses. Note also the jagged line at the foramen magnum level corresponding to the cut edge of the periosteal layer of the cranial dura. Below this line, a single-layered dural sheath continues around the spinal cord. (From Mettler FA: *Neuroanatomy*, ed 2, St. Louis, 1948, Mosby.)

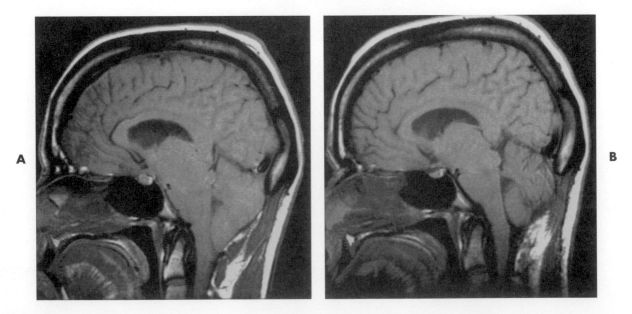

A

B

FIGURE 4-8
Headache caused by mechanical deformation of the meninges. This 40-year-old man had a several-year history of debilitating headaches that were relieved by lying down. He was found to have a meningeal diverticulum at the level of the second lumbar vertebra, through which CSF presumably drained. This interfered with the normal flotation effect of the CSF (described in Chapter 5), causing "sagging" of the brain (**A**) and consequent traction on the meninges. After ligation of the diverticulum, the brain assumed a nearly normal shape (**B**). [From Schievink WI et al: Spontaneous spinal cerebrospinal fluid leaks and intracranial hypotension, *J Neurosurg* 84:598, 1996.]

The Dura Mater Has Its Own Blood Supply

The arterial supply of the dura comes from a large number of meningeal arteries. These are somewhat misnamed because they travel in the periosteal layer of the dura and function mainly in supplying the bones of the skull; however, many small arterial branches penetrate the dura itself. The largest of the meningeal arteries is the **middle meningeal artery,** a branch of the maxillary artery, which ramifies over most of the lateral surface of the cerebral dura. Anteriorly the dura is supplied by branches of the ophthalmic artery, and posteriorly it is supplied by branches of the occipital and vertebral arteries. Meningeal veins, also located in the periosteal layer, generally parallel the arteries.

The Dura Mater Is Pain Sensitive

Remarkably, the brain itself, as well as the arachnoid and pia mater, is not sensitive to pain, and some neurosurgical procedures can be carried out without general anesthesia. The principal pain-sensitive intracranial structures are the dura mater and proximal portions of blood vessels at the base of the brain.

Most of the cranial dura, except for that of the posterior fossa, receives sensory innervation from the trigeminal nerve. Dural nerves follow the meningeal arteries and end near either the arteries or the dural sinuses. Areas of dura between branches of meningeal arteries are innervated poorly, if at all. Deformation of these endings causes pain and is presumably the cause of certain types of headache (Figure 4-8). Interestingly, the way the pain is perceived depends on whether endings near meningeal arteries or endings near dural sinuses are stimulated. In the former case, the pain is fairly accurately localized to the area of stimulation; in the latter case, the pain is referred to portions of the peripheral distribution of the trigeminal nerve, such as the eye, temple, or forehead.

The dura of the posterior fossa is supplied primarily by fibers of the vagus nerve and the second and third cervical nerves.* As in the case of supratentorial dural innervation, the pain-sensitive endings in the posterior fossa are mostly located near dural arteries and venous sinuses. Deformation in these areas causes pain referred to the area behind the ear or the back of the neck.

THE DURA MATER HAS AN ARACHNOID LINING

The arachnoid is a thin, avascular membrane composed of a few layers of cells interspersed with bundles of collagen. It is semitransparent and resembles a substantial cobweb, for which it is named (the Greek word *arachne* means "spi-

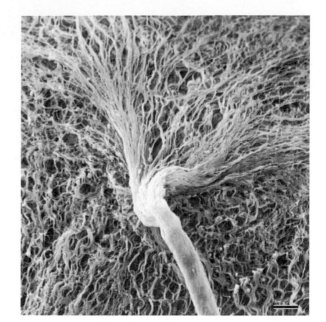

FIGURE 4-9
Scanning electron micrograph of a human arachnoid trabecula. The view is as though you were standing in the lateral sulcus looking out at the overlying arachnoid and dura mater. Collagen bundles spread out from the trabecula and merge with the arachnoid lining of the dura mater. Scale mark = 3 μm. [From Alcolado R et al: The cranial arachnoid and pia mater in man: anatomical and ultrastructural observations, *Neuropath Applied Neurobiol* 14:1, 1988.]

der's web"). The outer portion of the arachnoid consists of several layers of flattened cells adhering to the innermost cellular layer of the dura mater. This interface layer of cells, partially dura and partially arachnoid, contains no collagen and is only about 100 μm thick. Small strands of collagenous connective tissue called **arachnoid trabeculae** (Figure 4-9), covered with fibroblast-like arachnoid cells, leave this interface layer and extend to the pia, with which they merge. Arachnoid trabeculae help keep the brain suspended within the meninges, much the way the Lilliputians stabilized Gulliver's position.*

The Arachnoid Bridges Over CNS Surface Irregularities, Forming Cisterns

Because the arachnoid is attached to the inner surface of the dura mater, it (like the dura) conforms to the general shape of the brain but does not dip into sulci or follow the more intricate contours of the surface of the brain. Therefore there is a **subarachnoid space,** filled with CSF, between the arachnoid and the pia mater, because the pia closely covers all the external surfaces of the CNS. This is the only substantial fluid-filled space normally found around the brain. The subarachnoid space is very narrow over the surfaces of gyri, relatively small where the arachnoid bridges over small sulci, and much larger in certain locations where it bridges over large surface irregularities

---

*The first cervical nerve rarely has a sensory component.

*I thank Dr. Theodore J. Tarby for the analogy.

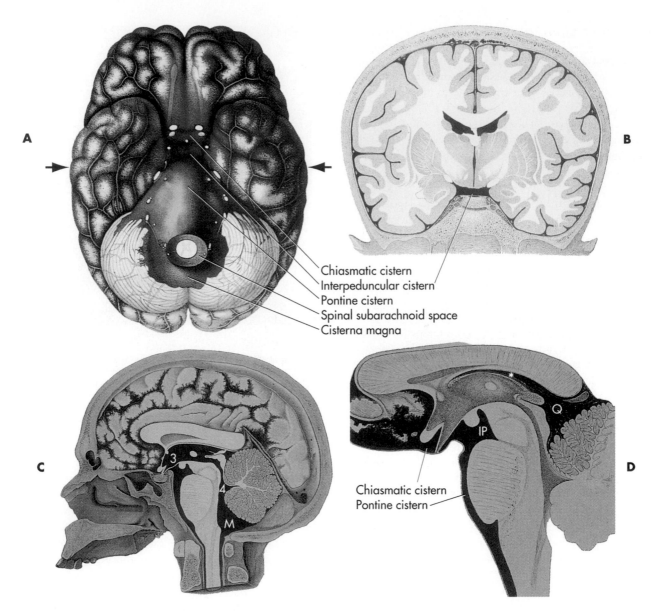

A

B

Chiasmatic cistern
Interpeduncular cistern
Pontine cistern
Spinal subarachnoid space
Cisterna magna

C

D

Chiasmatic cistern
Pontine cistern

FIGURE 4-10
Subarachnoid cisterns. **A,** Cisterns at the base of the brain, demonstrated by filling subarachnoid space with dyed gelatin. The dye fills prominent cisterns, as well as cerebral sulci, but is mostly excluded from the surface of gyri, where there is little subarachnoid space. **B,** A coronal section of a similar specimen, in the plane indicated by the arrows in **A.** Dye fills the ventricles and subarachnoid space, including the interpeduncular cistern. **C** and **D,** Low (**C**) and high (**D**) magnification views of the cisterns and ventricles near the midline, demonstrated by filling subarachnoid space (and in **C,** the ventricles as well) with dyed gelatin. As in **A** and **B,** the dye fills prominent cisterns, as well as cerebral sulci, but is mostly excluded from the surface of gyri. *3,* Third ventricle; *,* transverse cerebral fissure; *4,* fourth ventricle; *IP,* interpeduncular cistern; *M,* cisterna magna (cerebellomedullary cistern); *Q,* quadrigeminal (superior) cistern. (From Key A, Retzius G: *Studien in der Anatomie des Nervensystems und des Bindegewebes,* vol I, Stockholm, 1875, Norstad.)

(Figure 4-10). An example of such a location is the space between the inferior surface of the cerebellum and the posterior surface of the medulla. Regions such as this, which contain a considerable volume of CSF, are called **subarachnoid cisterns.** This particular example is called the **cerebellomedullary cistern** on anatomical grounds, and because it is the largest cranial cistern, it is also referred to as **cisterna magna.** Other prominent cisterns are indicated in Figure 4-10 and include (1) the **pontine cistern,** which is located around the anterior surface of the pons and medulla and is posteriorly continuous with the cerebellomedullary cistern; (2) the **interpeduncular cistern,** which is located between the cerebral peduncles and contains the posterior part of the arterial circle of Willis (see Figure 6-3); and (3) the **superior cistern** (also referred to as the **quadrigeminal cistern** and the **cistern of the great cerebral vein**), a radiological landmark above the midbrain (see Figure 5-14, C). The **transverse cerebral fissure,** a fingerlike extension of subarachnoid space between the fornix and the roof of the third ventricle, continues anteriorly from the superior cistern; it became trapped in this location as the cerebral hemispheres grew backward over the diencephalon during development. The superior cistern is continuous laterally with a thin, curved layer of subarachnoid space on each side that partially encircles the midbrain before opening into the interpeduncular cistern. The combination of the superior cistern and these sheetlike extensions is referred to as the **ambient cistern.**

Arachnoid trabeculae are particularly prominent in subarachnoid cisterns, sometimes coalescing into delicate membranes that partially occlude the subarachnoid space.

CSF Reaches the Venous Circulation Through Arachnoid Villi

The CSF contained in the subarachnoid space generally is separated from the venous blood in dural sinuses by a layer of arachnoid, a thick layer of dura, and the endothelial lining of the sinus. However, at many locations along dural sinuses, particularly along the superior sagittal sinus, small evaginations of the arachnoid, called **arachnoid villi,** protrude into the sinus. At these sites the connective tissue of the dura is lacking, and only a loose layer of arachnoid cells and a layer of endothelium intervene between subarachnoid space and venous blood (Figure 4-6). Large arachnoid villi are called **arachnoid granulations,** and those that become calcified with age are referred to as **pacchionian bodies.** The villi are especially numerous in laterally directed dilations of the superior sagittal sinus, called **venous lacunae** or **lateral lacunae** (Figure 4-11), but some are found along all the sinuses and even along some cerebral veins.

The arachnoid villi are the major sites of reabsorption of CSF into the venous system. Functionally, they behave like one-way valves, allowing flow from subarachnoid space into venous blood but not in the reverse direction.

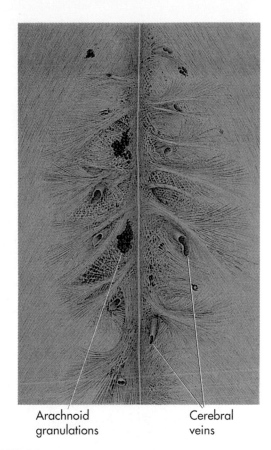

Arachnoid granulations   Cerebral veins

FIGURE 4-11
The floor of the superior sagittal sinus, penetrated by both arachnoid granulations and cerebral veins. (From Key A, Retzius G: *Studien in der Anatomie des Nervensystems und des Bindegewebes,* vol I, Stockholm, 1875, Norstad.)

Because CSF pressure is ordinarily greater than venous pressure, the villi normally allow continuous movement of CSF, more or less as though by bulk flow, into the sinuses; however, even if the pressure gradient reverses, the flow does not. The exact mechanism of this flow has been the subject of debate for many years. Some authors have described continuous open channels, micrometers in diameter, through the walls of the arachnoid villi, but others deny their existence. Some have suggested that giant vacuoles originating on the subarachnoid side of the endothelial cells, traveling across to the venous side, and sometimes being transiently open to both sides simultaneously, are responsible for the flow (Figure 4-12).

The Arachnoid Has a Barrier Function

The CNS is insulated in some respects from the rest of the body and lives in a tightly controlled environment (discussed in more detail in Chapters 5 and 6). This control is achieved partly by a system of barriers between the extracellular space in and around the nervous system and extracellular space elsewhere. One such barrier is between the CSF in the subarachnoid space and the extracellular

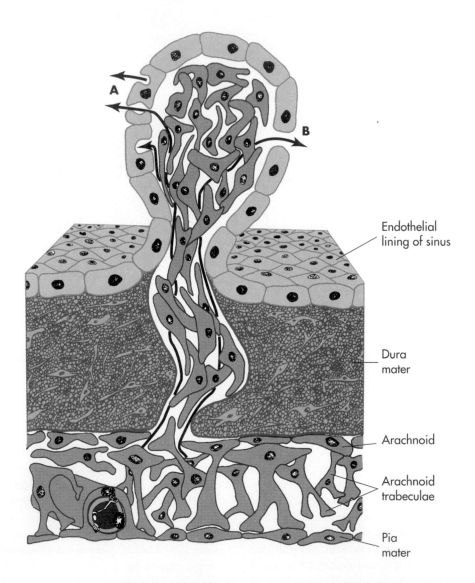

Endothelial
lining of sinus

Dura
mater

Arachnoid

Arachnoid
trabeculae

Pia
mater

FIGURE 4-12
An arachnoid villus, showing the passage of CSF from subarachnoid space into a dural venous sinus. **A**, Cerebrospinal fluid movement through large vacuoles in endothelial cells, as described by some workers. **B**, Movement through channels between cells, as described by other workers. [Modified from Shabo AL, Maxwell DS: The morphology of the arachnoid villi: a light and electron microscopic study in the monkey, *J Neurosurg* 29:451, 1968.]

fluids of the dura. Marker substances injected into the middle meningeal artery spread throughout the dura but do not enter the subarachnoid space. The barrier resides in those cellular layers of the arachnoid in the interface layer with the dura, where the cells are connected to each other by a series of tight junctions that occlude extracellular space (Figure 4-14).

PIA MATER COVERS THE SURFACE OF THE CNS

The pia mater (from the Latin word *pia,* meaning "tender") is a second delicate membrane that, unlike the arachnoid, closely invests all external surfaces of the CNS. Pia follows all the contours of the brainstem and all the folds of the cerebral and cerebellar cortices, abutting the layer of astrocyte end-feet at the surface of the CNS. Arachnoid trabeculae span the subarachnoid space and merge with the pia mater so subtly that it is difficult to decide where the arachnoid ends and the pia begins. For this reason, some speak of the entire leptomeningeal complex as one entity—the pia-arachnoid.

Cerebral arteries and veins travel in subarachnoid space, held against the pia by sheets and strands of connective tissue, before penetrating the brain. As each small vessel enters or leaves the brain, it carries with it a sleeve of **perivascular space** (or **Virchow-Robin space**). This space extends inward, filled with connective tissue and extracellular fluid, to the level at which the vessel becomes a capillary. The actual nature and extent of this microscopic space and the question of whether it provides a functional pathway of communication between the extracellular space around neurons and the subarachnoid space have been matters of controversy for decades. The traditional view holds that the connective tissue elements of the perivascular space arise as an inwardly directed cuff of pia that accompanies each vessel (as in Figure 4-6), but there are indications that in fact the pia may be left behind on the surface of the CNS. Similarly, some claim that perivascular space is small and restricted, although there are indications that it may provide an important route for movement of extracellular fluid that may even be continuous with the cervical lymphatics through the adventitia of larger vessels.

THE VERTEBRAL CANAL CONTAINS SPINAL EPIDURAL SPACE

The meningeal coverings of the spinal cord are fundamentally similar to those of the brain, but there are several important differences (Table 4-2).

The spinal dura mater is a single-layered membrane, lacking the periosteal component of the cranial dura. The

Table 4-2	Differences Between Cranial and Spinal Meninges	
	Cranial	**Spinal**
Dura mater	Double layered	Single layered
	Attached to inner calvarial surface	Suspended in vertebral canal
Epidural space	Potential space	Real space → *Veins + Fat*
	Between periosteum and calvaria	Between dura and vertebral periosteum
Arachnoid	Attached to inner surface of dura	Attached to inner surface of dura
Pia mater	Attached to CNS surface	Attached to CNS surface
		Expanded as dentate ligaments

inner layer of the cranial dura is continuous at the foramen magnum with the spinal dural sheath, which is separated from the vertebral periosteum by an epidural space (Figure 4-7). Thus there are two basic differences between cranial and spinal epidural spaces:

1. Cranial epidural space is a potential space, whereas spinal epidural space is an actual space.
2. Cranial epidural space, when present, is located between periosteum and cranium, whereas spinal epidural space is located between periosteum and dura. This spinal epidural space is filled with fatty connective tissue and a vertebral venous plexus.

The spinal arachnoid, like its cranial counterpart, is closely applied to the inner surface of the dura, leaving a CSF-filled subarachnoid space between itself and the spinal cord (Figure 4-13). The spinal dural sheath (and its arachnoid lining) ends at about the second sacral vertebra, whereas the spinal cord itself ends at about the level of the disk between the first and second lumbar vertebrae (see Figure 10-2). There is, therefore, a large subarachnoid cistern, the **lumbar cistern,** between these two points. This is the favored site for sampling CSF, because a needle can be inserted here with relatively little risk of damaging the CNS.

The pial covering of the spinal cord is relatively thick and gives rise to a toothed longitudinal projection on each side called the **dentate (denticulate) ligament.** The dentate ligament anchors the spinal cord to the arachnoid and through it to the dura. In addition, another pial projection, the **filum terminale,** anchors the caudal end of the spinal cord (the **conus medullaris**) to the caudal end of the spinal dural sheath (see Figure 10-2). The caudal end of the dural sheath, in turn, is anchored to the caudal end of the vertebral canal.

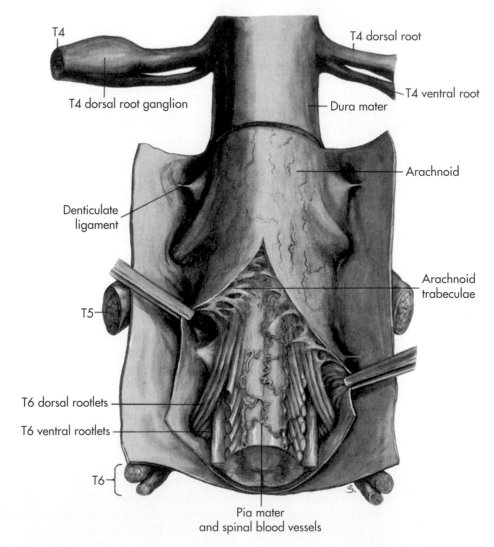

T4

T4 dorsal root ganglion

T4 dorsal root

T4 ventral root

Dura mater

Arachnoid

Denticulate
ligament

Arachnoid
trabeculae

T5

T6 dorsal rootlets

T6 ventral rootlets

T6

Pia mater
and spinal blood vessels

FIGURE 4-13
The spinal meninges, showing how dentate ligaments anchor the spinal cord to its dural sheath through the arachnoid. (From Mettler FA: *Neu-roanatomy*, ed 2, St. Louis, 1948, Mosby.)

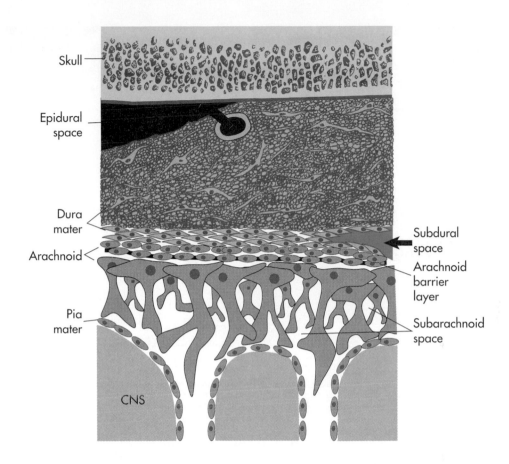

FIGURE 4-14
Actual spaces and potential spaces in and around the meninges. Epidural space (not normally present) between dura and skull may be opened up by blood from a ruptured meningeal artery or, less commonly, a torn dural venous sinus. Subdural space (not normally present), typically within the dura near the latter's junction with the arachnoid, may be opened up by blood from a vein that tears at its entrance into a dural sinus. Dark bars joining superficial arachnoid cells represent the tight junctions that are the basis of the barrier properties of this portion of the arachnoid.

Table 4-3 Locations of Hematomas	
Source of blood	**Nature of bleeding or hematoma**
Meningeal artery	Epidural hematoma
Dural venous sinus	Subdural or epidural hematoma
Vein at attachment to sinus	Subdural hematoma
Cerebral artery or vein	Subarachnoid hemorrhage Intraparenchymal hemorrhage Intraventricular hemorrhage

BLEEDING CAN OPEN UP POTENTIAL MENINGEAL SPACES

As discussed previously, the three meningeal coverings of the brain have various real or potential spaces associated with them (Figure 4-14). There is no space between the pia and the brain, but there is a subarachnoid space between the pia and the arachnoid, along with potential subdural and epidural spaces. Both of these potential spaces can become actual fluid-filled spaces under certain conditions (Table 4-3).

Tearing of Meningeal Arteries Can Cause an Epidural Hematoma

The meningeal arteries run in the periosteal layer of the dura. If one of these arteries is torn (typically as a result of traumatic skull injury), bleeding occurs between the periosteum and the skull, opening up the potential epidural space and causing an **epidural hematoma.** As the hematoma expands, it compresses and distorts the underlying brain (Figure 4-15) and is likely to be fatal unless promptly treated surgically. Less commonly, tearing of a dural venous sinus can cause an epidural hematoma (Figure 4-16).

Tearing of Veins Where They Enter Venous Sinuses Can Cause a Subdural Hematoma

Bleeding can also occur into the potential subdural space, resulting in a **subdural hematoma. T**he most common cause of subdural hematomas is tearing of a cerebral vein

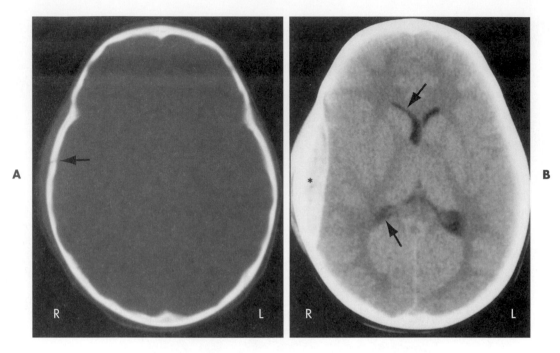

FIGURE 4-15

Epidural hematoma in a 3-year-old girl who hit her head in an automobile accident. About 2 hours after the accident she complained of a severe headache and nausea and became lethargic. CT set to show bony details (A) revealed a fracture of the right temporal bone *(arrow)*. CT set to reveal soft-tissue details (B) revealed a lens-shaped epidural hematoma (*) and compression of the right lateral ventricle *(arrows)*; *L*, left side, *R*, right side. After rapid neurosurgical treatment she made a full recovery. (Courtesy Dr. Raymond F. Carmody, Department of Radiology, The University of Arizona College of Medicine.)

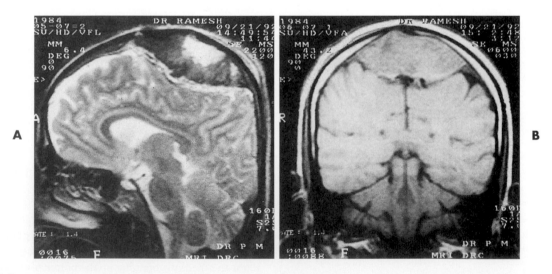

FIGURE 4-16

Epidural hematoma, seen in sagittal (A) and coronal (B) MRIs, resulting from laceration of the superior sagittal sinus several days previously. This very large hematoma has the characteristic lens shape of epidural hematomas and crosses the midline (B); *R*, right side. (Subdural hematomas typically are crescent shaped [Figures 4-17 and 4-18] and do not cross the midline.) In this case "a 43-year-old medical practitioner presented with severe generalized headache of 4 days' duration. Four days earlier, he had a fall from a scooter while trying to avoid collision with a cyclist. He had transient loss of consciousness lasting a few minutes, following which he was hospitalized elsewhere for a day and discharged." The patient was treated surgically and recovered. (From Ramesh VG, Sivakumar S: Extradural hematoma at the vertex: a case report, *Surg Neurol* 43:138, 1995.)

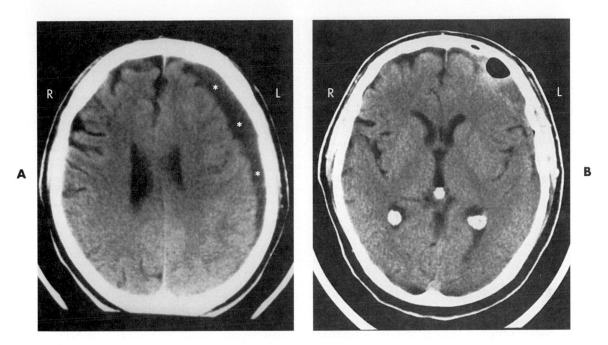

FIGURE 4-17

A, Crescent-shaped subdural hematoma (*) over the surface of the left cerebral hemisphere, compressing its subarachnoid spaces and lateral ventricle and shifting midline structures to the right; *L,* left side, *R,* right side. Although subdural hematomas are commonly caused by a blow to the head, they can also be caused by other mechanical disturbances (as in the shaken-baby syndrome). This is the case of a 64-year-old man whose "headaches developed gradually after he began riding a roller coaster at an amusement park. The roller coaster, he reported, 'swings people upside down as many as six times.'...He rode the roller coaster on 11 different occasions until his headaches became so severe that he was unable to continue." After surgical removal of the hematoma (**B**), subarachnoid spaces and ventricular symmetry returned and the patient recovered uneventfully. (**A** from Bo-Abbas Y, Bolton CF: Roller-coaster headache, *N Engl J Med* 332:1585, 1995. Copyright © 1995 Massachusetts Medical Society. All rights reserved. **B** courtesy Dr. Y. Bo-Abbas, Victoria Hospital, London, Ontario, Canada.)

as it enters a dural sinus. This can result from rapid accelerations or decelerations of the head (Figure 4-17): the venous sinuses are attached to the skull and move with it, but the brain can lag behind, so a vein extending from the brain to a sinus can tear loose. Some subdural hematomas are acute and produce symptoms much like those of an epidural hematoma, whereas others may progress very slowly and become surprisingly large before producing symptoms.

PARTS OF THE CNS CAN HERNIATE FROM ONE INTRACRANIAL COMPARTMENT INTO ANOTHER

Dural reflections such as the falx cerebri and the tentorium cerebelli are firmly attached to the cranium. These reflections are stretched rather taut, which allows them to perform their mechanical support function; but this very tautness can result in additional problems in cases of increasing intracranial pressure (for example, subdural hematoma or an expanding tumor). The midbrain may be pushed against the edge of the tentorium while passing through the tentorial notch (Figure 4-18), causing damage to a cerebral peduncle and one or more cranial nerves. Also, depending on where the expanding mass causing the increased pressure is located, certain portions of the brain may herniate from one side of a dural reflection to another (Figures 4-19 and 4-20). For example, increased pressure on the lateral surface of one cerebral hemisphere can cause the hemisphere to be displaced inferiorly and medially, in turn causing the uncus and adjacent portions of the temporal lobe to herniate through the tentorial notch and compress the midbrain. Such pressure could also cause one cingulate gyrus to herniate under the falx. Similarly, downward pressure can cause portions of the cerebellum to herniate into the foramen magnum and compress the medulla. Herniations that compress the brainstem are likely to have grave consequences.

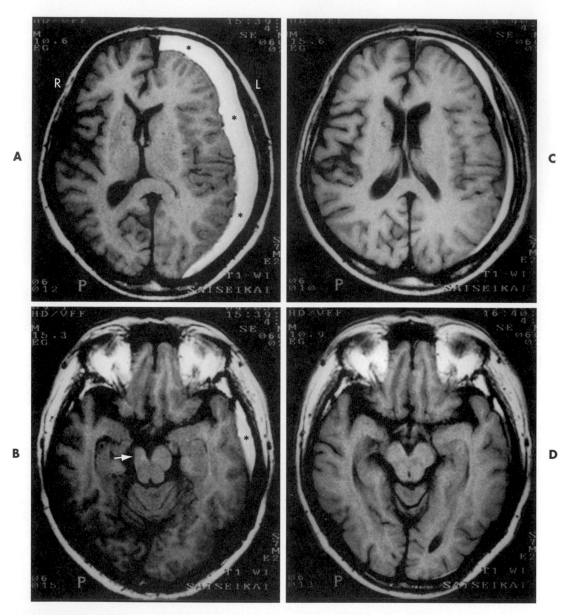

FIGURE 4-18
Chronic subdural hematoma (*) over the surface of the left cerebral hemisphere, compressing its subarachnoid spaces and lateral ventricle (**A**), shifting midline structures to the right and deforming the right cerebral peduncle (*arrow*, **B**) by pressing it against the edge of the tentorium cerebelli; *L*, left side, *R*, right side. This deformation of the cerebral peduncle caused left-sided weakness, which improved when surgical removal of the hematoma resolved the compression (**C** and **D**). (From Itoyama Y, Fukioka S, Ushio Y: Kernohan's notch in chronic subdural hematoma: findings on magnetic resonance imaging, *J Neurosurg* 82:645, 1995.)

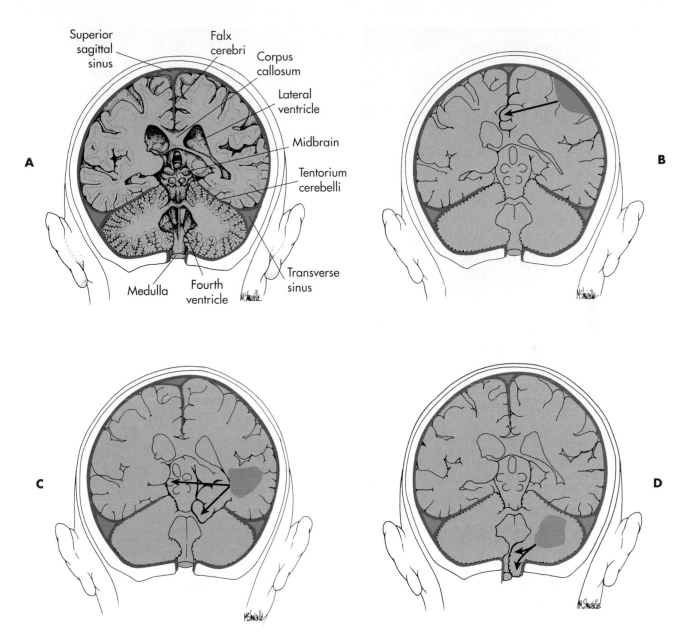

FIGURE 4-19

The three most common ways in which portions of the brain herniate from one compartment into another. **A,** The normal configuration in a plane approximately parallel to the long axis of the brainstem. **B,** As a result of pressure from a subdural hematoma, one cingulate gyrus has slipped under the falx cerebri and is pressing on the opposite cingulate gyrus; this can happen with no serious neurological consequences. **C,** As a result of pressure from an expanding tumor in one temporal lobe, part of the medial temporal lobe has herniated through the tentorial notch and is pressing the midbrain against the free edge of the tentorium. The midbrain contains structures essential for consciousness, and this type of herniation typically produces coma, often followed by death. **D,** As a result of pressure from a cerebellar tumor, one tonsil of the cerebellum has herniated through the foramen magnum, compressing the medulla against the margin of the foramen. The medulla contains respiratory and cardiovascular centers, and pressure on it is usually rapidly fatal.

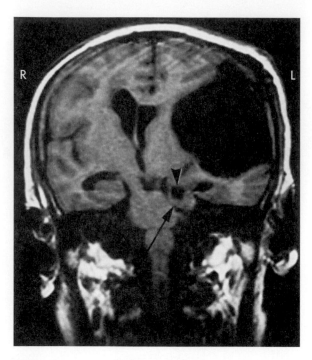

FIGURE 4-20
Magnetic resonance image of uncal herniation; *L*, left side, *R*, right side. A 62-year-old woman experienced slowly progressive weakness over a period of 2 years. She was found to have a large cyst that distended the left lateral sulcus. This pushed the left uncus, adjacent portions of the parahippocampal gyrus, and part of the inferior horn of the lateral ventricle *(arrowhead)* through the tentorial notch. Notice how the herniated temporal lobe distorts the midbrain and rostral pons *(arrow)*, and how the large cyst pushed the bodies of both lateral ventricles to the right. Uncal herniation is usually a neurosurgical emergency, so images like this can rarely be obtained. (From Iwama T et al: MRI demonstration of uncal herniation caused by arachnoid cyst in the Sylvian fissure, *Neuroradiol* 33:346, 1991.)

SUGGESTED READINGS

Alcolado R et al: The cranial arachnoid and pia mater in man: anatomical and ultrastructural observations, *Neuropathol Applied Neurobiol* 14:1, 1988. *Argues that cerebral vessels enter the brain beneath the pia, rather than through subarachnoid space.*

Bisaria KK: Anatomic variations of venous sinuses in the region of the torcular Herophili, *J Neurosurg* 62:90, 1985.

Bo-Abbas Y, Bolton CF: Roller-coaster headache, *New Engl J Med* 332:1585, 1995. *One way that rapid accelerations and decelerations can cause subdural hematoma.*

Coffey RJ, Rhoton AL Jr: *Pain-sensitive cranial structures.* In Dalession DJ, Silberstein SD, editors, *Wolff's headache and other head pain,* ed 6, New York, 1993, Oxford University Press. *A lucid review of sometimes conflicting reports.*

Davson H, Hollingsworth G, Segal MB: The mechanism of drainage of the cerebrospinal fluid, *Brain* 93:665, 1970. *Physiological experiments supporting the concept of bulk flow of CSF through arachnoid villi.*

Esiri MM, Gay D: Immunological and neuropathological significance of the Virchow-Robin space, *J Neurol Sci* 100:3, 1990. *Reviews the evidence for a connection between Virchow-*

Robin *spaces and the lymphatic system and the idea that this connection can be significant in CNS diseases involving the immune system.*

Fox RJ et al: Anatomic details of intradural channels in the parasagittal dura: a possible pathway for flow of cerebrospinal fluid, *Surg Neurol* 39:84, 1996.

Itoyama Y, Fujioka S, Ushio Y: Kernohan's notch in chronic subdural hematoma: findings on magnetic resonance imaging, *J Neurosurg* 82:645, 1995. *Kernohan's notch is the impression made in the midbrain in situations where it is pressed against the free edge of the tentorium by an expanding mass.*

Keller JT et al: Innervation of the posterior fossa dura of the cat, *Brain Res Bull* 14:97, 1985.

Krahn V: The pia mater at the site of the entry of blood vessels into the central nervous system, *Anat Embryol* 164:257, 1982.

Laine FJ et al: Acquired intracranial herniations: MR imaging findings, *AJR Am J Roentgenol* 165:967, 1995. *A nice pictorial review of conditions causing herniation under the falx, through the tentorial notch, or through the foramen magnum.*

Liliequist B: The subarachnoid cisterns: an anatomic and roentgenologic study, *Acta Radiol Suppl* 185, 1959.

Livingston RB: *Mechanics of cerebrospinal fluid.* In Ruch TC, Patton HD, editors: *Physiology and biophysics,* ed 19, Philadelphia, 1965, WB Saunders. *Explains why a brain suspended in CSF has an effective weight of only 50 g.*

May PRA et al: Woodpecker drilling behavior: an endorsement of the rotational theory of impact brain injury, *Arch Neurol* 36:370, 1979. *Not closely related to the meninges but an interesting discussion of suspension of the brain within the cranium and protection of the brain from injury. Imagine what would happen to you if you banged your beak on a tree as often and as hard as a woodpecker does.*

Meyer A: Herniation of the brain, *Arch Neurol Psychiatr* 4:387, 1940.

Millen JW, Woollam DHM: On the nature of the pia mater, *Brain* 84:514, 1961. *A lucid discussion of the appearance of the pia at the light microscopic level.*

Nabeshima S et al: Junctions in the meninges and marginal glia, *J Comp Neurol* 164:127, 1975. *Ultrastructural appearance of the meninges, the arachnoid barrier layer, and subdural space.*

Pease DC, Schultz RL: Electron microscopy of rat cranial meninges, *Am J Anat* 102:301, 1958.

Penfield W, McNaughton F: Dural headache and innervation of the dura mater, *Arch Neurol Psychiatr* 44:43, 1940. *A long but interesting account of the gross anatomy of dural innervation, headaches resulting from dural distortion, and the surgical relief of such headaches.*

Ramesh VG, Sivakumar S: Extradural hematoma at the vertex: a case report, *Surg Neurol* 43:138, 1995. *An example of epidural hematoma caused by laceration of a venous sinus.*

Ray BS, Wolff HG: Experimental studies on headache: pain-sensitive structures of the head and their significance in headache, *Arch Surg* 41:813, 1940.

Schachenmayr W, Friede RL: The origin of subdural neomembranes. I. Fine structure of the dura-arachnoid interface in man, *Am J Pathol* 92:53, 1978.

Schievink WI et al: Spontaneous spinal cerebrospinal fluid leaks and intracranial hypotension, *J Neurosurg* 84:598, 1996. *An illustration of the painful consequences of partial loss of the buoyant effect of CSF.*

Shabo AL, Maxwell DS: The morphology of the arachnoid villi: a light and electron microscopic study in the monkey, *J Neurosurg* 29:451, 1968.

Tripathi BJ, Tripathi RC: Vacuolar transcellular channels as a drainage pathway for cerebrospinal fluid, *J Physiol* 239:195, 1974.

Upton ML, Weller RO: The morphology of cerebrospinal fluid drainage pathways in human arachnoid granulations, *J Neurosurg* 63:867, 1985.

Vandenabeele F, Creemers J, Lambrichts I: Ultrastructure of the human spinal arachnoid mater and dura mater, *J Anat* 189:417, 1996.

Vinas FC et al: Microsurgical anatomy of the infratentorial trabecular membranes and subarachnoid cisterns, *Neurol Res* 18:117, 1996.

Waggener JD, Beggs J: The membranous coverings of neural tissues: an electron microscopy study, *J Neuropathol Exp Neurol* 26:417, 1967.

Yaśargil MG: *Microneurosurgery, vol I: Microsurgical anatomy of the basal cisterns and vessels of the brain, diagnostic techniques, general operative techniques and pathological considerations of the intracranial aneurysms*, Stuttgart, 1984, Georg Thieme Verlag.

Zhang ET, Inman CBE, Weller RO: Interrelationships of the pia mater and the perivascular (Virchow-Robin) spaces in the human cerebrum, *J Anat* 170:111, 1990.

Zouaoui A, Hidden G: Cerebral venous sinuses: anatomical variants or thrombosis? *Acta Anat* 133:318, 1988.

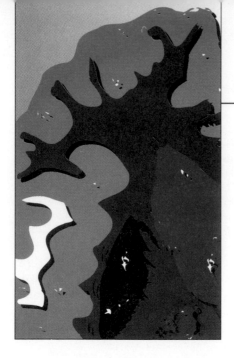

VENTRICLES AND CEREBROSPINAL FLUID

The hollow core of the embryonic neural tube develops into a continuous, fluid-filled system of ventricles lined with **ependymal cells** in the adult; each division of the CNS contains a portion of this ventricular system. Cerebrospinal fluid (CSF) is formed within the ventricles, fills them, and emerges from apertures in the fourth ventricle to fill the subarachnoid space. CSF is responsible for suspension of the brain through its partial flotation, as discussed in Chapter 4, but it does much more than this—it is an important component of the system that regulates the composition of the fluid bathing the neurons and glial cells of the CNS and provides a route through which certain chemical messengers can be widely distributed in the nervous system.

THE BRAIN CONTAINS FOUR VENTRICLES

Within each cerebral hemisphere is a relatively large **lateral ventricle.** The paired lateral ventricles communicate with the **third ventricle** of the diencephalon through the **interventricular foramina (foramina of Monro).** The third ventricle in turn communicates with the **fourth ventricle** of the pons and medulla through the narrow **cerebral aqueduct (aqueduct of Sylvius)** of the midbrain. The fourth ventricle continues caudally as the tiny **central canal** of the caudal medulla and spinal cord; this canal is usually not patent over much of its extent.

A Lateral Ventricle Curves Through Each Cerebral Hemisphere

Each lateral ventricle follows a long C-shaped course through all the lobes of the cerebral hemisphere in which it resides. It is customarily divided into five parts (Figures 5-1 and 5-2): (1) an **anterior** (or **frontal**) **horn** in the frontal lobe anterior to the interventricular foramen; (2) a **body** in the frontal and parietal lobes, extending posteriorly to the region of the splenium of the corpus callosum; (3) a **posterior** (or **occipital**) **horn** projecting backward into the occipital lobe; (4) an **inferior** (or **temporal**) **horn** curving down and forward into the temporal lobe; and (5) an **atrium**, or **trigone,** the region near the splenium where the body and the posterior and inferior horns meet. The body and inferior horn of the ventricle represent the original C-shaped development of the lateral ventricle; the anterior and posterior horns are extensions from this basic shape.

Various structures form the borders of the lateral ventricle in its course through the cerebral hemisphere; many of them can be seen easily in coronal sections (see Figures 3-17 to 3-22) or in brains dissected from above (Figure 5-3). The similarly C-shaped caudate nucleus (see Figure 3-16) is a constant feature in sections through the ventricle. Its enlarged head forms the lateral wall of the anterior horn

(see Figure 3-17), its somewhat smaller body is most of the lateral wall of the body of the ventricle (see Figure 3-19), and its attenuated tail lies in the roof of the inferior horn (see Figures 3-20 and 5-7, *C*). Proceeding posteriorly, as the caudate nucleus becomes smaller, the thalamus becomes larger and forms the floor of the body of the ventricle (compare Figures 3-18 and 3-20). The corpus callosum and **septum pellucidum** give a good indication of the size and location of the anterior horn and body of the ventricle. The body of the corpus callosum forms the roof of these parts of the ventricle, and the genu of the corpus callosum curves down to form the anterior wall of the anterior horn. The septum pellucidum forms the medial wall of the body and anterior horn, and its termination near the splenium marks the site where the bodies of the ventricles diverge from the midline and begin to curve around into the inferior horns (compare Figures 3-19 and 3-21).

The posterior horn is phylogenetically the most recently developed part of the lateral ventricle and is also the most variable in size, sometimes being rudimentary. A number of asymmetries between the cerebral hemispheres of the human brain have been discovered (or rediscovered) in recent years, and it appears that the left posterior horn tends to be longer than the right, particularly in right-handed individuals. The two lateral ventricles are otherwise quite symmetrical.

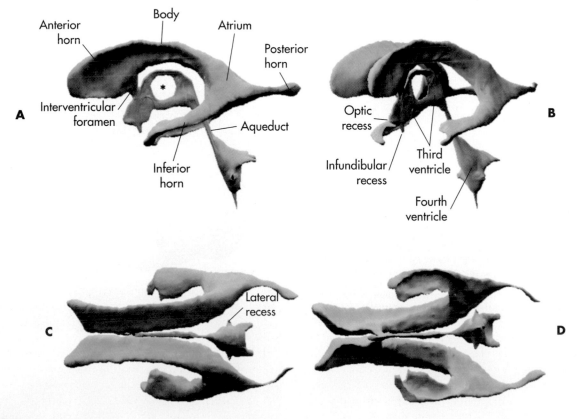

FIGURE 5-1
Three-dimensional reconstruction of the ventricular system, seen from the left (**A**), the left and front (**B**), above (**C**), and below (**D**). The location of the interthalamic adhesion is indicated by an asterisk (*).

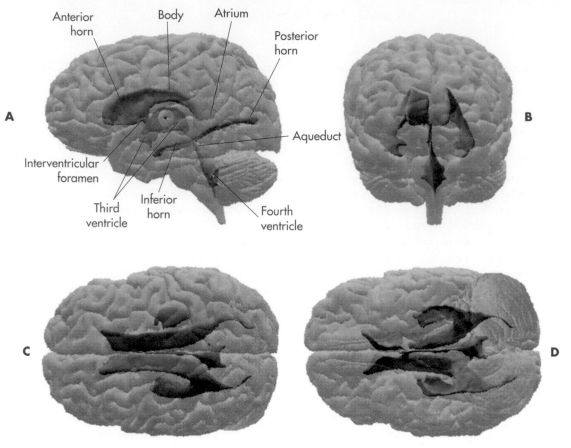

FIGURE 5-2
Three-dimensional reconstruction of the ventricular system inside a translucent CNS, seen from the left (**A**), front (**B**), above (**C**), and below (**D**). The location of the interthalamic adhesion is indicated by an asterisk (*).

FIGURE 5-3
Dissection demonstrating the lateral ventricles, viewed from above and to the right. **A,** A horizontal cut was made to expose the ventricles, and most of the corpus callosum was removed. Some white matter was removed on both sides to expose the posterior horns. The superior portions of the right temporal lobe and most of the insula were also removed so that the inferior horn could be seen on that side. **B,** Continuous choroid plexus follows a C-shaped course from the inferior horn through the atrium, through the body of the lateral ventricle, and into the interventricular foramen (not visible from this angle). There is no choroid plexus in the anterior or posterior horn.

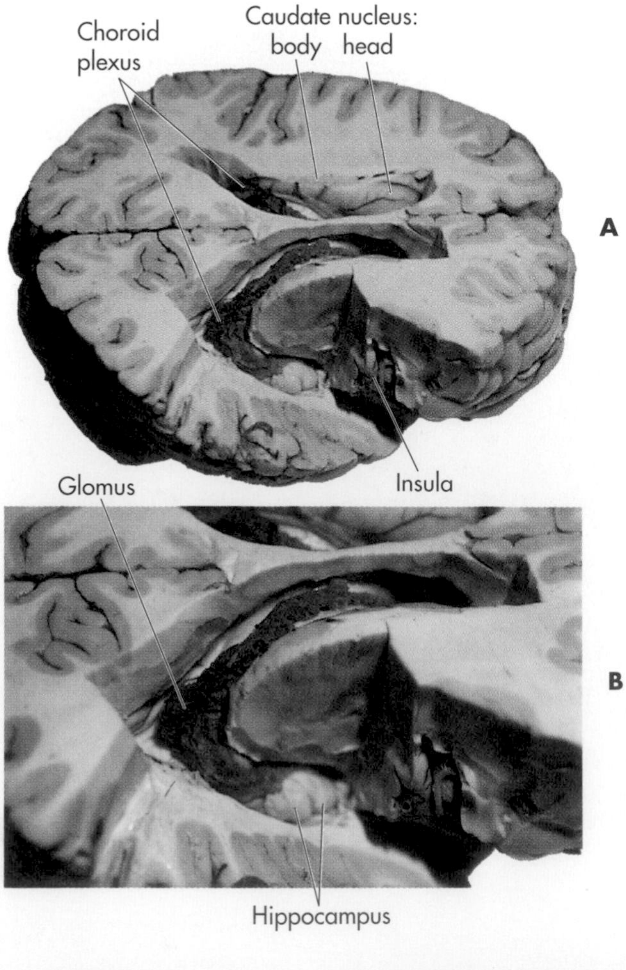

The hippocampus forms most of the floor and medial wall of the inferior horn (see Figure 5-7, *C*), which ends anteriorly at about the level of the uncus.

The Third Ventricle Is a Midline Cavity in the Diencephalon

The narrow, slit-shaped third ventricle occupies most of the midline region of the diencephalon (Figures 5-1 and 5-2), and so its entire outline can be seen in a hemisected brain (see Figure 3-13). It often looks like a misshapen doughnut in casts or reconstructions of the ventricular system (Figure 5-1). The hole in the doughnut corresponds to the **interthalamic adhesion,** which crosses the ventricle in most human brains.

Anteriorly the third ventricle ends at the **lamina terminalis,** the adult remnant of the rostral end of the neural tube. Much of the medial surface of the thalamus and hypothalamus forms the wall of the third ventricle, and part of the hypothalamus forms its floor. It has a thin, membranous roof containing choroid plexus (discussed in the next section). At the posterior end of the mammillary bodies, the third ventricle narrows fairly abruptly to become the **cerebral aqueduct (aqueduct of Sylvius),** which traverses the midbrain. The interventricular foramen, in the anterior part of each wall of the third ventricle, is an important radiological landmark because its location can be visualized by several different methods and it bears a known anatomical relationship to a number of deep structures.

An outline of the third ventricle reveals four protrusions, called **recesses** (Figure 5-1), corresponding to structures that have evaginated from the diencephalon. Inferiorly the **optic recess** lies in front of the optic chiasm at the base of the lamina terminalis; the **infundibular recess** lies just behind the chiasm. Superiorly the **pineal recess** invades the stalk of the pineal gland, and the **suprapineal recess** lies just anterior to this stalk.

The Fourth Ventricle Communicates With Subarachnoid Cisterns

The fourth ventricle is sandwiched between the cerebellum posteriorly and the pons and rostral medulla anteriorly (Figure 5-2). It is shaped like a tent with a doubly peaked roof, the peaks protruding into the cerebellum. The floor is relatively flat, and because it narrows rostrally into the aqueduct and caudally into the central canal, it is somewhat diamond-shaped (see Figure 11-3, *A*). For this reason, the floor is sometimes referred to as the **rhomboid fossa.** At the location where the lateral point of the diamond would be expected, the entire ventricle becomes a narrow tube that proceeds anteriorly and curves around the brainstem, ending adjacent to the flocculus of the cerebellum. This tubular prolongation is the **lateral recess** of the fourth ventricle (Figure 5-1). The portion of the roof of the ventricle rostral to the peak is the **superior medullary velum,** and the portion caudal to the peak is the **inferior medullary velum.** The superior medullary velum is a thin layer of white matter related to the cerebellum, whereas the inferior medullary velum is a membrane containing choroid plexus, similar to the roof of the third ventricle.

The lateral and third ventricles are nearly-closed cavities, communicating only with other parts of the ventricular system. In contrast, there are three apertures in the fourth ventricle through which the ventricular system communicates freely with subarachnoid space. These are the unpaired **median aperture** (or **foramen of Magendie**) and the two **lateral apertures** (or **foramina of Luschka**) of the fourth ventricle (Figures 5-9 and 5-10). The median aperture is simply a hole in the inferior medullary velum (Figure 5-4); it is as though the caudal end of the membrane, where it should have closed off the ventricle at its junction with the central canal, had instead been lifted up and attached to the inferior surface of the cerebellar vermis. The result is a funnel-shaped opening from the subarachnoid space (the cerebellomedullary cistern, or cisterna magna) into the ventricle. The inferior medullary velum also covers the lateral recess, and at the end of each recess is another opening in the velum, the lateral aperture.

The Ventricles Contain Only a Fraction of the CSF

The ventricles are both smaller and more variable in size than one might expect. Although there is an average total of approximately 130 ml of CSF within and around the brain and spinal cord, only about 25 ml of this fluid is contained within the ventricles. The rest occupies subarachnoid space. The third and fourth ventricles together have a volume of only about 2 ml, and the volumes of the aqueduct and central canal are negligible, so the lateral ventricles contain nearly all the ventricular CSF. The total volume of 25 ml is only an average figure, and the ventricles of some apparently normal brains have been found to have total volumes of less than 10 ml or more than 50 ml (however, volumes greater than 30 ml are usually considered suspicious).

CHOROID PLEXUS IS THE SOURCE OF MOST CSF

All four ventricles contain strands of highly convoluted and vascular membranous material **(choroid plexus)** that secretes most of the CSF. The composition of choroid plexus can be appreciated by first considering, for example, the anatomy of the roof of the third ventricle (see Figures 2-18 and 5-4). This roof is simply a layer of ependymal cells over-

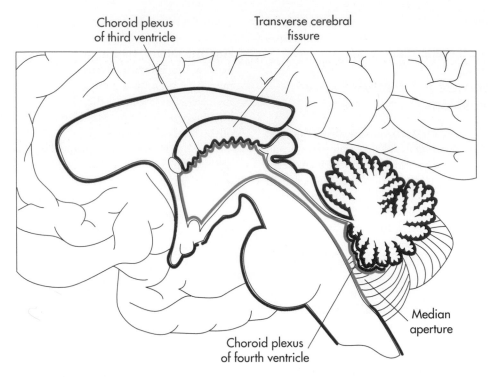

Choroid plexus
of third ventricle

Transverse cerebral
fissure

Median
aperture

Choroid plexus
of fourth ventricle

FIGURE 5-4
Disposition of the pia mater and ependyma in and around the third and fourth ventricles. Edges of the pia mater and ependymal lining that would have been cut during hemisection are indicated as colored lines. Areas where pia and ependyma are directly applied to one another form part of the choroid plexus.

laid by a layer of pia. As in all other locations, the pial layer also faces subarachnoid space, where the brain's blood supply is located. At certain locations this pia-ependyma complex invaginates into the ventricle with a collection of arterioles, venules, and capillaries (Figure 5-5). Here the ependymal layer appears as cuboidal epithelium **(choroid epithelium)** and functions as a secretory epithelium; the whole ependyma-pia-capillary complex is the choroid plexus. There is a long, continuous band of choroid plexus reflecting the original C-shaped course of each lateral ventricle, extending from near the tip of the inferior horn, through the body of the ventricle, and reaching the interventricular foramen (Figures 5-3 and 5-6). There is no choroid plexus in the anterior or posterior horn. The plexus is enlarged in the region of the atrium, and here it is called the **glomus** (Latin for "ball of thread"). Choroid plexus tends to become calcified with age, and the glomus can often be seen in x-ray studies (Figure 5-14, *D*). The choroid plexus of each lateral ventricle grows through the interventricular foramen, forming part of its posterior wall, and becomes one of the two narrow strands of choroid plexus in the roof of the third ventricle (Figure 5-6). It does not continue through the aqueduct, which is completely surrounded by neural tissue.

The choroid plexus of the fourth ventricle is formed from a similar invagination of the inferior medullary velum into the caudal half of the ventricle. It is T-shaped, with the vertical part of the T consisting of two adjacent longitudinal strands of plexus. These frequently extend as far as the median aperture, where they would be directly exposed to subarachnoid space (Figure 5-4). The transverse portion of the T consists of one strand of plexus, which extends into each lateral recess. Each end reaches a lateral aperture, where a small tuft of choroid plexus generally protrudes through the aperture and is exposed directly to subarachnoid space.

Because one side of pia mater always faces subarachnoid space, choroid plexus must always be adjacent to subarachnoid space on its pial side and to intraventricular space on its choroid epithelial side. Although this may seem contrary to the plexus's apparent location deep within each cerebral hemisphere (Figure 5-3), it can be easily demonstrated in coronal sections (Figure 5-7). The location of the invagination of choroid plexus into the lateral ventricle is called the **choroid fissure.** The choroid fissure is a C-shaped slit of subarachnoid space that accompanies the fornix system of fibers from the inferior horn to the interventricular foramen. By the same reasoning, the space above the roof of the third ventricle, which continues laterally into the choroid fissure, is also subarachnoid space (Figures 5-4 and 5-7). This is the **transverse cerebral fissure,** a long finger of subarachnoid space trapped in the middle of the cerebrum by the growth of the cerebral hemispheres posteriorly over the diencephalon and brainstem. The transverse cerebral fissure continues posteriorly into the superior cistern.

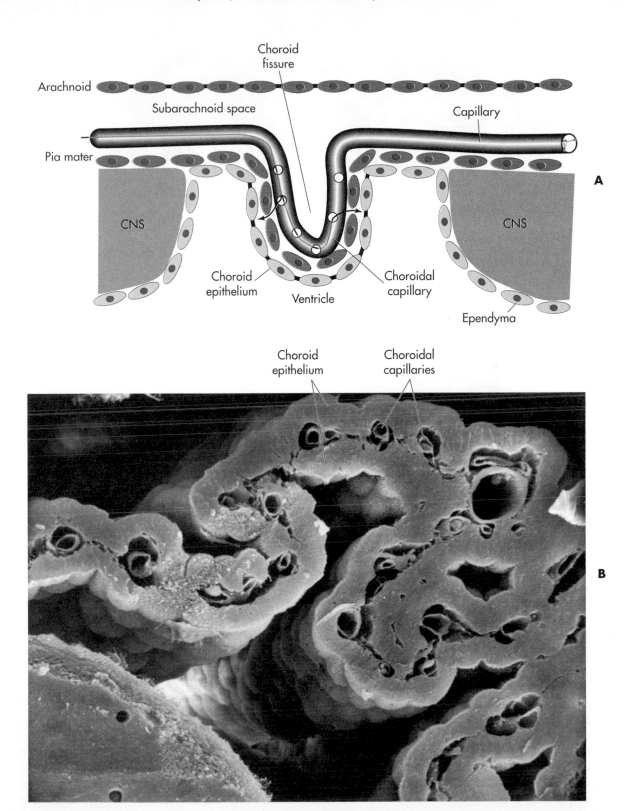

FIGURE 5-5
A, Composition of choroid plexus. Fenestrations are shown in the choroidal segment of a capillary as opposed to those of ordinary cerebral capillaries, indicating that substances can escape from blood into the choroid plexus. However, they are stopped by arrays of tight junctions (represented here as dark bars) between choroid epithelial cells. **B,** Scanning electron micrograph of a freeze-fractured preparation of choroid plexus. Note that choroid epithelium almost completely surrounds the choroidal capillaries, being separated from the capillaries only by attenuated pial elements. (**B** from Kessel RG, Kardon RH: *Tissues and organs: a text–atlas of scanning electron microscopy,* New York, WH Freeman & Co. Copyright 1979.)

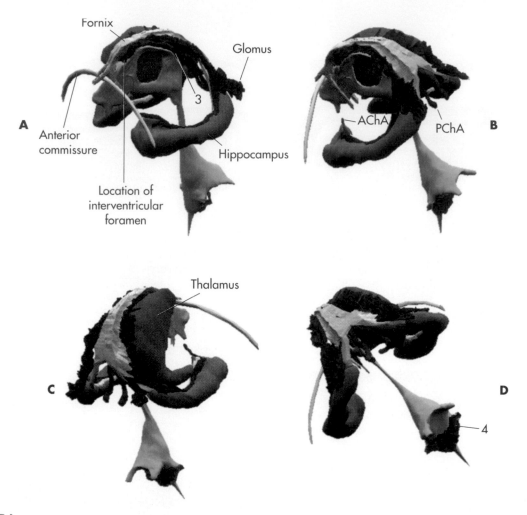

FIGURE 5-6

Three-dimensional reconstruction showing the location of choroid plexus, seen from the left and front **(A)**, the left and rear **(B)**, right and rear **(C)**, and obliquely from above and behind **(D)**. The cerebral hemispheres, lateral ventricles, and left thalamus were removed for clarity. A C-shaped strand of choroid plexus curves around with the medial wall of the inferior horn and body of each lateral ventricle, forms part of the wall of the interventricular foramen, and continues into the roof of the third ventricle (3). Separate strands of choroid plexus invaginate the roof of the fourth ventricle (4). The arterial supply of cerebral choroid plexus, as described further in Chapter 6, is provided mainly by the anterior and posterior choroidal arteries (AChA, PChA).

The Ependymal Lining of Choroid Plexus Is Specialized as a Secretory Epithelium

Choroid plexus is functionally a three-layered membrane between blood and CSF (Figure 5-8). The first layer is the endothelial wall of the choroidal capillary. This wall is fenestrated, allowing easy movement of substances out of the capillary (in contrast to capillary walls elsewhere in the brain, which, as discussed in Chapter 6, are tightly sealed). The second layer, consisting of scattered pial cells and some collagen, is very incomplete. The third layer, derived from the same layer of cells that forms the ependymal lining of the ventricles, is the choroid epithelium. The choroid epithelial cells look as though they are specialized for secretion because they have many basal infoldings, numerous microvilli on the side facing

the CSF, and abundant mitochondria. In addition, adjacent cells are connected to one another by arrays of tight junctions that occlude the extracellular space around them. As in the case of the arachnoid barrier layer discussed in Chapter 4, these junctions help to limit the movement of substances across the choroid epithelium; some ions are able to diffuse across these tight junctions, but peptides and other larger molecules are impeded.

The surface area of the choroid plexus is increased not only by the folding of individual cell membranes into microvilli but also by the macroscopic folding of the choroid plexus itself into numerous fronds and villi (Figure 5-7). This folding is so extensive that the total surface area of the human choroid plexus, neglecting the contribution of

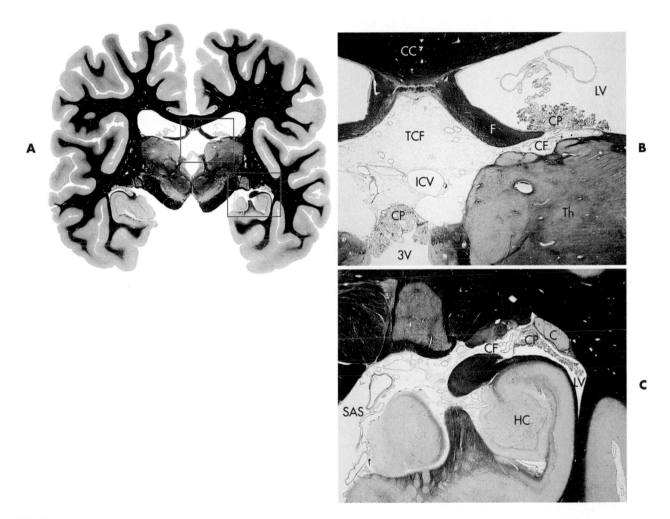

FIGURE 5-7
Coronal sections at different magnifications demonstrating the relationship of choroid plexus to subarachnoid space on one side and ventricular space on the other. The areas outlined in **A** are enlarged in **B** and **C.** In **B,** choroid plexus *(CP)* separates the subarachnoid space of the transverse cerebral fissure *(TCF)* from the intraventricular spaces of the lateral *(LV)* and third ventricles *(3V).* Similarly, in **C** choroid plexus *(CP)* separates subarachnoid space *(SAS)* adjacent to the interpeduncular cistern from the intraventricular space of the inferior horn of the lateral ventricle *(LV).* The site of invagination of the choroid plexus in the medial wall of the lateral ventricle is the choroid fissure *(CF). C,* Tail of the caudate nucleus; *CC,* corpus callosum; *F,* fornix; *HC,* hippocampus; *ICV,* internal cerebral vein (see Chapter 6); *Th,* thalamus. (**A** from Nolte J, Angevine JB Jr: *The human brain in photographs and diagrams,* St. Louis, 1995, Mosby.)

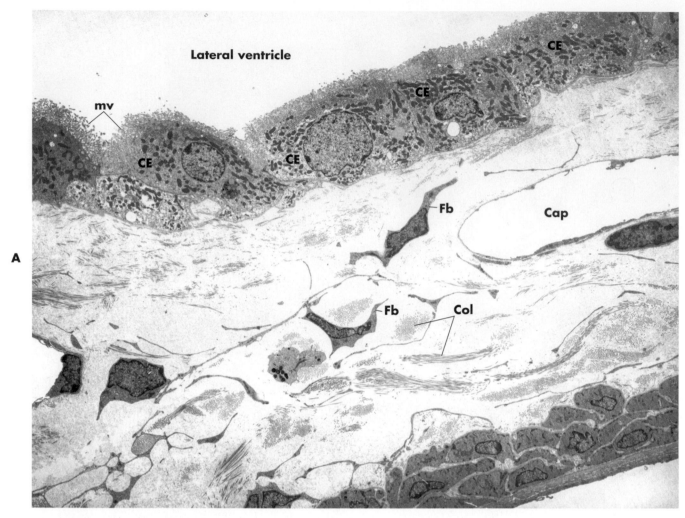

FIGURE 5-8
Electron micrographs of choroid plexus. **A,** Low magnification view showing the single layer of choroid epithelial cells *(CE),* covered with microvilli *(mv)* that protrude into the ventricle. Near the basal surfaces of the choroid epithelial cells are thin-walled, fenestrated capillaries *(Cap)* embedded in a loose connective tissue matrix *(Col,* collagen; *Fb,* fibroblast) derived from the pia mater.

the microvilli, is more than 200 cm², or about two thirds of the total ventricular surface area.

CSF IS A SECRETION OF THE CHOROID PLEXUS

CSF is a clear, colorless liquid, low in cells and proteins, but generally similar to plasma in its ionic composition. For this reason, it was considered for some time to be an ultrafiltrate of blood. However, careful analysis of the composition of CSF reveals that its content of various ions differs from that of plasma in a way that is not consistent with its being an ultrafiltrate. For example, compared with plasma, CSF contains an excess of magnesium and chloride ions and a deficiency of potassium and calcium ions. Furthermore, these concentrations are maintained at very stable levels in the face of changes in plasma concentra-

tions—a constancy that would not be expected if CSF were an ultrafiltrate.★ Finally, the formation of new CSF is depressed by certain metabolic inhibitors, as would be expected if it were formed by an active, energy-requiring process. From these and other observations, it is clear that CSF is an actively secreted product whose composition is dictated by specific transport mechanisms.

Most of the CSF is produced within the ventricles by their choroid plexuses. Production of fluid by the choroid plexus was demonstrated rather directly by the neurosurgeon Cushing early in the twentieth century. During procedures in which it was necessary to open

---

★Because the composition of CSF is so constant in health, changes in its composition can be very helpful in diagnosing neurological disease. For example, meningitis can be either viral or bacterial in origin. In the latter case, the glucose concentration in the CSF is markedly reduced (the bacteria eat the glucose), and the protein concentration is elevated. In viral meningitis, glucose is normal and protein slightly elevated or normal.

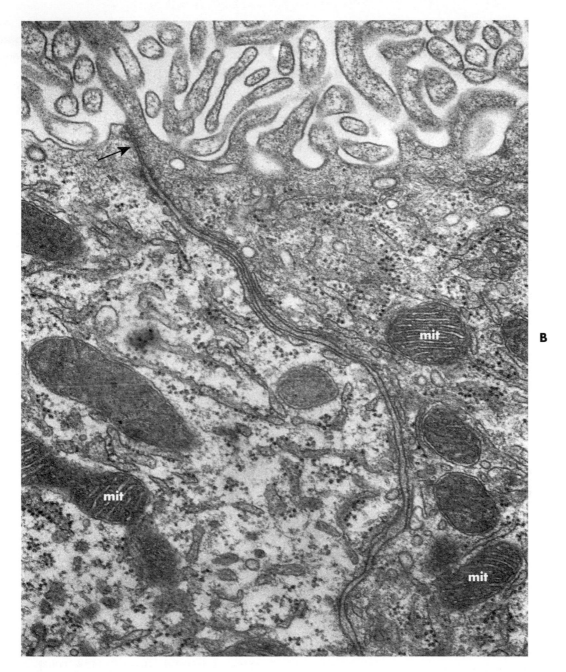

FIGURE 5-8—cont'd
B, Higher-magnification view of two adjacent choroid epithelial cells, joined near their ventricular surfaces by a tight junction (*arrow*). Abundant mitochondria (*mit*) subserve the energy requirements of CSF secretion. (**A** from Peters A, Palay SL, Webster H deF: *The fine structure of the nervous system: neurons and their supporting cells,* ed 3, New York, 1991, Oxford University Press. **B** from Pannese E: *Neurocytology: fine structure of neurons, nerve processes, and neuroglial cells,* New York, 1994, Thieme Medical Publishers, Inc.)

and drain a lateral ventricle, he noted that fluid could be seen accumulating on the surface of the choroid plexus; if he put a small silver clip on the artery supplying the choroid plexus, the fluid stopped appearing. A basically similar procedure has been used since then to study the composition of newly formed CSF: a micropipette in contact with oil-covered choroid plexus can collect the fluid as it is formed. Chemical analysis has shown that it is identical in composition to bulk CSF in normal ventricles.

CSF is formed by filtration of blood through the fenestrations of the choroidal capillaries, followed by the active transport of substances (particularly sodium ions) across the choroid epithelium into the ventricle. Water then flows passively across the epithelium to maintain osmotic balance. The barrier properties of the choroid epithelium prevent substances from diffusing across it in an uncontrolled manner. The total process is actually more complicated than this and involves a balance between active transport and some passive diffusion of ions and other substances either through or between the choroid epithelial cells. It is also known that some substances are transported in the reverse direction (i.e., from CSF to blood) and that there are specific transporters for certain nutrients, vitamins, and other substances.

Although CSF is secreted primarily by choroid plexus, there is also evidence that this is not its only source. This has been shown most directly in monkeys from whose lateral ventricles all the choroid plexus had been removed; these ventricles still produced substantial quantities of CSF, although less than normal. The source of this extrachoroidal CSF is generally considered to be fluid movement from CNS capillaries into the parenchyma of the brain, and from there across the ependymal lining into the ventricle. The proportion of CSF normally arising from this source is not known accurately, but most researchers agree that well over half is made by the choroid plexus.

The rate of formation of new CSF (an average of about 350 μl/minute—half a liter/day—in humans) is relatively constant and little affected by systemic blood pressure or intraventricular pressure. This means that the total volume of CSF is renewed more than three times per day.

One way this rate of formation can be modified is by the autonomic nervous system. Both sympathetic and parasympathetic fibers end not only on choroidal blood vessels, but also near the bases of the choroid epithelial cells. Experimental activation of these fibers can cause substantial changes in CSF production, mainly through direct effects on the secretory rate of the choroid epithelial cells. Stimulating the sympathetic fibers, for example, causes a reduction of about 30% in the rate of CSF production. Little is known, however, about the significance of this autonomic innervation under ordinary circumstances.

CSF Circulates Through and Around the CNS, Eventually Reaching the Venous System

If the CSF is turned over several times per day, it must circulate from its site of formation to a site of removal. We have already discussed all the elements of the system involved (Figures 5-9 and 5-10): CSF formed in the lateral ventricles passes through the interventricular foramina into the third ventricle, from there through the cerebral aqueduct into the fourth ventricle, and then through the median and lateral apertures into cisterna magna and the pontine cistern. From these basal cisterns, the fluid slowly moves through the tentorial notch, up over the cerebral hemispheres, through the arachnoid villi, and into the superior sagittal sinus. The flow should not be thought of as slow and steady because arterial pulsations cause a constant ebb and flow, with a small net movement toward the

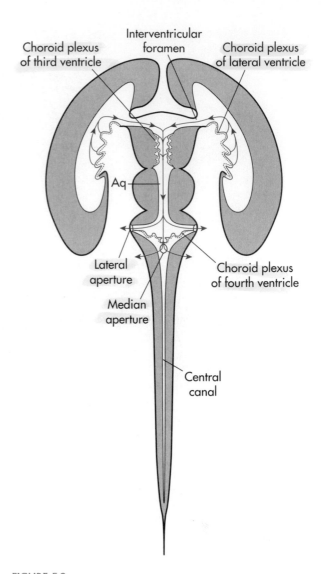

FIGURE 5-9
Path followed by CSF through the ventricles. *Aq,* Cerebral aqueduct. [Redrawn from Hamilton WJ, editor: *Textbook of human anatomy,* ed 2, St. Louis, 1976, Mosby.]

superior sagittal sinus with each heartbeat. As would be expected from the rate of CSF formation, it takes several hours for new CSF to complete the journey.

In addition to this basic pattern of circulation, some CSF moves from the cisterns around the fourth ventricle into the subarachnoid space around the spinal cord. It slowly makes its way caudally to the lumbar cistern, and then some of it slowly makes its way back rostrally. Along the way, most of this fluid is returned to the venous system through arachnoid villi that are found in the dural sleeves accompanying spinal nerve roots.

CSF Has Multiple Functions

The CSF in the subarachnoid space plays a mechanically supportive role because of the buoyant effect discussed previously. In addition, CSF serves as part of a

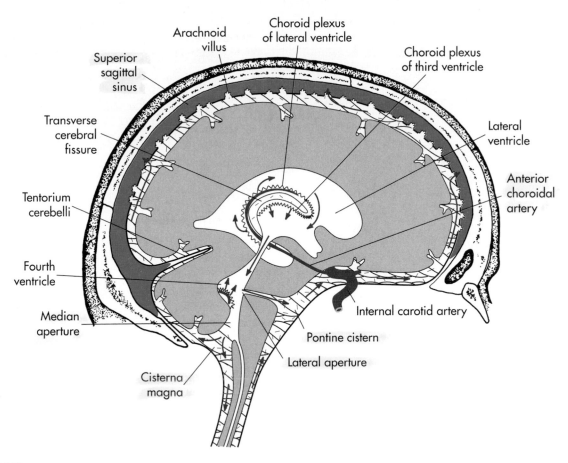

FIGURE 5-10

Path of circulation of CSF from its formation in the ventricles to its absorption into the superior sagittal sinus. (Redrawn from Hamilton WJ, editor: *Textbook of human anatomy,* ed 2, St. Louis, 1976, Mosby.)

spatial buffering system necessitated by the fact that the brain lives inside a rigid skull: something inside the skull can enlarge only if something else leaves. For example, the heart pumps arterial blood into the brain with each beat. Space is made for this arterial blood partly by venous blood leaving and partly by CSF leaving, either through the arachnoid villi or into spinal subarachnoid space. Hence a small volume of CSF sloshes back and forth through the foramen magnum with each heartbeat. Similarly, but over a longer time scale, an expanding mass such as a tumor can be accommodated to some extent by decreased CSF volume.

It seems apparent, however, that an actively secreted, constantly renewed fluid with a closely regulated composition must have other functions as well. Most of the functions that have been suggested involve the regulation of the extracellular environment of neurons. This could happen in either or both of two ways. First, the CSF is in free communication with the extracellular fluid of the brain, so secretion of controlled CSF by the choroid plexus will secondarily control, to some extent, the composition of this extracellular fluid. Second, the CSF system probably exerts a reverse sort of control by acting as a "sink" for substances produced by the brain, which are then selec-

tively absorbed from CSF by the choroid plexus or nonselectively removed by flow through arachnoid villi. It is also likely that the CSF is a route for the spread of neuroactive hormones through the nervous system.

IMAGING TECHNIQUES ALLOW BOTH CNS AND CSF TO BE VISUALIZED*

The neurological examination of a patient can often reveal a great deal about any underlying pathology, particularly its probable anatomical location. However, much additional information, sometimes critically important, can be provided in images of the CNS or its surroundings. Until fairly recently, the CNS of live, unopened people could not be imaged at all, and it was necessary to make images of things within or around the brain and infer the shape of the brain from these images.

Conventional skull x-ray studies, the first clinical imaging modality used to provide indirect information about the brain, work by directing x-rays through a patient's

---

*Parts of this discussion were adapted from Nolte J, Angevine JB Jr: *The human brain in photographs and diagrams,* St. Louis, 1995, Mosby.

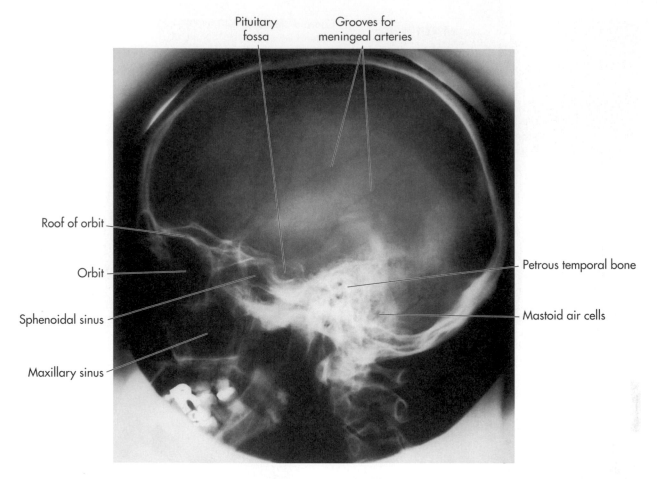

Pituitary fossa

Grooves for meningeal arteries

Roof of orbit

Orbit

Sphenoidal sinus

Maxillary sinus

Petrous temporal bone

Mastoid air cells

FIGURE 5-11
Normal skull x-ray image (67-year-old man). The CNS cannot be distinguished, and the x-ray densities of multiple spatially separated structures (e.g., sella turcica, both temporal bones) are collapsed onto one plane. (Courtesy Dr. Raymond F. Carmody, Department of Radiology, The University of Arizona College of Medicine.)

head and using photographic film to record what comes out the other side; areas that are particularly x-ray dense (e.g., temporal bones) block a lot of transmission and are recorded as light areas on the film. This procedure has two major disadvantages: (1) it can only record differences between things that vary fairly substantially in x-ray density (e.g., bone vs. brain vs. air), so different parts of the brain cannot be distinguished from each other; (2) all of the x-ray density between the source and the film gets "collapsed" into a single plane (Figure 5-11). Both of these problems have been overcome by the tomographic techniques described a little later.

One of the few ways to get hints about the shape of the brain using skull x-rays is to introduce air into the subarachnoid space or ventricles. (Another is to record the configuration of intracranial arteries and veins, as described in Chapter 6.) Air is much less dense to x-ray beams than is CSF, so the shape of air-filled ventricles can be recorded by x-ray photography in a procedure called **pneumoencephalography** (Figure 5-12). The shape of the ventricles can yield information not only about the ventricles themselves (e.g., the presence and location of

hydrocephalus, as discussed a little later) but also about masses pushing against the brain and distorting the ventricles. Pneumoencephalography is painful and dangerous, and fortunately has been replaced by more recent imaging techniques.

Tomography Produces Images of Two-Dimensional "Slices"

The Greek word *tomos* means "slice" (as in a microtome used to cut brain sections), and **tomography** means "constructing pictures of slices." There are some photographic tricks that can be used to get one plane of someone's skull in better focus than the rest of the skull—this is what tomography originally referred to—but the use of computers to reconstruct slices using signals coming from or through the brain has revolutionized neuroradiology. Computed tomography can be based on any measurable parameter that varies in different parts of the brain.

The method of computation is beyond the scope of this book, but its essence can be appreciated from the following example. If an x-ray source and an x-ray de-

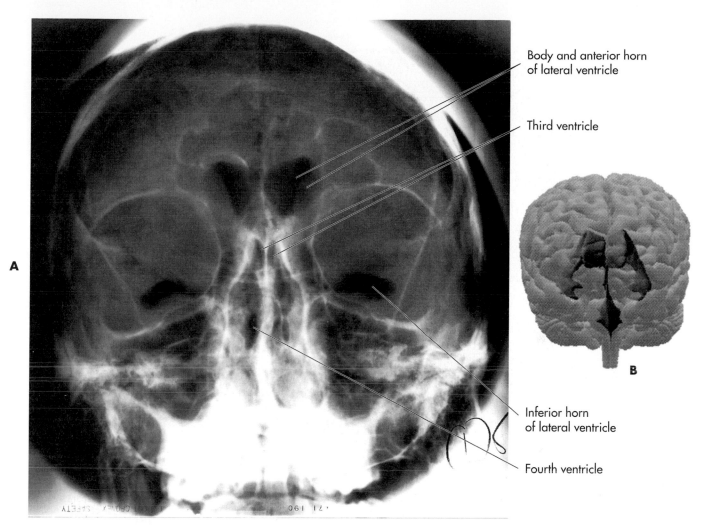

Body and anterior horn
of lateral ventricle

Third ventricle

Inferior horn
of lateral ventricle

Fourth ventricle

FIGURE 5-12

A, Normal pneumoencephalogram, anterior-posterior view (as though you were looking into the patient's face). The body and inferior horn of each lateral ventricle are particularly dark because they are viewed approximately end-on, so that the x-rays traverse a relatively long path through air. **B,** Three-dimensional reconstruction of the ventricular system inside a translucent CNS, seen in a similar orientation. (**A** provided by Dr. John Stears, University of Colorado Health Sciences Center.)

tector were coupled together and rotated around some-one's head at ear level, the x-ray beam would be attenuated by varying amounts as the source/detector pair rotated. For example, the beam would be attenuated a lot when it passed through the temporal bones, less when it was oriented at other angles. The only x-ray density that would be present at *every* angle would be the density of the spot inside the head where all the beams intersected (Figure 5-13); this would be a constant, to which a varying density that depended on x-ray angle is added. By repeating this procedure with many different centers of rotation and, in essence, subtracting the variable density each time, it is possible to compute the density at each point in the plane of rotation.

There are multiple techniques that produce reconstructed "slices" using some variant of this calculation. The parameter mapped, as described further in this and the next chapter, can be x-ray density or the concentration of water or a variety of other substances.

CT Produces Maps of X-Ray Density

X-ray computed tomography (usually referred to simply as **CT**) is based on variations in x-ray density at different points in the head or body, as in the example just described. CT was the first of the new wave of techniques that have overcome the limitations referred to earlier: it can produce a picture of brain itself, and it can do so in slices (rather than collapsing the whole brain into a single plane). CSF, gray matter, white matter, and bone can all be distinguished from each other (Figure 5-14). Because CT provides images based on x-ray density, structures such as bone that attenuate x-rays appear light; structures such as air and CSF that do not attenuate x-rays as much appear darker; blood and brain are intermediate. The spatial reso-

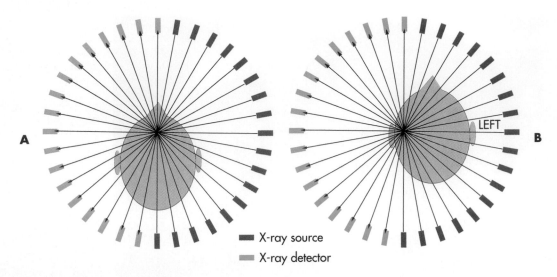

FIGURE 5-13
Principle of computed tomography. The only x-ray density encountered by *all* the beams in **A** is that at their point of intersection. Moving the sources and detectors (**B**) results in a change in the common density encountered by all beams. (By convention, images are constructed as though you were looking from below the patient's head, so the patient's left side is on the right side of the image.)

lution of CT is not as good as that of skull x-rays, but for most purposes its advantages far outweigh this limitation.

The range of x-ray densities in someone's head is much greater than can be displayed in a single gray-scale image,★ so if the contrast "window" of the CT apparatus is set to display CSF/gray matter/white matter differences, bone will be solid white with little detail visible. The window can be reset to emphasize bone detail, turning soft tissue a more or less uniform dark gray (Figure 5-15; see also Figure 4-15, *A*). Because x-ray CT produces maps of x-ray density, radiopaque dyes (called *contrast agents*) can be injected intravenously and the portions of blood vessels in any given slice can be visualized (see Figure 6-11, *A*).

MRI Produces Maps of Water Concentration

Because X-ray computed tomography reconstructs images based on spatial variations in x-ray density, the relatively small density differences between gray and white matter limit its ability to differentiate between different areas of the brain. In addition, the much greater x-ray density of bone can overwhelm these small gray-white differ-

ences and cause artifacts in bony areas such as the posterior fossa (Figure 5-14, *B*).

Magnetic resonance imaging (MRI) overcomes these problems by being exquisitely sensitive to spatial variations in the concentration and physicochemical situation of particular atomic nuclei (almost always hydrogen nuclei). Nuclei with an odd number of protons or neutrons, such as hydrogen nuclei, behave like tiny magnets. Imposing a powerful magnetic field on something containing these nuclei (such as someone's head) causes a net tendency for the nuclei to align themselves with the external field. Once so aligned, the nuclei preferentially absorb and then emit electromagnetic energy at a particular frequency (the resonant frequency for that nucleus in that situation). Hence applying radiofrequency pulses to a subject in a strong, static magnetic field, and then measuring the spatial distributions of various time constants with which the absorbed energy is re-emitted, can provide the data for construction of extraordinarily detailed images (Figure 5-16) based on different tissue properties. In addition, images can be reconstructed not only in approximately horizontal planes similar to those used for CT but also in coronal and parasagittal planes (Figure 5-17).

Two time constants—T1 and T2—are important in clinical MRI (Figure 5-18). T1 is the time constant with which nuclei return to alignment with the static field. T2 is the time constant with which nuclei, all perturbed at the same time by radiofrequency pulses, lose alignment with each other. T1- and T2-weighted images emphasize different tissue parameters in different ways. For example, CSF is dark in T1 images and light in T2 images; white matter is light in T1, dark in T2. Both types of image can be used to demonstrate various kinds of intracranial pathology, often in ways that could not be accomplished with x-ray CT (Figures 5-19 and 20).

★Our visual system can only distinguish a few hundred levels of gray between the parts of an image that are completely black and those that are completely white. The gray scale in printed images, for example, uses 256 levels of gray, so two things that differ in brightness by less than about 0.4% will look the same. The difference in x-ray density between gray matter and white matter accounts for less than 0.2% of the range from air to dense bone; even the difference between brain and CSF accounts for less than 1%. Hence CT images are constructed so that the available levels of gray are devoted to a restricted range of the x-ray densities present. In typical images, gray matter, white matter, and CSF are the center of attention; CSF and everything significantly less dense (e.g., fat, air) appears black, everything significantly more dense than blood (e.g., all kinds of bone) appears white.

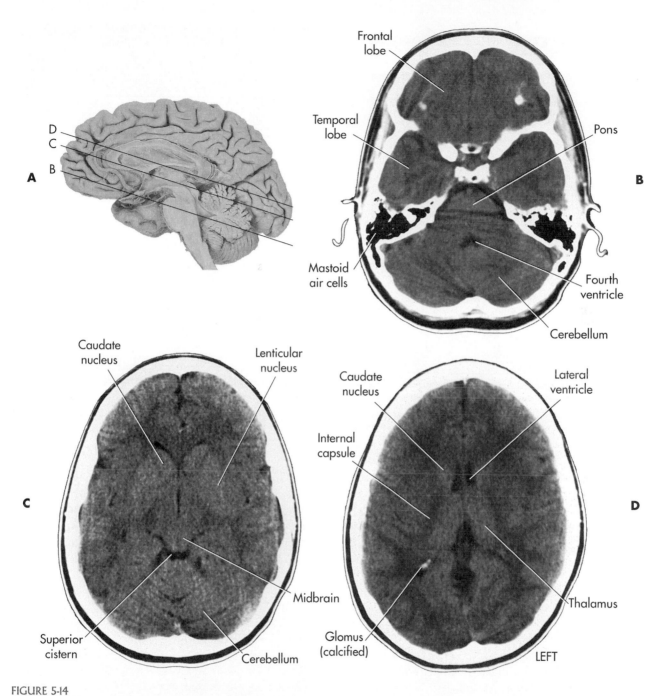

FIGURE 5-14
Examples of CT scans. CSF is dark in these scans and fills the ventricular system, subarachnoid cisterns, and cerebral sulci around the edge of the brain. Bone is white, air is black, and gray matter is slightly less gray than white matter. **A,** Planes of section produced by the computer and displayed as **B, C,** and **D.** The streaks cutting across the brainstem and cerebellum in **B** are artifacts reflecting the dense bone surrounding these regions. [From Nolte J, Angevine JB Jr: *The human brain in photographs and diagrams*, St. Louis, 1995, Mosby.]

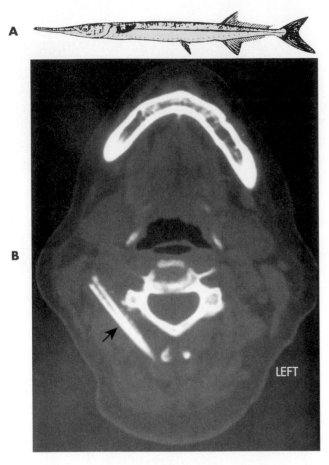

A

B

LEFT

FIGURE 5-15
Imaging of calcified objects using CT. A 53-year-old woman was
swimming in the Red Sea when a needlefish (*Tylosorus crocodilus*, **A**)
leaped from the water about 20 m away, flew through the air, and
struck her on the neck. A neck x-ray at the time revealed nothing
abnormal, so her wound was dressed and she was released. She had
neck pain of increasing intensity, and a bone-window CT of her
neck (**B**) a month later revealed the calcified beak of the needlefish
(arrow) adjacent to the transverse process of the C4 vertebra. The
beak was removed successfully. (From Bendet E et al: Penetrating cervical injury caused by a needlefish, *Ann Otol Rhinol Laryngol* 104:248,
1995.)

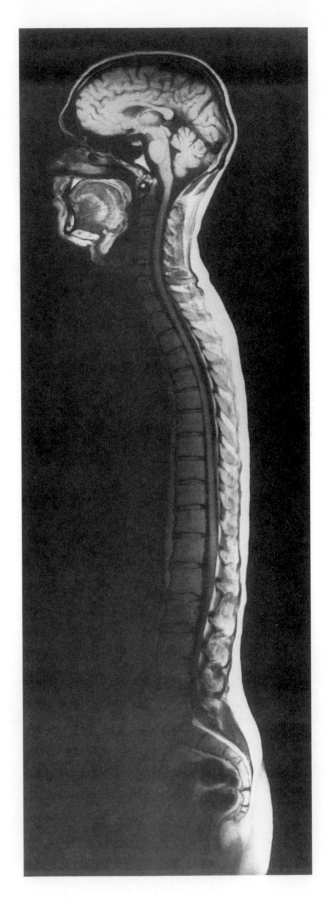

FIGURE 5-16
Midsagittal MRI, demonstrating the extraordinary anatomical detail
possible with this technique. So much can be seen that the figure was
left unlabeled (a difficult task for an anatomist). I feared that once I
started, the lines and arrows would multiply uncontrollably and obscure the anatomy. (Courtesy Philips Medical Systems.)

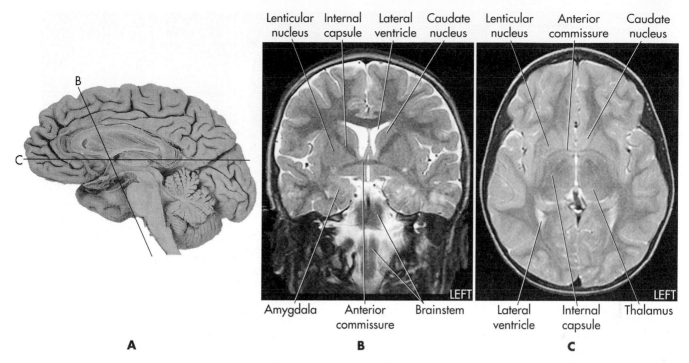

Lenticular nucleus   Internal capsule   Lateral ventricle   Caudate nucleus   Lenticular nucleus   Anterior commissure   Caudate nucleus

Amygdala   Anterior commissure   Brainstem   Lateral ventricle   Internal capsule   Thalamus

A   B   C

FIGURE 5-17

Examples of MR images (T2 weighted). **A,** Planes of section produced by the computer and displayed as **B** and **C.** Magnetic resonance images can be produced not only in horizontal planes, but also in coronal and parasagittal planes. By convention, coronal images are constructed as though you were looking at the patient's face, so the patient's left side is on the right side of the image. [Modified from Nolte J, Angevine JB Jr: *The human brain in photographs and diagrams,* St. Louis, 1995, Mosby.]

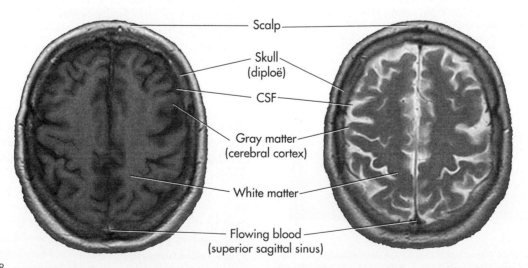

Scalp

Skull (diploë)

CSF

Gray matter (cerebral cortex)

White matter

Flowing blood (superior sagittal sinus)

FIGURE 5-18

T1-weighted and T2-weighted MR images (left and right, respectively). In T1-weighted images, white matter is lighter than gray matter, and CSF is dark. Conversely, in T2-weighted images, white matter is darker than gray matter, and CSF is bright and prominent. In both, air and dense bone, which contain relatively few hydrogen nuclei, are dark. (The part of the skull indicated in these images is the spongy, marrow-containing diploic layer.) The appearance of flowing blood depends on a number of technical parameters, but in many instances (such as the T2-weighted image on the right) perturbed nuclei have left the area before the imaging measurement is made, so the blood vessel appears dark, as though no hydrogen nuclei were present. [From Nolte J, Angevine JB Jr: *The human brain in photographs and diagrams,* St. Louis, 1995, Mosby.]

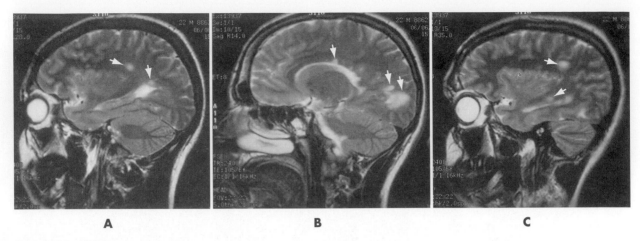

FIGURE 5-19
Multiple sclerosis demonstrated by MRI. The hallmark of multiple sclerosis is multiple areas of demyelination, separated in space and typically in time. The demyelinated plaques appear as areas of increased signal intensity *(arrows)* in T2-weighted magnetic resonance images, seen in the left hemisphere **(A)**, midline **(B)**, and right hemisphere **(C)** of this 22-year-old man. (Courtesy Dr. Raymond F. Carmody, Department of Radiology, The University of Arizona College of Medicine.)

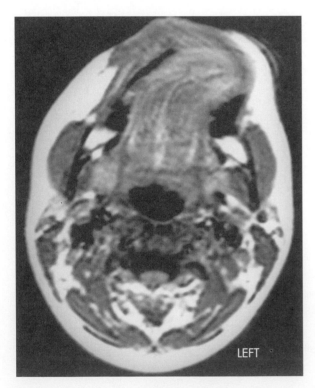

FIGURE 5-20
An unusual case of linguobuccal dislocation demonstrated by MRI. In this case, "a 48-year-old, 160-pound white man was admitted to our hospital for evaluation of a distended left cheek and pain in his neck. The man reported that while dining, his head became entangled in the purse strap of a female diner walking behind his chair. The force of the strap pulled his head backward, overturning the chair, and forcing his head against the bowling bag belonging to another diner. He was dragged a distance of 14 ft before the woman realized she had snared him. In the emergency room, a protrusion of the left cheek was noted and evaluated with a 0.5-T magnetic resonance (MR) scanner . . . [which] revealed the patient's tongue in his cheek." (From IM Fasesjas, Jess Kidden: A linguobuccal dislocation studied with MR, *AJNR Am J Neuroradiol* 16:777, 1995.)

DISRUPTION OF CSF CIRCULATION CAN CAUSE HYDROCEPHALUS

Because the rate of production of CSF is relatively independent of blood pressure and intraventricular pressure, the fluid will continue to be produced even if the path of its circulation is blocked or is otherwise abnormal. When this happens, CSF pressure rises and ultimately the ventricles expand at the expense of surrounding brain, creating a condition known as **hydrocephalus** (Figure 5-21). In principle, hydrocephalus can result from excess production of CSF, from blockage of CSF circulation, or from a deficiency in CSF reabsorption. All three types occur, but that caused by a blockage of circulation is by far the most common.

Tumors of the choroid plexus, called *papillomas,* are sometimes associated with hydrocephalus. In some of these cases, a much greater than normal production of CSF has been shown directly and is believed to be the cause of the hydrocephalus.

Circulation of CSF can be obstructed at any point in the pathway. A tumor can occlude one interventricular foramen (or both of them), in which case the lateral ventricle involved becomes hydrocephalic and the remainder of the ventricular system remains normal. Tumors of the pineal gland sometimes push down on the midbrain, squeeze the aqueduct shut, and cause hydrocephalus of the third ventricle and both lateral ventricles. In some congenital abnormalities, all three apertures of the fourth ventricle may either fail to develop or be occluded, resulting in hydrocephalus of the entire ventricular system. (Occlusion of only one or two of these apertures apparently has no effect.) Finally, circulation may be obstructed outside the ventricular system in subarachnoid space. For exam-

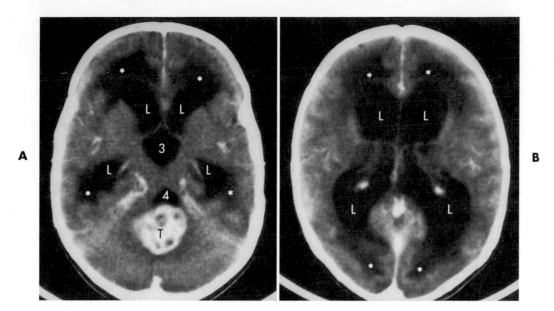

FIGURE 5-21

Hydrocephalus demonstrated by CT. **A** and **B,** A tumor (*T,* an ependymoma) in the fourth ventricle of this 2-year-old girl obstructed CSF outflow pathways and caused noncommunicating hydrocephalus involving the third (*3*), fourth (*4*), and lateral (*L*) ventricles. The increased intraventricular pressure also caused areas of edema (*) adjacent to the lateral ventricles. (Courtesy Dr. Raymond F. Carmody, Department of Radiology, The University of Arizona College of Medicine.)

ple, meningitis is sometimes followed by meningeal adhesions around the base of the brain that block the flow of CSF through the tentorial notch. (CSF passes from the fourth ventricle into the posterior fossa, so it must ordinarily pass through the tentorial notch before reaching the arachnoid villi of the superior sagittal sinus.) This too causes hydrocephalus of the entire ventricular system.

Persistent defects in the reabsorption of CSF are not common, but rare cases have been reported in which apparent congenital absence of arachnoid villi was associated with hydrocephalus. Also there are occasional reports that obstruction of the superior sagittal sinus can cause hydrocephalus, presumably because venous pressure becomes high enough to prevent CSF movement through the arachnoid villi.★

Clinically, hydrocephalus is divided into **communicating** and **noncommunicating** types, depending on whether both lateral ventricles are in communication with subarachnoid space. Thus blockage of flow through the tentorial notch would cause communicating hydrocephalus; stenosis of the aqueduct or occlusion of the apertures of the fourth ventricle would cause noncommunicating hydrocephalus. Note that in both situations the basic cause of hydrocephalus is the same: an obstruction in the circulation path of CSF. Terminology such as *communicating* and *noncommunicating* is just a partial specification of the location of the blockage.

Once diagnosed, many cases of hydrocephalus can be treated surgically by implanting a shunt that extends from the locus of increased pressure to sites such as the peritoneal cavity or the right atrium. The implanted catheter must contain a valve to prevent reverse flow. There were many early attempts to treat hydrocephalus by removing the choroid plexus, but they were generally unsuccessful, probably because of the continued extrachoroidal production of CSF.

SUGGESTED READINGS

Atlas SW (editor): *Magnetic resonance imaging of the brain and spine,* ed 2, Philadelphia, 1996, Lippincott-Raven.

Brightman MW, Reese TS: Junctions between intimately apposed cell membranes in the vertebrate brain, *J Cell Biol* 40:648, 1969. *An interesting paper that discusses, among other things, the barrier properties of the choroid epithelium.*

Bruni JE, DelBigio MR, Clattenburg RE: Ependyma: normal and pathological—a review of the literature, *Brain Res Rev* 9:1, 1985.

Bull JWD: The volume of the cerebral ventricles, *Neurol* 11:1, 1961.

Cushing H: *Studies in intracranial physiology and surgery,* London, 1926, Oxford University Press. *Contains the classic account of the direct observation of CSF forming on the surface of human choroid plexus.*

Cutler RWP et al: Formation and absorption of cerebrospinal fluid in man, *Brain* 91:707, 1968. *Direct measurement of the rate of formation of CSF in humans.*

Dandy WE: Experimental hydrocephalus, *Ann Surg* 70:129, 1919. *The classic description of the production of hydrocephalus by obstruction of an interventricular foramen, the cerebral aqueduct, or subarachnoid space around the base of the brain. It appears in the light of subsequent work that some of the experiments were technically flawed, but the conclusions are basically sound.*

★The fact that occlusion of the superior sagittal sinus is only rarely (if ever) accompanied by hydrocephalus has been taken as evidence that the arachnoid villi are not the sole route by which CSF can leave the subarachnoid space. Possible alternate routes include movement along the adventitia of blood vessels and the sheaths of cranial and spinal nerves

Davson H, Segal MB: *Physiology of the CSF and blood-brain barriers*, Boca Raton, 1996, CRC Press Inc.

De Rougemont J et al: Fluid formed by choroid plexus, *J Neurophysiol* 23:485, 1960. *Experiments in which droplets of CSF were collected, under oil, from the surface of the choroid plexus, and their composition analyzed.*

DiChiro G: Observations on the circulation of the cerebrospinal fluid, *Acta Radiol (Diagn)* 5:988, 1966. *Description of the time course and pattern of movement of tracer substances through subarachnoid space on their way toward the venous system.*

Dohrmann GJ: The choroid plexus: a historical review, *Brain Res* 18:197, 1970.

Dohrmann GJ, Bucy PC: Human choroid plexus: a light and electron microscopic study, *J Neurosurg* 33:506, 1970.

Eisenberg HM, McComb JG, Lorenzo AV: Cerebrospinal fluid overproduction and hydrocephalus associated with choroid plexus papilloma, *J Neurosurg* 40:381, 1974.

Fishman RA: *Cerebrospinal fluid in diseases of the nervous system*, ed 2, Philadelphia, 1992, WB Saunders.

Gudeman SK et al: Surgical removal of bilateral papillomas of the choroid plexus of the lateral ventricles with resolution of hydrocephalus, *J Neurosurg* 50:677, 1979.

Gutierrez Y, Friede RL, Kaliney WJ: Agenesis of arachnoid granulations and its relationship to communicating hydrocephalus, *J Neurosurg* 43:553, 1975.

Haaxma-Reiche H, Piers DO, Beekhuis H: Normal cerebrospinal fluid dynamics: a study with intraventricular injection of ^{111}In-DTPA in leukemia and lymphoma without meningeal involvement, *Arch Neurol* 46:997, 1989. *A discussion of the time course of tracer movement out of the ventricles and through subarachnoid space.*

Hewitt W: The median aperture of the fourth ventricle, *J Anat* 94:549, 1960.

Iwasaki S et al: Identification of pre- and postcentral gyri on CT and MR images on the basis of the medullary pattern of cerebral white matter, *Radiol* 179:207, 1991.

Kier EL: *The cerebral ventricles: a phylogenetic and ontogenetic study.* In Newton TH, Potts DG, editors: *Radiology of the skull and brain, vol 3: anatomy and pathology*, St. Louis, 1977, Mosby. *A long but fascinating and beautifully illustrated account.*

Lindvall M, Owman C: Autonomic nerves in the mammalian choroid plexus and their influence on the formation of cerebrospinal fluid, *J Cereb Blood Flow Metab* 1:245, 1981.

Lowhagen P, Johansson BB, Nordborg C: The nasal route of cerebrospinal fluid drainage in man: a light-microscope study, *Neuropath Applied Neurobiol* 20:543, 1994.

Matsumae M et al: Age-related changes in intracranial compartment volumes in normal adults assessed by magnetic resonance imaging, *J Neurosurg* 84:982, 1996. *Measurements of age-related and gender-related differences in brain volume, ventricular volume, and total CSF volume.*

Matsushima T, Rhoton AL Jr, Lenkey C: Microsurgery of the fourth ventricle, Part 1. Microsurgical anatomy, *Neurosurgery* 11:631, 1982. *Finely detailed and beautifully illustrated.*

McConnell H, Bianchine J, editors: *Cerebrospinal fluid in neurology and psychiatry*, London, 1994, Chapman and Hall.

McRae DL, Branch CL, Milner B: The occipital horns and cerebral dominance, *Neurol* 18:95, 1968.

Milhorat TH: Choroid plexus and cerebrospinal fluid production, *Sci* 166:1514, 1969. *An account of the continued production of CSF in the lateral ventricles of monkeys after removal of the choroid plexus.*

Nagata S, Rhoton AL Jr, Barry M: Microsurgical anatomy of the choroidal fissure, *Surg Neurol* 30:3, 1988.

Naidich TP, Valvanis AG, Kubik S: Anatomic relationships along the low-middle convexity: Part I—normal specimens and magnetic resonance imaging, *Neurosurg* 36:517, 1995. *A beautifully illustrated paper showing techniques for identifying gyri and sulci in parasagittal MR images.*

Nilsson C, Lindvall-Axelsson M, Owman C: Neuroendocrine regulatory mechanisms in the choroid plexus-cerebrospinal fluid system, *Brain Res Rev* 17:109, 1992. *Choroid epithelial cells have receptors for a host of hormones and neurotransmitters, the function of which is just beginning to be understood.*

Oka K et al: An observation of the third ventricle under flexible fiberoptic ventriculoscope: normal structure, *Surg Neurol* 40:273, 1993. *Peering into the ventricles during neurosurgery.*

Oldendorf WH: *The quest for an image of brain*, New York, 1980, Raven Press. *A thoroughly delightful, nontechnical book by one of the founders of computed tomography, tracing the history of various imaging techniques.*

Pollay M, Curl F: Secretion of cerebrospinal fluid by the ventricular ependyma of the rabbit, *Am J Physiol* 213:1031, 1967. *Technically admirable experiments demonstrating the production of CSF within the aqueduct and rostral fourth ventricle.*

Schurr PH, Polkey CE, editors: *Hydrocephalus*, New York, 1993, Oxford University Press.

Spector R, Johanson CE: The mammalian choroid plexus, *Sci Am* 261(5):68, 1989.

Timurkaynak E, Rhoton AL Jr, Barry M: Microsurgical anatomy and operative approaches to the lateral ventricle, *Neurosurg* 19:685, 1986. *Finely detailed and beautifully illustrated.*

Voetmann E: On the structure and surface area of the human choroid plexus, *Acta Anat Suppl* 10, 1949.

Welch K, Pollay M: The spinal arachnoid villi of the monkeys *Cercopithecus aethiops sabaeus* and *Macaca irus*, *Anat Rec* 145:43, 1963.

Yamamoto I, Rhoton AL Jr, Peace DA: Microsurgery of the third ventricle. Part 1. Microsurgical anatomy, *Neurosurg* 8:334, 1981. *Finely detailed and beautifully illustrated.*

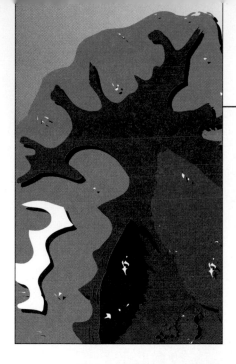

BLOOD SUPPLY OF THE BRAIN

Turtles can walk around for hours with no oxygen supply to their brains. In contrast, our brains are absolutely dependent on a continuous supply of well-oxygenated blood. After just 10 seconds of brain ischemia, we lose consciousness. After 20 seconds, electrical activity ceases; and after just a few minutes, irreversible damage *3 min* usually begins. Corresponding to this metabolic dependence, blood vessels in the CNS, particularly in gray matter, are arranged in a dense meshwork (Figure 6-1). Obviously, an understanding of the brain's blood supply is essential to an understanding of its normal function and of the consequences of cerebrovascular disease. This chapter provides a general overview of the circulatory system of the CNS. Many subsequent chapters include a more de-

tailed discussion of the arterial supply of individual portions of the CNS.

THE INTERNAL CAROTID ARTERIES AND VERTEBRAL ARTERIES SUPPLY THE BRAIN

The arterial supply of the brain and much of the spinal cord is derived from two pairs of vessels, the **internal carotid arteries** and the **vertebral arteries** (Figure 6-2). The internal carotid system supplies most of the telencephalon and much of the diencephalon (Table 6-1). The vertebral system supplies the brainstem and cerebel-

Arteries

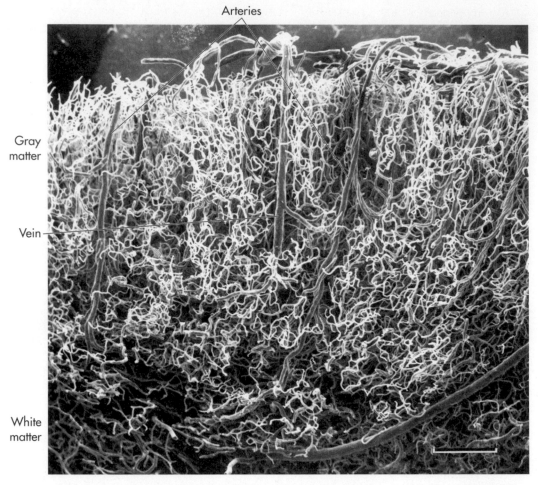

Gray matter

Vein

White matter

FIGURE 6-1

Arrangement of blood vessels in the cerebral cortex of the temporal pole of a 66-year-old man. The blood vessels were injected with plastic, the surrounding tissues were dissolved away, and the resulting cast was observed with a scanning electron microscope; the scale mark corresponds to 500 μm. Notice that the meshwork of vessels is more dense in gray matter than in white matter, corresponding to the greater metabolic needs of neuronal cell bodies. In gray matter, the vessels are so tightly packed that no neuron is more than 100 μm or so from a capillary. (From Duvernoy HM, Delon S, Vannson JL: Cortical blood vessels of the human brain, *Brain Res Bull* 7:519, 1981.)

lum, as well as parts of the diencephalon, spinal cord, and occipital and temporal lobes (Table 6-1).

The Internal Carotid Arteries Supply Most of the Cerebrum

The internal carotid artery ascends through the neck, traverses the petrous temporal bone, passes through the cavernous sinus, and finally reaches the subarachnoid space at the base of the brain (Figure 6-10). Just as it leaves the cavernous sinus, it gives rise to the **ophthalmic artery,** which travels along the optic nerve to the orbit, where it supplies the eyeball, other orbital contents, and some nearby structures. The internal carotid artery then proceeds superiorly alongside the optic chiasm (Figure 6-3) and bifurcates into the **middle** and **anterior cerebral arteries.** Before bifurcating, it gives rise to two smaller branches, the **anterior choroidal artery** and the **poste-**

rior communicating artery. The anterior choroidal artery is a long, thin artery that can be significant clinically because it supplies a number of different structures and is not infrequently involved in cerebrovascular accidents. Along its course (Figure 6-6), it supplies the optic tract, the choroid plexus of the inferior horn of the lateral ventricle, part of the cerebral peduncle, and some deep structures such as portions of the internal capsule, thalamus, and hippocampus (Figure 6-20). The posterior communicating artery passes posteriorly, inferior to the optic tract and toward the cerebral peduncle, and joins the **posterior cerebral artery** (part of the vertebral artery system).

The anterior cerebral artery runs medially, superior to the optic nerve, and enters the longitudinal fissure (Figure 6-3). It and its branches then arch posteriorly, following the corpus callosum, to supply the medial aspect of the frontal and parietal lobes (Figure 6-4, *A*). Some of the smaller branches extend onto the dorsolateral surface of

Look at grouping of areas

Table 6-1 Arterial Supply of the CNS*			
Anatomical area	Artery	Anatomical area	Artery
CEREBRAL HEMISPHERE		**CEREBRAL HEMISPHERE—CONT'D**	
Cortical areas		Limbic structures	
Frontal lobe		Amygdala	AChA
Lateral surface	MCA	Hippocampus	PCA, AChA
Medial surface	ACA	Internal capsule	MCAp, AChA, ACAp
Inferior surface	ACA, MCA	Corpus callosum	
Parietal lobe		Genu, body	ACA
Lateral surface	MCA	Splenium	ACA, PCA
Medial surface	ACA		
Occipital lobe		**DIENCEPHALON**	
Lateral surface	MCA, PCA	Thalamus	PCAp, AChA
Medial, inferior surfaces	PCA	Hypothalamus	ACAp, MCAp, PCAp
Temporal lobe			
Lateral surface	MCA	**CEREBELLUM**	
Medial, inferior surfaces	PCA	Superior surface	SCA
Temporal pole	MCA	Inferior, anterior surfaces	PICA, AICA
Limbic lobe			
Cingulate gyrus	ACA	**BRAINSTEM**	
Parahippocampal gyrus	PCA	Midbrain	PCA, SCA, BA
Insula	MCA	Pons	BA, AICA
Basal ganglia		Medulla	VA, PICA
Caudate nucleus (head)	ACAp, MCAp		
Putamen	MCAp, ACAp	**SPINAL CORD**	
Globus pallidus	AChA	Anterior two thirds	ASpA
		Posterior third	PSpA

*Includes major arteries only, and does not include areas of overlap such as ACA/MCA overlap on the lateral surface near the longitudinal fissure. More details on particular areas of supply are included in subsequent chapters. *ACA,* Anterior cerebral artery; *AChA,* anterior choroidal artery; *AICA,* anterior inferior cerebellar artery; *ASpA,* anterior spinal artery; *BA,* basilar artery; *MCA,* middle cerebral artery; *PCA,* posterior cerebral artery; *PICA,* posterior inferior cerebellar artery; *PSpA,* posterior spinal artery; *SCA,* superior cerebellar artery; *VA,* vertebral artery. "p" denotes perforating branches of the artery.

the hemisphere (Figure 6-4, *B*). Along this course, the anterior cerebral artery commonly divides into two particularly prominent branches, the **pericallosal artery,** which stays immediately adjacent to the corpus callosum, and the **callosomarginal artery,** which follows the cingulate sulcus (Figure 6-4, *A*). The two anterior cerebral arteries, near their entrance into the longitudinal fissure, are connected by the **anterior communicating artery.** Parts of the precentral and postcentral gyri extend onto the medial surface of the frontal and parietal lobes, so occlusion of an anterior cerebral artery causes restricted contralateral motor and somatosensory deficits.

The large middle cerebral artery proceeds laterally into the lateral sulcus (Figure 6-3). It divides into a number of branches that supply the insula, emerge from the lateral sulcus, and spread out to supply most of the lateral surface of the cerebral hemisphere (Figures 6-4, *B* and 6-5). Most of the precentral and postcentral gyri are within this area

of supply, so occlusion of a middle cerebral artery causes major motor and somatosensory deficits. In addition, if the left hemisphere is the one involved, language deficits are almost invariably found.

Small perforating arteries supply deep cerebral structures

Along its course toward the lateral sulcus, the middle cerebral artery gives rise to many very small branches that penetrate the brain near their origin and supply deep structures of the diencephalon and telencephalon (Figures 6-6 and 6-7). These particular arteries are called the **lateral striate** (or **lenticulostriate**) **arteries,** but similar small branches arise from all the arteries around the base of the brain (Figure 6-8). They are referred to collectively as **perforating** or **ganglionic** branches. Perforating arteries are particularly numerous in the area adjacent to the optic chiasm and

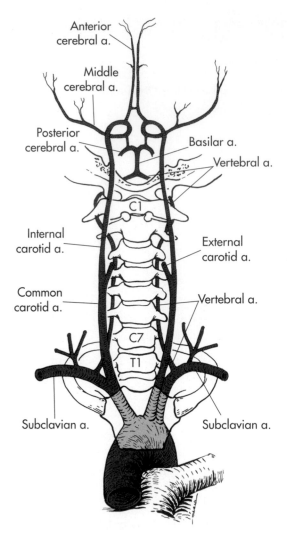

FIGURE 6-2
Origins of the arterial supply of the brain. *a,* artery. (From Osborn AG: *Introduction to cerebral angiography,* Hagerstown, 1980, Harper & Row.)

Imaging Techniques Allow Arteries and Veins to be Visualized*

Blood vessels can be visualized with most imaging techniques by finding a way to make the blood contained within them differ in some way from surrounding structures. Cerebral angiography utilizes the intravenous injection of iodinated dyes to make blood much more opaque than brain to x-rays. A cerebral angiogram is typically produced by introducing a catheter into the femoral artery, threading it (under fluoroscopic guidance) up the aorta and into the aortic arch, then steering the catheter tip into the artery of interest. In this way, the contrast material can be introduced into a single vertebral or internal carotid artery. Once the dye has been introduced, a rapid series of x-ray pictures can follow it as it flows through the artery, into capillaries, and then into veins (Figure 6-9). Finally, photographic† (as in Figure 6-9) or digital techniques can be used to remove bone images and reveal blood vessels in relative isolation.

Angiography was the first technique developed for making images of normal and diseased vessels, and for decades it was also a major tool for inferring changes in the brain that caused distortion of the vasculature. It still produces the most detailed images of cerebral vasculature available (Figure 6-10). CT and MRI, however, are less invasive and can simultaneously show the CNS itself. Hence they have become widely used for imaging studies of blood vessels (Box 6-1).

The Vertebral-Basilar System Supplies the Brainstem and Parts of the Cerebrum and Spinal Cord

The two vertebral arteries run rostrally alongside the medulla and fuse at the junction between the medulla and pons to form the midline **basilar artery,** which proceeds rostrally along the anterior surface of the pons (Figure 6-3).

Before joining the basilar artery, each vertebral artery gives rise to three branches: the **posterior spinal artery, anterior spinal artery,** and **posterior inferior cerebellar artery.** The posterior spinal artery runs caudally along the dorsolateral aspect of the spinal cord and supplies the posterior third of that half of the cord. The anterior spinal artery joins its counterpart from the opposite side, forming a single anterior spinal artery that runs cau-

Text continued on p. 127

in the area between the cerebral peduncles; for this reason these are called the **anterior** and **posterior perforated substances,** respectively. The narrow, thin-walled vessels of the anterior perforated substance are involved frequently in strokes. The deep cerebral structures they supply are such that damage to these small vessels can cause neurological deficits out of proportion to their size. For example, the somatosensory projection from the thalamus to the postcentral gyrus must pass through the internal capsule; damage to a small part of the internal capsule, from rupture or occlusion of a perforating artery, can cause deficits similar to those resulting from damage to a large expanse of cortex.

---

*Parts of this discussion were adapted from Nolte J, Angevine JB Jr: *The human brain in photographs and diagrams,* St. Louis, 1995, Mosby.
† An x-ray image is made before injection of the iodinated dye and its contrast is reversed (i.e., a positive image is made, so that bone is dark). The reverse-contrast image is stacked on top of the image made after dye injection and a print made of both together. The reciprocally contrasting portions of the two images thus provide a relatively uniform background from which the blood vessels stand out.

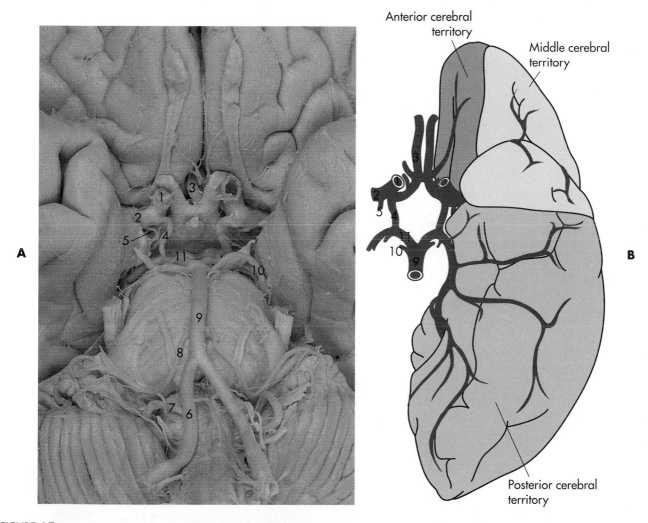

FIGURE 6-3

Arteries on the inferior surface of the brain **(A)** and sources of arterial supply to cortical areas **(B).** The internal carotid artery *(1)* divides into the middle *(2)* and anterior *(3)* cerebral arteries after giving rise to the posterior communicating *(4)* and anterior choroidal *(5)* arteries. Collectively these vessels supply anterior and lateral parts of the cerebrum. The vertebral arteries *(6)* join to form the basilar artery *(9)* after giving rise to the posterior inferior cerebellar artery *(7).* The basilar artery in turn gives rise to the anterior inferior *(8)* and superior *(10)* cerebellar arteries before bifurcating into the posterior cerebral arteries *(11).* Collectively the vertebral-basilar system supplies the brainstem, much of the diencephalon, and inferior and posterior parts of the cerebral hemispheres. [**A** from Nolte J, Angevine JB Jr: *The human brain in photographs and diagrams, St. Louis,* 1995, Mosby. **B** modified from Mettler FA: *Neuroanatomy,* ed 2, St. Louis, 1948, Mosby.]

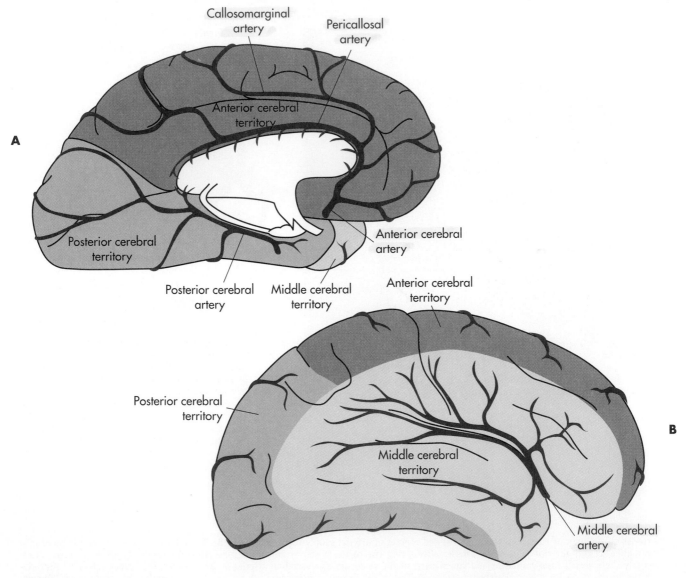

FIGURE 6-4
Arteries on the medial (**A**) and lateral (**B**) surfaces of the brain, with their areas of supply indicated. (Modified from Mettler FA: *Neuroanatomy,* ed 2, St. Louis, 1948, Mosby.)

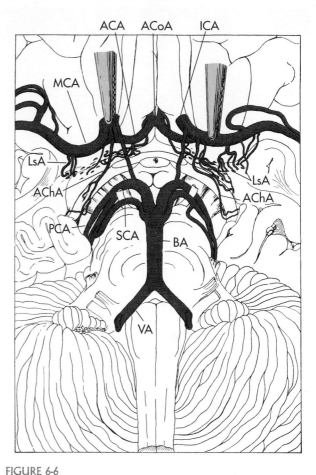

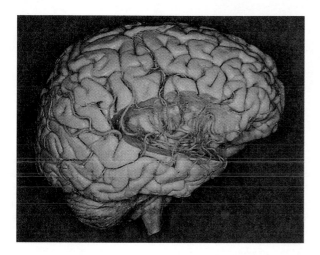

FIGURE 6-5

Branches of the right middle cerebral artery on the surface of the insula, revealed by removing the opercula of the right hemisphere. (From Yaşargil MG: *Microneurosurgery, vol IV, A: CNS tumors: surgical anatomy, neuropathology, neuroradiology, neurophysiology, clinical considerations, operability, treatment options*, New York, 1994, Thieme Medical Publishers, Inc.)

FIGURE 6-6

Lateral striate arteries, together with ganglionic branches of the anterior cerebral and anterior choroidal arteries, entering the anterior perforated substance. Similar perforating branches arise from other arteries of the circle of Willis and from the basilar artery (see Figures 6-9 and 6-10), but these are not included in this drawing. *ACA,* Anterior cerebral artery; *AChA,* anterior choroidal artery; *ACoA,* anterior communicating artery; *BA,* basilar artery; *ICA,* internal carotid artery; *LsA,* lateral striate arteries; *MCA,* middle cerebral artery; *PCA,* posterior cerebral artery; *SCA,* superior cerebellar artery; *VA,* vertebral artery. (From Alexander L: The vascular supply of the strio-pallidum, *Res Pub Assoc Res Nerv Ment Dis* 21:77, 1942.)

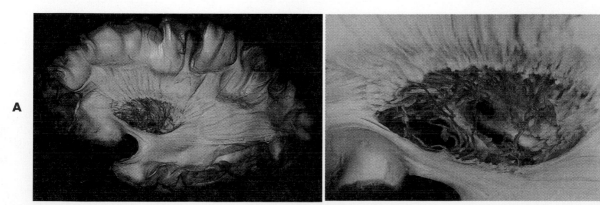

FIGURE 6-7

Low (**A**) and high (**B**) magnification views of a dissection in which the insula and lenticular nucleus were removed. Lateral striate arteries remain, crossing the space formerly occupied by the lenticular nucleus and entering the internal capsule. (From Yaşargil MG: *Microneurosurgery, vol IV, A: CNS tumors: surgical anatomy, neuropathology, neuroradiology, neurophysiology, clinical considerations, operability, treatment options*, New York, 1994, Thieme Medical Publishers, Inc.)

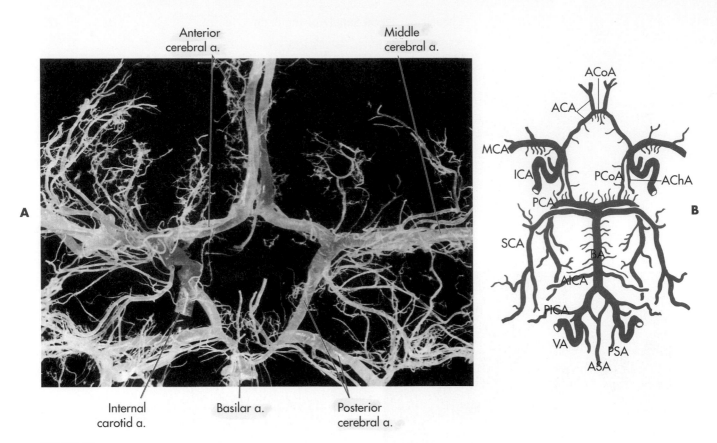

Anterior cerebral a.

Middle cerebral a.

ACoA

ACA

MCA

ICA   PCoA   AChA

PCA

SCA   BA   B

AICA

PICA

VA   PSA

ASA

A

Internal carotid a.

Basilar a.

Posterior cerebral a.

FIGURE 6-8

Ganglionic branches arising from the circle of Willis. **A,** A cast of a human circle of Willis, demonstrating many of the small ganglionic or perforating arteries that arise from major vessels in or adjacent to the circle. The internal carotid and basilar arteries were injected with plastic, after which the surrounding tissues were dissolved away. This circle of Willis is somewhat unusual in that both posterior cerebral arteries arise from an internal carotid rather than the basilar artery (Figure 6-15, *D*). **B,** A drawing of the arteries on the base of the cerebrum and anterior surface of the brainstem, showing the small perforating branches of many of these vessels. Those arising in and near the circle of Willis are commonly divided into groups: an anteromedial group from the anterior cerebral and anterior communicating arteries (*ACA, ACoA*), an anterolateral group (including the lateral striate arteries) from the middle cerebral artery (*MCA*) and most proximal part of the anterior cerebral artery, a posteromedial group from the posterior communicating artery (*PCoA*) and the part of the posterior cerebral artery (*PCA*) in the circle of Willis, and a posterolateral group from the posterior cerebral artery distal to the circle of Willis. *AChA,* Anterior choroidal artery; *AICA,* anterior inferior cerebellar artery; *ASA,* anterior spinal artery; *BA,* basilar artery; *ICA,* internal carotid artery; *PICA,* posterior inferior cerebellar artery; *PSA,* posterior spinal artery; *SCA,* superior cerebellar artery; *VA,* vertebral artery. (**A** from Marinković SV, Milisavljević MM, Marinković ZD: The perforating branches of the internal carotid artery: the microsurgical anatomy of their extracerebral segments, *Neurosurg* 26:472, 1990. **B** from Mettler FA: **Neuroanatomy,** ed 2, St. Louis, 1948, Mosby.)

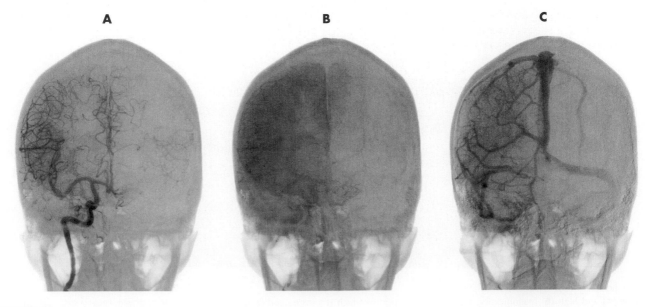

A   B   C

FIGURE 6-9

Movement of contrast material through the intracranial vasculature, as seen in a series of anterior-posterior views (as though you were looking down at the patient's forehead) after injection of the right internal carotid artery. **A,** About 2 seconds after injection, the arteries are filled. **B,** About 5 seconds after injection, the contrast agent has moved out of the arteries and into capillary beds, resulting in a diffuse image. **C,** About 7 seconds after injection, the contrast agent has moved into veins and venous sinuses. (From Nolte J, Angevine JB Jr: *The human brain in photographs and diagrams,* St. Louis, 1995, Mosby.)

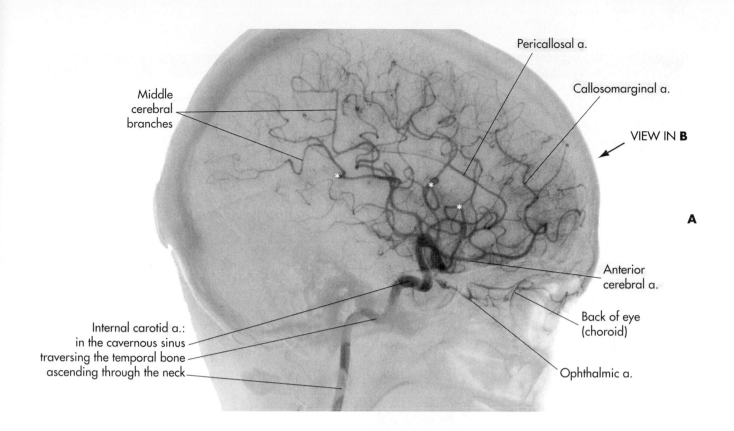

Pericallosal a.

Callosomarginal a.

Middle
cerebral
branches

VIEW IN **B**

A

Anterior
cerebral a.

Back of eye
(choroid)

Internal carotid a.:
in the cavernous sinus
traversing the temporal bone
ascending through the neck

Ophthalmic a.

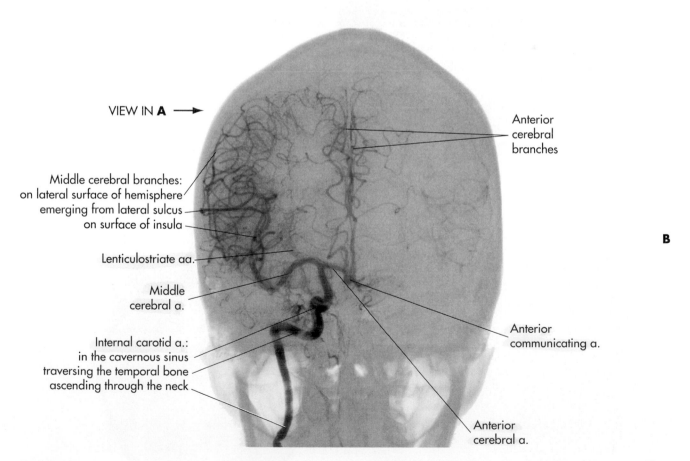

VIEW IN **A**

Anterior
cerebral
branches

Middle cerebral branches:
on lateral surface of hemisphere
emerging from lateral sulcus
on surface of insula

Lenticulostriate aa.

Middle
cerebral a.

Internal carotid a.:
in the cavernous sinus
traversing the temporal bone
ascending through the neck

B

Anterior
communicating a.

Anterior
cerebral a.

FIGURE 6-10

The arterial phase of a right internal carotid angiogram. **A,** A lateral view; anterior is to the right. Asterisks indicate sites where middle cerebral branches turn dorsally or ventrally as they emerge from the lateral sulcus. **B,** An anterior-posterior view; the view is as though you were looking at the patient's forehead. (From Nolte J, Angevine JB Jr: *The human brain in photographs and diagrams,* St. Louis, 1995, Mosby.)

Box 6-1   Imaging Blood Vessels With CT and MRI

CT and MRI techniques can be used to produce not only images of CNS planes but also images of the cerebral vasculature. The x-ray density of blood is not different enough from that of CNS to allow imaging of blood vessels in ordinary CTs. However, prior intravenous injection of an x-ray dense contrast agent such as those used in angiography allows images of both CNS and blood vessels to be created (Figure 6-11). The spatial resolution of **contrast-enhanced CTs** is not as good as in the case of angiography, but the need to thread catheters into places such as the aortic arch is avoided.

In addition, computer processing can remove the CNS from the images and allow three-dimensional reconstructions of arteries or veins (Figures 6-21 and 6-29). Various MRI parameters can be adjusted to emphasize the intrinsic properties of flowing blood, making vessels visible even without the use of an intravenous contrast agent (Figure 6-12). As in the case of contrast-enhanced CTs, three-dimensional reconstructions—**magnetic resonance angiograms**—can be produced (Figure 6-13).

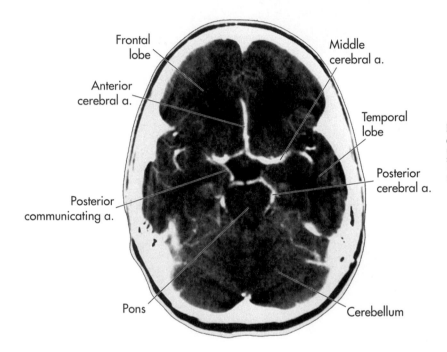

FIGURE 6-11
CT scan of a normal brain, made after the injection of an iodinated contrast agent. (From Nolte J, Angevine JB Jr: *The human brain in photographs and diagrams,* St. Louis, 1995, Mosby.)

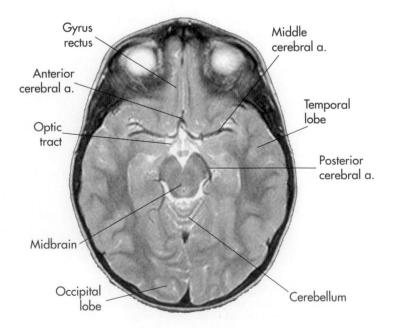

FIGURE 6-12
T2-weighted MRI in which the major arteries of the circle of Willis can be seen, even without injection of a contrast agent. (Modified from Nolte J, Angevine JB Jr: *The human brain in photographs and diagrams,* St. Louis, 1995, Mosby.)

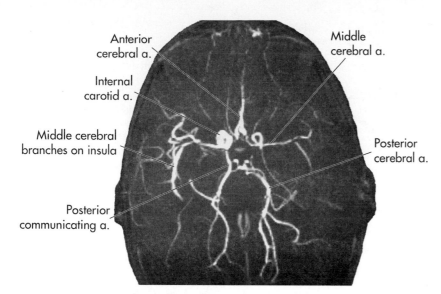

Anterior
cerebral a.

Middle
cerebral a.

Internal
carotid a.

Middle cerebral
branches on insula

Posterior
cerebral a.

Posterior
communicating a.

FIGURE 6-13
Magnetic resonance angiogram (MRA), demonstrating most of the arterial supply of the brain. The view is as though you were looking up from the patient's feet; anterior is toward the top of the image. (From Nolte J, Angevine JB Jr: *The human brain in photographs and diagrams,* St. Louis, 1995, Mosby.)

dally along the ventral midline of the spinal cord, supplying the anterior two thirds of the cord. These spinal arteries cannot carry enough blood from the vertebral arteries to supply more than the cervical segments of the spinal cord and must be reinforced at various points caudal to this (discussed in Chapter 10). The posterior inferior cerebellar artery (often referred to by the acronym **PICA**), as its name implies, supplies much of the inferior surface of the cerebellar hemisphere (Figure 6-14); however, it sends branches to other structures on its way to the cerebellum. As it curves around the brainstem, the artery supplies the choroid plexus of the fourth ventricle and much of the lateral medulla. This is a uniform occurrence in the large named branches of the vertebral-basilar system, quite analogous to the perforating branches of the circle of Willis: on their way to their major area of supply, these arteries send branches to brainstem structures. By knowing the brainstem level at which these large named branches emerge, one can make reasonably accurate inferences about the blood supply of any given region of the brainstem (see Figures 11-25 and 11-26).

The basilar artery proceeds rostrally and, at the level of the midbrain, bifurcates into the two **posterior cerebral arteries.** Before this bifurcation, it gives rise to numerous unnamed branches and two named branches, the **anterior inferior cerebellar artery** and the **superior cerebellar artery.**

The anterior inferior cerebellar artery (often referred to by the acronym **AICA**) arises just rostral to the formation point of the basilar artery and supplies the more anterior portions of the inferior surface of the cerebellum (e.g., the flocculus), as well as parts of the caudal pons. The superior cerebellar artery arises just caudal to the bifurcation of the basilar artery and supplies the superior surface of the cerebellum and much of the caudal midbrain and rostral pons. The many smaller branches of the basilar artery, collectively called **pontine arteries** (Figure 6-8,

B), supply the remainder of the pons. One of these, the **internal auditory** or **labyrinthine artery** (which often is actually a branch of the AICA), though hard to distinguish from the others by appearance, is functionally important because it also supplies the inner ear. Its occlusion can lead to vertigo and ipsilateral deafness.

The posterior cerebral artery curves around the midbrain and passes through the superior cistern; its branches spread out to supply the medial and inferior surfaces of the occipital and temporal lobes (Figures 6-3; 6-4, *A;* and 6-14). Along the way, it sends branches to the rostral midbrain and caudal diencephalon. It also gives rise to several **posterior choroidal arteries,** which supply the choroid plexus of the third ventricle and of the body of the lateral ventricle. The anterior and posterior choroidal arteries form anastomoses in the vicinity of the glomus. The primary visual cortex is located in the occipital lobe, so occlusion of a posterior cerebral artery at its origin leads to visual field losses in addition to other deficits referable to the midbrain and diencephalon.

The Circle of Willis Interconnects the Internal Carotid and Vertebral-Basilar Systems

The posterior cerebral artery is connected to the internal carotid artery by the posterior communicating artery. This completes an arterial polygon called the **circle of Willis,** through which the anterior cerebral, internal carotid, and posterior cerebral arteries of both sides are interconnected. Normally, there is little or no blood flow around this circle because the appropriate pressure differentials are not present: the arterial pressure in the internal carotid arteries is about the same as that in the posterior cerebral arteries, so little or no blood flows through the posterior communicating arteries. However, if one major vessel becomes occluded, either within the circle of Willis or proximal to it,

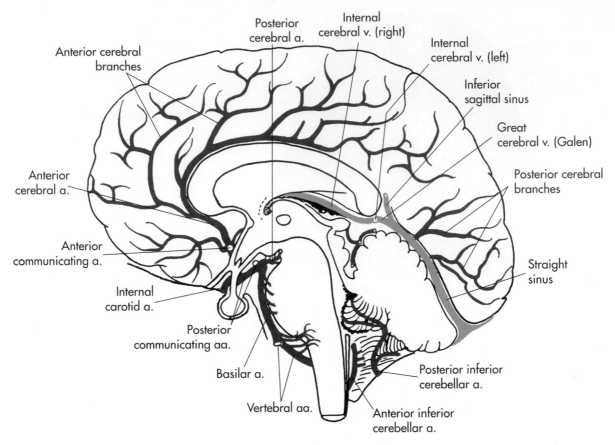

FIGURE 6-14
A hemisected brain, showing the arterial supply to its medial surface. (Modified from Mettler FA: *Neuroanatomy,* ed 2, St. Louis, 1948, Mosby.)

the communicating arteries may allow critically important anastomotic flow and prevent neurological damage. By such a mechanism it would be theoretically possible (though highly unlikely) for the entire brain to be perfused by just one of the four major arteries that normally supply it. The anterior and posterior communicating arteries are quite variable in size (see below), and so the establishment of effective anastomotic flow in the event of an arterial occlusion may also depend on the time course of the occlusion. A small communicating artery can enlarge slowly to compensate for a slowly developing occlusion, but in such a case an abrupt blockage might cause serious damage.

Designating the circle of Willis shown in Figure 6-3, *B* as "normal" represents to a great extent a nod to an aesthetic need because fewer than half the circles have this appearance. Some frequently seen "abnormalities" are indicated in Figure 6-15. Asymmetries are common; one or more of the communicating arteries may be very small; one anterior cerebral artery may be much smaller at its origin than the other; one posterior cerebral artery may retain its embryological origin from the internal carotid and may be connected to the basilar artery through a posterior communicating artery. In rare cases, one of the communicating arteries may be missing, resulting in an incomplete circle.

Other routes of collateral circulation are available, although the circle of Willis is likely to be the most important. There are anastomoses at the arteriolar and capillary levels between terminal branches of the cerebral arteries. These are usually inadequate in the adult for maintaining the entire territory of a major cerebral artery if it becomes occluded, but occasionally they may be sufficient for maintaining a large part of this territory. In addition, well-defined arterial anastomoses may enlarge to a remarkable degree to compensate for slowly developing occlusions. For example, there have been documented cases in which the territory of one posterior cerebral artery was supplied by the internal carotid artery of that side by means of flow through the anterior choroidal artery and from there through a posterior choroidal artery and into the posterior cerebral artery.

Finally, there are a limited number of intracranial-extracranial anastomoses that can enlarge to a functional degree. The most important are anastomoses in the orbit between the ophthalmic artery and branches of the external carotid artery. If an internal carotid artery becomes occluded, it is possible for blood from the external carotid artery to flow backward through the ophthalmic artery to reach internal carotid territory.

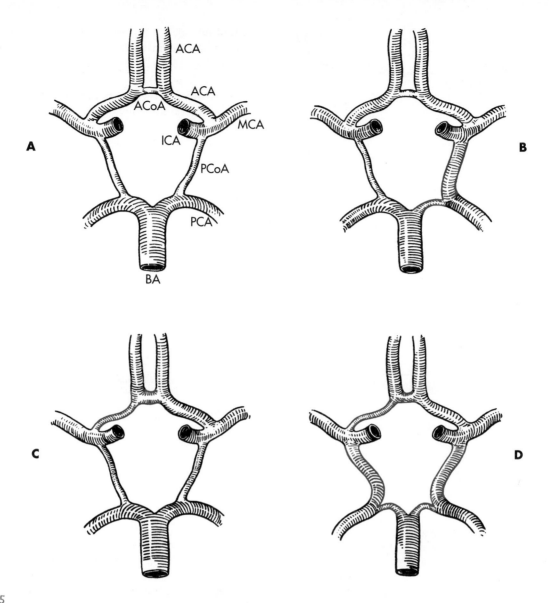

FIGURE 6-15

Normal circle of Willis (**A**) compared with some common "abnormalities" (indicated in color in **B, C,** and **D**). **B,** One posterior cerebral artery arises from an internal carotid artery in 30% to 40% of brains. **C,** Both anterior cerebral arteries are perfused primarily from one internal carotid artery in 10% to 15% of brains. **D,** Various combinations of hypoplastic and asymmetrical arteries are also found, but the circle of Willis is almost always complete. *ACA,* Anterior cerebral artery; *ACoA,* anterior communicating artery; *BA,* basilar artery; *ICA,* internal carotid artery; *MCA,* middle cerebral artery; *PCA,* posterior cerebral artery; *PCoA,* posterior communicating artery. (Modified from Hodes PJ et al: Cerebral angiography: fundamentals in anatomy and physiology, *Am J Roentgenol* 70:61, 1953.)

Blood Flow to the CNS Is Closely Controlled

The brain is very active metabolically but has no effective way to store oxygen or glucose. A stable and copious blood supply is therefore required, and the brain, which represents only 2% of the total body weight, uses about 15% of the normal cardiac output and accounts for nearly 25% of the body's oxygen consumption. The overall flow rate is normally maintained at a very constant level, but this rate may increase or decrease in particular regions of the brain, in a pattern correlated with neural activity.

The overall flow rate is constant, but there are regional changes in blood flow

The mechanisms that control cerebral blood flow are not completely understood, but at least three factors seem to be involved. The first is a process termed **autoregulation** (Figure 6-16), by which cerebral blood vessels themselves act to maintain constant flow; the vessels constrict (thus increasing their resistance) in response to increased blood pressure, and they relax in response to decreased pressure.

The second factor may be generally thought of as a response of the cerebral vessels to metabolites, of which

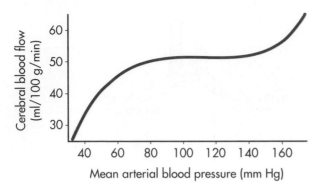

FIGURE 6-16
Autoregulation of cerebral blood flow. Over a broad range of blood pressure, cerebral vessels dilate as pressure decreases, thus keeping flow constant. Outside of the range in which autoregulation functions, increases or decreases in pressure cause increases or decreases in flow.

carbon dioxide is the best studied. Increases of carbon dioxide tension in brain extracellular fluid cause dilation of the cerebral vessels and increased blood flow; decreases of carbon dioxide tension have opposite effects. Changes in oxygen tension have reciprocal effects to those of carbon dioxide. Local changes in metabolite concentration in response to neuronal activity are at least part of the basis for regional variations in blood flow. Because blood flow increases in active areas of the brain, measuring these regional changes in blood flow during various mental activities is, in a very real sense, watching the mind at work. A number of methods for doing this are now available (Box 6-2). The same methods can be used to study regional metabolic or vascular abnormalities, in some cases when CT and MRI studies appear normal.

Box 6-2   Watching Changes in Blood Flow: Images of the Brain at Work

The electrical signals generated by neurons as they communicate with each other are difficult to localize from outside the head. Hence there has been great interest in indirect measures of neuronal activity, such as increases in blood flow to active areas of the brain. Methods are now available for measuring the regional blood flow in normal human cerebral hemispheres and, by inference, measuring the varying levels of metabolic activity of different areas of the brain during different types of mental activity. An early, conceptually straightforward technique involves the injection of a small amount of an inert, radioactive gas (such as ^{133}Xe, a gamma-emitting isotope of xenon) into the cerebral circulation. After the injection, a bank of gamma-ray cameras records the inflow and washout of the gas while the patient performs various tasks. The spatial resolution of this method is not very good, and it suffers from one of the same drawbacks as plain skull x-rays: the signals from all parts of the three-dimensional brain are collapsed onto a plane. The latter difficulty can be addressed by using intravenously injected gamma-emitting isotopes, a ring of gamma-ray detectors, and tomographic calculations similar to those used in x-ray CT. Because the signal used to construct the tomographic images consists of gamma-ray photons, the process is referred to as **single photon emission computed tomography (SPECT)**. Although technical limitations of SPECT imaging result in a spatial resolution of only 10 mm or so, it is nevertheless a useful clinical method for demonstrating regional changes in brain blood flow.

Positron emission tomography (or **PET scanning**) is related to SPECT, but has twice the spatial resolution. PET scanning relies on the fact that certain isotopes decay by emitting a positron. The emitted positron quickly combines with a nearby electron, and the two particles are annihilated, producing two gamma rays that travel in opposite directions.

By surrounding a patient's head with a ring of gamma-ray detectors, it is possible to localize the positron-emitting isotope within the brain. One way to utilize this phenomenon is to label deoxyglucose with the positron emitter ^{18}F and inject the resulting compound. Active neurons take up deoxyglucose as readily as glucose but metabolize it much more slowly. Therefore the ^{18}F remains in the active neurons long enough for computer-generated tomographic images to be formed (Figures 6-17). Although expensive and technologically complex, the potential for PET scanning is exciting. Many different compounds can be labeled with positron-emitting isotopes, making it possible to map out not only glucose metabolism but also oxygen consumption, blood flow, and the locations of receptors for neurotransmitters and hormones. It is even possible to combine PET and MRI data from single individuals to produce remarkable images of brain activity (Figure 6-18).

Finally, magnetic resonance imaging protocols can be adjusted to emphasize changes in blood flow. One method takes advantage of the differences between the paramagnetic properties of hemoglobin and deoxyhemoglobin. Active areas of brain receive an even greater increase in blood flow than they need, so blood leaving active areas actually has a higher concentration of oxygen than blood leaving inactive areas. Hence MRI signals that reflect hemoglobin/deoxyhemoglobin ratios can provide a measure of regional changes in blood flow. Other methods utilize precisely timed signals to emphasize the intrinsic properties of flowing blood. Because these images (Figure 6-19) demonstrate areas of brain activity, the process is referred to as **functional magnetic resonance imaging (fMRI)**. FMRI is the newest of the activity-imaging techniques and is still under development, but it has the major advantage that it, like MRI in general, is completely noninvasive.

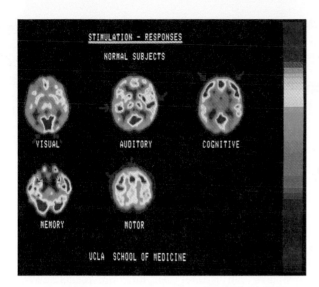

FIGURE 6-17
Use of PET and ¹⁸F-fluorodeoxyglucose (FDG) to map increased glucose consumption in distinctive areas of the brain during different kinds of tasks. All images are in CT planes, with anterior at the top. A checkerboard visual stimulus activates the medial parts of the occipital lobes. An auditory stimulus causes increased glucose consumption in the superior parts of the temporal lobes; the areas of increase have different shapes in the two hemispheres, reflecting the anatomical asymmetry of the surface of the superior temporal gyrus (see Chapter 22). When an individual is involved in an active, cognitive task rather than passive perception of stimuli, glucose consumption increases in the frontal lobes. Subjects trying to remember information from a verbal stimulus (a story) show increased glucose consumption in the medial parts of the temporal lobes, consistent with increased metabolism in the hippocampus and amygdala (see Chapter 23). Sequential movements of the fingers of the right hand activate motor cortex on the left, as well as the supplementary motor area (*vertical arrow*). (Courtesy Drs. Michael E. Phelps and John C. Mazziotta, UCLA School of Medicine.)

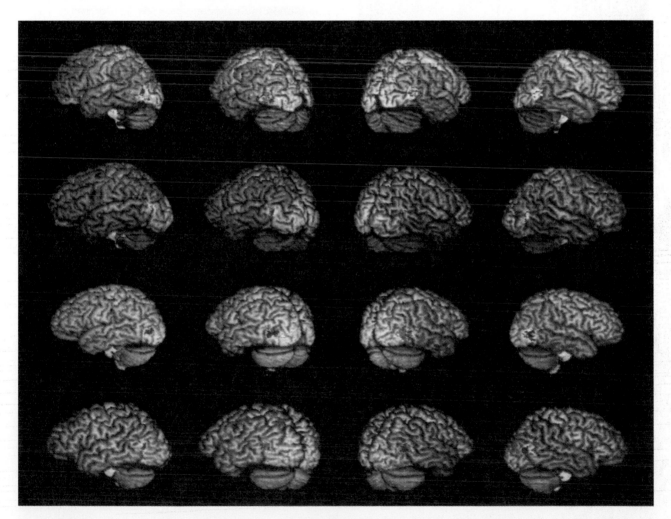

FIGURE 6-18
Combined use of PET and MRI to demonstrate changes in blood flow as subjects watched moving visual stimuli (vs. stationary stimuli); each row of four images is from a different subject. Blood flow was mapped using PET scanning after intravenous injection of $H_2^{15}O$ (^{15}O is a positron-emitting isotope of oxygen), an image of the surface of each subject's brain was reconstructed from T1-weighted MRIs, and the two sets of data coregistered. Moving visual stimuli particularly activate an area on the lateral surface of each occipital lobe, near its junction with the temporal lobe (see Chapter 17). (From Watson JDG et al: Area V5 of the human brain: evidence from a combined study using positron emission tomography and magnetic resonance imaging, *Cerebral Cortex* 3:79, 1993.)

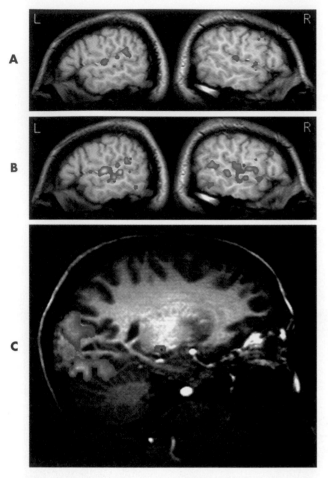

FIGURE 6-19

Functional magnetic imaging demonstration of human auditory and visual cortex. fMRI data from a 30-year-old man listening to white noise (**A**) and to spoken words (**B**) were superimposed on TI-weighted parasagittal slices of his left (L) and right (R) hemispheres. Yellow and orange areas correspond to areas of increased blood flow. Both stimuli activate the superior temporal gyrus, but spoken words activate a more extensive area of this gyrus. **C**, fMRI data from another subject watching a red and black checkerboard in which the squares reversed color 8 to 10 times per second, again superimposed on a TI-weighted parasagittal slice. The stimulus activates not only occipital cortex above and below the calcarine sulcus, but also the principal thalamic nucleus relaying visual information (*, lateral geniculate nucleus). (**A** and **B** from Binder JR et al: Functional magnetic resonance imaging of human auditory cortex, *Ann Neurol* 35:662, 1994. **C** from Chen W et al: Mapping of lateral geniculate nucleus activation during visual stimulation in human brain using fMRI, *Magn Reson Med* 39:89, 1998.

Finally, cerebral vessels are innervated, both by standard autonomic fibers and by fibers from several locations within the brain. The evidence concerning the roles of this innervation is incomplete and somewhat conflicting, but the current consensus is that neural control is of relatively minor importance. It may play a part in adaptation to stress of various sorts and in sustaining the extremes of the autoregulation range, but under ordinary circumstances, metabolic and direct autoregulatory mechanisms seem to predominate.

Strokes Result From Disruption of the Vascular Supply

Cerebrovascular disease and accidents constitute the most common cause of neurological deficits. Normally, about 50 ml of blood flows through each 100 g of CNS per minute. This is a little more than the CNS needs to survive, but significant reduction of this perfusion rate rapidly causes malfunction or even death of neurons. Reduction of the flow rate to about 20 ml/100 g/min causes neurons to stop generating electrical signals. Neurons can survive in this condition for a while, and timely restoration of normal flow can restore their function. Reduction to about 10 ml/100 g/min for more than a few minutes sets in motion multiple destructive cascades of events that result in necrosis of the involved brain tissue. A necrotic region of tissue is called an **infarct.** An abrupt incident of vascular insufficiency or of bleeding into or immediately adjacent to the brain is called a **stroke.**

The exact mechanism whereby ischemia causes neuronal death is not completely understood and involves multiple processes. Given the brain's metabolic needs, one might expect that total ischemia would be more detrimental than partial ischemia and that increased blood glucose during partial ischemia would be helpful. In fact, exactly the opposite is observed. Apparently, neurons are damaged less by total ischemia and a total halt of metabolism than they are by lactic acidosis and other consequences of anaerobic metabolism and the inability of the vasculature to remove waste products. The fact that neurons are more tolerant of anoxia than was believed previously has given rise to some hope for treatments that can ameliorate the effects of stroke.

Ischemic strokes (those caused by sudden vascular insufficiency) are most commonly caused by a **thrombus** (a blood clot formed within a vessel) or an **embolus** (a bit of foreign matter, such as part of a blood clot or an atherosclerotic plaque, that is carried along in the bloodstream). Either can cause occlusion of an artery supplying the brain, and both are highly correlated with atherosclerosis (although this is by no means the only cause). If the occlusion occurs within or proximal to the circle of Willis, there is some possibility of adequate collateral circulation, particularly if the involved artery had slowly become occluded before the stroke. On the other hand, anastomoses between arteries distal to the circle of Willis are variable, and collateral circulation is less likely to be adequate, so occlusion of one of these vessels typically results in an infarct in a predictable territory (Figure 6-20). The size of the infarct is obviously related to the size of the occluded vessel, ranging from tiny lesions (called **lacunes**) caused

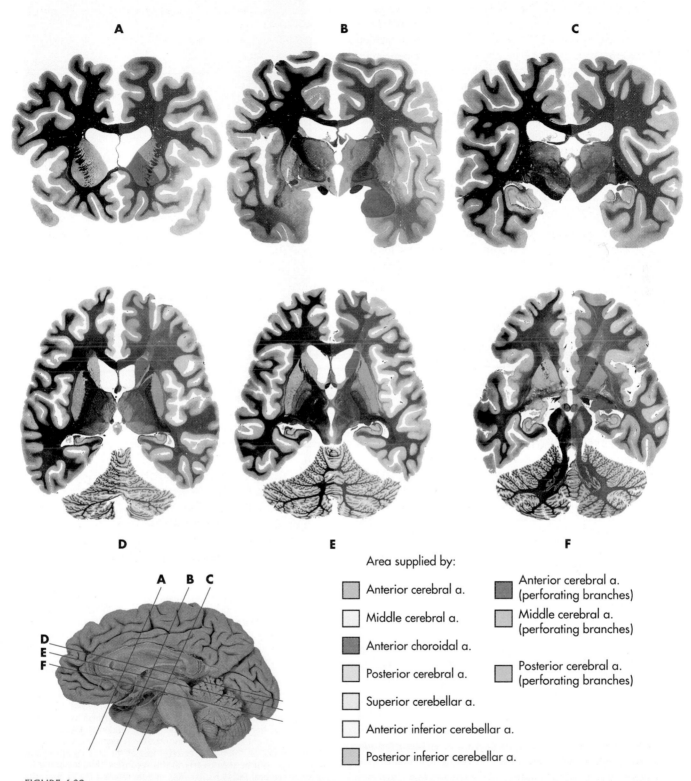

A   B   C

D   E   F

Area supplied by:

- Anterior cerebral a.
- Middle cerebral a.
- Anterior choroidal a.
- Posterior cerebral a.
- Superior cerebellar a.
- Anterior inferior cerebellar a.
- Posterior inferior cerebellar a.

- Anterior cerebral a. (perforating branches)
- Middle cerebral a. (perforating branches)
- Posterior cerebral a. (perforating branches)

FIGURE 6-20
Areas of the cerebrum and cerebellum supplied by major arteries and their perforating branches, shown in coronal (**A-C**) and horizontal (**D-F**) sections.

by occlusion of a small perforating artery to infarcts that affect large expanses of a cerebral hemisphere. However, as pointed out earlier in this chapter, the magnitude of a neurological deficit is not necessarily related to the size of the infarct causing it. A very small lesion in the brainstem or internal capsule can have a much more devastating effect than damage to certain relatively large areas of the cerebellum or cerebral hemispheres. The size and distribution of the infarct is also related to the location of the occlusion along the course of an artery. For example, occlusion of a middle cerebral artery in the lateral sulcus would cause a large cortical infarct; occlusion of the same artery as it leaves the circle of Willis would also block flow into the lenticulostriate arteries on that side, damaging deep structures as well.

Another vascular event with symptoms somewhat similar to an ischemic stroke is a **transient ischemic attack (TIA).** The crucial difference between a transient ischemic attack and an ischemic stroke is that the deficits associated with a transient ischemic attack (as the name implies) persist for only a few minutes to a few hours and are followed by an essentially complete recovery. Transient ischemic attacks are usually caused by minute emboli that originate from atherosclerotic plaques or thrombi, partially occlude brain arteries, and are then broken down by normal body mechanisms.

Hemorrhagic strokes most commonly result from the rupture of small perforating arteries or the rupture of an aneurysm (see next paragraph). The lateral striate (lenticulostriate) arteries are the most frequent site of the former type of hemorrhage. These are particularly thin-walled vessels, and the likelihood of their spontaneous rupture is increased greatly in individuals suffering from hypertension. The lateral striate arteries supply some important deep cerebral structures, and hemorrhage here can be rapidly fatal.

Aneurysms are balloon-like swellings of arterial walls. They occur most frequently at or near the place where an artery bifurcates. Those close to the brain usually occur in or near the anterior half of the circle of Willis (Figure 6-21, A), although they also are found at other locations (Figure 6-21, B). An aneurysm can cause neurological deficits in two ways. As it grows (and some become huge), it can push against and compress brain structures, much as a growing tumor would. It also can rupture (Figure 6-22) and, depending on its size and location, have disastrous consequences. Many aneurysms, particularly if they are detected before they become too large, can be corrected surgically.

Another type of vascular problem is an **arteriovenous malformation (AVM).** This is a congenital malformation in which large anastomoses exist between arteries and veins in a relatively circumscribed area (Figure 6-23). These malformations may become larger with age and can cause neurological problems, either by "stealing" blood from adjacent normal brain tissue as a result of their low resistance or by hemorrhaging.

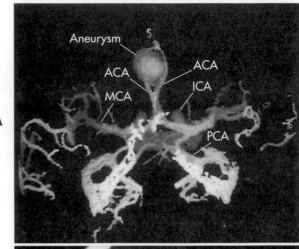

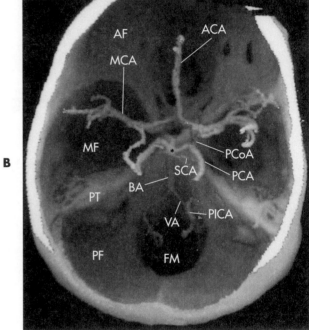

FIGURE 6-21

Intracranial aneurysms. **A,** An aneurysm near the anterior half of the circle of Willis. The patient was a 58-year-old woman who presented with headache and altered mental status. CT studies without contrast revealed subarachnoid hemorrhage, and a three-dimensional rendering of the circle of Willis reconstructed from contrast-enhanced CTs demonstrated an aneurysm of the left anterior cerebral artery. *ACA,* Anterior cerebral artery; *ICA,* internal carotid artery; *MCA,* middle cerebral artery; *PCA,* posterior cerebral artery; *R,* the patient's right side. **B,** An aneurysm in a less typical location, the posterior half of the circle of Willis. The patient was a 46-year-old woman being evaluated for what she described as the worst headache of her life. A three-dimensional rendering reconstructed from contrast-enhanced CTs demonstrated a small aneurysm (*) at the rostral end of the basilar artery. Most of the arteries at the base of the brain can be seen clearly in this reconstruction, including the anterior cerebral (*ACA*), basilar (*BA*), middle cerebral (*MCA*), posterior cerebral (*PCA*), posterior communicating (*PCoA*), posterior inferior cerebellar (*PICA*), superior cerebellar (*SCA*), and vertebral (*VA*) arteries. Features of the base of the skull are also apparent, including the anterior, middle, and posterior fossae (*AF, MF, PF*), the foramen magnum (*FM*), and the petrous temporal bone (*PT*). (Courtesy Dr. Sean O. Casey, University of Minnesota Medical School.)

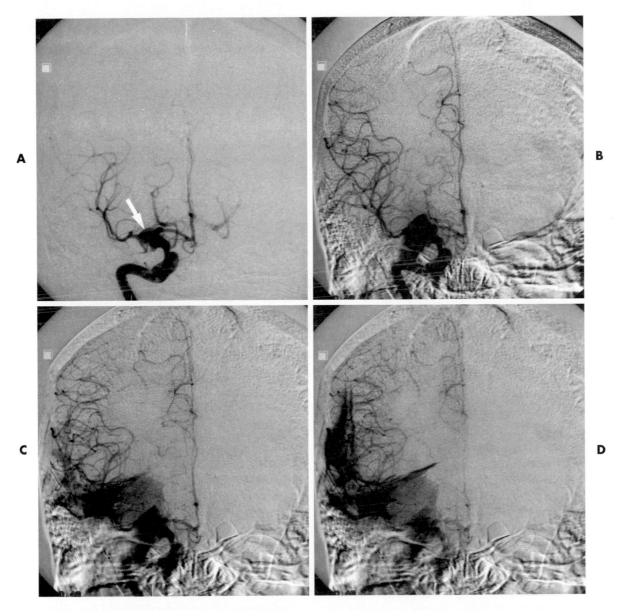

FIGURE 6-22
Four consecutive images obtained at 0.5-second intervals, showing subarachnoid bleeding from an aneurysm. Angiography of the right internal carotid artery of a 48-year-old woman being evaluated for the sudden onset of severe headache revealed an aneurysm of the internal carotid artery (*arrow* in **A**). As the angiographic procedure began, blood and contrast agent escaped from the aneurysm and spread through subarachnoid space (**B-D**). [From Franke CL, Engelshove H: Subarachnoid haemorrhage, *J Neurol Neurosurg Psych* 60:140, 1996.]

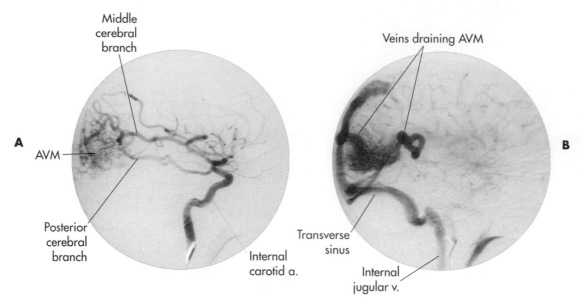

Middle cerebral branch

Veins draining AVM

A

AVM

B

Posterior cerebral branch

Internal carotid a.

Transverse sinus

Internal jugular v.

FIGURE 6-23

An occipital lobe arteriovenous malformation; lateral view, anterior to the right. The AVM is supplied **(A)** by enlarged branches of the middle and posterior cerebral arteries and drains **(B)** through distended venous channels into the straight and superior sagittal sinuses. (From Nolte J, Angevine JB Jr: *The human brain in photographs and diagrams,* St. Louis, 1995, Mosby.)

A SYSTEM OF BARRIERS PARTIALLY SEPARATES THE NERVOUS SYSTEM FROM THE REST OF THE BODY

The concept of a **blood-brain barrier** arose from the early observation that many substances, when injected into the bloodstream, do not gain access to the brain. Such a barrier must consist of more than just an impediment at the junction between blood vessels and brain, because this alone would not prevent substances in tissues around the brain from diffusing into it. The term *blood-brain barrier* therefore is commonly used in a more general sense to refer to the anatomical and physiological complex that controls the movement of substances from the general extracellular fluid of the body to the extracellular fluid of the brain. Using the term in this way, the barrier includes the arachnoid barrier layer and the blood-CSF barrier (Figure 6-24). It also includes a true blood-brain barrier, which consists of rows of tight junctions between adjacent endothelial cells of cerebral capillaries together with a lack of pinocytotic vesicles in these endothelial cells (Figure 6-25). As in the case of the blood-CSF barrier, this barrier is selective. Lipid-soluble substances can diffuse across it, glucose can cross it by a process of facilitated diffusion, but other molecules of similar size and solubility cannot. In addition, various substances can be actively transported in both directions across this endothelial wall. The permeability and transport properties of the barrier are under a degree of neural control.

This complex barrier system can be a mixed blessing. For example, it is rather efficient at keeping microorganisms out of the brain, but it is equally efficient at keeping many antibiotics out. An intracranial infection therefore can be difficult to treat. The development of techniques for reversibly opening the blood-brain barrier and the synthesis of therapeutic agents that can cross an intact blood-brain barrier are both active areas of research.

As discussed in Chapter 5, the capillaries of the choroid plexus are fenestrated, and substances can leave them, only to be stopped by the arrays of tight junctions between adjacent choroid epithelial cells. There are several other locations where the cerebral capillaries are fenestrated and allow free communication between the blood and the brain's extracellular fluid. These additional sites are in contact with the walls of the ventricular system and collectively are termed the **circumventricular organs** (Figures 6-26 and 6-27). They include the pineal gland, portions of the hypothalamus, and a few other structures. Each circumventricular organ probably has either a secretory function or a role in monitoring the composition of the general extracellular fluid; in both cases, free access to the bloodstream seems reasonable in terms of efficient operation. The ependymal cells overlying each circumventricular organ form a partial barrier between the organ and the ventricular CSF, but there is no particular barrier between the organs and the surrounding neural tissue. In this sense, the circumventricular organs appear to be small holes in the blood-brain barrier.

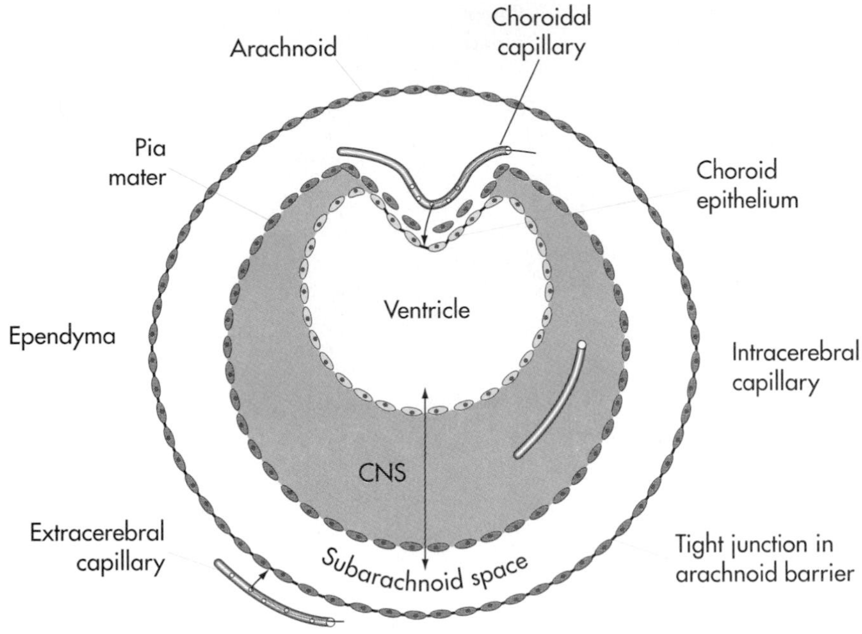

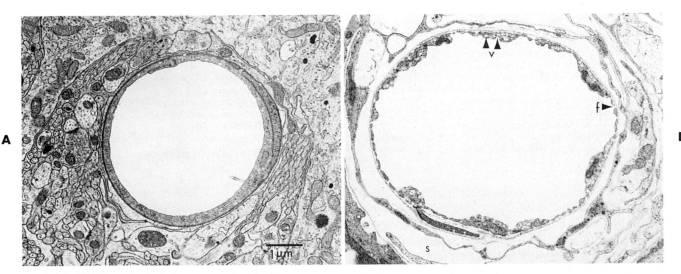

FIGURE 6-24
Barrier systems in and around the brain. Substances can leave extracerebral capillaries but are then blocked by the arachnoid barrier. They can also leave choroidal capillaries but are then blocked by the choroid epithelium. They cannot leave any other capillaries that are inside the arachnoid barrier (except for those in the circumventricular organs). The ventricular and subarachnoid spaces are in free communication with each other, and both communicate with the extracellular space of the brain.

FIGURE 6-25
Capillaries inside and outside the blood-brain barrier. **A,** Capillary in a hypothalamic nucleus (the supraoptic nucleus) of a rat. The continuous endothelial wall and the lack of pinocytotic vesicles are apparent; tight junctions are also present between endothelial cells, but cannot be seen at this magnification. **B,** Capillary in the subfornical organ, which is a circumventricular organ in the roof of the third ventricle near the interventricular foramen. The walls of this capillary are quite permeable and are characterized by fenestrations *(f),* pinocytotic vesicles *(v),* and substantial spaces *(s)* around the capillary. (From Gross PM: The subfornical organ as a model of neurohumoral integration, *Brain Res Bull* 15:65, 1985.)

SUPERFICIAL AND DEEP VEINS DRAIN THE BRAIN

The principal route of venous drainage of the brain is through a system of cerebral veins that empty into the dural venous sinuses and ultimately into the internal jugular veins (Figure 6-28). These veins, like cerebral arteries, can be visualized by angiographic (Figure 6-9, *C*) or dig-

ital (Figure 6-29) techniques. There is also a collection of **emissary veins** connecting extracranial veins with dural sinuses, and a **basilar venous plexus** around the base of the brain that communicates with the **epidural venous plexus** of the spinal cord. These play a relatively minor role in the normal circulatory pattern of the brain, but emissary veins can be important clinically as a path for the spread of infection into the cranial cavity.

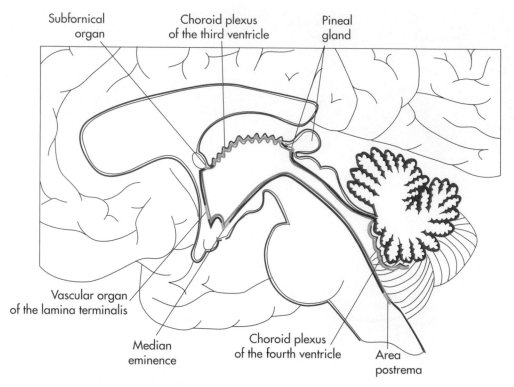

Subfornical organ · Choroid plexus of the third ventricle · Pineal gland · Vascular organ of the lamina terminalis · Median eminence · Choroid plexus of the fourth ventricle · Area postrema

FIGURE 6-26

Sites in the walls of the third and fourth ventricles where a blood-brain barrier is lacking. *Blue* and *green* represent pia mater and ependyma, as in Figure 5-4. *Red* represents areas where capillaries in the ventricular wall are part of the blood-brain barrier, and *pink* represents areas where the capillaries are leaky. The **subfornical organ** is a small nodule in the anterior, superior corner of the third ventricle, adjacent to the interventricular foramina; it has been implicated in the control of fluid balance and drinking behavior. The **vascular organ of the lamina terminalis,** as its name implies, is embedded in the lamina terminalis; it may participate in the control of fluid balance and may be involved in neuroendocrine functions as well. The **median eminence** and the **posterior lobe of the pituitary** (not shown) are major elements of the neuroendocrine system and are discussed further in Chapter 23. The **pineal gland** secretes melatonin, which participates in the control of reproductive behavior in many animals; its role in humans is less clear, but dysfunction of this system may be involved in some affective disorders. The **area postrema,** located in the walls of the caudal end of the fourth ventricle, monitors blood for the presence of toxins and triggers vomiting when appropriate. Some authors also include the choroid plexuses of the lateral, third, and fourth ventricles in the list of circumventricular organs because they lack a blood-brain barrier and are located in ventricular walls.

Cerebral veins are conventionally divided into **superficial** and **deep** groups. In general, the superficial veins lie on the surface of the cerebral hemispheres and most empty into the superior sagittal sinus, whereas the deep veins drain internal structures and eventually empty into the straight sinus. The **basal vein,** described later in this section, drains some cortical areas but is nevertheless considered a deep vein because it also drains some deep structures and eventually empties into the straight sinus.

Cerebral veins are valveless and, in contrast to cerebral arteries, are interconnected by numerous functional anastomoses, both within a group and between superficial and deep groups.

Most Superficial Veins Empty Into the Superior Sagittal Sinus

The superficial veins are quite variable and consist of a superior group that empties into the superior and inferior sagittal sinuses and an inferior group that empties into the transverse and cavernous sinuses (Figure 6-30). Only three

of these veins are reasonably constant from one brain to another. These are (1) the **superficial middle cerebral vein,** which runs anteriorly and inferiorly along the lateral sulcus, draining most of the temporal lobe into the cavernous sinus or into the nearby sphenoparietal sinus; (2) the **superior anastomotic vein** (or **vein of Trolard**), which typically travels across the parietal lobe and connects the superficial middle cerebral vein with the superior sagittal sinus; and (3) the **inferior anastomotic vein** (or **vein of Labbé**), which travels posteriorly and inferiorly across the temporal lobe and connects the superficial middle cerebral vein with the transverse sinus.

Deep Veins Ultimately Empty Into the Straight Sinus

The deep veins are more constant in configuration than are the superficial veins. Because they are found deep in the brain in locations where arteries are small, the deep veins form clinically useful radiological landmarks.

The major deep vein is the **internal cerebral vein** (Figure 6-31), which is formed at the interventricular

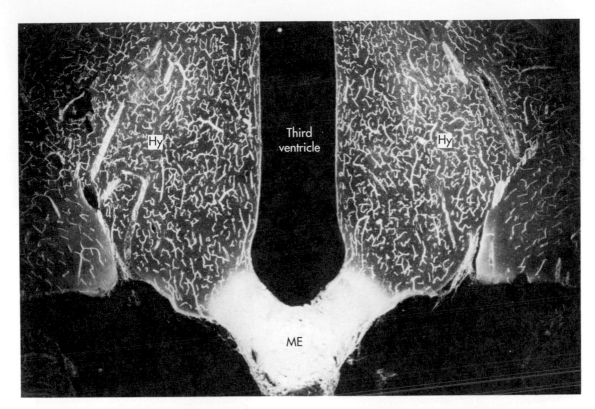

FIGURE 6-27
Macroscopic demonstration of capillaries inside and outside the blood-brain barrier. Horseradish peroxidase was administered intravenously to a monkey, demonstrated histochemically, and viewed in coronal sections using darkfield microscopy. Reaction product fills the median eminence *(ME)*, an area of the hypothalamus that has no blood-brain barrier and is one of the circumventricular organs. However, no reaction product is seen around the numerous capillaries in the remainder of the hypothalamus *(Hy)*. (From Broadwell RD et al: Angioarchitecture of the CNS, pituitary gland, and intracerebral grafts revealed with peroxidase cytochemistry, *J Comp Neurol* 260:47, 1987.)

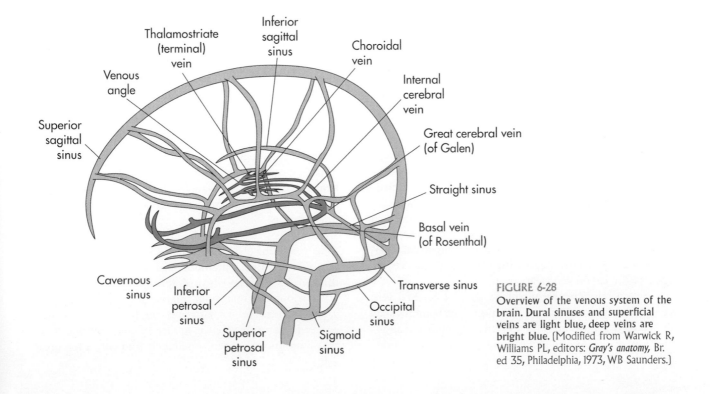

FIGURE 6-28
Overview of the venous system of the brain. Dural sinuses and superficial veins are light blue, deep veins are bright blue. (Modified from Warwick R, Williams PL, editors: *Gray's anatomy*, Br. ed 35, Philadelphia, 1973, WB Saunders.)

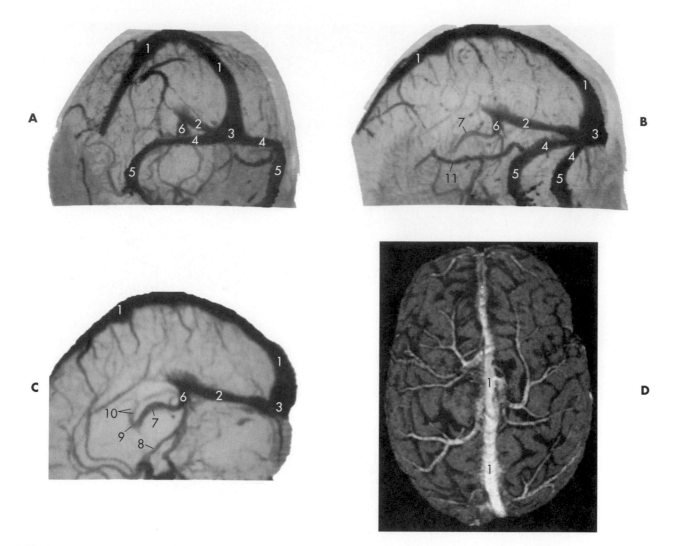

FIGURE 6-29

Cerebral veins reconstructed from contrast-enhanced CTs (**A-C**) or MRIs (**D**) and viewed from the left and behind (**A, B**), from the left (**C**) and from above (**D**). Blood in the superior sagittal *(1)* and straight *(2)* sinuses reaches the confluence of the sinuses *(3)* and flows from there into the transverse *(4)* and sigmoid *(5)* sinuses. Most superficial cortical veins empty into the superior sagittal sinus (**D**) although some empty into other sinuses, as in the vein of Labbé *(11)* joining the transverse sinus. Deep cerebral veins empty into the great vein *(6)*, which in turn joins the straight sinus. The internal cerebral *(7)* and basal *(8)* veins are major tributaries of the great vein. The choroidal, thalamostriate *(10)*, and other veins join at the interventricular foramen and turn posteriorly in the venous angle *(9)* to form the internal cerebral vein of each side. (**A** and **D** courtesy Dr. Sean O. Casey, University of Minnesota Medical School. **B** and **C** from Casey SO et al: Cerebral CT venography, *Radiol* 198:163, 1996.)

foramen by the confluence of two smaller veins, the **septal vein** (so named because it runs posteriorly across the septum pellucidum) and the **thalamostriate** (or **terminal**) **vein** (which travels in the groove between the thalamus and the caudate nucleus (Figure 6-32), draining much of both these structures). Near the interventricular foramen, the thalamostriate vein receives the **choroidal vein,** a tortuous vessel that drains the choroid plexus of the body of the lateral ventricle.

Immediately after forming, the internal cerebral vein bends sharply in a posterior direction. This bend is called the **venous angle** and is used in imaging studies as an indication of the location of the interventricular foramen (Figure 6-29). The paired internal cerebral veins proceed

posteriorly through the transverse cerebral fissure and fuse in the superior cistern to form the unpaired **great cerebral vein** (or **vein of Galen**). The great vein turns superiorly and joins the inferior sagittal sinus to form the straight sinus.

Along its short course, the great vein receives the basal veins (or **veins of Rosenthal**). On each side the basal vein is formed near the optic chiasm by the **deep middle cerebral vein,** which drains the insula, and several other tributaries that drain inferior portions of the basal ganglia and the orbital surface of the frontal lobe. It then proceeds along the medial surface of the temporal lobe, curves around the cerebral peduncle, and enters the great vein.

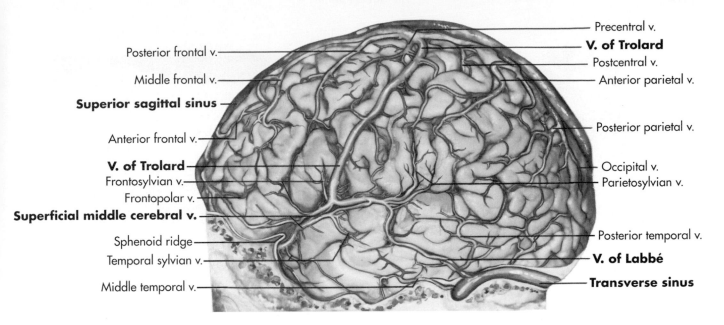

Posterior frontal v.

Middle frontal v.

Superior sagittal sinus

Anterior frontal v.

V. of Trolard
Frontosylvian v.
Frontopolar v.
Superficial middle cerebral v.
Sphenoid ridge
Temporal sylvian v.
Middle temporal v.

Precentral v.
V. of Trolard
Postcentral v.
Anterior parietal v.

Posterior parietal v.

Occipital v.
Parietosylvian v.

Posterior temporal v.
V. of Labbé
Transverse sinus

FIGURE 6-30
Superficial veins of the lateral surface of the brain. Anterior is to the left, and the names of the major veins mentioned in the text are shown in color. (From Oka K et al: Microsurgical anatomy of the superficial veins of the cerebrum, *Neurosurg* 17:711, 1985.)

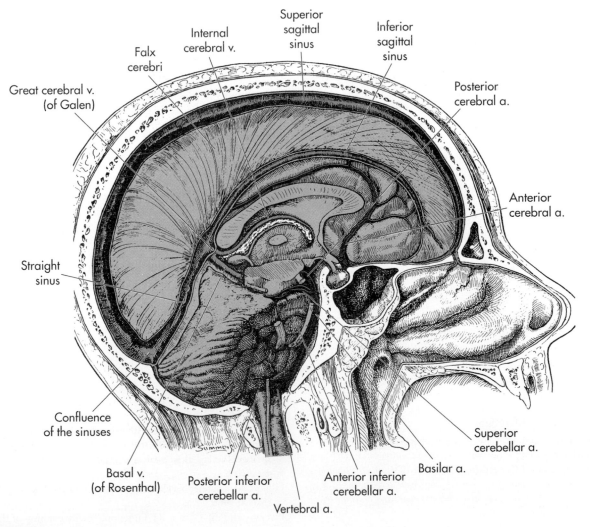

Falx
cerebri

Internal
cerebral v.

Superior
sagittal
sinus

Inferior
sagittal
sinus

Posterior
cerebral a.

Great cerebral v.
(of Galen)

Straight
sinus

Anterior
cerebral a.

Confluence
of the sinuses

Basal v.
(of Rosenthal)

Posterior inferior
cerebellar a.

Vertebral a.

Anterior inferior
cerebellar a.

Basilar a.

Superior
cerebellar a.

FIGURE 6-31
Major tributaries of the straight sinus. (Modified from Mettler FA: *Neuroanatomy*, ed 2, St. Louis, 1948, Mosby.)

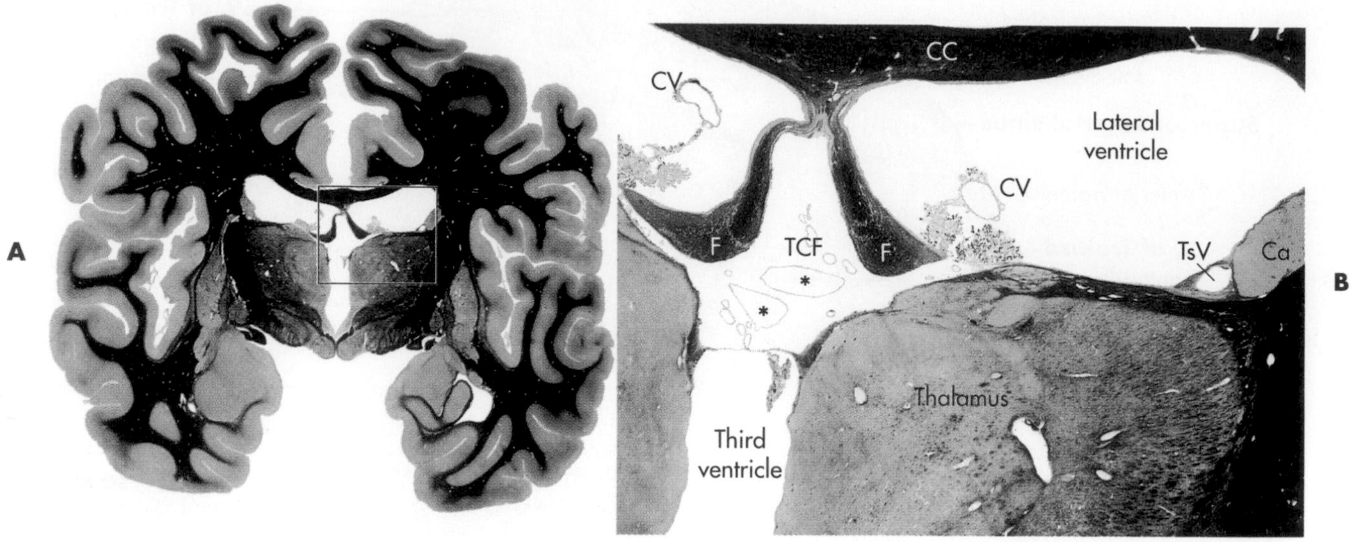

FIGURE 6-32

Deep cerebral veins; the area outlined in the coronal section in **A** is enlarged in **B**. The thalamostriate vein *(TsV)* of each hemisphere, in the groove between the thalamus and the caudate nucleus *(Ca)*, joins the choroidal vein *(CV)* and other deep veins at the interventricular foramen to form the internal cerebral vein. The paired internal cerebral veins (*) turn posteriorly, forming the venous angle, and travel through the transverse cerebral fissure *(TCF)* before joining to form the great vein. *CC*, corpus callosum; *F*, fornix.

In addition to the superficial and deep veins already described, there is a separate, complex collection of veins that serves the cerebellum and brainstem. These drain into the great vein and into the straight, transverse, and petrosal sinuses.

Vascular problems involving the venous system are not seen nearly as often as those involving the arterial supply. This is partly because occlusions and hemorrhages occur less often in the venous system and partly because of the large number of functional anastomoses. Thus a slowly developing occlusion of the anterior portion of the superior sagittal sinus probably would be asymptomatic. Even if such an occlusion developed rapidly, the symptoms might be no more than a transient headache. However, if the occlusion were in a more critical location, such as the posterior portion of the superior sagittal sinus, the consequences would be much more serious and might include headache (due to increased intracranial pressure), seizures, and motor problems. Occlusion of the great vein, although unusual, is particularly serious and can result in coma and death.

SUGGESTED READINGS

Balin BJ et al: Avenues for entry of peripherally administered protein to the central nervous system in mouse, rat and squirrel monkey, *J Comp Neurol* 251:260, 1986. *A discussion of the possible significance of circumventricular organs, peripheral nerve sheaths, endothelial transport, and other potential ways of circumventing the blood-brain barrier.*

Bogousslavsky J, Caplan L, editors: *Stroke syndromes*, New York, 1995, Cambridge University Press.

Borison HL: Area postrema: chemoreceptor circumventricular organ of the medulla oblongata, *Prog Neurobiol* 32:351, 1989. *"The area postrema is the prime body sensor of toxic chemical intrusion that results in nausea and vomiting."*

Brightman MW, Reese TS: Junctions between intimately apposed cell membranes in the vertebrate brain, *J Cell Biol* 40:648, 1969. *A classic paper describing the ultrastructural basis of the blood-brain barrier and blood-CSF barrier.*

Candelise L et al: Prognostic significance of hyperglycemia in acute stroke, *Arch Neurol* 42:661, 1985.

Caplan LR, editor: *Brain ischemia: basic concepts and clinical relevance*, New York, 1995, Springer-Verlag.

Casey SO et al: Cerebral CT venography, *Radiol* 198:163, 1996.

Chorobski J, Penfield W: Cerebral vasodilator nerves and their pathway from the medulla oblongata: with observations on the pial and intracerebral vascular plexus, *Arch Neurol Psychiatr* 28:1257, 1932.

Cobb S, Finesinger JE: Cerebral circulation. XIX. The vagal pathway of the vasodilator impulses, *Arch Neurol Psychiatr* 28:1243, 1932. *Although not all subsequent investigators agree with the findings, this paper provides a straightforward and convincing demonstration of a pathway through the vagus nerve into the brainstem and out through the facial nerve, causing dilation of cortical vessels.*

Damasio H: A computed tomographic guide to the identification of cerebral vascular territories, *Arch Neurol* 40:138, 1983.

Duvernoy HM: *Human brainstem vessels*, New York, 1978, Springer-Verlag. *A painstakingly detailed and magnificently illustrated book.*

Fisher CM: Lacunes: small, deep cerebral infarcts, *Neurol* 15:774, 1965.

Frackowiak RSJ, Friston KJ: Functional neuroanatomy of the human brain: positron emission tomography—a new neuroanatomical technique, *J Anat* 184: 211, 1994.

Galatius-Jensen F, Ringberg V: Anastomosis between the anterior choroidal artery and the posterior cerebral artery demonstrated by angiography, *Radiol* 81:942, 1963.

Gavrilescu T, Kase CS: Clinical stroke syndromes: clinical-anatomical correlations, *Cerebrovasc Brain Metab Rev* 7:218, 1995.

Harik SI: Blood-brain barrier sodium/potassium pump: modulation by central noradrenergic innervation, *Proc Nat Acad Sci US* 83:4067, 1986.

Helgason C et al: Anterior choroidal artery-territory infarction: report of cases and review, *Arch Neurol* 43:681, 1986.

Humberstone MR, Sawle GV: Functional magnetic resonance imaging in clinical neurology, *Eur Neurol* 36:117, 1996.

Kapp JP, Schmidek HH: *The cerebral venous system and its disorders*, Orlando, Fla, 1984, Grune & Stratton.

Koroshetz WJ, Moskowitz MA: Emerging treatments for stroke in humans, *Trends Pharmacol Sci* 17:227, 1996. *A concise review of the multiple fronts on which research into stroke treatment is progressing; conveys a sense of the cautious optimism current in this field.*

Lassen NA, Ingvar DH, Skinhøj E: Brain function and blood flow, *Sci Am* 239(4):62, 1978. *One of the original techniques for studying the activity of different areas of the brain by measuring, with an external gamma-ray camera, the amounts of radioactive isotope delivered to different areas through the arterial circulation.*

Long JB, Holaday JW: Blood-brain barrier: endogenous modulation by adrenal-cortical function, *Science* 277:1580, 1980.

McCulloch J: Perivascular nerve fibers and the cerebral circulation, *Trends Neurosci* 7:135, 1984.

McKinley MJ, Oldfield BJ: *Circumventricular organs*. In Paxinos G, editor: *The human nervous system*, San Diego, 1990, Academic Press.

Millen JW, Woollam DHM: Vascular patterns in the choroid plexus, *J Anat* 87:114, 1953.

Miller AD, Leslie RA: The area postrema and vomiting, *Frontiers Neuroendocrinol* 15:301, 1994.

Newelt EA, editor: *Implications of the blood-brain barrier and its manipulation, vol 1: basic science aspects; vol 2: clinical aspects*, New York, 1989, Plenum Publishing.

O'Connell JEA: Some observations on the cerebral veins, *Brain* 57:484, 1934. *A lucid description of the developmental patterns of the superficial cerebral veins and their relationship to the superior sagittal sinus.*

Oka K et al: Microsurgical anatomy of the superficial veins of the cerebrum, *Neurosurg* 17:711, 1985.

Ono M et al: Microsurgical anatomy of the deep venous system of the brain, *Neurosurg* 15:621, 1984.

Posner MI, Raichle ME: *Images of mind*, New York, 1994, Scientific American Library. *A recent review of contemporary imaging techniques and how they are now being used to study complex mental functions.*

Pullicino PM, Caplan LR, Hommel M, editors: *Cerebral small artery disease (Adv Neurol vol 62)*, New York, 1993, Raven Press.

Rhoton Jr AL, Fujii K, Fradd B: Microsurgical anatomy of the anterior choroidal artery, *Surg Neurol* 12:171, 1979. *Finely detailed and beautifully illustrated.*

Riggs HE, Rupp C: Variation in form of circle of Willis, *Arch Neurol* 8:8, 1963.

Robin ED: The evolutionary advantages of being stupid, *Perspect Biol Med* 16:369, 1972/73. *Turtles may not be very smart, but they don't need much oxygen either and they've been around for a long, long time.*

Saeki N, Rhoton Jr AL: Microsurgical anatomy of the upper basilar artery and posterior circle of Willis, *J Neurosurg* 46:563, 1977.

Sawle GV: Imaging the head: functional imaging, *J Neurol Neurosurg Psych* 58:132, 1995. *A succinct review of the experimental and clinical uses and limitations of PET, SPECT, and functional MRI.*

Scheinberg P: Transient ischemic attacks: an update, *J Neurol Sci* 101:133, 1991.

Sengupta RP, McAllister VL: *Subarachnoid haemorrhage*, Berlin, 1986, Springer-Verlag. *Includes discussions of normal anatomy and its variations, aneurysms, and arteriovenous malformations.*

Siesjö BK, Wieloch T, editors: *Cellular and molecular mechanisms of ischemic brain damage (Adv Neurol vol 71)*, Philadelphia, 1996, Lippincott-Raven Publishers.

Smith PM, Beninger RJ, Ferguson AV: Subfornical organ stimulation elicits drinking, *Brain Res Bull* 38:209, 1995.

Stephens RB, Stilwell DL: *Arteries and veins of the human brain*, Springfield, Ill., 1969, Charles C Thomas. *A well-photographed series of dissections of brains in which the arteries or veins had been injected.*

Sweeney MI et al: Cellular mechanisms involved in brain ischemia, *Can J Physiol Pharmacol* 73:1525, 1995.

Tatu L et al: Arterial territories of human brain: brainstem and cerebellum, *Neurol* 47: 1125, 1996.

Toole JF: *Cerebrovascular disorders*, ed 4, New York, 1990, Raven Press.

Tsukada H et al: Regulation of cerebral blood flow response to somatosensory stimulation through the cholinergic system: a positron emission tomography study in unanesthetized monkeys, *Brain Res* 749:10, 1997.

Van den Bergh R, Vander Eecken H: Anatomy and embryology of cerebral circulation, *Prog Brain Res* 30:1, 1968.

Vander Eecken HM, Adams RD: The anatomy and functional significance of the meningeal arterial anastomoses of the human brain, *J Neuropath Exp Neurol* 12:132, 1953.

Wackenheim A, Braun JP: *The veins of the posterior fossa*, New York, 1978, Springer-Verlag.

Welch K et al: The collateral circulation following middle cerebral branch occlusion, *J Neurosurg* 12:361, 1955. *Discussion of two cases in which much of the middle cerebral artery filled through the anterior cerebral artery.*

Yaşargil MG: *Microneurosurgery, vol IIIA: AVM of the brain, history, embryology, pathological considerations, hemodynamics, diagnostic studies, microsurgical anatomy; vol IVA: CNS tumors: surgical anatomy, neuropathology, neuroradiology, neurophysiology, clinical considerations, operability, treatment options*, Stuttgart, 1987 and 1994, Georg Thieme Verlag. *Beautifully illustrated books with extensive discussions of cerebrovascular anatomy.*

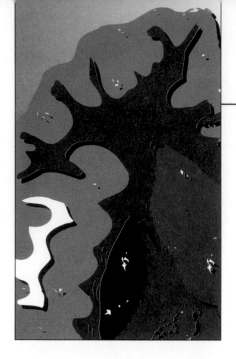

ELECTRICAL SIGNALING BY NEURONS

All they need to know is, it starts at the bottom and goes to the top, and little things come in, and there you go.

Anonymous pediatrician

W e depend on our brains to process and convey huge quantities of information rapidly and reliably using neurons and their axons and synapses, rather than things such as wires and transistors. This is a difficult task, in part because it is substantially more difficult to move electrical signals around in the aqueous medium inside and surrounding neurons than in more conventional electronic devices.★ The solution used by neurons is for current to be carried not by electrons, but rather by the movement of ions, driven by the energy stored in ionic concentration gradients and controlled by molecular switches.

Neurons, as described in Chapter 1, have a complement of organelles comparable to that of other cells, but arrayed in a fashion supporting their signaling functions and their unusual shapes. Like other cells, neurons also are bounded by a semipermeable membrane that is electrically polarized, in this case to a **resting membrane potential** of typically about -65 mv. (By convention the extracellular fluid is considered to be at 0 mv, so a resting potential of -65 mv means the inside of the cell is 65 mv negative to the outside.) Neurons, however, are masters at

moment-to-moment modulation of this membrane potential and use the changes as a signaling mechanism. They use a combination of (1) graded, often relatively slow, local potential changes (e.g., **synaptic potentials, receptor potentials**) that can be compared and summed, and (2) actively propagated potentials **(action potentials)** for conveying information over long distances (Figure 7-1). This chapter describes the biophysical bases for the resting potential, the spread of slow potentials, and the generation and propagation of action potentials. Synaptic potentials are discussed in Chapter 8, and the potentials produced by sensory receptors are addressed in Chapter 9.

A LIPID/PROTEIN MEMBRANE SEPARATES INTRACELLULAR AND EXTRACELLULAR FLUIDS

The electrical signaling properties of neurons are based on ionic concentration gradients between the intracellular and extracellular compartments (Table 7-1). The cell membrane, a complex of a bilayer of lipid molecules with an assortment of protein molecules embedded in it (Figure 7-2), separates these two compartments. Concentration gradients are maintained by a combination of selective permeability characteristics and active pumping mechanisms.

★For example, Hodgkin (1964) pointed out that an axon 1 μm in diameter and 1 m long has the same electrical resistance as 10^{10} miles of 22-gauge copper wire—a length of wire 10 times the distance from here to Saturn!

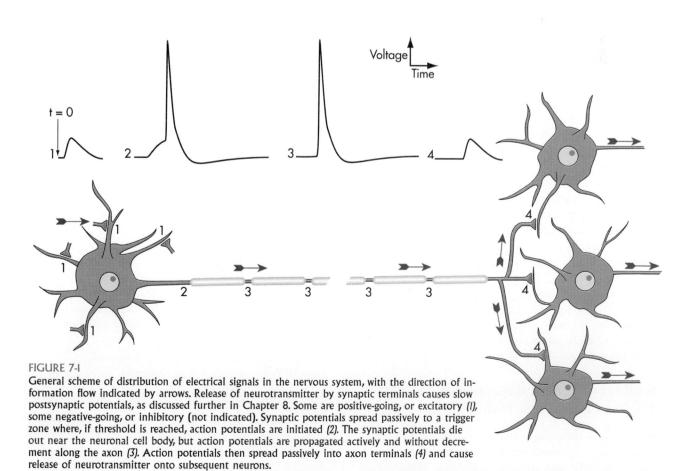

FIGURE 7-1
General scheme of distribution of electrical signals in the nervous system, with the direction of information flow indicated by arrows. Release of neurotransmitter by synaptic terminals causes slow postsynaptic potentials, as discussed further in Chapter 8. Some are positive-going, or excitatory (1), some negative-going, or inhibitory (not indicated). Synaptic potentials spread passively to a trigger zone where, if threshold is reached, action potentials are initiated (2). The synaptic potentials die out near the neuronal cell body, but action potentials are propagated actively and without decrement along the axon (3). Action potentials then spread passively into axon terminals (4) and cause release of neurotransmitter onto subsequent neurons.

Table 7-1   Extracellular and Intracellular Ionic Concentrations for Typical Mammalian Neurons

	Extracellular concentration (mM)	Intracellular concentration (mM)	Equilibrium potential* (37° C)
Na⁺	140	15	+60 mv
K⁺	4	130	-94 mv
Ca²⁺	2.5	.0001†	+136 mv
Cl-	120	5	-86 mv

★The potential at which the electrical gradient balances the concentration gradient. See Appendix 7-B for details.

† The total intracellular Ca^{2+} concentration is 1 to 2 mM, but almost all of it is bound or sequestered. The free cytoplasmic Ca^{2+} concentration is $\leq 10^{-7}$ M.

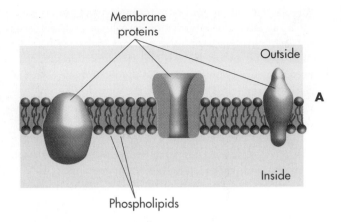

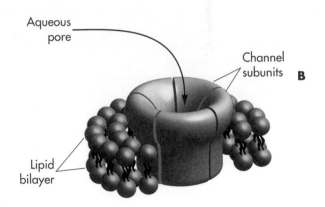

FIGURE 7-2

A, Schematic view of part of a neuronal cell membrane, with membrane proteins embedded in a phospholipid bilayer. **B,** An ion channel consisting of multiple subunits, embedded in the lipid bilayer.

The Lipid Component of the Membrane Is a Diffusion Barrier

The lipid component of the membrane is a double sheet of phospholipids, elongated molecules with polar groups at one end and fatty acid chains at the other (Figure 7-2). This structure leads to differential activities of the two parts of the molecule when exposed to water (itself a polar molecule): the polar groups are **hydrophilic,** interacting with water, and the fatty acid tails are **hydrophobic,** interacting with each other. The consequence is a lipid arrangement in which the fatty acid tails face each other in the center of the membrane and the polar groups face the aqueous solutions inside and outside the neuron. This was a pivotal event in the evolution of life, because the hydrophobic core prevents diffusion of water-soluble substances and allows the maintenance of concentration gradients across the membrane. The ions that carry the currents used for neuronal signaling are among these water-soluble substances, so the lipid bilayer is also an insulator, the barrier across which membrane potentials develop (Figure A-3 in Appendix 7-A). In biophysical terms, the lipid bilayer is not **permeable** to ions. In electrical terms, it functions as a **capacitor,** able to store charges of opposite sign that are attracted to each other but unable to cross the membrane (Appendix 7-A).

Membrane Proteins Regulate the Movement of Solutes Across the Membrane

Embedded in the lipid bilayer is a large assortment of proteins, some exposed on the outer or inner surface, most completely spanning the membrane (Figure 7-2). Different categories of these proteins have distinctive

functions. Some serve as anchor points for cytoskeletal elements; some are surface recognition molecules, participating in physical interactions between neurons and their neighbors or other elements of their extracellular surroundings; some facilitate the movement of lipid-insoluble nutrients such as glucose into neurons. Most important for the purposes of this chapter are proteins that regulate the passage of ions into or out of the cell. A lipid bilayer by itself, as indicated above, does not allow ions to cross and so cannot be the entire basis for electrical signaling. Certain membrane-spanning proteins confer this ability, either by allowing selected ions to flow down electrical or concentration gradients or by pumping them across.

Ions diffuse across the membrane through pores in protein molecules

Some membrane-spanning proteins consist of several subunits surrounding a central aqueous pore (Figure 7-2, B). Ions whose size and charge "fit" the pore can diffuse through it, allowing these proteins to serve as **ion channels.** Hence unlike the lipid bilayer, ion channels have an

Box 7-1   Methods of Measuring Voltages and Currents Across Neuronal Membranes

Our knowledge of the mechanism of electrical signaling by neurons has grown during the twentieth century with the development of more and more sophisticated techniques. Very early work depended on indirect methods, measuring currents and voltages in extracellular spaces outside neurons. In the 1930s Hodgkin, Huxley, Katz, Cole, and others began to take advantage of the huge axons contained in certain invertebrates (Figure 7-21), devising methods to thread wires longitudinally through these axons and record currents and voltages directly across the axon membrane.

At about the same time, other workers found that controlled heating and stretching of capillary tubing until it snaps can produce micropipettes with tip diameters smaller than 1 μm. Filled with a salt solution, these micropipettes can be used as electrodes for recording voltages and currents across

neuronal membranes; the tip diameter is small enough to puncture many kinds of relatively large neurons without damaging them too much (Figure 7-4, *A*).

Micropipette electrodes were a mainstay of neurophysiologists for decades, but they always had shortcomings. They damaged small cells and processes, and even when successful it was only possible to record events across expanses of membranes. A technique that opened up new horizons appeared in the late 1970s, when Neher and Sakmann developed patch clamping (Figure 7-4, *B*). Patch clamping makes it possible to record events across the membrane of small cells and processes, but more remarkably it allows recordings of the activity of individual ion channels in patches of membrane (Figure 7-17)!

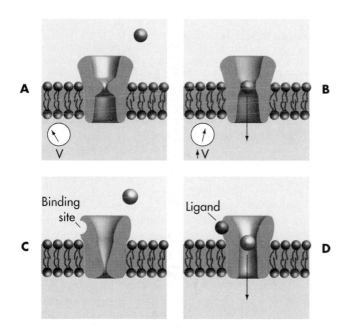

FIGURE 7-3
Gating properties of ion channels. Voltage-gated channels respond to appropriate voltage changes (in this example, to decreased negativity inside the cell, as in the case of voltage-gated sodium channels) by switching from a closed (**A**) to an open (**B**) state. Ligand-gated channels bind specific ligands when available and switch from a closed (**C**) to an open (**D**) state.

appreciable permeability (or **conductance★**) to at least some ions. In electrical terms, they function as **resistors,†** allowing a predictable amount of current flow in response to a voltage across them (Appendix 7-A). Although many different ion channels have been described, they have some characteristics in common:

1. **Multiple states.** Most or all ion channels can exist in two or more different, stable conformations. The different conformations fall into two general categories: open, in which the pore is available for ions to traverse, and closed, in which the pore is occluded enough to prevent ion flow. Open channels have high conductance and closed channels have low conductance, so ion channels are variable resistors; this is the key to their role in membrane potential changes. Remarkably, the transitions between these different conductance states can be observed directly using **patch–clamp** techniques (Box 7-1, Figure 7-17). Most channels in resting neuronal membranes are closed and respond to particular stimuli by opening.

2. **Gating.** The opening and closing of an individual ion channel is a probabilistic event, and the channel can flip between these states nearly instantaneously. Each type of channel is tuned to certain factors that affect the probability of its being open or closed.★ Some channels open in response to changes in membrane potential and are referred to as **voltage-gated** channels (Figure 7-3, *A* and *B*). The best understood of these is the voltage-gated sodium channel that underlies the action potential (Figure 7-10). Others open or close in response to the binding of signal molecules (Figure 7-3, *C* and *D*). The bound molecule is called a **ligand,** so these are **ligand-gated** channels. The best known of these are postsynaptic receptors that bind specific neurotransmitters and change their permeability in response (see Chapter 8),

---

★*Conductance* and *permeability* technically have slightly different meanings but are commonly used interchangeably. A membrane permeable to a given ion easily conducts currents carried by that ionic species.
†Resistance is simply the inverse of conductance. A channel with high conductance has little resistance to current flow and vice versa.

★Discussions in this and other chapters may seem to imply that populations of channels as a whole open or close (slowly or suddenly) in response to some stimulus. The individual channels in such populations, however, exist in an equilibrium state, flipping back and forth between different states; the only thing that changes is the probability of being in one or another state. A population of channels, each with a slowly increasing probability of being open, would seem macroscopically like a population of channels all opening slowly at the same time.

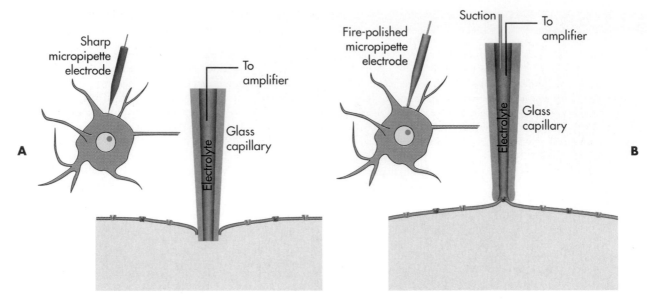

FIGURE 7-4
Recording electrical activity across neuronal membranes using sharp microelectrodes (**A**) and patch-clamp electrodes (**B**). If the tip of a sharp micropipette electrode is small enough, it can be used to impale relatively large neurons with minimal injury. The punctured cell membrane seals around the electrode, and transmembrane potentials and potential changes such as those shown in Figure 7-1 can be recorded. Patch-clamp electrodes are generally larger and are prepared with smooth, fire-polished tips. Contact with the surface of a neuron, combined with gentle suction, causes the neuronal membrane to seal onto the pipette tip. Once the seal is established, a series of additional maneuvers allow various recording arrangements: current passing through the attached area of membrane can be measured (Figure 7-17); the attached area of membrane can be perforated, creating electrical continuity between the pipette and the cell's interior and allowing measurement of voltage changes across the cell membrane (referred to as *whole–cell recordings* (Figure 7-13); or the attached membrane patch can be torn away from the cell and exposed to controlled solutions of various sorts while measuring current flows.

but other channels bind intracellular ligands released in response to various stimuli. Some channels are **thermally gated,** allowing the neurons that contain them to function as miniature thermometers or as thermal injury detectors (see Chapters 9 and 23). Finally, some channels are **mechanically gated.** A prominent example is the receptor cells of the inner ear (see Figure 14-6), but others are known.

3. **Selectivity.** The central pores of ion channels are not wide enough to let any and all ions traverse them. Rather, the size of the pore and the nature of the amino acid residues lining it are such that some ions can diffuse through more easily than others. Some channels are minimally selective and may simply distinguish between small anions and small cations. Others are highly selective and may be, for example, hundreds of times more permeable to sodium ions than to potassium ions. Small differences in amino acid sequences are sufficient to change the selectivity of a channel, and many channel types are closely related to each other. All the voltage-gated channels are the products of one closely related family of genes, and ligand-gated postsynaptic receptors are the products of two other families.

The many different types of ion channels for the most part are not distributed uniformly in neuronal membranes.

Rather, neurons somehow manage to place them preferentially in sites that make functional sense. For example, although the channels that determine the resting membrane potential are widely distributed, voltage-gated sodium channels are grouped so that only certain regions of the neuron can generate action potentials. Similarly, appropriate ligand-gated channels are located in postsynaptic membranes across from presynaptic terminals and not in other locations. This regional distribution of channels and other membrane proteins forms much of the basis for the functional specialization of different parts of each neuron.

The chemical differences between channel types, although often subtle, are nevertheless sufficient to allow pharmacological manipulation of particular channels. This is commonly exploited in the treatment of disease states. It has also become increasingly clear in recent years that some diseases are themselves the result of abnormal functioning of particular channel types.

The number and selectivity of ion channels determine the membrane potential

The importance of ion channels in the development of the resting membrane potential is indicated in Figure 7-5. A lipid bilayer separating intracellular and extracellular fluids with the ionic concentrations shown in Table 7-1

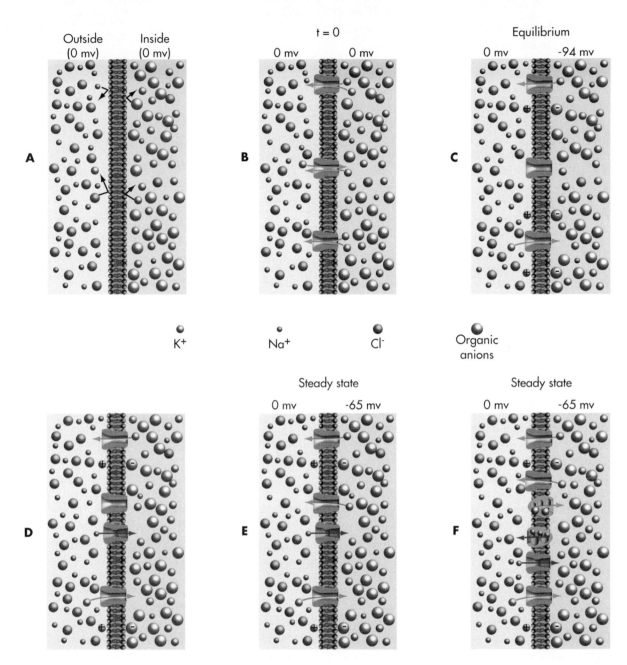

FIGURE 7-5

Development and maintenance of a resting membrane potential. **A,** A lipid bilayer by itself is impermeable, allowing no charge separation to develop. **B,** Adding K+ channels initially results in net movement of K+ ions out of the cell (K+ ions are free to move in either direction, but because there are more inside the cell more will move from inside to outside than in the opposite direction). **C,** At equilibrium, a small number of excess K+ ions on the outside of the membrane, counterbalanced by anions on the inner surface of the membrane, account for the resting membrane potential. K+ ions still flow through their channels, but now equal numbers move out (down the concentration gradient) and in (down the voltage gradient). **D,** Addition of a small number of Na+ channels causes a small inward movement of Na+ ions down their concentration gradient. **E,** A steady state is reached in which equal numbers of cations move inward and outward across the membrane. However, there is a net inward movement of Na+ and outward movement of K+. **F,** The Na+/K+ ATPase is an exchange pump that compensates for the net Na+ and K+ fluxes in **E.**

would not be expected to develop a membrane potential. Even though all the ion species involved (including Ca^{2+}, which is not indicated in Figure 7-5 for reasons of simplicity) are unequally distributed, the impermeability of the membrane would prevent them from moving down their concentration gradients (Figure 7-5, *A*). The number of positive charges and negative charges on each side of the membrane would be identical.

Consider what would happen if ion channels selectively permeable only to K^+ were added to such a membrane (Figure 7-5, *B*). K^+ ions would be equally free to diffuse into or out of the cell through these channels. However, simply because there are so many more K^+ ions inside the cell than outside, more K^+ ions would move out than in, that is, K^+ ions would flow out of the cell down the K^+ concentration gradient). This would leave behind a number of intracellular negative charges. Because opposite charges attract each other, the excess intracellular negative charges would attract K^+ ions back into the cell. At a time determined by the number of channels available for K^+ ion movement, the concentration gradient driving K^+ out of the cell would be exactly counterbalanced by the intracellular negativity; the K^+ current moving out of the cell would be equal and opposite to the K^+ current moving into the cell (Figure 7-5, *C*). The system at this point is in **equilibrium:** no energy is required to maintain it in this state. The membrane potential at which this equilibrium is reached is the **potassium equilibrium potential (V_K);** its value can be calculated using a logarithmic relationship called the **Nernst equation,** knowing only the intracellular and extracellular K^+ concentrations, the temperature, and some physical constants (Appendix 7-B). Each ion species that is unequally distributed across the membrane has an equilibrium potential that can be calculated in the same way (Table 7-1); this indicates the membrane potential that would develop if the membrane were permeable solely to this type of ion.

The initial net outward movement of K^+ ions required to establish this membrane potential is actually extremely small—just enough to charge up the membrane capacitance—and no significant change in intracellular or extracellular K^+ concentration results. For example, the net outward movement of only about 175 million K^+ ions is enough to establish the predicted membrane potential of -94 mv across the membrane of a spherical cell 100 μm in diameter. Although this sounds like a lot of ions, a cell this size with an intracellular K^+ concentration of 130 mM contains about 4×10^{13} K^+ ions, so the net loss of K^+ ions required to establish this membrane potential is less than 0.001% of the starting number! This is a common theme in electrical signaling by neurons: substantial electrical signals can be generated by moving relatively minuscule numbers of ions, so that intracellular and extracellular ionic concentrations change little over brief periods of time. (As will be seen a little later in this chapter, however, active pumping mechanisms are required to maintain ionic concentration gradients over long periods.)

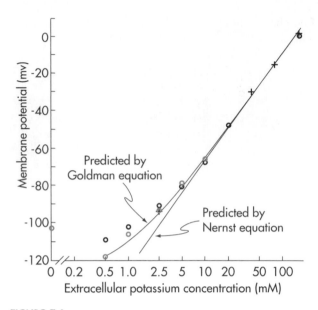

FIGURE 7-6
The membrane potential of frog muscle fibers at different K^+ concentrations in the bathing solution. (The membranes of skeletal muscle fibers have properties similar to those of neurons.) *Crosses* indicate measurements made after the muscle fiber had equilibrated with a new K^+ concentration for 10 to 60 minutes, *blue circles* 20 to 60 seconds after an abrupt increase in K^+ concentration, and *green circles* 20 to 60 seconds after an abrupt decrease. The curves fitted to the data are provided by equations described in Appendix 7-B. (Redrawn from Hodgkin AL, Horowicz P: The influence of potassium and chloride ions on the membrane potential of single muscle fibers, *J Physiol* 148:127, 1959.)

The resting membrane potential of typical neurons is heavily influenced, but not completely determined, by the potassium concentration gradient

The scenario just developed is actually close to the situation in typical neurons, whose membrane at rest is dominated by a steady potassium conductance. Hence the resting membrane potential of typical neurons is near the potassium equilibrium potential. Increases in extracellular potassium concentration cause the membrane potential to become less negative, almost by the amount predicted by the Nernst equation (Figure 7-6). However, the membrane is never quite as negative as the potassium equilibrium potential, and the deviation becomes greater the lower the extracellular potassium concentration becomes.

The basis for this deviation from the membrane potential predicted by the Nernst equation is the additional presence of a relatively small resting permeability to Na^+ ions, as indicated in Figure 7-5, *D* and *E*. If one imagines this permeability being added to the K^+-permeable membrane of Figure 7-5, *C*, an inward flow of Na^+ ions results, driven not only by the interior negativity of the cell but also by the Na^+ concentration gradient (Figure 7-5, *D*). The inward Na^+ current would be small because the Na^+ conductance is small, but it would nevertheless move positive charges into the cell, making its interior less negative. This in turn would cause the membrane potential to move slightly away from V_K, creating a small voltage gradient that drives K^+ ions out of the cell. Assuming for a moment that concentrations remain constant, a **steady state** is reached in which the small inward Na^+ current (small because the Na^+ conductance is small) is exactly counterbalanced by a small outward K^+ current (small because the conductance is relatively large but the voltage gradient is small). The exact membrane potential at this steady state is somewhere between V_K and V_{Na}, dictated by the relative magnitudes of the K^+ and Na^+ permeabilities (Appendix 7-B). Typical neurons have resting Na^+ permeabilities that are 1% to 10% as great as the resting K^+ permeability, so the resting membrane potential is a weighted average of V_K and V_{Na}, around -65 mv.

Concentration gradients are maintained by membrane proteins that pump ions

There is a major difference between the equilibrium condition that exists when the membrane is permeable only to one ion (Figure 7-5, C) and the steady state that is achieved when the membrane is permeable to more than one ion (Figure 7-5, E). In the equilibrium condition the equal and opposite current flows involve the same ion (e.g., K^+), so no concentration changes ensue and no energy is required to maintain the condition. In the steady state condition the equal and opposite current flows involve different ions and eventually result in concentration changes. In the typical neuronal situation, the small but constant inward Na^+ and outward K^+ currents, if uncompensated, would slowly dissipate the Na^+ and K^+ concentration gradients across the membrane. The equilibrium potential for ions with no concentration gradient is 0 mv, so the membrane potential would slowly fade away. Another class of membrane proteins called **ion pumps** allows this dilemma to be circumvented by neurons, and indeed by all cells. The best studied of these is a membrane-spanning **Na^+/K^+ ATPase,** so called because it uses the energy released by hydrolysis of ATP to move Na^+ ions out of the cell and K^+ into the cell (Figure 7-5, F). However, Ca^{2+} ions or Cl^- ions can also move into cells in response to certain kinds of stimuli, and specific membrane pumps are available to redistribute them as well. All of them pump at concentration-sensitive rates, so they speed up when there are more ions to be extruded or recaptured.

INPUTS TO NEURONS CAUSE SLOW, LOCAL POTENTIAL CHANGES

We think of conventional electronic devices as designed *not* to distort, but rather to transmit signals over long distances unchanged, accurately amplifying them as necessary. Neurons do not seem to be very well designed for

transmitting information over long distances—axons, relative to metal wires, are poor conductors; their insulation (except where myelin is present) is not very good; and the input signals to neurons become smeared out over space and time because of membrane resistance and capacitance. As will be seen in this chapter and the next, however, these apparent shortcomings are precisely what allows neurons to compare and summate numerous inputs and make determinations about appropriate outputs.

Changes in the relative permeabilities of the membrane to ions such as K^+ and Na^+ (and Ca^{2+} and Cl^-) are the basis for electrical signaling by neurons. Increasing the Na^+ permeability, for example, would cause an increased inward Na^+ current and **depolarization**★ of the membrane (i.e., decreased internal negativity). Increasing the K^+ permeability would **hyperpolarize** the membrane (i.e., make the inside more negative by moving its potential even closer to V_K). Such permeability changes may be caused by the action of ligand-gated channels at postsynaptic sites (Chapter 8) or by the action of stimulus-gated channels in the membranes of sensory receptors (Chapter 9). In either case, the net effect is a change in current flow through the affected channels for as long as the probability of their being open remains altered. The consequences of a local current injection such as this are dictated largely by the passive electrical properties of adjacent areas of neuronal membrane—their resistance and capacitance. These passive electrical properties are referred to as the **cable properties** of neurons.

Membrane Capacitance and Resistance Determine the Speed and Extent of the Response to a Current Pulse

Abruptly increasing the membrane conductance to some ions causes an abrupt change in the rate at which it crosses the membrane (i.e., it causes a rapid change in current flow either into or out of the neuron's cytoplasm). The time course and spatial distribution of the voltage changes caused by this current flow depend on the properties of both the cytoplasm and the membrane of the neuron, with major implications for the way signals spread along neuronal membranes. The following discussion of applicable principles is based on inward current flow (e.g., of Na^+ ions), but the same considerations apply for outward current flow.

Membranes have a time constant, allowing temporal summation

In the simple (though unlikely) case of uniform conductance changes over the entire surface of a spherical cell, the current flow and voltage changes across all parts of the

---

★Strictly speaking, *depolarization* should mean a movement of the membrane potential toward 0 mv. As the terms are commonly used, however, depolarization and hyperpolarization mean changes of the membrane potential in a positive or negative direction from some starting point.

membrane will be identical. A step increase in conductance, producing a step increase in current flow, will cause an exponential increase in membrane voltage because of the parallel resistance and capacitance of the membrane (Figure 7-7). The final value of the voltage change is determined by the product of the current and the membrane resistance (V = IR), whereas the **time constant** for reaching this final voltage is determined by the product of the membrane resistance and capacitance (τ = RC; Appendix 7-A). Hence membranes with many open channels (high conductance, low resistance) will have relatively short time constants, and membranes with few open channels will have longer time constants. Ten msec would be a typical neuronal time constant, although shorter and longer values are common.

The membrane capacitance similarly slows the decay of voltage at the end of the conductance change, with a similar time constant. A brief conductance change may cause only partial charging of the membrane capacitance (Figure 7-7, C). This seemingly disadvantageous slowing of electrical signals actually has an important function. Because signals are spread out over time, multiple inputs that occur at not quite the same time can partially reinforce each other. This phenomenon is called **temporal summation,** and its limits are dictated largely by the membrane time constant.

Larger diameter neuronal processes have longer length constants

Conductance changes in real neurons are usually localized (e.g., to a postsynaptic site on a dendrite), so the effects of distance from the conductance change must also be considered in determining the resulting potential changes. The effects of just the resistive elements are indicated in Figure 7-8, *A*. Current entering a dendrite (or any other part of a neuron) begins to leak out immediately and cause a voltage change across the membrane, so less is present a few μm from the site of entry. At this point a few μm away, some percentage of the remaining current leaks out (causing a smaller voltage change), so even less remains. The amount of current remaining at any given point declines exponentially with distance from the site of entry, until eventually all the current leaks out. The distance required for the current (and for the voltage change) to decline to 1/e (37%) of the value at the site of entry is called the **length constant.** Typical length constants for neuronal processes are a few hundred μm, and constants of more than a millimeter or two are unusual. Hence the passive spread of signals in neurons (called **electrotonic spread** or **electrotonic conduction**) is said to be **decremental,** indicating that the signal becomes smaller with distance.

The factors influencing the length constant of a neuronal process can be appreciated by considering the lo-

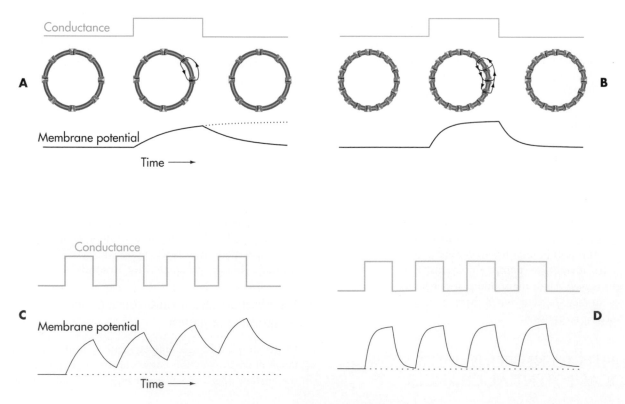

FIGURE 7-7
Membrane time constants and temporal summation. **A,** High membrane resistance results in a long time constant; the membrane capacitance may not be completely charged *(dashed line)* at the end of a relatively brief conductance change. **B,** Low membrane resistance results in a short time constant. Neurons or neuronal processes with long time constants **(C)** display more temporal summation than neurons with short time constants **(D).**

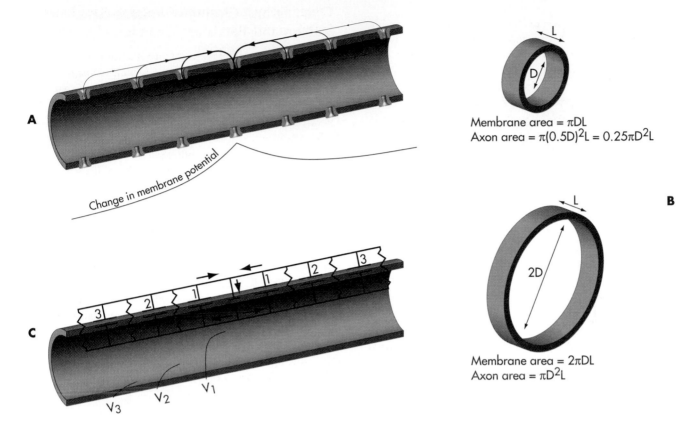

Membrane area = πDL
Axon area = π(0.5D)²L = 0.25πD²L

Membrane area = 2πDL
Axon area = πD²L

FIGURE 7-8
Passive spread of voltage changes in neuronal processes. **A,** Progressively less of a steady current entering a neuronal process at one location remains with increasing distance from the point of entry. Hence the voltage change declines exponentially with distance from the point of entry. **B,** Influence of the diameter of a neuronal process on its length constant. Membrane area (and conductance) increases directly with the diameter, whereas cross-sectional area (and conductance) increases with its square. Hence doubling the diameter doubles the membrane conductance but quadruples the longitudinal conductance. **C,** Effects of membrane capacitance on the longitudinal spread of voltage changes. The final value of the voltage change at any given point is dictated by membrane and longitudinal (not indicated) resistances. However, the rate of reaching this final value becomes progressively slower with distance, as more and more capacitance is added.

cations of conductance in the path of current flow (Figure 7-8, *B*). At any given point along the interior of the process, current has two alternative paths: it can either cross the membrane and leave, or it can continue along longitudinally through the process. The higher the membrane conductance, the more likely the current is to leave; the higher the longitudinal conductance of the process, the more likely the current is to continue flowing longitudinally. For a given length of neuronal process, the conductance of the membrane is determined by the number of available ion channels, which in turn is proportional to the area of membrane covering the process. The membrane area, and therefore its conductance, is proportional to the *diameter* of the process. In contrast, each little cross-sectional bit of cytoplasm represents a longitudinal path for current flow, so the longitudinal conductance increases with the cross-sectional area of the process and is proportional to the *square of the diameter*. Hence as dendrites and axons get larger, the longitudinal conductance increases more than the mem-

brane conductance does, so the length constant increases. (Alternatively, keeping the diameter of the process constant and decreasing the number of ion channels would also increase the length constant.★)

Membrane capacitance, as in the case of uniform current flow, does not affect the final value of the voltage change at any point along the dendrite. It does, however, cause the rate of change of the voltage to diminish progressively with distance because the total capacitance increases with distance (Figure 7-8, *C*).

Just as multiple inputs that are temporally close to each other can summate, so too can inputs that are physically close to each other exhibit **spatial summation** (Figure 7-9).

★Continuing with the water-flow analogy used in Appendix 7-A, a dendrite with a very short length constant is like a garden hose with many gaping holes in its walls; a dendrite with a very long length constant is like a fire hose with a few pinholes.

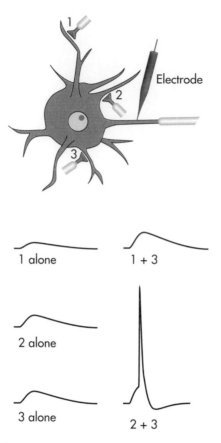

Electrode

1 alone   1 + 3

2 alone

3 alone   2 + 3

FIGURE 7-9
Spatial summation. Multiple simultaneous voltage changes (in this example, synaptic potentials) add to each other, to a degree determined by their relative proximity to each other and by various space constants. Summation may be sufficient to bring the neuron's trigger zone to threshold.

ACTION POTENTIALS CONVEY INFORMATION OVER LONG DISTANCES

Spatial summation has computational advantages for neurons because the degree of interaction between signals can be influenced by their relative locations. On the other hand, it comes at a price. The decremental conduction of slow potentials, such as synaptic potentials, means that they will die out completely within a few millimeters of the site where they are generated. Some neurons that are small and only need to convey information over distances that are short relative to their length constants can rely on electrotonic conduction. Most neurons, however, must convey signals over distances equal to hundreds or even thousands of length constants. **Action potentials** (commonly referred to as **spikes** or **nerve impulses** because of their shape in time), actively propagated over long distances and mediated by special voltage-gated ion channels, take care of this part of the signaling process (Figure 7-1).

Opening and Closing of Voltage-Gated Sodium and Potassium Channels Underlies the Action Potential

We are accustomed to thinking about voltages much larger than membrane potentials, as in the 110-volt circuits that run U.S. household appliances and the 1.5- to 9-volt batteries that power portable electronic devices. By comparison, a membrane potential of -65 mv seems puny. However, the membrane potential is developed across a membrane only 5 to 10 nm thick, resulting in a very large electric field across the membrane (130,000 volts/cm across a 5-nm membrane!). Neuronal membranes contain an assortment of ion channels whose conformation changes in response to fluctuations in this electric field, changing their probability of being open or closed. Two of these in particular, a voltage-gated Na^+ channel and a voltage-gated K^+ channel, are centrally involved in the generation of action potentials. (Neurons also contain several varieties of voltage-gated Ca^{2+} channels, but these are usually not major factors in carrying the current for electrical signaling. Instead, they often admit sufficient Ca^{2+} to trigger other intracellular processes.)

The voltage-gated Na^+ channels have three states (Figure 7-10). In their "resting" state at the normal neuronal resting potential, the probability of being open is very low. Membrane depolarization rapidly increases their probability of being open. After a millisecond or so in this mostly-open state, the channels spontaneously move into an inactivated state in which they are closed and will not reopen in response to further depolarization. Repolarizing the membrane toward resting potential moves the channels from this inactivated state back to the original resting state. Voltage-gated K^+ channels also open in response to depolarization, but more slowly. Once open, however, they do not inactivate; their probability of being open remains high as long as the membrane is depolarized.

Membranes with sufficient densities of these channels have the special property of **electrical excitability** (Figures 7-11). In response to hyperpolarizing current, they show normal charging curves, but depolarization is different. In a membrane without voltage-gated Na^+ channels, depolarization draws K^+ ions out of the cell, at a rate determined by the resting K^+ conductance and the magnitude of the depolarization. In an excitable membrane, depolarization begins to cause the voltage-gated Na^+ channels to open and a small inward Na^+ current develops. For small depolarizations, the expected outward K^+ current is equal and opposite and balances the Na^+ influx. At some level of depolarization, the inward Na^+ current exceeds the driving force for the compensating K^+ current and adds a little extra depolarization of its own. Reaching this **threshold** causes more voltage-gated Na^+ channels to open and more depolarization, initiating an explosive increase in Na^+ conductance. In less than a millisecond, most available Na^+ channels enter the mostly-open state, Na^+ conductance

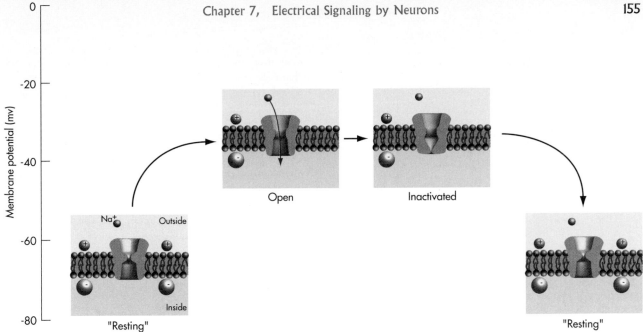

FIGURE 7-10

The Na$^+$ channel cycle. At the normal resting membrane potential, most voltage-gated Na$^+$ channels are closed. Depolarization increases the probability of opening. Once open, the channels enter a closed, inactivated state until the membrane is repolarized.

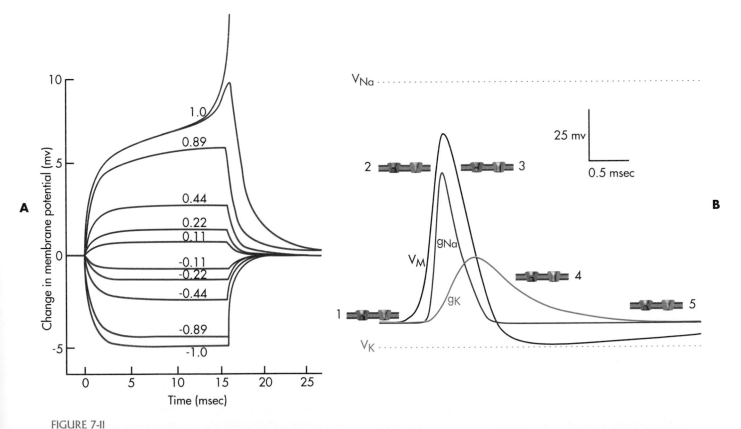

FIGURE 7-11

Generation of action potentials. **A,** Small hyperpolarizing (negative numbers) current pulses delivered to an unmyelinated axon (from a crab) result in smooth charging curves. Depolarizing current pulses result in mirror-image charging curves until a critical level of depolarization is reached (current magnitude = 1.0). At this threshold level, half the current pulses are followed by a return to baseline and half induce an action potential that drives the membrane potential off scale. The magnitude of each current pulse is indicated as a fraction of the threshold value. **B,** Changes in Na$^+$ and K$^+$ conductance (g_{Na}, g_K) and in channel states underlying action potentials. At rest (1) most voltage-gated Na$^+$ channels and many voltage-gated K$^+$ channels are closed; many more K$^+$ channels than Na$^+$ channels are open, however, so the membrane potential (V_M) is near the K$^+$ equilibrium potential (V_K). Suprathreshold depolarization causes most voltage-gated Na$^+$ channels to open (2), and the membrane potential moves toward the sodium equilibrium potential (V_{Na}). Thereafter (3) the Na$^+$ channels inactivate, and voltage-gated K$^+$ channels begin to open. The resulting decrease in Na$^+$ conductance and increase in K$^+$ conductance repolarizes the membrane, and the voltage-gated Na$^+$ channels revert to their resting state (4); extra K$^+$ channels open during this period cause an afterhyperpolarization until the baseline state is reached again (5). [**A** redrawn from Hodgkin AL, Rushton WAH: The electrical constants of a crustacean nerve fibre, *Proc Royal Soc* B133:444, 1946. Voltage and conductance records in **B** redrawn from Hodgkin AL, Huxley AF: A quantitative description of membrane current and its application to conduction and excitation in nerve, *J Physiol* 117:500, 1952.]

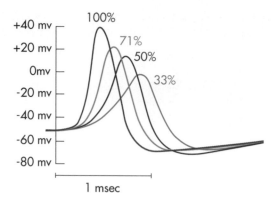

FIGURE 7-12
Dependence of the peak voltage reached during action potentials on the extracellular Na^+ concentration. The number accompanying each record is the percentage of sea water in a sea water–isotonic dextrose solution bathing a squid axon. (Redrawn from Hodgkin AL, Katz B: The effect of sodium ions on the electrical activity of the giant axon of the squid, *J Physiol* 108:37, 1949.)

reaches a level as much as 50 times greater than the K^+ conductance, and the membrane potential moves past 0 mv and almost reaches V_{Na} (Figure 7-12). As the membrane potential moves toward V_{Na}, two things happen to terminate the action potential: the voltage-gated Na^+ channels inactivate and close, and the voltage-gated K^+ channels open. The K^+ channels stay open for a few milliseconds, causing a brief **afterhyperpolarization,** during which the membrane potential moves even closer to V_K than it is in the resting state. This repolarization allows the voltage-gated Na^+ channels to return to the resting state, ready for the initiation of another action potential.

Action potentials are stereotyped, **all–or–none** events— if threshold is reached they occur, if not they don't. They are always depolarizing events, and for a given neuronal type they are all the same size and duration. In these and several other ways they are fundamentally different from the slow potentials discussed earlier in this chapter (Table 7-2). Neurons use both kinds of potential changes to perform their information-processing roles. They receive a variety of inputs that spread electrotonically, summing spatially and temporally, eventually reaching a zone with a low threshold for generating action potentials (Figure 7-13). The low-threshold zone (assumed in most instances to be the initial segment of the axon) is a kind of analog-to-digital converter, the site where slowly fluctuating membrane potential changes are converted into a series of brief action potentials separated by varying intervals.

Action Potentials Are Followed by Brief Refractory Periods

The two-part repolarization process used by neurons to terminate an action potential has consequences for the production of subsequent action potentials. For a brief pe-

riod after the peak of an action potential, so many Na^+ channels are inactivated that another impulse cannot be generated, no matter how much the membrane is depolarized. This is the **absolute refractory period** (Figure 7-14, *A*). This grades into a **relative refractory period** during which some but not all Na^+ channels have returned to the resting state. A larger percentage of this reduced population of Na^+ channels must be activated to initiate an impulse, and this in turn requires more depolarization than after full recovery. In addition, the voltage-gated K^+ channels are still open. This shortens the time constant and the length constant, making it more difficult to depolarize the membrane to threshold. Both refractory periods together last only a few milliseconds, but they have important implications for the production and propagation of action potentials.

Refractory periods limit the repetition rate of action potentials

Continued depolarization of a neuron, by current injection through an electrode (Figure 7-15) or through a post-synaptic ion channel, causes the production of repetitive action potentials. The greater the depolarization, the more frequent the action potentials. At low frequencies, the firing rates of some neurons are remarkably linear functions of the depolarizing stimulus (Figure 7-16, *A*); others may fire in bursts or have other nonlinear characteristics (Figure 7-16, *B* and *C*). The refractory periods, however, set upper limits on firing frequency (Figure 7-14, *B* and *C*). A second impulse cannot be generated during the rising phase of an action potential (because all the voltage-gated Na^+ channels are already in the process of opening) or during most of the falling phase (the absolute refractory period). Because these two phases together typically last about 1 msec, the absolute upper limit on action potential frequency is about 1 kHz. In addition, the relative refractory period makes it difficult to reach this upper limit, and most neurons have maximum firing frequencies considerably lower than 1 kHz.

Toxins and Disease Processes Can Selectively Affect Voltage-Gated Channels

The dependence of electrical processes in neurons on particular ion channels makes them vulnerable to genetic mutation, disease processes, and toxins. It has become clear in recent years, for example, that certain genetic diseases of muscle (which has an action potential mechanism similar to that of neurons) are caused by mutations affecting voltage-gated Na^+ channels. Patients with *periodic paralysis* have episodes of weakness during which affected muscle fibers are depolarized by 30 to 40 mv and unable to fire action potentials. A percentage of their voltage-gated Na^+ channels do not inactivate after depolarization (Figure

Table 7-2   Contrasting Properties of Slow Potentials and Action Potentials

	Slow potentials	Action potentials
Amplitude	Graded, typically a few mv	All-or-none, typically about 100 mv
Duration	Graded according to stimulus	1-2 ms
Polarity	+ or −	Always +
Threshold	None (graded)	10-20 mv above resting potential
Summation	Temporal and spatial	None
Conduction	Decremental, passive	Nondecremental, active
Direction of propagation	All directions from stimulus	Unidirectional

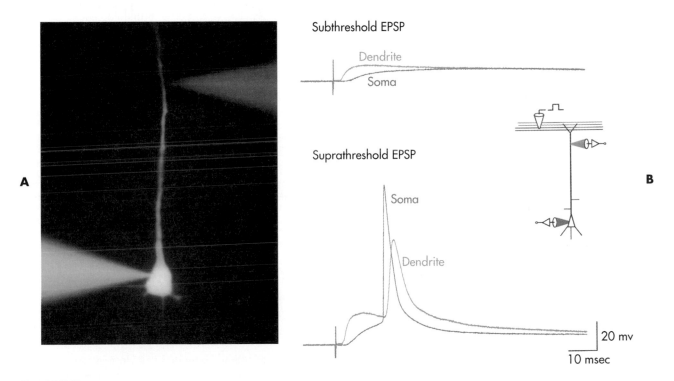

FIGURE 7-13

Spread of synaptic potentials and action potentials through the dendrites and soma. **A,** Simultaneous whole-cell recordings were made from the soma and apical dendrite of a pyramidal neuron in rat cerebral cortex, using patch-clamp electrodes filled with two different fluorescent dyes. **B,** Weak stimulation of the superficial layer of cortex (arrangement shown in inset) caused a depolarizing synaptic potential in the dendrite, which spread passively into the soma and arrived there later, slower, and smaller. **C,** Stronger stimulation of the superficial layer of cortex caused a large depolarizing synaptic potential in the dendrite, in this case large enough by the time it reached the action potential trigger zone (in the axon) to trigger an action potential that could be recorded in the soma. The action potential in turn spread back into the dendrite, arriving there later, slower, and smaller. (The dendritic action potential is actually larger than would be expected based on passive electrical properties because the dendrites of these neurons contain some voltage-gated Na^+ channels. However, there are not enough to initiate action potentials, just enough to "boost" signals that would otherwise spread passively.) (From Sakmann B, Neher E: *Single-channel recording,* ed 2, New York, 1995, Plenum Press.)

7-17). This causes a small but constant inward Na^+ current that depolarizes the fiber and is thought to inactivate normal channels.

Toxins that affect voltage-gated channels would obviously be powerful weapons for animals that dispense them. They also are powerful tools for studying neuronal

physiology and for developing pharmacological agents useful for treating neurological problems. One of the best known neurotoxins is **tetrodotoxin,** which is concentrated in the liver and ovaries of some species of puffer fish and found in a few other animal species as well. Tetrodotoxin binds tightly to the extracellular part of

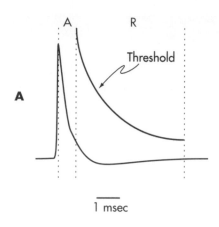

1 msec

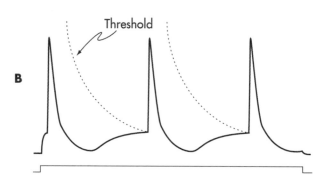

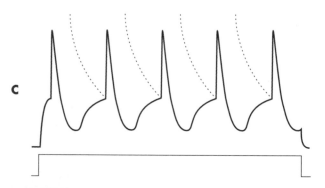

FIGURE 7-14
Refractory periods and their effects on neuronal firing rates. **A,** Threshold during the absolute refractory period (*A,* infinite) and the relative refractory period (*R*). **B** and **C,** Ideal neurons fire repetitively in response to a sustained depolarization, at a rate determined by the time it takes for the membrane potential to reach the declining threshold during the relative refractory period.

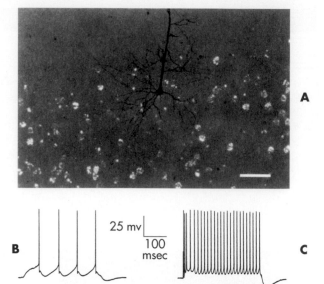

25 mv
100 msec

current   current

FIGURE 7-15
Repetitive action potentials recorded from a corticospinal neuron. **A,** The cell bodies of corticospinal neurons were labeled by retrograde transport of a fluorescent marker injected into the spinal cord. One of the resulting fluorescent neurons was impaled with a dye-filled micropipette and stained. **B,** A small amount of depolarizing current injected into the neuron in **A** caused repetitive firing at a slow regular rate. **C,** A larger current injection in the same neuron caused a brief burst of action potentials followed by repetitive firing at a regular rate faster than that in **B.** (From Tseng G-F, Parada I, Prince DA: Double-labelling with rhodamine beads and biocytin: a technique for studying corticospinal and other projection neurons in vitro, *J Neurosci Meth* 37:121, 1991.)

Action Potentials Are Propagated Without Decrement Along Axons

The series of channel openings and closings just described not only generates an all-or-none action potential, but also triggers the propagation of the action potential along adjacent areas of membrane that contain similar voltage-gated channels—primarily down the axon to ultimately cause the release of neurotransmitter from its synaptic terminals.

Propagation is continuous and relatively slow in unmyelinated axons

Propagation of action potentials along unmyelinated axons is straightforward, though relatively slow. The inward current flowing through voltage-gated Na$^+$ channels during the action potential spreads longitudinally in both directions from the trigger zone, depolarizing adjacent areas of membrane (Figure 7-19, *A*). What happens next depends on the density of voltage-gated Na$^+$ channels in these adjacent regions. If the density is high enough to sustain an action potential, the electrotonically conducted

voltage-gated Na$^+$ channels, preventing Na$^+$ ions from entering. As might be expected, this makes tetrodotoxin a potent poison (Box 7-2), but it has also proven invaluable in experimental studies. For example, tritium-labeled tetrodotoxin has been used to map out the locations of Na$^+$ channels in neuronal membranes. Plants and animals have developed a host of other toxins that affect various aspects of Na$^+$ channels and other channels.

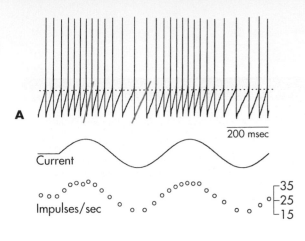

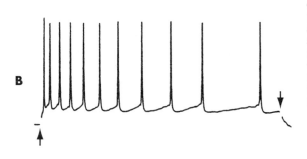

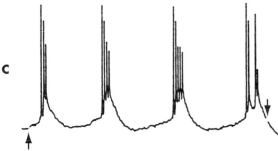

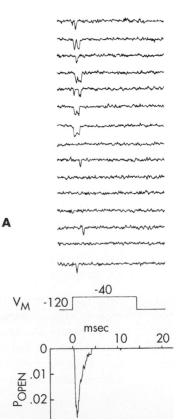

FIGURE 7-16

Varying patterns of repetitive firing in different types of neuron. **A,** A neuron in one of the vestibular nuclei whose firing rate varied linearly with the amount of depolarizing current injected into it. The action potentials were all of uniform size, and threshold *(dashed line)* remained constant, but the rate at which the membrane potential reached threshold *(green lines)* varied with the amount of current injected. **B** and **C,** Some cortical neurons respond to steady depolarization (beginning and end indicated by arrows) with a declining frequency **(B)** or a series of bursts **(C).** (**A** from du Lac S, Lisberger SG: Cellular processing of temporal information in medial vestibular nucleus neurons, *J Neurosci* 15:8000, 1995. **B** and **C** from Agmon A, Connors BW: Correlation between intrinsic firing patterns and thalamocortical synaptic responses of neurons in mouse barrel cortex, *J Neurosci* 12:319, 1992.)

FIGURE 7-17

Abnormal voltage-gated Na+ channels in a patient with periodic paralysis. Repeated patch-clamp recordings of the current flowing through single channels of normal muscle membranes **(A)** and those of the patient **(B)** during depolarization from −120 mv to −40 mv indicate that the patient's channels do not inactivate rapidly. Averages of many such records were used to calculate the probability of channels being open (P_{OPEN}) over time. The continued, albeit reduced, probability of the patient's channels being open corresponds to a small but constant inward Na+ current that depolarizes the fiber. (From Cannon SC: Ion-channel defects and aberrant excitability in myotonia and periodic paralysis, *Trends Neurosci* 19:3, 1996.)

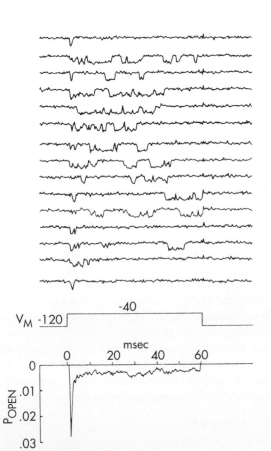

Box 7-2   Puffer Fish and Sodium Channels

Puffer fish (Figure 7-18) are scaleless, spiny fish, mostly living in warm tropical seas. They get their name from a striking ability to inflate themselves when provoked, by sucking large amounts of water or air into a sac connected to their stomach. Some species of puffer fish have been known in Asia for thousands of years to be poisonous, so much so that one Chinese proverb says "To throw away life, eat puffer fish." Despite this warning, puffer fish are also considered a culinary delicacy, particularly in Japan, where they are called *fugu*. Because tetrodotoxin, the active ingredient in puffer fish poison, is concentrated in internal organs such as the liver and gonads and is not destroyed by cooking, puffer fish is served publicly in Japan only by specially trained fugu chefs who are skilled at avoiding contamination of the meal.

Europeans were unaware of the poisonous nature of puffer fish until the seventeenth century. One of the first recorded European victims of tetrodotoxin poisoning was Captain James Cook, more widely known for naval explorations of the Pacific Ocean. On September 8, 1774, during his second voyage to the Pacific, he was offered some puffer fish by the inhabitants of New Caledonia. Two naturalists on board tried to convince Cook not to eat it, but he insisted that he had eaten such fish before and that they all should have some. All three had a taste—fortunately a small taste—of the liver and roe late that evening. Captain Cook, in his journal, described what happened next:

> About three o'clock in the morning we found ourselves seized with an extraordinary weakness and numbness all over our limbs. I had almost lost the sense of feeling; nor could I distinguish between light and heavy bodies of such as I had strength to move, a quart pot full of water and a feather being the same in my hand... *

Late in the last century it was demonstrated that crude extracts containing puffer fish poison block the responses of frog motor nerves to stimulation. In the 1960s intracellular recordings during the application of purified tetrodotoxin demonstrated that it selectively blocks current flow through voltage-gated Na^+ channels. Blocking the Na^+ channels of the peripheral nerves of victims explains tetrodotoxin's effects; larger doses than those consumed by Captain Cook can cause respiratory paralysis and death in minutes. Tetrodotoxin was the first-studied of a long line of naturally occurring toxins that selectively affect various aspects of electrical signaling by neurons. Collectively they have been extremely helpful in unraveling the multiple processes involved in bioelectric phenomena.

*From Cook J: *A voyage towards the South Pole and around the world*, vol 2, London, 1777, Straham and Cadell; quoted in Kao, 1966)

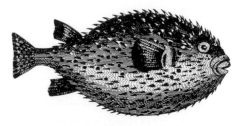

FIGURE 7-18
A puffer fish. (From Heck JG: *Heck's pictorial archive of nature and science*, New York, 1851, Rudolph Garrigue.)

depolarization will reach threshold and trigger one; if it is not, the depolarization will diminish with distance according to the space constant of the neuronal process. Most neuronal cell bodies and dendrites are thought not to be electrically excitable (although some contain enough Na^+ channels to propagate impulses under some circumstances). Axons, however, contain such channels in relative abundance, either distributed uniformly along unmyelinated axons or concentrated at the nodes of Ranvier along myelinated axons. Hence, the initial action potential will propagate along the axon toward its distal terminals, each segment of axonal membrane depolarizing the next segment to threshold Figure 7-19, *B*). Unlike electrotonically conducted slow potentials, action potentials move down the axon in a **nondecremental** fashion.

The rate at which the action potential propagates down the axon—the **conduction velocity**—is directly related to the length constant of the axon: the longer the length constant, the farther down the axon the depolarization reaches and the sooner the next segment of membrane will reach threshold (Figure 7-19, *C* and *D*). Because larger diameter axons have longer length constants, they also have faster conduction velocities. The thinnest unmyelinated axons in our peripheral nerves are 0.2 μm in diameter and conduct at 0.5 m/sec; the largest are 1.5 μm and conduct at 2.5 m/sec. Some invertebrates have taken the strategy of speeding conduction velocity by increasing axonal diameter to extremes, typically in axons that mediate rapid escape responses. The most celebrated example is the giant axons that innervate the mantle muscle of squid. They may be up to 500 μm in diameter, allowing them to conduct at 25 m/sec (Figure 7-21).

Refractory periods ensure that action potentials are propagated in only one direction

Action potentials can propagate from their point of initiation into any nearby excitable membrane. Initiation of an action potential midway along an axon, for example, would cause impulses to propagate not only **orthodromically** toward the distal terminals of the axon, but also **antidromically** toward the cell body (Figure 7-20, *A*).

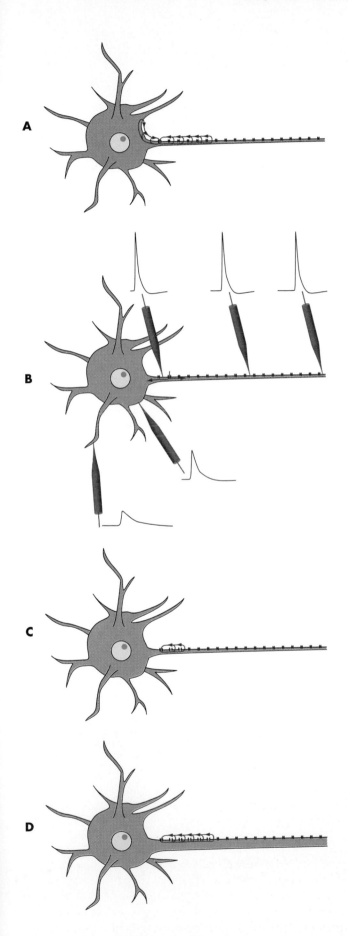

Under normal physiological conditions, however, impulses only travel orthodromically. This is the second major consequence of the refractory periods that follow production of an action potential. Action potentials typically are initiated at a trigger zone in the axon near the cell body and then spread antidromically into the inexcitable cell body and propagate orthodromically down the axon. As an impulse travels down an axon, inward Na^+ current travels both orthodromically and antidromically. However, the part of the axon most recently traversed by the impulse is refractory, and an antidromic impulse cannot be initiated (Figure 7-20, B).

Action potentials jump rapidly from node to node in myelinated axons

Although the giant axons of invertebrates are effective at propagating impulses rapidly, this speed has a cost—they take up a lot of space (Figure 7-21). (If the million axons in a human optic nerve were all 500 μm in diameter, then the nerve would need to be larger than a typical human neck!) Vertebrates take the alternative approach to increasing conduction velocity: rather than simply increasing the diameter of the axon, they increase the length constant by adding myelin, which prevents longitudinal current from leaking out. The result is a major saving of space because a myelinated axon with a conduction velocity of 25 m/sec only needs to be 4 to 5 μm in diameter (including the myelin). Our largest myelinated fibers are about 20 μm in diameter and conduct at about 100 m/sec.

Even though the addition of myelin greatly increases the length constant of the axon, some current still leaves and an action potential, if initiated only at a trigger zone such as the axon initial segment, would die out after a few millimeters. This is prevented by the presence of nodes of Ranvier (see Figures 1-23 and 1-27, B) every millimeter or so. The nodal membrane contains a very high concentration of voltage-gated Na^+ channels (Figure 7-22, A; see also Figure 1-23, A). Action potentials spread electrotonically along internodal parts of the axon, depolarize one node after another to threshold, and are regenerated at

FIGURE 7-19
Propagation of action potentials along unmyelinated axons. **A,** Initiation of an action potential in the axonal trigger zone close to the cell body causes the spread of depolarizing current in both directions—into the electrically inexcitable cell body and into adjacent, electrically excitable parts of the axon. **B,** The action potential waveform spreads passively into the cell body and dendrites, becoming progressively later, slower, and smaller. In contrast, each successive part of the axon reaches threshold and generates its own action potential, so the spike becomes progressively later but not slower or smaller. **C,** Thin axons have relatively short space constants, so a shorter length of axon is depolarized to threshold at any given time (i.e., conduction velocity is relatively slow). **D,** Thick axons have relatively long space constants, so a greater length of axon is depolarized to threshold at any given time (i.e., conduction velocity is relatively rapid).

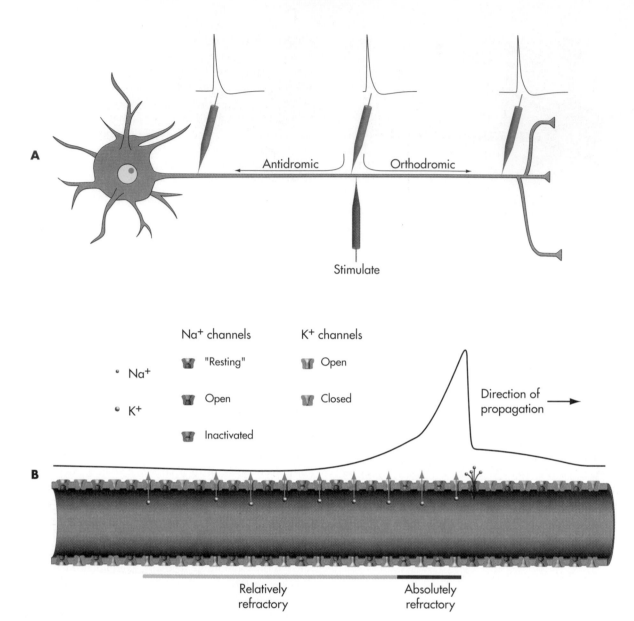

FIGURE 7-20

Normally unidirectional propagation of action potentials. **A,** An action potential artificially induced part way along an axon would encounter excitable membrane in both directions and so would propagate both orthodromically and antidromically. Because the typical zone where action potentials begin under normal physiological conditions is flanked on one side by inexcitable membrane (the cell body) and on the other side by excitable membrane (the rest of the axon), propagation normally proceeds only in the orthodromic direction. **B,** An action potential "frozen" in one instant of time as it propagates orthodromically. Na+ ions rush in at the site of action potential generation and depolarize membrane segments in both directions. However, the trailing zones of absolutely and relatively refractory membrane ensure that the action potential continues to propagate only orthodromically. (This drawing is a schematic representation and is not to scale. In the case of an unmyelinated axon with a typical conduction velocity of 1 m/sec, and an action potential and afterhyperpolarization of 3-msec total duration, the action potential and its afterhyperpolarization would be spread out along 3 mm of axon [1 m/sec x 10^{-3} sec]. Because a typical unmyelinated axon might be 1 μm in diameter, on the scale of this figure the action potential should be spread out over 60 meters!)

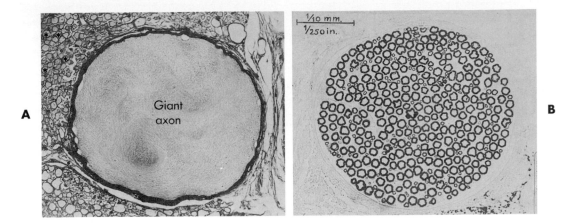

FIGURE 7-21
Space-saving benefits of myelin. **A,** A squid giant axon, surrounded by axons of more typical size (*). The giant axon, because of its size, conducts at 20 to 25 m/sec and is used by the squid to make its mantle muscle contract quickly when trying to escape. Also because of their size, squid giant axons were the subject of most early experiments on the mechanism of action potential generation and conduction. They were, for example, the source of the data in Figure 7-11, *B*. **B,** The motor nerve to a rabbit's gastrocnemius, at the same magnification as the squid nerve in **A.** About 400 myelinated fibers fit into the space occupied by a single giant axon and, because of their myelin, are able to conduct at speeds up to 90 m/sec. (From Young JZ: *Doubt and certainty in science,* New York, 1960, Oxford University Press.)

each node sequentially (Figure 7-22, *B*). The electrotonic spread is very rapid, but the regeneration at each node takes a little time, so the action potential appears to skip from one node to the next (Figure 7-22, *B*). Hence this is called **saltatory conduction** (from a Latin word meaning "to leap" or "to dance"). The larger the diameter of a myelinated axon, the more rapidly it conducts (Figure 7-23), in part because of lower longitudinal resistance and also because of the more widely spaced nodes of Ranvier this allows.

Demyelinating diseases can slow or block conduction of action potentials

Some disease processes selectively affect myelin, either in the PNS or CNS. Nodal membrane contains 1000 to 2000 voltage-gated Na^+ channels/μm^2; internodal axonal membrane contains fewer than 25/μm^2. The membrane of unmyelinated axons contains from 100 to 200 channels/μm^2, so loss of myelin slows conduction drastically and may even cause failure of propagation. The two following examples in which the patient's own immune system attacks and destroys myelin are illustrative.

Guillain-Barré syndrome is an inflammatory process that typically begins a week or two after a viral infection, which is thought to trigger an immune response. Infiltrating macrophages selectively attack and damage PNS myelin, mainly that of motor nerves. Over a period of a week or so patients become progressively weaker, often in an ascending pattern, and may become almost completely paralyzed and require ventilatory assistance. Conduction in proximal parts of motor nerves is slowed and may be blocked. Fortunately, most patients recover completely over a period of weeks to months.

Multiple sclerosis is named for the multiple **plaques** of demyelinated CNS white matter (see Figure 5-19) that often wax and wane over time. The plaques are the result of an autoimmune attack on focal areas of CNS myelin. The demyelination can occur at any CNS site, but some selected locations are more common than others: in the optic nerve, in the deep cerebral white matter (especially around the ventricles), in the cerebellar peduncles, and in particular parts of the brainstem and spinal cord. A genetic predisposition, together with unknown environmental exposures, are thought to trigger the immune response. Multiple sclerosis is relatively common, particularly in young adults, and can be a seriously debilitating chronic disorder. A variety of immunosuppression strategies are being studied as possible approaches to treatment.

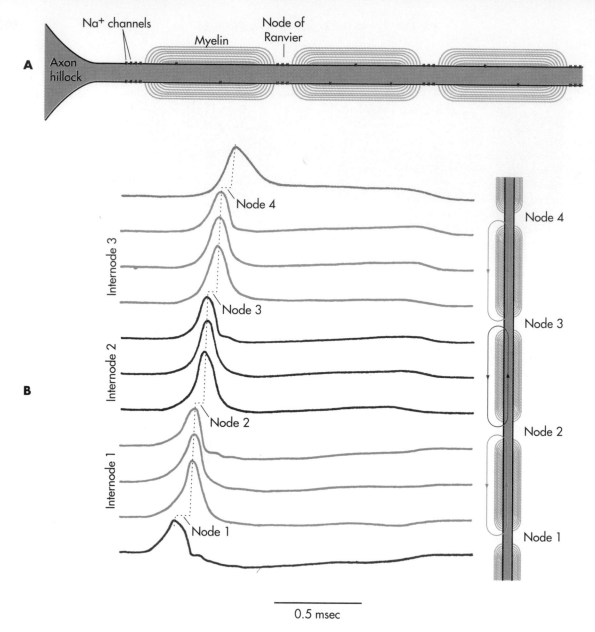

FIGURE 7-22

Propagation of action potentials along myelinated axons. **A,** Voltage-gated Na+ channels are concentrated in areas of the axon near the cell body and at nodes of Ranvier. **B,** Measurements of extracellular current flow as an action potential propagates along a myelinated axon from a frog. Little current leaks across myelin, and current flows almost instantaneously along each internode. A little time is required at each internode for the voltage-gated Na+ channels to open and regenerate the action potential, which therefore appears to "skip" from node to node. (**B** modified from Huxley AF, Stämpfli R: Evidence for saltatory conduction in peripheral myelinated nerve fibres, *J Physiol* 108:315, 1949.)

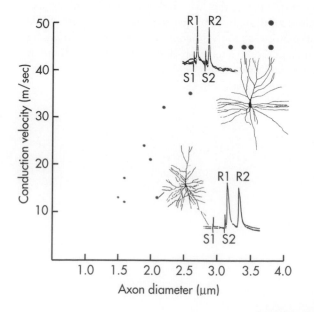

FIGURE 7-23

Conduction velocity of myelinated corticospinal axons as a function of axon diameter. Reconstructions of two of the corticospinal neurons are shown; larger-diameter axons generally arise from larger cell bodies. The electrical records accompanying the reconstruction of each neuron show pairs of antidromically conducted action potentials *(R)* recorded in the neuronal cell body in response to pairs of brief shocks *(S)* delivered to the corticospinal tract. The time between a stimulus and a response (e.g., from S1 to R1) provides a measure of conduction velocity. (Modified from Sakai H, Woody CD: Relationships between axonal diameter, soma size, and axonal conduction velocity of HRP-filled, pyramidal tract cells of awake cats, *Brain Res* 460:1, 1988.)

SUGGESTED READINGS

Adams ME, Swanson G: Neurotoxins, ed 2, *Trends Neurosci* 19(Suppl), 1996. *An extensive listing of toxins that affect a variety of ion channels.*

Black JA, Kocsis JD, Waxman SG: Ion channel organization of the myelinated fiber, *Trends Neurosci* 13:48, 1990.

Cannon SC: Sodium channel defects in myotonia and periodic paralysis, *Ann Rev Neurosci* 19:141, 1996.

Colbert CM, Johnston D: Axonal action-potential initiation and Na+ channel densities in the soma and axon initial segment of subicular pyramidal neurons, *J Neurosci* 16:6676, 1996. *Standard teaching for a long time has been that the trigger zone for action potential initiation is in the axon initial segment. This paper provides evidence that it is actually more distal—at the beginning of the myelin sheath or at the first node of Ranvier.*

Forsythe ID, Redman SJ: The dependence of motoneuron membrane potential on extracellular ion concentrations studied in isolated rat spinal cord, *J Physiol* 404:83, 1988.

Fuhrman FA: Tetrodotoxin, tarichatoxin, and chiriquitoxin: historical perspectives, *Ann NY Acad Sci* 479:1, 1986.

Greenberg DA: Calcium channels in neurological disease, *Ann Neurol* 42:275, 1997.

Hille B: *Ionic channels of excitable membranes*, ed 2, Sunderland, Mass, 1992, Sinauer.

Hodgkin AL: *The conduction of the nervous impulse*, Liverpool, 1964, Liverpool University Press.

Hodgin AL, Huxley AF: A quantitative description of membrane current and its application to conduction and excita-tion in nerve, *J Physiol* 117:500, 1952. *The Nobel prize-winning work that first established the ionic basis of the action potential, taking advantage of the large size of squid giant axons.*

Johnston D et al: Active properties of neuronal dendrites, *Ann Rev Neurosci* 19:165, 1996.

Kandel ER, Schwartz JH, Jessell TM: *Essentials of neural science and behavior*, Norwalk, Conn, 1995, Appleton and Lange.

Kao CY: Tetrodotoxin, saxitoxin and their significance in the study of excitation phenomena, *Pharmacol Rev* 18:997, 1966.

Katz B: *Nerve, muscle and synapse*, New York, 1966, McGraw-Hill. *A lucid introduction to neurophysiology by a Nobel laureate who did much of the early work on action potentials and on neuro-muscular transmission.*

Liem LK et al: The patch clamp technique, *Neurosurg* 36:382, 1995.

Neher E, Sakmann B: Single-channel currents recorded from membrane of denervated frog muscle fibres, *Nature* 260:799, 1976. *The introduction of the patch-clamp technique.*

Nicholls JG, Martin AR, Wallace BG: *From neuron to brain: a cellular and molecular approach to the function of the nervous system*, ed 3, Sunderland, Mass, 1992, Sinauer Associates.

Sakai H, Woody CD: Relationships between axonal diameter, soma size, and axonal conduction velocity of HRP-filled, pyramidal tract cells of awake cats, *Brain Res* 460:1, 1988.

Unwin N: The structure of ion channels in the membranes of excitable cells, *Neuron* 3:665, 1989.

Waxman SG, Kocsis JD, Stys PK, editors: *The axon: structure, function, and pathophysiology*, New York, 1995, Oxford University Press.

RESISTORS, CAPACITORS, AND NEURONAL MEMBRANES

Most of the voltage and current changes that develop across biological membranes can be understood and described in terms of simple electrical circuits made up of batteries, switches, resistors, and capacitors. These electrical circuits themselves are a lot like networks of fluid-filled pipes, in which water pressure is equivalent to voltage, water flow to current, switches to valves, and resistors to constrictions in pipes (the analogy becomes a little strained in the case of capacitors).

Just as water pressure drives water flow through pipes, so does voltage drive electrical current through wires or across biological membranes. (In the latter case, the voltage source is the energy stored in the form of concentration gradients across the membrane.) For a pipe of a given size or a membrane of a given resistance, flow (current) increases linearly with pressure (voltage). This is Ohm's Law:

(A-1)
$$V = IR$$

or

(A-2)
$$V = \frac{I}{G}$$

where V = voltage, I = current, R = resistance, and G = conductance (1/R).

Current always flows in complete circuits (so does water, although sometimes all the parts of the circuit may not be obvious), and all the voltage is dissipated in moving current through the resistances of the circuit (Figure A-1). Two resistors strung end to end (in series) present more of an impediment to current flow than does a single resistor, so resistors in series add:

(A-3)
$$R_{series} = R_1 + R_2 + R_3, \text{etc}$$

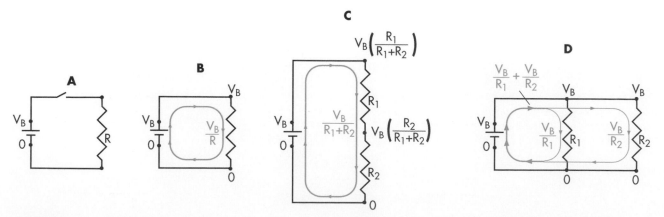

FIGURE A-I

Voltages and current flows in purely resistive circuits. **A,** With a switch open, the battery voltage (V_B) drives no current flow around the circuit and there is no voltage across resistor (R). **B,** Closing the switch allows current flow according to Ohm's Law, and the entire battery voltage is seen across the resistor. **C,** Resistors in series add, and the total current flow through both is predicted by Ohm's Law. The battery voltage is divided between the resistors, in a proportion again predicted by Ohm's Law. **D,** Resistors in parallel add as reciprocals. In this case the voltage across both resistors is the same, but the current is divided between them as predicted by Ohm's Law.

In contrast, two resistors connected side by side (in parallel) offer two paths through which current can flow simultaneously, so the total resistance diminishes. In other words, *conductances* (reciprocals of resistance) in parallel add:

(A-4)

$$G_{parallel} = G_1 + G_2 + G_3, \text{ etc}$$

or

(A-5)

$$\frac{1}{R_{parallel}} = \frac{1}{R_1} + \frac{1}{R_2} + \frac{1}{R_3}, \text{ etc}$$

Voltage changes in response to current flows in purely resistive networks happen almost instantaneously. Capacitors add a dimension of time. As an electrical device, a capacitor is simply two plates of conducting material separated by an insulating layer—say, two sheets of aluminum foil separated by a sheet of plastic film. If the two conducting sheets are connected to a circuit in which current is flowing, positive charges collect on one sheet and repel positive charges on the other. Therefore current, at least initially, continues to flow in the circuit, even though none actually crosses the insulating layer of the capacitor (Figure A-2). The separation of charges across the plates of the capacitor constitutes a voltage across the capacitor, which continues to increase as long as current continues to flow (in real-life situations, until the voltage across the capacitor is equal and opposite to the battery voltage). Once accumulated on the plates of the capacitor, charge stays there until given a path through which to leak away (Figure A-2). Hence, capacitors store charge and build up voltage in response to current flow:

(A-6)

$$V = \frac{Q}{C}$$

and

(A-7)

$$\Delta V/\Delta t = \frac{\Delta Q/\Delta t}{C} = \frac{I}{C}$$

where V = voltage, Q = charge, C = capacitance, ΔV = change in voltage, and ΔQ/Δt = change in charge over time (i.e., ΔQ/Δt = current).

Capacitors act like a very low resistance when a voltage change is first applied, allowing current to flow easily in the circuit, and behave like an open switch once they are charged up. Connecting two capacitors side by side is like having one capacitor with larger plates, so capacitors in parallel add:

(A-8)

$$C_{parallel} = C_1 + C_2 + C_3, \text{ etc}$$

Conversely, capacitors in series add reciprocally and the total capacitance diminishes:

(A-9)

$$\frac{1}{C_{series}} = \frac{1}{C_1} + \frac{1}{C_2} + \frac{1}{C_3}, \text{ etc}$$

Biological membranes, like real electrical circuits, include combinations of resistances and capacitances. In the case of a patch of membrane, the lipid bilayer acts like a capacitor and the ion channels act like resistors in parallel with this capacitor (Figure A-3). Parallel resistor-capacitor combinations change the time course of signals. An injection of constant current, for example, initially flows easily through the capacitor, causing a change in voltage dictated by I/C (Equation A-7). As soon as voltage begins to develop across the capacitor, the same voltage is present across the resistor. Some of the current then begins flowing through the resistor, slowing the rate at which the capacitor charges. Eventually the capacitor is charged and all

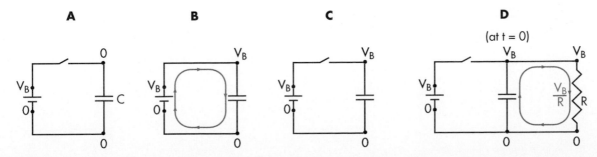

FIGURE A-2

Storage of charge by capacitors. **A,** With a switch open, the battery voltage *(V$_B$)* drives no current flow around the circuit and there is no voltage across capacitor *(C)*. **B,** Closing the switch allows rapid current flow until the capacitor is charged to the battery voltage. The charge remains stored on the capacitor even if the switch is reopened **(C). D,** Addition of a leakage path (resistor *R*) allows charge to leave the capacitor, initially at a rate (i.e., current flow) predicted by Ohm's Law. As charge progressively leaves the capacitor, its voltage declines (Equation A-7), so the current through and voltage across the resistor declines exponentially.

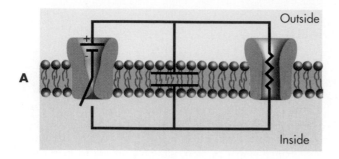

A

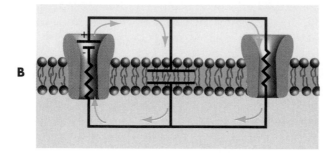

B

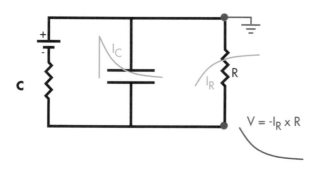

C

the current flows through the resistor. The voltage across both at this point is dictated by IR (Equation A-1). The rate at which the current flow moves from the capacitor to the resistor is influenced by the size of both. The larger the capacitance, the longer the duration of current flow required to charge it. The larger the resistance, the less current flows through it at a given capacitor voltage, so the longer it takes for all the current flow to move to the resistor (i.e., if the resistance is large, the final voltage change will also be large, but it will take a long time to get there). Thus membranes do not respond instantaneously to changes in current flow. Instead they have exponential charging curves with a **time constant:**

(A-10)

$$\tau = RC$$

where τ is the time constant, the time required for the voltage to reach 63% ($1-1/e$) of its final value.

FIGURE A-3

Neuronal membranes as parallel circuits of resistors and capacitors. **A,** The lipid bilayer is electrically equivalent to a series of capacitors and ion channels to resistors. Considering only the voltages and currents attributable to the channel on the left, when the channel is closed no current flows through the membrane resistance or capacitance. **B,** Opening this channel initiates current flow through the membrane resistance and capacitance, dictated by a voltage corresponding to the gradient for the ion passing through this channel. **C,** An electrical equivalent circuit (neglecting extracellular and cytoplasmic resistances). At time = 0 the capacitors act like very small resistances, so initial current flow is through the membrane capacitance (I_C), no current flows through the membrane resistance (I_R), and no change in membrane potential develops. At steady state, the capacitance is fully charged and an amount of current predicted by Ohm's Law flows through the membrane resistance. The time course of the voltage change (V) between time = 0 and steady state is an exponential curve whose duration depends on both membrane resistance and capacitance.

CALCULATING THE MEMBRANE POTENTIAL*

Walther Nernst in 1888 studied quantitatively the equilibrium condition for membranes permeable to only one ion, deriving an equation that still bears his name. The conceptual basis for the Nernst equation is simply that at equilibrium the work required to move a given ion across the electrical potential gradient is equal and opposite to the work required to move it against its concentration gradient. The work (W_e) required to move a mole of an ion across voltage V is:

(B-1)

$$W_e = zFV$$

where z is the valence of the ion and F is Faraday's constant (the charge in one mole of monovalent ions). Hence it takes work to move positive ions to a more positive potential, whereas moving them to a less positive potential can be a source of work.

The work (W_c) required to change the concentration of a mole of the same ion (X) from $[X]_1$ to $[X]_2$ is:

(B-2)

$$W_c = RT \ln \frac{[X]_2}{[X]_1}$$

where R is the gas constant and T is the temperature in °K. Hence it takes work to concentrate the ion ($[X]_2 > [X]_1$), whereas diluting a solution can be a source of work ($[X]_2 < [X]_1$).

At equilibrium $W_e + W_c = 0$, so

(B-3)

$$zFV_X = -RT \ln \frac{[X]_2}{[X]_1} = RT \ln \frac{[X]_1}{[X]_2}$$

Rearranging terms yields the Nernst equation:

(B-4)

$$V_X = \frac{RT}{zF} \ln \frac{[X]_1}{[X]_2}$$

Combining all the constants (at $T = 37°$ C $= 310°$ K) and converting natural logs to $\log_{10}$ yields

(B-5)

$$V_X = 62 \log_{10} \frac{[X]_1}{[X]_2}$$

for monovalent cations such as Na^+ and K^+. For Cl^- the lumped constant would be -62 (because of the negative valence) and for Ca^{2+} it would be 31.

If we consider the example of a membrane permeable only to K^+, make $[K^+]_1$ and $[K^+]_2$ respectively the extracellular and intracellular K^+ concentrations ($[K^+]_o$ and $[K^+]_i$) and use the values in Table 7-1, then

(B-6)

$$V_K = 62 \log_{10} \frac{[K^+]_o}{[K^+]_i} = 62 \log_{10} \frac{4}{130} = -94 \ mv$$

Once it became apparent that real membranes are permeable not just to K^+, but also to some extent to Na^+ and Cl^-, Goldman, and at about the same time Hodgkin and Katz, developed an equation describing the predicted membrane potential (V_m):

(B-7)

$$V_m = 62 \log_{10} \frac{P_K[K^+]_o + P_{Na}[Na^+]_o + P_{Cl}[Cl^-]_i}{P_K[K^+]_i + P_{Na}[Na^+]_i + P_{Cl}[Cl^-]_o}$$

where P_K, P_{Na}, and P_{Cl} are the permeabilities of the membrane to K^+, Na^+, and Cl^-, respectively.

Although this equation initially looks terrifying, it simply describes a weighted average of V_K, V_{Na}, and V_{Cl}, with permeability as the weighting factor. As the permeability to a particular ion increases, the membrane potential will move closer to the equilibrium potential for that ion. This is shown most dramatically during an action potential, when a large but transient increase in Na^+ permeability causes the membrane potential transiently to approach V_{Na} (Figure 7-11, *B*). In situations where the membrane is permeable to only one ion, the Goldman-Hodgkin-Katz equation reduces directly to the Nernst equation. Hence the equation indicates limiting conditions for the membrane potential: no combination of permeability changes

---

*This account draws on the excellent discussion by Katz (1966).

to Na^+, K^+, or Cl^- can make the membrane potential more negative than V_K or more positive than V_{Na}.

The ratio of $P_K:P_{Na}:P_{Cl}$ in a typical resting neuronal membrane might be 1:0.1:0.25, although there is considerable variation among different types of neurons. P_K is always substantially greater than P_{Na}, however, so the resting membrane potential is closer to V_K than to V_{Na} and is determined by the Na^+ and K^+ concentration gradients maintained by the Na^+/K^+ ATPase. In some neurons Cl^- is passively distributed across the membrane, adjusting its concentration gradient to counterbalance the membrane potential. Others, however, contain a Cl^- pump that pumps Cl^- out of the cell. In neurons such as these, the resulting Cl^- concentration gradient contributes to the resting membrane potential and alterations in Cl^- conductance can cause changes in the membrane potential. Some neurotransmitters, for example, cause an increase in the Cl^- conductance of the postsynaptic membrane and consequent inward Cl^- movement and hyperpolarization.

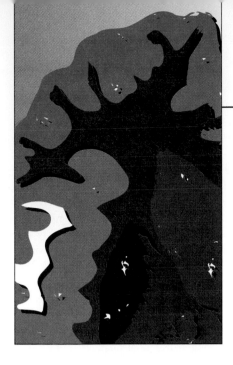

CHAPTER 8

SYNAPTIC TRANSMISSION BETWEEN NEURONS

E arly in this century, Ramón y Cajal and others used the Golgi stain to demonstrate that the nervous system is a collection of individual neurons (e.g., Figure 1-14, *A*) rather than a vast syncytial network, as some had alleged. An obvious corollary of this demonstration is that neurons must have mechanisms by which they communicate with each other. Although there are some instances in which neurons are directly coupled, allowing ionic currents to flow from one into another, in most cases neurons communicate with each other by releasing neuroactive chemical transmitters, typically at specialized sites called **synapses.**★

The first insights into how synapses between neurons might work came from studies of the **neuromuscular**

★*Synapse* started out as a noun, derived from two Greek words meaning "to fasten together." It is now also used commonly as a verb, referring to one neuron making a synaptic contact with another.

junction. Here the endings of motor neurons release a small-molecule transmitter (**acetylcholine**), which diffuses across the cleft between neuronal ending and muscle fiber, attaches to receptor molecules in the muscle fiber membrane, and initiates permeability changes and consequent rapid depolarization (Figures 8-1, 8-9, and 8-10). The depolarization is short-lived because an enzyme (acetylcholinesterase) simultaneously competes for acetylcholine and hydrolyzes it. It is now apparent that the neuromuscular junction is representative of only one type of synaptic interaction. Dozens of **neurotransmitters** have been described to date. Some are small molecules such as acetylcholine (Figures 8-17, 8-18, 8-20, and 8-21), whereas others are larger peptide molecules or diffusible gases; some produce brief depolarizing or hyperpolarizing changes in membrane potential, whereas others produce prolonged potential changes (Figure 8-2)

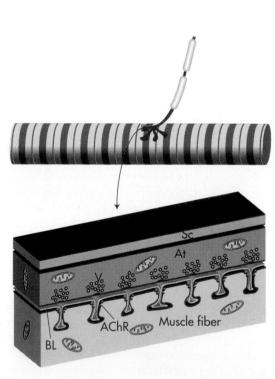

FIGURE 8-1

General arrangement of a neuromuscular junction (Figure 8-10 for a scanning electron micrograph). A motor axon loses its myelin sheath and divides into several terminal branches *(At)* covered by processes of Schwann cells *(Sc,* not indicated in the upper drawing). Each terminal contains a series of clusters of vesicles *(V)* filled with acetylcholine. Invasion of a terminal by an action potential causes some of the vesicles to merge with the terminal membrane and dump their contents into the cleft between terminal and muscle fiber. The liberated acetylcholine diffuses across the cleft, through the basal lamina *(BL),* and reaches acetylcholine receptor molecules *(AChR)* at the entrance to troughs in the muscle surface across from each vesicle cluster. These acetylcholine receptors are ligand-gated cation channels, and binding acetylcholine causes depolarization of the muscle fiber (Figure 8-9). The action of acetylcholine is temporally limited by the enzyme acetylcholinesterase, associated with the basal lamina, which competes for and hydrolyzes acetylcholine.

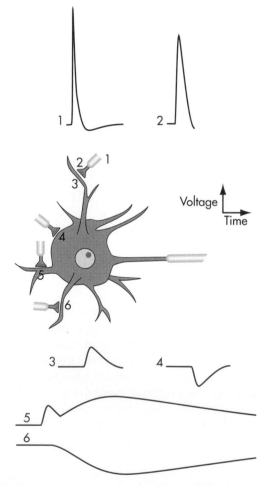

FIGURE 8-2

Schematic overview of the electrical events at typical chemical synapses. Action potentials *(1)* spread electrotonically into axon terminals *(2)* and cause release of neurotransmitter molecules. Neurotransmitter then diffuses to postsynaptic membranes and elicits electrical responses determined by postsynaptic receptors; these include brief depolarizing *(3)* and hyperpolarizing *(4)* responses as well as slower responses, either preceded by a brief response *(5)* or not *(6).* Release and diffusion of neurotransmitter takes a millisecond or so, and as a result postsynaptic signals are delayed slightly.

or changes in membrane properties that last days or longer.★

MOST CHEMICAL SYNAPSES SHARE CERTAIN STRUCTURAL AND FUNCTIONAL FEATURES

Although chemical synapses come in a variety of shapes and sizes, they all include as their essential components a **presynaptic** ending and a **postsynaptic** element, separated by a 10 to 20 nm **synaptic cleft** (see Figure 1-19). The presynaptic elements are usually either terminal expansions of axons (Figure 8-2) or expansions of axons as they pass by other neuronal elements (referred to as **boutons terminaux** and **boutons en passage,** respectively—French for "terminal buttons" and "buttons along the way"). In some instances, however, dendrites or even parts of neuronal cell bodies can be presynaptic elements. Similarly, the postsynaptic element is usually part of the surface of a dendrite, but alternatively can be located on a cell body, axon initial segment, or another synaptic terminal (Figure 8-3; see also Figure 1-20). All of these locations have functional implications, as described a little later in this chapter.

Presynaptic Endings Release Neurotransmitters That Bind to Postsynaptic Receptors

Although portions of the membranes of both presynaptic and postsynaptic elements appear thickened (as **presynaptic** and **postsynaptic densities**), the presynaptic element is distinguished by the presence of a swarm of neurotransmitter-filled **synaptic vesicles.** This anatomical asymmetry corresponds to the functional unidirectionality of synaptic transmission: in response to depolarization, the presynaptic ending releases the neurotransmitter contents of one or more vesicles, the transmitter diffuses across the synaptic cleft and binds to receptor molecules embedded in the postsynaptic membrane, and the postsynaptic neuron responds in some way. Although, as described a little later in this chapter, chemical messages can also move in a retrograde direction across synapses, the direction of *electrical* signaling is from presynaptic to postsynaptic.

All presynaptic endings contain small (about 40 nm) vesicles, and many also contain less numerous but larger (about 100 nm) vesicles. Depending on the preparation conditions used for electron microscopy, some of the small

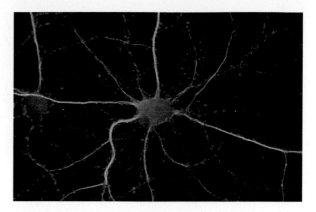

FIGURE 8-3
Synapses densely distributed over the surface of hippocampal neurons developing in tissue culture. The cell bodies and dendrites were stained with a fluorescent antibody directed against MAP2, a microtubule-associated protein restricted to the perikaryal-dendritic region of neurons *(green fluorescence)*. Axon terminal projections originating from other neurons not visible in this field form a dense network of synaptic contact sites and were stained with a fluorescent antibody directed against synaptotagmin *(red fluorescence)*, an integral membrane protein of synaptic vesicles. Overlapping red and green fluorescence, from sites where an axon terminal is superimposed on part of dendrite, appears yellow. (Courtesy Drs. Olaf Mundigl and Pietro De Camilli, Yale University School of Medicine.)

vesicles may appear dark and others clear but flattened; each large vesicle contains a dark core (Figure 8-4). These differences in appearance correspond to differences in neurotransmitter content. For example, endings with clear, flattened vesicles are usually inhibitory.

Release of neurotransmitter is a Ca^{2+}-mediated secretory process. Each presynaptic density, or **active zone,** contains an abundance of voltage-gated Ca^{2+} channels, together with anchoring sites for a cluster of small vesicles that are held there ("docked") by a Ca^{2+}-sensitive system of proteins. Depolarization of the presynaptic terminal, as by propagation of an action potential down the axon and subsequent electrotonic spread into the terminal, causes opening of the voltage-gated Ca^{2+} channels. Because the free intracellular Ca^{2+} concentration is only about 10^{-7} M, Ca^{2+} ions flow in through these channels and momentarily elevate the Ca^{2+} concentration near the active zone by as much as 1000-fold. During the brief period before the excess Ca^{2+} diffuses away or is sequestered, one of the vesicles docked nearby may fuse with the presynaptic membrane and discharge its contents into the synaptic cleft in a process called **exocytosis** (Figure 8-5). The whole process, from the arrival of an action potential to the release of a small vesicle's contents, takes as little as 100 μsec. Because the large, dense-cored vesicles are not located adjacent to active zones, repetitive action potentials, additional Ca^{2+} entry, and more time (tens of msec) are typically required for their exocytosis (Figure 8-5, *B*). This exocytotic addition of membrane clearly could not continue for very long, or else presynaptic endings would expand continuously. In fact, vesicle membranes are taken

---

★Alternate terms such as *neuromodulator* or *neurohormone* are used by many authors to refer to neuroactive substances that have long-lasting effects or diffuse from sites that are not typical synapses. However, there is not yet general agreement on how these terms should be defined, and a number of intermediate cases are known. Hence for the sake of simplicity, all such molecules are referred to as *neurotransmitters* in this chapter.

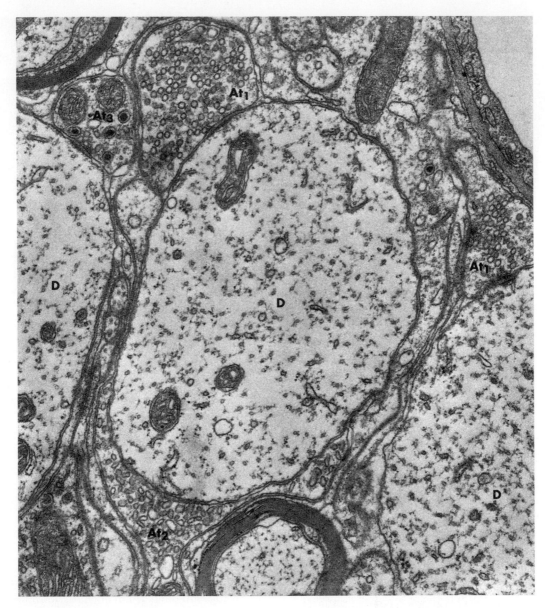

FIGURE 8-4
Types of synaptic vesicles in axon terminals (At) making synaptic contact with transversely sectioned dendrites (D) in the anterior horn of rat spinal cord. Two of the terminals (At₁) contain clear, round vesicles; one (At₂) contains clear, flattened vesicles; and one (At₃) contains a mixture of small, round vesicles and large, dense-cored vesicles. The actual size of the dendrite in the center of the micrograph is about 2.5 μm x 1.5 μm. [From Pannese E: *Neurocytology: fine structure of neurons, nerve processes, and neuroglial cells,* New York, 1994, Thieme Medical Publishers, Inc.]

back up (by **endocytosis**) and can be recycled in less than a minute (Figure 8-5).

Neurotransmitters released from small vesicles find postsynaptic receptor molecules waiting for them directly across the synaptic cleft (Figure 8-6). For this reason, it takes the contents of such vesicles very little time to exert their effects. The total synaptic delay, from presynaptic action potential to postsynaptic effect, can be as little as 200 μsec. The contents of large vesicles, in contrast, take longer to be released and often diffuse to receptors relatively far away (Figure 8-8), so their effects develop more slowly.

Neurotransmitter action is terminated by uptake, degradation, or diffusion

Neurotransmitter molecules need to be removed quickly once they have had a chance to bind to receptors so that the postsynaptic membrane will be prepared for subsequent releases of transmitter. This is accomplished by virtually every means imaginable (Figure 8-7). Binding of neurotransmitter and receptor is a reversible event, so receptors and removal mechanisms compete for transmitter. Some transmitter simply diffuses away, but this is too slow a process to be the principal mechanism. In some

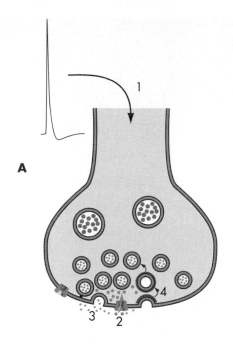

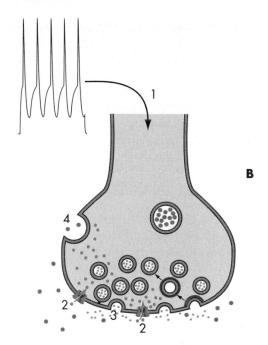

FIGURE 8-5

Ca²⁺-triggered release of neurotransmitter. **A,** Invasion of a presynaptic terminal by a single action potential (*1*) causes brief opening of voltage-gated Ca²⁺ channels (*2*) and a local increase in Ca²⁺ concentration. One or more nearby small vesicles may fuse with the presynaptic membrane (*3*) and discharge their contents into the synaptic cleft; they then are recycled (*4*) in the synaptic terminal. **B,** Repetitive action potentials (*1*) cause opening of more voltage-gated Ca²⁺ channels for longer periods (*2*) and a correspondingly more widespread increase in Ca²⁺ concentration. This causes fusion not only of small vesicles docked at active zones (*3*), but also of larger vesicles away from active zones (*4*).

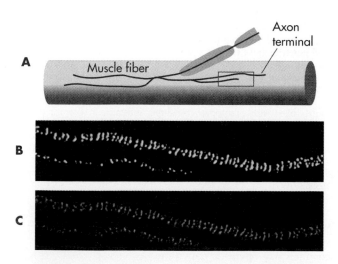

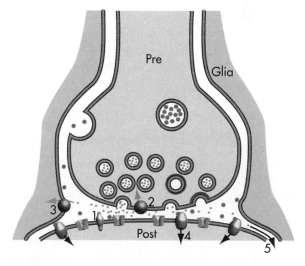

FIGURE 8-6

Juxtaposition of presynaptic voltage-gated Ca²⁺ channels and postsynaptic neurotransmitter receptors, shown at a neuromuscular junction by using toxins coupled to fluorescent dyes. The area of a frog neuromuscular junction outlined in **A** is enlarged in **B** and **C**. **B,** A marine snail toxin (ω-conotoxin) that binds selectively to voltage-gated Ca²⁺ channels demonstrates their locations in the presynaptic terminal. **C,** Staining the same area with a snake toxin (α-bungarotoxin) that binds to nicotinic acetylcholine receptors (the type found at neuromuscular junctions) demonstrates that these have an almost exactly parallel distribution in the postjunctional muscle **membrane.** [From Robitaille R, Adler EM, Charlton MP: Strategic location of calcium channels at transmitter release sites of frog neuromuscular synapses, *Neuron* 5:773, 1990.]

FIGURE 8-7

Mechanisms for removing neurotransmitters from the vicinity of postsynaptic receptors. Although all of these mechanisms are unlikely to be used at a single synapse, different synapses use various combinations of enzymatic inactivation of neurotransmitter (*1*), reuptake of neurotransmitter by the presynaptic terminal (*2*) or nearby glial cells (*3*), and uptake by the postsynaptic terminal (*4*). Finally, some neurotransmitter simply diffuses out of the synaptic cleft (*5*).

synapses, enzymes in the synaptic cleft degrade free transmitter. In others, transmitter is reabsorbed into the presynaptic ending, into neighboring glial cells, or even into the postsynaptic process. Reabsorbed transmitters or their metabolic products, like vesicle membranes, are often recycled for use in a subsequent synaptic event.

Different kinds of neurotransmitters have different preferred mechanisms of removal. For example, acetylcholine is split into acetate and choline by acetylcholinesterase in the synaptic cleft; the choline is then transported back into the presynaptic ending and used for the synthesis of more acetylcholine. Norepinephrine, on the other hand, is rapidly transported back into the presynaptic ending for repackaging in synaptic vesicles. Neuropeptides are either degraded by extracellular peptidases or swallowed up by the postsynaptic cell while still attached to their receptors (Figure 8-8).

Synaptic Transmission Can Be Rapid and Point-to-Point, or Slow and Often Diffuse

Postsynaptic events in response to transmitter-receptor binding fall into two general categories—fast and slow. Some postsynaptic responses involve electrically silent metabolic or membrane changes, but most involve depolarizing or hyperpolarizing potential changes across the postsynaptic membrane. A depolarizing response brings the postsynaptic element closer to its threshold for firing an action potential and so is referred to as an **excitatory postsynaptic potential** (or **EPSP**). Conversely, a hyperpolarizing response moves the membrane away from the threshold and so is referred to as an **inhibitory postsynaptic potential** (or **IPSP**). Hence there are fast and slow EPSPs, and fast and slow IPSPs.

Rapid synaptic transmission involves transmitter-gated ion channels

Early studies of synaptic transmission demonstrated that a single action potential in the motor nerve ending at a neuromuscular junction causes a large but brief EPSP,★ sufficient to cause an action potential and contraction in the muscle fiber (Figure 8-9, *B*). Closer analysis revealed small, brief depolarizing events in the postjunctional muscle membrane during the periods between action potentials (Figure 8-9, *A*), each corresponding to a brief period of channel opening and depolarizing current flow. We now know that each of these small depolarizing events is the response of the postsynaptic membrane to the spontaneous release of one synaptic vesicle. Each vesicle contains about 10,000 acetylcholine molecules, which diffuse across the synaptic cleft and bind briefly to acetylcholine receptors, which themselves are ligand-gated ion channels permeable

---

★Often referred to as an **end-plate potential** because **motor end plate** is another term for neuromuscular junction.

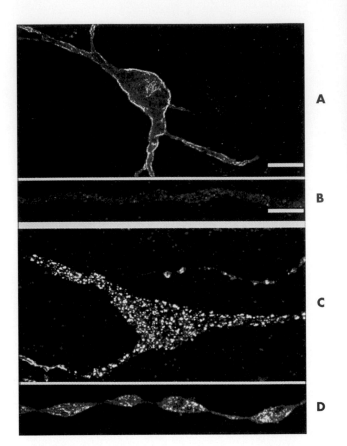

FIGURE 8-8

Endocytotic removal of a neuropeptide (substance P) and its receptor by postsynaptic neurons, demonstrated by staining substance P receptors using a fluorescent antibody technique. In the absence of stimulation, substance P receptors coat the somatic and dendritic membranes of pain-sensitive second-order neurons in the spinal cord posterior horn (**A**, red and yellow fluorescence) and the distal dendrites of these cells have a uniform diameter (**B**). Five minutes after a painful stimulus on the ipsilateral side most of the substance P receptor has left the surface membranes and is found intracellularly (**C**), and distal dendrites have a beaded appearance with varicosities filled with endosomes containing substance P receptor (**D**). Over about the next hour, the internalized substance P receptor molecules are recycled to the cell surface. The scale mark in **A** (also applies to **C**) is 20 μm. The scale mark in **B** (also applies to **D**) is 10 μm. (From Mantyh PW et al: Receptor endocytosis and dendritic reshaping in spinal neurons after somatosensory stimulation, *Science* 268:1629, 1995.)

to both Na^+ and K^+ ions. Acetylcholinesterase competes with the receptors for the released acetylcholine, so the channels stay open for only a millisecond or two. During this time, they allow a current flow that tries to move the membrane potential to a value around 0 mv (between the Na^+ and K^+ equilibrium potentials; see Appendix 7-B, equation B-7). Because 2 msec is considerably less than the time constant of the muscle membrane, the membrane potential never reaches 0 mv. Instead, it rises rapidly at the beginning of the postsynaptic current flow and then decays slowly at the end of the current flow (Figure 8-9, *A*). Entry of depolarizing current is localized to the site of the receptors, so the postsynaptic potential decays electrotonically (Figure 8-9, *C* and *D*). However, the presynaptic

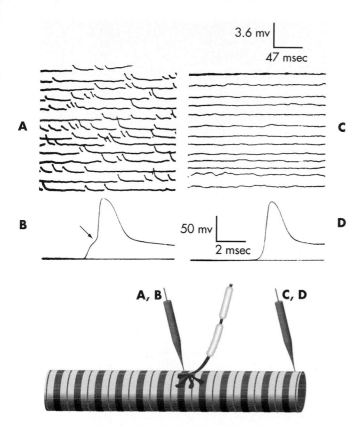

FIGURE 8-9

Intracellular recordings of muscle membrane potential at the motor endplate of a frog muscle fiber (**A** and **B**) and about 2 mm away from the endplate (**C** and **D**), demonstrating the localization of postjunctional potentials to the region of the neuromuscular junction. At rest, small depolarizing events (referred to as *miniature endplate potentials*), each corresponding to the release of a single acetylcholine-filled vesicle, can be recorded at the endplate (**A**). Two mm away, they have almost completely died out because of electrotonic spread (**C**). An action potential in the motor axon elicits a large postjunctional potential at the endplate (**B**, note the different time and voltage scale), rapidly reaching threshold (*arrow*) and triggering a muscle action potential. Two mm away (**D**), only the propagated action potential remains. (Electrical recordings from Fatt P, Katz B: Spontaneous subthreshold activity at motor nerve endings, *J Physiol* 117:109, 1952.)

ending at each neuromuscular junction contains upwards of a thousand active zones (Figures 8-6 and 8-10), so a single action potential in the motor axon causes the nearly simultaneous release of hundreds of vesicles full of acetylcholine at closely spaced sites, which in turn causes the large EPSP normally seen (Figure 8-9, *B*).

The basic elements of neuromuscular transmission have proved to be generally true of fast synaptic transmission throughout the nervous system (Figure 8-11, *A*). Depolarization-induced Ca^{2+} entry causes the release of packets of neurotransmitter, called **quanta,** each one generally assumed to be the contents of a single vesicle docked at an active zone. The neurotransmitter then diffuses across the synaptic cleft and binds transiently to a **transmitter-gated** (i.e., ligand-gated) **ion channel.** The selectivity of the channel determines the postsynaptic effect. Opening channels selective for monovalent cations, as in the exam-

ple of the neuromuscular junction, causes an EPSP. Opening channels selective for Cl⁻, on the other hand, moves the membrane potential toward the Cl⁻ equilibrium potential; this is the most common basis of fast IPSPs in the CNS. The selective concentration of receptors on the postsynaptic membrane ensures that fast postsynaptic potentials are localized spatially.

Slow synaptic transmission involves postsynaptic receptors linked to G proteins

Slow synaptic potentials are also caused by changes in current flow through membrane ion channels, but in this case a multistep process is involved in which binding of neurotransmitter leads to altered concentrations of **second messengers,** which in turn modulate channel conductance. The receptors for most such events are membrane-spanning proteins linked to adjacent guanine nucleotide–binding proteins **(G proteins).** Transmitter binding by a **G protein–coupled receptor** causes dissociation of a subunit of the G protein, which is then able to move laterally in the postsynaptic membrane and exert other effects (Figure 8-11, *B*).

In the simplest scenario, the G protein subunit directly influences the state of ion channels, for example, causing K^+ or Ca^{2+} channels to open; in this instance, the G protein subunit itself is the second messenger. In most cases, however, the G protein subunit increases or decreases the activity of an enzyme, which in turn causes changes in the concentration of something else.

Multistep pathways such as this are slow and seem unwieldy, but they actually have considerable advantages. Synaptic inputs can be amplified, because a single receptor can cause the dissociation of multiple G proteins, and changing the activity of an enzyme can cause the synthesis or degradation of thousands of second messenger molecules. In addition, because there are many types of G protein–coupled receptors and many types of G proteins, a wide array of postsynaptic effects can result. Some, as indicated previously, are as simple as opening or closing an ion channel. Others may actually be electrically silent, causing things such as changes in sensitivity to other transmitters or changes in gene transcription. This kind of strategy is so versatile that it is not restricted to synapses. G proteins and second messengers are the basis for potentials generated by retinal rods and cones and by olfactory sensory neurons (see Chapter 9).

The postsynaptic receptor determines the effect of a neurotransmitter

There is nothing intrinsically "excitatory" or "inhibitory" about any neurotransmitter. The effect of a transmitter at any given synapse is instead determined by the nature of the receptor to which it binds. Because there are multiple types of receptors for most or all neurotransmitters, most

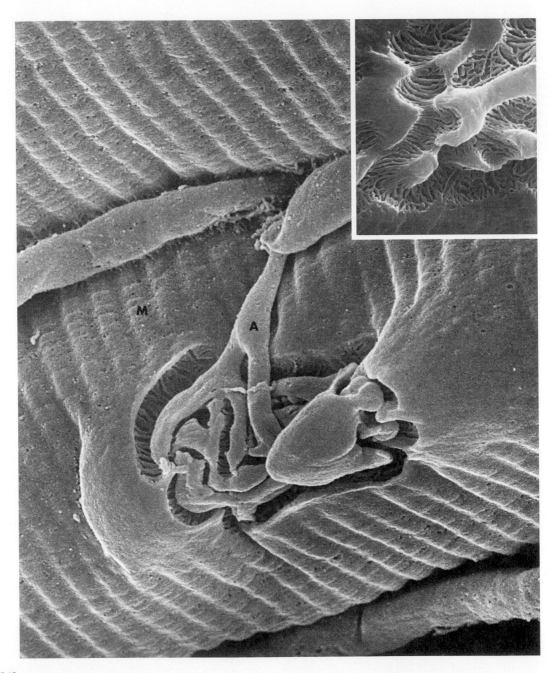

FIGURE 8-10

Three-dimensional structure of a neuromuscular junction. This scanning electron micrograph shows a motor axon *(A)* approaching a muscle fiber *(M)* in a calf muscle (peroneus longus) of a hamster. The axon divides into a series of terminal branches that occupy grooves in the surface of the muscle fiber. Removing these branches from a similar neuromuscular junction reveals a series of troughs traversing the grooves, each corresponding to one of the troughs in Figure 8-1 and containing acetylcholine receptors. The actual size of the endplate is about 7 μm × × 12 μm. (From Pannese E: *Neurocytology: fine structure of neurons, nerve processes, and neuroglial cells*, New York, 1994, Thieme Medical Publishers, Inc.)

transmitters can have more than one effect. This is well illustrated by acetylcholine, which causes fast excitatory events at some synapses and slow excitatory or inhibitory events at others. The reason for these differences is the fact that there are two categories of acetylcholine receptors. **Nicotinic** acetylcholine receptors (so called because they bind nicotine as well as acetylcholine), the kind found at neuromuscular junctions, are transmitter-gated ion channels. **Muscarinic** acetylcholine receptors

(which bind muscarine, a substance derived from the mushroom *Amanita muscaria*), found on smooth and cardiac muscle fibers and elsewhere, are G protein–coupled receptors. Acetylcholine applied to cardiac muscle, for example, causes increased opening of K^+ channels and a slow IPSP.

Not only are there two categories of acetylcholine receptors, there are also multiple subtypes in each category—at least three different nicotinic receptors and five

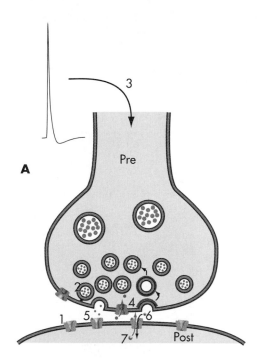
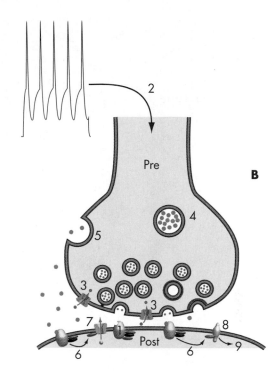

FIGURE 8-11
Basic events in typical fast (**A**) and slow (**B**) synaptic transmission. **A,** At rest, ligand-gated ion channels in the postsynaptic membrane are closed (*1*) and vesicles are docked in the presynaptic terminal (*2*) awaiting release. Depolarization of the terminal (*3*) causes Ca^{2+} influx (*4*), transmitter exocytosis, binding of transmitter to postsynaptic ligand-gated ion channels (*5*) and opening of the channels. In this example, open channels allow Na^+ influx (*6*) and K^+ efflux (*7*), depolarizing the postsynaptic membrane. **B,** Most slow synaptic responses involve receptors coupled at rest to a G protein (*1*), and may involve transmitters in large, dense-core vesicles or in certain small vesicles. Prolonged or repetitive depolarization (*2*) of the presynaptic terminal causes widespread Ca^{2+} influx (*3*), exocytosis of transmitter from large, dense-core vesicles (*4, 5*), and binding to G protein–coupled receptors (some of which may be located some distance from the presynaptic terminal [see Figure 8-8]). This binding causes dissociation of the G protein into subunits (*6*) that can have a variety of effects. They may bind to ion channels and alter their conductance (*7*), activate an enzyme (*8*) that in turn alters the concentration of a second messenger (e.g., cyclic AMP, inositol triphosphate, arachidonic acid metabolites), or have even more complex effects (*9*), such as altering gene expression.

different muscarinic receptors—with different distributions. For example, the nicotinic receptor of skeletal muscle fibers is different from that of parasympathetic ganglion cells. This multiplicity of subtypes, which is true of neurotransmitter receptors in general, has made it possible to begin designing drugs that target very specific neuronal subsystems (Figure 8-23).★

The Size, Location, and History of a Synaptic Ending Influence the Magnitude of Its Effects

Neurons usually receive hundreds or even thousands of synaptic inputs from other neurons (Figure 8-3), combining their effects at the trigger zone to determine whether and how often to fire an action potential. This ability of neurons to compare and combine many different inputs is in great part responsible for the computational power of the nervous system. The net impact of any individual

synapse will obviously depend on the amount of transmitter released there, as well as on the distance from there to the trigger zone. In addition, the strength of a synapse can be influenced, sometimes profoundly and for long periods, by the history of activity at that synapse.

Synapses with many active zones have a greater effect

Muscle fibers do not need to do much computing—it makes functional sense for every action potential in the motor axon to trigger a twitch of the muscle fiber. Release of a single quantum of neurotransmitter has only a small effect (Figure 8-9, *A*), so neuromuscular transmission calls for a very large presynaptic ending with many active zones at the neuromuscular junction (Figures 8-6 and 8-10). There are a few other instances in the PNS or CNS where one input is of overwhelming functional importance and the presynaptic ending is very large (Figure 8-12). Most synapses, however, are minute—less than 1 μm in diameter (Figure 8-4; see also Figure 1-21)—and individually release just a few quanta and produce very small postsynaptic potentials, usually less than a mv. Hence concerted activity at many synapses, and spatial and temporal

---

★Nature, of course, has a head start on pharmacologists in this regard. A wide variety of toxins and other naturally occurring substances—nicotine and muscarine, for example—interact with specific receptor types or even subtypes

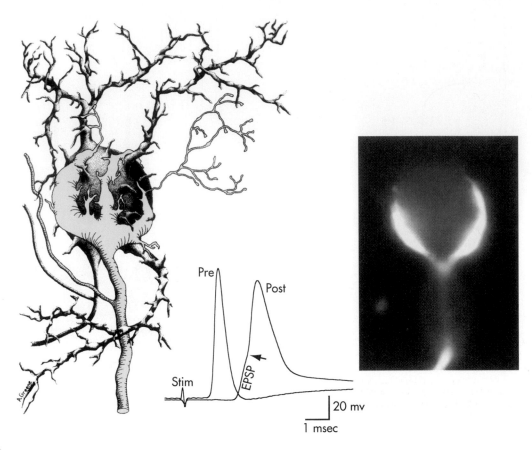

FIGURE 8-12
Simultaneous recordings from the presynaptic and postsynaptic elements at a CNS synapse with many active zones. Certain afferents to a brainstem nucleus in the auditory pathway form large, cuplike presynaptic endings (called *calyces of Held*) that partially envelop the neurons on which they synapse, as indicated in the drawing on the left. Two patch-clamp electrodes filled with different fluorescent materials were used to record from and stain both elements. This yielded the electrical records in the center and the photograph on the right, in which the presynaptic ending is yellow and the postsynaptic neuron is blue. After stimulation of the afferent axon *(Stim)* it takes about 1 msec for an action potential to be conducted to the presynaptic ending and spread into it *(Pre)*. After about another msec for Ca^{2+} influx and transmitter exocytosis and diffusion, a rapidly rising EPSP is recorded in the postsynaptic neuron *(Post)*, quickly bringing it to threshold *(arrow)*. This type of CNS synapse is unusual in terms of the magnitude of the postsynaptic potential elicited—a reflection of the large number of active zones in the presynaptic terminal. (Drawing from Morest DK et al: Stimulus coding at caudal levels of the cat's auditory nervous system. II. Patterns of synaptic organization. In Møller AR, editor: *Basic mechanisms in hearing,* New York, 1973, Academic Press. Electrical records and photograph from Borst JGG, Helmchen F, Sakmann B: Pre- and postsynaptic whole-cell recordings in the medial nucleus of the trapezoid body of the rat, *J Physiol* 489:825, 1995.)

summation of their effects, is likely to be required to substantially alter the firing frequency of most neurons.

Synapses closer to the action potential trigger zone have a greater effect

Synaptic potentials are generated focally at sites where neurotransmitter receptors are located, and spread electrotonically from their point of origin. Hence things such as time constants and space constants become critical determinants of the effects that synaptic potentials cause in other parts of the postsynaptic neuron. A synapse on an axon's initial segment (see Figure 1-15), close to the trigger zone, will have a relatively powerful effect. In contrast, postsynaptic potentials generated far out on a distal dendrite would be expected to decay during electrotonic spread toward the trigger zone. In fact, some dendritic membranes have a sprinkling of voltage-gated channels—not enough to generate action potentials on their own, but enough to

give postsynaptic potentials a little boost along the way.

Synapses on neuronal cell bodies and initial segments are often inhibitory, making them particularly influential for two reasons. They are not only close to the trigger zone in an electrotonic sense, but they are also in a position to diminish the effects of EPSPs generated more distally (Figure 8-13) by, in effect, shortening the length constant of the neuron. In contrast, synapses on dendrites are often excitatory.

Presynaptic endings can themselves be postsynaptic

Presynaptic terminals themselves contain the same kinds of receptors found in postsynaptic membranes. These receptors are involved in two different kinds of processes that control the amount of transmitter released by the terminal.

Some presynaptic terminals receive axoaxonic synaptic inputs that oppose the entry of Ca^{2+} into the presynaptic

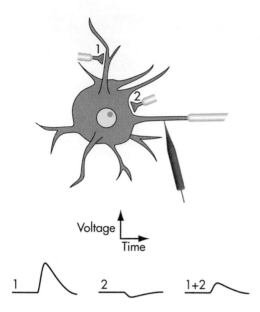

FIGURE 8-13

Interactions of a dendritic excitatory synapse (1) and a somatic inhibitory synapse (2), as recorded at the initial segment. The inhibitory synapse by itself produces a small IPSP, typically the result of increased conductance to K^+ or Cl^-, ions whose equilibrium potential is close to the resting membrane potential. However, simultaneous activation of both synapses causes a marked diminution of the EPSP because much of the current flowing in at the excitatory synapse flows out at the inhibitory synapse and never reaches the initial segment.

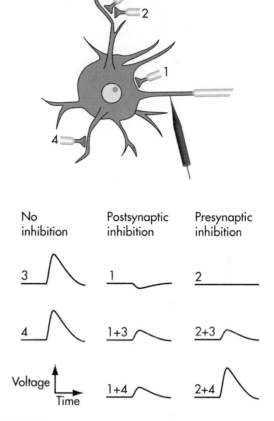

FIGURE 8-14

Presynaptic and postsynaptic inhibition. Standard inhibitory synapses (1), as indicated in Figure 8-13, generate an IPSP in the postsynaptic neuron and diminish the effect of all excitatory synapses on the same neuron (1 + 3, 1 + 4). Presynaptic inhibition, in contrast, results in no IPSP (2), except perhaps in the inhibited terminal, and diminishes the effect of only a subset of excitatory synapses (2 + 3 vs. 2 + 4).

terminal (Figure 8-14). Because Ca^{2+} entry is the critical element in vesicle exocytosis, this will decrease the amount of transmitter released in response to an action potential arriving at the terminal. This in turn will decrease the likelihood of depolarizing the postsynaptic neuron to threshold, almost as though it had received an inhibitory input. The critical difference is that there is no IPSP in the postsynaptic neuron and no effect on its other inputs. In addition, only the terminal receiving the axoaxonic synapse has its transmitter release affected. Thus **presynaptic inhibition** is a clever mechanism for affecting only selected branches of an axon, and for selectively depressing only certain inputs to a postsynaptic neuron. Other axoaxonic synapses enhance the entry of Ca^{2+} into presynaptic terminals, mediating an analogous process of **presynaptic facilitation.**

Many presynaptic terminal membranes also contain receptors for their own transmitters, called **autoreceptors.** Some fraction of the transmitter released into the synaptic cleft binds to these autoreceptors. The most common effect is inhibition of further transmitter release.

Synaptic strength can be facilitated or depressed

An action potential arriving at a presynaptic terminal does not necessarily always produce the same postsynaptic response. Presynaptic inhibition or facilitation can alter the effectiveness of a terminal temporarily to meet specific functional needs, but in addition the properties of both a terminal and its postsynaptic process can vary depending on the history of activity at that synapse.

Given the molecular workings of synapses, it is easy to imagine that a brief, high-frequency burst of action potentials arriving at a synaptic terminal could cause entry of too much Ca^{2+} to diffuse away or be sequestered for a few seconds, or alternatively that a high-frequency burst could deplete the terminal's supply of available vesicles. An elevated Ca^{2+} concentration would cause release of extra transmitter the next time an action potential arrived at the terminal, and a depleted vesicle pool would cause release of fewer vesicles than normal. Both of these phenomena, called **potentiation** and **depression,** respectively, occur to varying degrees at many synapses, depending on the pattern of stimulation and the characteristics of a particular synapse. These effects usually last no more than seconds.

Learning and memory (see Chapter 23) involve long-term, even permanent, changes in the way neurons respond to particular stimuli. Short-lived changes such as brief periods of synaptic potentiation and depression are clearly inadequate for this kind of role. Other, much

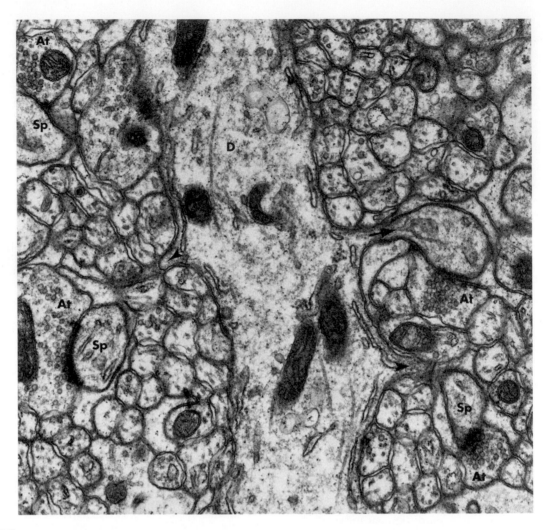

FIGURE 8-15
Synapses on spines of cerebellar Purkinje cells. A Purkinje cell dendrite *(D)* runs vertically through the micrograph, and the narrow neck *(arrow)* of one spine leads to an enlargement on which an axon terminal *(At)* ends. The necks of two other spines *(arrowheads)* can also be seen, as can sections through parts of other spines *(Sp)* contacted by axon terminals. The actual diameter of this dendrite is about 1 μm. (From Pannese E: *Neurocytology: fine structure of neurons, nerve processes, and neuroglial cells*, New York, 1994, Thieme Medical Publishers, Inc.)

longer lasting changes in synaptic efficacy are thought to be critical for this function. **Long-term potentiation,** lasting for days, weeks, or even longer after a tetanic input delivered to some synaptic terminals, has taken center stage as a model for learning and memory. Long-term potentiation depends on activation of a particular receptor for the neurotransmitter **glutamate,** as described a little later in this chapter, and may involve long-term increases in transmitter release, postsynaptic sensitivity, or both. Synaptic spines (see Figure 1-14) have long been candidates as sites for the synaptic changes of learning and memory, in part because of the cells on which they occur (e.g., cortical neurons) and in part because of their geometry (Figure 8-15). Spines are connected to the main shaft of the dendrite by a narrow neck, and small changes in something such as the diameter of the neck could produce large changes in the spine's electrical properties or its ability to maintain altered concentrations of second messengers. In support of a role of spines in long-term changes in the CNS are the observations that they are favored sites

for the development of long-term potentiation (or the complementary phenomenon of **long-term depression**), and that their shapes and numbers can change when learning occurs.

Messages Also Travel Across Synapses in a Retrograde Direction

The preceding account makes it sound as though all information flow at chemical synapses is unidirectional, and indeed for electrical signaling this is the case. However, postsynaptic elements have several electrically silent, nonvesicular mechanisms at their disposal to influence the properties of presynaptic terminals and neurons. For example, binding of transmitter at some G protein–coupled receptors activates enzymes that produce **nitric oxide** (NO) or **carbon monoxide** (CO). These gases can diffuse easily through neuronal membranes, so even though they have a short lifetime they can enter nearby presynaptic terminals, where they influence subsequent transmitter release. In addition, **growth factors** released by postsynaptic cells and transported back to the cell bodies of presynaptic neurons are important for the development and maintenance of synaptic connections.

MOST NEUROTRANSMITTERS ARE SMALL AMINE MOLECULES, AMINO ACIDS, OR NEUROPEPTIDES

Nearly all of the known or suspected neurotransmitters fall into one of two general categories: some are small amine molecules or amino acids, and the others are peptides. There are only about 10 known small-molecule transmitters (of which seven are particularly prominent [Table 8-1]), whereas there are dozens of neuroactive pep-

tides. Each kind of transmitter has a characteristic major role (Table 8-2).

Small synaptic vesicles contain small-molecule transmitters; large dense-core vesicles contain neuropeptides and may contain one or more small-molecule transmitters as well. The two kinds of vesicles are manufactured and recycled differently (Figure 8-16). Small-molecule transmitters are synthesized by cytoplasmic enzymes and can therefore be manufactured and packaged for release in individual synaptic endings. Peptide transmitters, in contrast, are manufactured in the neuronal cell body, where they are cleaved from larger precursor proteins, packaged for release, and dispatched by axonal transport to synaptic endings. Small synaptic vesicles can therefore be recycled entirely within a presynaptic ending, whereas large dense-core vesicles must be created anew in the cell body.

Table 8-1   Major Neurotransmitters

Type	Major Transmitters
Amines	Acetylcholine
	Cetecholamines
	Dopamine
	Norepinephrine
	Serotonin
Amino Acids	Glutamate (and asparate)
	GABA (γ-aminobutyric acid)
	Glycine
Neuropeptides	Angiotensin II
	β-Endorphin
	Cholecystokinin
	Enkephalin
	Neuropeptide Y
	Neurotensin
	Somatostatin
	Substance P
	And many others

Table 8-2   Typical Effects of Major Transmitters

Effect	Major transmitter(s)
Fast excitatory	PNS:acetylcholine (nicotinic receptor)
	CNS: glutamate (and aspartate)
Fast inhibitory	GABA (mostly in the brain)
	Glycine (mostly in the spinal cord)
Second-messenger effects	Catecholamines
	Serotonin
	Acetylcholine (muscarinic receptor)
	Neuropeptides

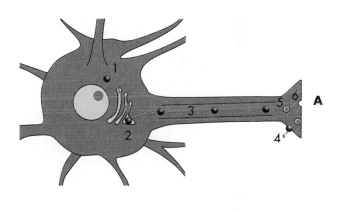

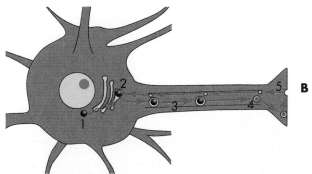

FIGURE 8-16
Life cycles of small-molecule neurotransmitters **(A)** and neuropeptides **(B)**. **A,** The enzymes required for the synthesis and packaging of small-molecule neurotransmitters are themselves synthesized in the cell body *(I),* released from the Golgi apparatus *(2),* and conveyed to presynaptic terminals by slow axonal transport *(3).* The neurotransmitters are then synthesized from substrates transported into the terminals *(4)* and packaged into vesicles *(5)* that were either recycled from the presynaptic membrane *(6)* or assembled from components transported from the cell body. **B,** Precursors of neuropeptides are synthesized in the cell body *(I)* and packaged in the Golgi apparatus into vesicles *(2),* which are conveyed to presynaptic terminals by fast axonal transport along microtubules *(3).* Either in the cell body or on the journey down the axon, the precursor proteins are modified and become neuropeptides *(4).* After exocytosis, the membranes of large, dense-core vesicles are returned to the cell body for recycling *(5).*

Acetylcholine Mediates Rapid, Point-to-Point Transmission in the PNS

Acetylcholine (Figure 8-17) was the first neurotransmitter to be discovered. It plays an especially prominent role in the PNS as the transmitter released by motor neurons at neuromuscular junctions and by many neurons of the autonomic nervous system (Table 8-3). Its distribution in the CNS is more restricted, and its role is quite different. Other than motor neurons, the **cholinergic** neurons of the CNS (see Figure 11-24) are concentrated in parts of the brainstem, the base of the forebrain, and the basal ganglia (Table 8-3). The brainstem and basal forebrain cholinergic neurons have extensively branching axons that innervate wide areas of the CNS, a pattern not suited for the point-to-point transfer of information. They are thought instead to play a role in regulating the general level of activity of CNS neurons, especially during different phases of the sleep-wake cycle and during learning.

The physiological action of acetylcholine is different at central and peripheral endings. As noted earlier, there are nicotinic and muscarinic acetylcholine receptors. Nicotinic receptors are transmitter-gated ion channels that me-

diate fast EPSPs, and muscarinic receptors are G protein–coupled receptors that mediate a variety of second-messenger effects. Nicotinic receptors are more common in the PNS and muscarinic receptors in the CNS, although there is overlap. For example, single autonomic ganglion cells may possess both nicotinic and muscarinic receptors, and acetylcholine produces both fast and slow postsynaptic potentials in these cells.

Amino Acids Mediate Rapid, Point-to-Point Transmission in the CNS

Certain amino acids serve double duty, involved not only in intermediary metabolism and protein synthesis but also as neurotransmitters. The most important of these are **glutamate** and its derivative **γ-aminobutyric acid,** which is commonly referred to by its acronym **GABA** (Figure 8-18). Glutamate is the major transmitter for brief, point-to-point, excitatory synaptic events in the CNS, playing a role analogous to that of acetylcholine in the periphery. Conversely, GABA is the major transmitter for brief, point-to-point, inhibitory synaptic events in the CNS. In addition to these two amino acids, **aspartate** is the probable transmitter at some excitatory CNS synapses, and **glycine** is the transmitter at some inhibitory CNS synapses. The distributions of GABA and glycine synapses overlap, but glycine is particularly prominent in the spinal cord.

As might be expected from these roles, neurons containing glutamate or GABA are very widespread in the nervous system (Tables 8-4 and 8-5). For example, the endings of primary afferents in the spinal cord, the endings of ascending pathways in the thalamus, and the myriad outputs from the cerebral cortex all use glutamate as an excitatory neurotransmitter. Inhibitory connections using GABA are similarly abundant, and will be noted in a number of subsequent chapters.

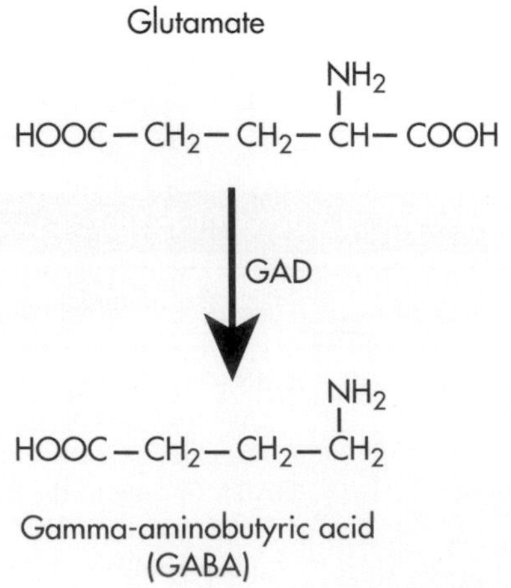

Table 8-3	Locations of Cholinergic Neurons and Synapses	
Location of neurons	Location of terminals	Principal receptor
Motor neurons	Skeletal muscle	Nicotinic
Preganglionic autonomics*	Autonomic ganglia	Nicotinic, muscarinic
Parasympathetic ganglia*	Smooth and cardiac muscle, glands	Muscarinic
Reticular formation†	Thalamus	Muscarinic
Basal nucleus†‡	Cerebral cortex, amygdala	Muscarinic
Septal nuclei†‡	Hippocampus	Muscarinic
Caudate nucleus, putamen	Local connections	Muscarinic

*Chapter 10.
†Chapter 11.
‡Chapter 23.

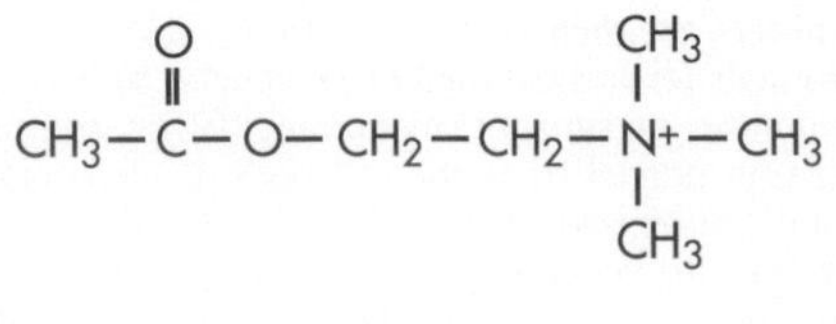

FIGURE 8-17
Acetylcholine, which is manufactured by the acetylation of choline, a reaction catalyzed by the enzyme choline acetyltransferase.

Glutamate

$$HOOC-CH_2-CH_2-\overset{\overset{\displaystyle NH_2}{|}}{CH}-COOH$$

GAD

$$HOOC-CH_2-CH_2-\overset{\overset{\displaystyle NH_2}{|}}{CH_2}$$

Gamma-aminobutyric acid (GABA)

FIGURE 8-18
The two most prominent amino acid neurotransmitters, glutamate and γ-aminobutyric acid (GABA). GABA is synthesized from glutamate via a decarboxylation catalyzed by glutamic acid decarboxylase (GAD).

Table 8-4	Major Locations of Neurons and Synapses That Use Glutamate (or Aspartate)	
Location of neurons	**Location of terminals**
Interneurons in many CNS sites	Local connections
Primary sensory neurons	Second-order neurons in CNS
Pyramidal cells of cerebral cortex★	Basal ganglia, thalamus, spinal cord, other cortical areas

★Chapter 22.

Table 8-5	Major Locations of Neurons and Synapses That Use GABA	
Location of neurons	**Location of terminals**
Interneurons in many CNS sites	Local connections
Cerebellar cortex (Purkinje cells★)	Deep cerebellar nuclei★
Caudate nucleus, putamen	Globus pallidus, substantia nigra
Globus pallidus, substantia nigra	Thalamus, subthalamic nucleus‡
Thalamic reticular nucleus†	Other thalamic nuclei

★Chapter 20.
†Chapter 16.
‡Chapter 19.

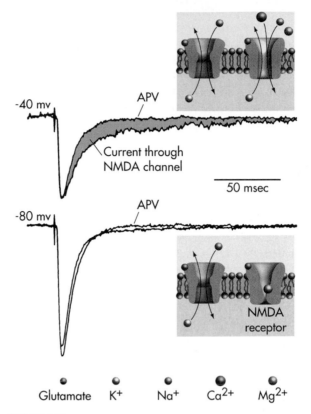

FIGURE 8-19

Properties of NMDA receptors, shown in patch-clamp recordings of postsynaptic currents in hippocampal pyramidal neurons. Near the normal resting membrane potential (-80 mv), most of the postsynaptic current in response to electrical stimulation of presynaptic fibers flows through non-NMDA channels, because the NMDA channels are blocked by Mg^{2+}. Hence application of the NMDA receptor antagonist 2-amino-5-phosphonovalerate (APV) causes no change in the postsynaptic current. Depolarization to -40 mv removes the Mg^{2+} block, and the same stimulus elicits an additional, slower, Na^+-K^+-Ca^{2+} current, blocked by APV, to flow through the NMDA channels. (Electrical recordings from Hestrin S et al: Analysis of excitatory synaptic action in pyramidal cells using whole-cell recording from rat hippocampal slices, J Physiol 422:203, 1990.)

Although some glutamate receptors are coupled to G proteins, most are transmitter-gated ion channels. One of the latter, called the **NMDA receptor** because it also binds the compound N-methyl-D-aspartate, has both transmitter-gated and voltage-gated properties (Figure 8-19) and is the channel responsible for long-term potentiation. NMDA receptors are found side by side on postsynaptic membranes with the more conventional glutamate-gated cation channels responsible for fast EPSPs. At the normal resting potential, a Mg^{2+} ion occupies the NMDA receptor channel and prevents current flow, even in the presence of glutamate. Depolarizing the postsynaptic membrane, for example as a result of repetitive presynaptic activity and release of neuropeptides as well as substantial glutamate, expels the Mg^{2+} ion and allows the NMDA channel to open. Open NMDA receptor channels are also unusual in that they permit the passage not only of Na^+ and K^+ ions, but also of large numbers of Ca^{2+} ions. The resulting postsynaptic increase in Ca^{2+} concen-

tration activates second-messenger cascades that in turn augment transmission at the synapse. NMDA receptors are found in other locations as well, such as the presynaptic terminals of some sensory neurons, and they may be widely involved in adjusting the strength of synapses.

As in the case of acetylcholine, there are two categories of GABA receptors. **GABA_A receptors** (as well as glycine receptors) are transmitter-gated ion channels, structurally similar to nicotinic receptors except for the fact that when open they are permeable to Cl^- ions. The less numerous **GABA_B receptors** are G protein–coupled receptors that cause slow IPSPs by opening K^+ channels.

Excessive levels of glutamate are toxic

Most neurons have receptors for glutamate, the principal excitatory neurotransmitter in the CNS, and this amino acid is available in high concentrations in excitatory synaptic terminals. Ordinarily, glutamate released at synapses is taken back up rapidly into the presynaptic terminal or surrounding glial cells, so that postsynaptic membranes are exposed to this amino acid only briefly. This is important, because more than a brief dose is toxic—prolonged exposure to glutamate triggers a sequence of events that can injure or even kill neurons, a phenomenon called **excitotoxicity.** Excessive Ca^{2+} entry through NMDA receptor channels is thought to initiate many aspects of the toxicity. Overexposure to glutamate could arise either from excessive release or from deficient reuptake, and both mechanisms may play a role in some forms of neuropathology. Part of the mechanism of brain damage in stroke may involve the release of toxic amounts of glutamate in response to anoxia, and some degenerative diseases of the nervous system may result from localized defects in glutamate reuptake.

Amines and Neuropeptides Mediate Slow, Diffuse Transmission

The other amine transmitters, called **monoamines,** are derived fairly directly from amino acids. Two of the three most prominent of these molecules, **norepinephrine** and **dopamine** (Figure 8-20), are derived from tyrosine.

(They are also referred to as **catecholamines** because of the catechol nucleus that forms part of each.) The third major monoamine transmitter, **serotonin** (Figure 8-21), is derived from tryptophan. Nearly all monoamine receptors are G protein–coupled receptors. The only exception is one type of serotonin receptor, which is a transmitter-gated ion channel.

Monoamine-containing CNS neurons are concentrated in the brainstem (Table 8-6). Despite this restricted distribution, these neurons, like those of some central cholinergic nuclei, have far-flung connections (see Figures 11-20, 11-22, and 11-23), suggesting that they too are involved in regulating or tuning the activity of large portions of the CNS. Nevertheless, there are characteristic differences between the termination patterns of fibers containing acetylcholine, norepinephrine, dopamine, and serotonin. This, together with consistent associations between certain transmitter systems and neurological syndromes (for example, dopamine and Parkinson's disease, as discussed in Chapter 19), suggests strongly that each of these four transmitters plays a distinctive role in the CNS.

There were demonstrations more than half a century ago that some neurons secrete hormones, as in the cases of neurosecretory neurons of the hypothalamus that produce oxytocin and vasopressin. These observations were ex-

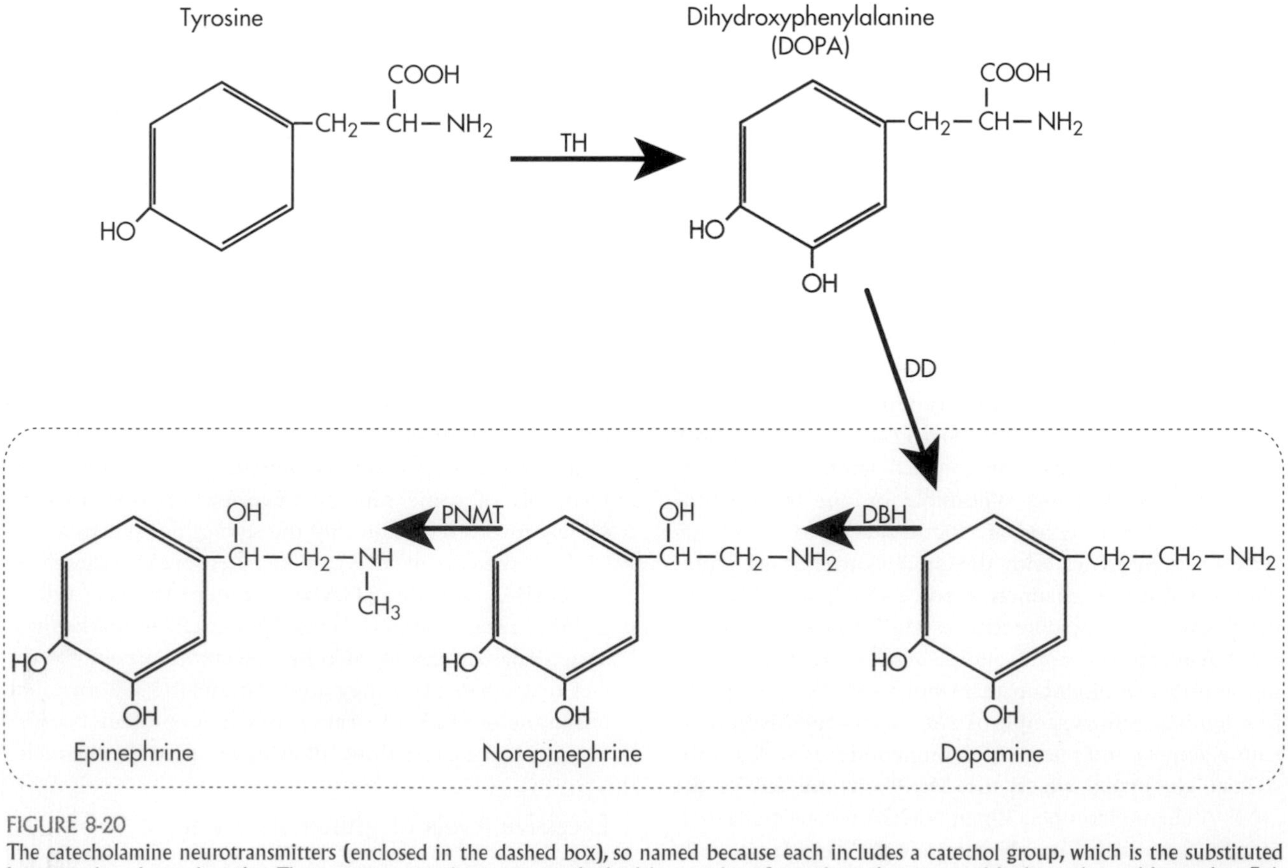

FIGURE 8-20
The catecholamine neurotransmitters (enclosed in the dashed box), so named because each includes a catechol group, which is the substituted benzene ring shown in color. These neurotransmitters are synthesized in a series of reactions that starts with the amino acid tyrosine. Epinephrine plays a relatively minor role as a neurotransmitter in the human brain, but dopamine and norepinephrine are widely distributed. *DBH,* dopamine β-hydroxylase; *DD,* DOPA decarboxylase; *PNMT,* phenylethanolamine-*N*-methyltransferase; *TH,* tyrosine hydroxylase (the rate-limiting enzyme for the whole pathway).

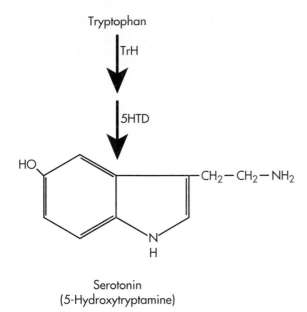

FIGURE 8-21
Structure and synthesis of serotonin. The pathway begins with the amino acid tryptophan, which is hydroxylated in a rate-limiting step catalyzed by tryptophan hydroxylase *(TrH)*. The resulting 5-hydroxytryptophan is decarboxylated in a reaction catalyzed by 5-hydroxytryptophan decarboxylase *(5HTD)*, resulting in serotonin.

Table 8-6	Major Locations of Neurons and Synapses That Use Monoamines	
Transmitter	Location of neurons	Location of terminals
Norepinephrine	Sympathetic ganglia★	Smooth and cardiac muscle, glands
	Locus ceruleus,† reticular formation†	Widespread CNS areas
Dopamine	Substantia nigra†‡ (compact part)	Caudate nucleus, putamen
	Ventral tegmental area†§	Limbic structures, cerebral cortex
	Hypothalamus	Infundibulum‡
	Retina (some amacrine cells) ‖	Local connections
	Olfactory bulb	Local connections
Serotonin	Raphe nuclei†	Widespread CNS areas

★Chapter 10.
†Chapter 11.
‡Chapter 19.
§Chapter 23.
‖ Chapter 17.

tended when, beginning in the early 1970s, the factors released by the hypothalamus to control the pituitary gland were isolated and characterized as short chains of amino acids, or peptides. Work since that time, using more recently available experimental techniques, has fundamentally transformed our view of the relationship between peptides and the function of the nervous system. It is now apparent that there are far more kinds of neuroactive peptides (or **neuropeptides**) in the brain than previously imagined—the number now stands at more than 50—and that most or all of them can function as neurotransmitters. For example, the 14-amino-acid peptide **somatostatin** was originally described as the hypothalamic inhibiting factor that controls the secretion of growth hormone by the anterior pituitary. It was subsequently found that hormonally released somatostatin accounts for only about 10% of the somatostatin in the brain, and that this peptide is localized primarily in the synaptic endings of neurons in many different CNS locations. Another example is the 11-amino acid peptide **substance P,** originally described as a smooth muscle relaxant isolated from gut, which has been localized in the synaptic endings of some basal ganglia neurons, dorsal root ganglion cells, and other neurons.

Some neuropeptides are widely distributed and presumably have multiple or general functions. Others have a more restricted distribution and may be associated with a specific function. For example, the octapeptide **angiotensin II** is a blood-borne hormone produced as part of the kidney's response to dehydration; it acts in the kidney and elsewhere outside the nervous system to promote water retention. Blood-borne angiotensin II also acts as a neurohormone by entering the CNS in the walls of the third ventricle and activating neurons in the subfornical organ (see Figure 6-26). Finally, a system of neurons (including those of the subfornical organ) that apparently use angiotensin II as a transmitter orchestrate vasopressin secretion, blood pressure adjustments, and a search for water.

Neuropeptides are metabolically expensive for cells to make and transport, so they are present and effective at very low concentrations. In addition, their initial synthesis from larger precursor proteins allows neurons to get some extra mileage: the precursor may contain multiple copies of a smaller neuropeptide or copies of multiple neuropeptides with different effects.

Most or all neurons that contain a neuropeptide also contain one or more of the "classical" small-molecule transmitters. This means that there are often separate subpopulations of neurons in a CNS area, each with its own chemical signature. For example, GABA-containing neurons of the putamen that project to one part of the globus pallidus also contain enkephalin; those that project to another part of the globus pallidus also contain substance P. The functional consequences of this coexistence of transmitter substances are unknown in most

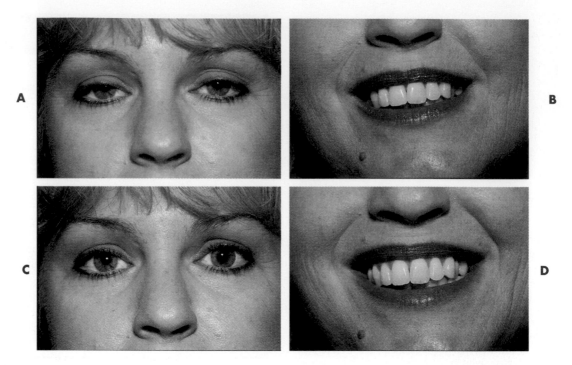

FIGURE 8-22
The eyes and smile of a patient with myasthenia gravis. When looking straight ahead (**A**), her eyelids drooped. Looking to either side (not shown) caused diplopia because of weakness of her eye muscles. Facial movements were also somewhat limited when she tried to smile (**B**). Minutes after the administration of an acetylcholinesterase inhibitor (which enhances the activity of acetylcholine at the neuromuscular junction by preventing its breakdown), her eyes were open wider (**C**), her diplopia resolved, and her smile was much broader (**D**).

cases, but it seems clear that single synapses can mediate multiple effects with different time courses and sensitivities.

Drugs and Toxins Can Selectively Affect Particular Parts of Individual Neurotransmitter Systems

Synaptic transmission involves a much wider array of proteins and processes than does generation and conduction of action potentials, and there is a correspondingly enormous array of toxins, disease processes, and drugs that affect different aspects of synaptic transmission. For example, one would predict that a molecule that binds to nicotinic receptors and prevents them from opening would cause weakness or paralysis by blocking neuromuscular transmission. This is in fact the mechanism of action of **curare,** the active ingredient of the plant extracts used for centuries on poisoned arrow tips to paralyze prey. A similar partial block occurs in patients with **myasthenia gravis,** who produce antibodies to their own nicotinic receptors (Figure 8-22). Although the plethora of transmitters, receptors, and receptor subtypes may seem at times like a curse of enormous proportions, it is actually a huge blessing. As we learn more about each, it becomes progressively more feasible to design pharmaceutical agents that precisely target particular neural processes (Figure 8-23).

GAP JUNCTIONS MEDIATE DIRECT CURRENT FLOW FROM ONE NEURON TO ANOTHER

Many cells in the body are electrically coupled to each other by junctions that allow the passage not only of ions, but also of a variety of small molecules. The morphological substrate is the **gap junction** (Figure 8-24), a site at which the normal separation between cells is narrowed to only about 3 nm. Cylindrical transmembrane protein assemblies called **connexons** butt up against one another at gap junctions, so that their aqueous centers are aligned and form a continuous channel interconnecting the two cells. The central pore is larger than in the case of ion channels, allowing the easy passage of small molecules.

Gap junctions between neurons form **electrical synapses,** allowing the direct spread of current from one neuron into another. This would seem to have considerable advantages—duplication of the presynaptic signal in the postsynaptic cell, no delay in the transmission of electrical information, and no need to synthesize vesicles and transmitters. However, the overriding disadvantage is a partial loss of the functional individuality of the coupled neurons. Chemical transmission allows neurons to be separate computational units, each one potentially doing something entirely different from its neighbor. Presumably for this reason, gap junctions are relatively rare in mammalian nervous systems. They are more common during

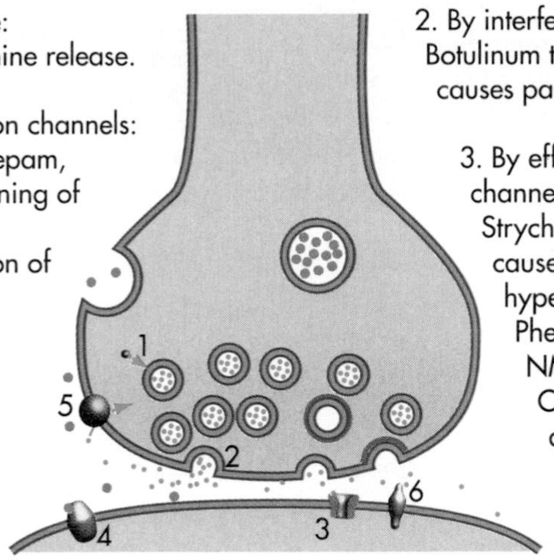

DRUGS OR TOXINS THAT ENHANCE TRANSMISSION

1. By enhancing synthesis or packaging of neurotransmitter: L-dopa crosses the blood-brain barrier and is metabolized into dopamine, compensating for lower dopamine levels in Parkinson's disease.

2. By enhancing neurotransmitter release: Amphetamine causes increased monoamine release.

3. By effects on neurotransmitter-gated ion channels: Benzodiazepine tranquilizers (e.g., diazepam, or Valium) increase the frequency of opening of GABA-gated Cl^- channels. Barbiturate sedatives increase the duration of opening of GABA-gated Cl^- channels.

4. By effects on G protein–coupled neurotransmitter receptors: Morphine mimics opioid peptides, binds to their receptors, causes analgesia and other effects.

5. By blocking removal of neurotransmitter: Fluoxetine (Prozac), an antidepressant, blocks serotonin reuptake. Cocaine blocks monoamine reuptake.

6. By blocking degradation of neurotransmitter: Pyridostigmine (Mestinon) blocks acetylcholinesterase, is used to treat patients with myasthenia gravis.

DRUGS OR TOXINS THAT DEPRESS TRANSMISSION

1. By interfering with synthesis or packaging of neurotransmitter: Reserpine blocks transport of monoamines into synaptic vesicles.

2. By interfering with neurotransmitter release: Botulinum toxin blocks release of acetylcholine, causes paralysis.

3. By effects on neurotransmitter-gated ion channels: Strychnine blocks glycine-gated Cl^- channels, causes convulsions and other signs of hyperexcitability. Phencyclidine (PCP, "angel dust") blocks NMDA receptors. Curare (arrow tip poison) blocks nicotinic acetylcholine receptors, causes paralysis.

4. By effects on G protein–coupled neurotransmitter receptors: Haloperidol (Haldol), an antipsychotic, blocks some dopamine receptors. Atropine blocks muscarinic acetylcholine receptors, causes autonomic changes.

FIGURE 8-23
Examples of agents that affect different aspects of synaptic transmission.

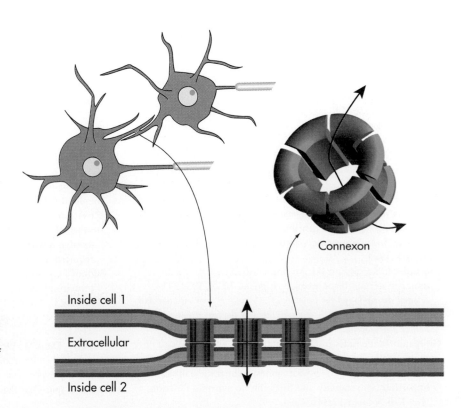

FIGURE 8-24
Schematic illustration of the structure of a gap junction. Each connexon is made up of six subunits surrounding a central pore, allowing diffusion of small molecules (typically, but not always, in both directions).

Connexon

Inside cell 1

Extracellular

Inside cell 2

development, probably allowing populations of cells to share metabolic information and signaling molecules. In adult nervous systems, they are found in some groups of neurons that tend to fire action potentials synchronously, and rarely are found in networks of cells designed to spread information electrotonically over long distances. Horizontal cells of the retina (see Chapter 17) are one example of the latter. The conductance of gap junctions may not be static; many can be modulated by second-messenger effects, allowing some control over the coupling between neurons.

SUGGESTED READINGS

Adams ME, Swanson G: Neurotoxins, ed 2, *Trends Neurosci* 19(suppl), 1996. *An extensive listing of toxins that affect a variety of ion channels.*

Agnati LF et al: Intercellular communication in the brain: wiring versus volume transmission, *Neurosci* 69:711, 1995. *In this context, "wiring" means anatomically defined synapses, and "volume transmission" means diffusion of transmitters through extracellular space to receptors in nonsynaptic locations.*

Attwell D, Barbour B, Szatkowski M: Nonvesicular release of neurotransmitter, *Neuron* 11:401, 1993. *There may be a little, in some special situations.*

Beal MF, Martin JB: Neuropeptides in neurological disease, *Ann Neurol* 20:547, 1986.

Bennett MVL et al: Gap junctions: new tools, new answers, new questions, *Neuron* 6:305, 1991.

Bliss TVP, Collingridge GL: A synaptic model of memory: long-term potentiation in the hippocampus, *Nature* 361:31, 1993.

Brown AM, Birnbaumer L: Ionic channels and their regulation by G protein subunits, *Ann Rev Physiol* 52:197, 1990.

Calakos N, Scheller RH: Synaptic vesicle biogenesis, docking, and fusion: a molecular description, *Physiol Rev* 76:1, 1996.

Choi DW, Rothman SM: The role of glutamate neurotoxicity in hypoxic-ischemic neuronal death, *Ann Rev Neurosci* 13:171, 1990.

Clapham DE: Direct G protein activation of ion channels, *Ann Rev Neurosci* 17:441, 1994.

Cooper JR, Bloom FE, Roth RH: *The biochemical basis of neuropharmacology*, ed 7, New York, 1996, Oxford University Press. *A concise, easily readable review.*

Dawson TM, Snyder SH: Gases as biological messengers: nitric oxide and carbon monoxide in the brain, *J Neurosci* 14:5147, 1994.

Eccles JC: *The physiology of synapses*, New York, 1964, Academic Press. *A review by one of the pioneers of synaptic physiology.*

Egberongbe YI et al: The distribution of nitric oxide synthase immunoreactivity in the human brain, *Neurosci* 59:561, 1994.

von Euler US, Gaddum JH: An unidentified depressor substance in certain tissue extracts, *J Physiol* 72:74, 1931. *The original description of the isolation of substance P from intestine and brain. Unbeknownst to the authors, this was the first recorded isolation of a neuropeptide.*

Guillemin R: Peptides in the brain: the new endocrinology of the neuron, *Science* 202:390, 1978.

Harris KM, Kater SB: Dendritic spines: cellular specializations imparting both stability and flexibility to synaptic function, *Ann Rev Neurosci* 17:341, 1994.

Herkenham M: Mismatches between neurotransmitter and receptor localization in brain: observations and implications, *Neurosci* 23:1, 1987.

Heuser JE: Review of electron microscopic evidence favouring vesicle exocytosis as the structural basis for quantal release during synaptic transmission, *Quart J Exp Physiol* 74:1051, 1989.

Isaacson JS, Walmsley B: Counting quanta: direct measurement of transmitter release at a central synapse, *Neuron* 15:875, 1995.

Jessell TM, Kandel ER: Synaptic transmission: a bidirectional and self-modifiable form of cell-cell communication, *Cell* 72/*Neuron* 10(Suppl):1, 1993. *An overview article introducing a special issue about synaptic transmission.*

Katz B: *Nerve, muscle and synapse*, New York, 1966, McGraw-Hill. *A lucid introduction to neurophysiology by a Nobel laureate who did much of the early work on neuromuscular transmission.*

Kostyuk P, Verkhratsky A: Calcium stores in neurons and glia, *Neurosci* 63:381, 1994. *A review of the elaborate mechanisms used by the nervous system to control intracellular levels of free Ca^{2+}.*

Lipton SA, Rosenberg PA: Excitatory amino acids as a final common pathway for neurological disorders, *New Engl J Med* 330:613, 1994.

Liu H et al: Synaptic relationship between substance P and the substance P receptor: Light and electron microscopic characterization of the mismatch between neuropeptides and their receptors, *Proc Natl Acad Sci* 91:1009, 1994.

Lundberg JM, Hökfelt T: Coexistence of peptides and classical neurotransmitters, *Trends Neurosci* 6:325, 1983.

Matthews G: Neurotransmitter release, *Ann Rev Neurosci* 19:219, 1996.

Nicoll R, Malenka R, Kauer J: Functional comparison of neurotransmitter receptor subtypes in the mammalian nervous system, *Physiol Rev* 70:513, 1990.

Olney JW: Inciting excitotoxic cytocide among central neurons. In Schwartz RW, Ben-Ari Y: Excitatory amino acids and epilepsy (*Adv Exp Med Biol*) vol 203, New York, 1986, Plenum Press. *"One of my major research goals in recent years has been to answer a simple question: 'Can one CNS neuron excite another CNS neuron to death?'"*

Sabatini BL, Regehr WG: Timing of neurotransmission at fast synapses in the mammalian brain, *Nature* 384:170, 1996. *Direct measurements of the remarkable speed of transmitter release at mammalian CNS synapses.*

Schwartz J-C et al: Histaminergic transmission in the mammalian brain, *Physiol Rev* 71:1, 1991. *One more amine neurotransmitter, this one prominent in hypothalamic neurons.*

Shepherd GM: The dendritic spine: a multifunctional integrative unit, *J Neurophysiol* 75:2197, 1996.

Stevens CF, Tsujimoto T: Estimates for the pool size of releasable quanta at a single central synapse and for the time required to refill the pool, *Proc Natl Acad Sci* 92:846, 1995.

Südhof TC: The synaptic vesicle cycle: a cascade of protein-protein interactions, *Nature* 375:645, 1995.

Walmsley B, Alvarez FJ, Fyffe REW: Diversity of structure and function at mammalian central synapses, *Trends Neurosci* 21:81, 1998.

Yuste R, Denk W: Dendritic spines as basic functional units of neuronal integration, *Nature* 375:682, 1995. *Technically extraordinary experiments in which Ca^{2+} concentration changes in individual spines are observed directly.*

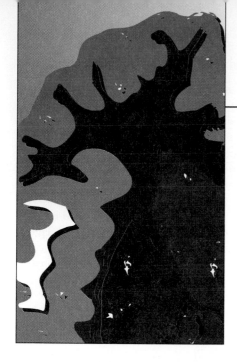

SENSORY RECEPTORS AND THE PERIPHERAL NERVOUS SYSTEM

RECEPTORS ENCODE THE NATURE, INTENSITY, DURATION, AND LOCATION OF STIMULI

Each Sensory Receptor Has an Adequate Stimulus, Allowing It to Encode the Nature of a Stimulus

Many sensory receptors have a receptive field, allowing them to encode the location of a stimulus

Receptor Potentials Encode the Intensity and Duration of Stimuli

Sensory receptors utilize stimulus-gated ion channels and G protein–coupled ion channels to produce receptor potentials

Most sensory receptors adapt to maintained stimuli, some more rapidly than others

Sensory Receptors All Share Some Organizational Features

Some sensory receptors do not produce action potentials

SOMATOSENSORY RECEPTORS DETECT MECHANICAL OR CHEMICAL CHANGES

Cutaneous Receptors Have Free Nerve Endings or Encapsulated Endings

Some cutaneous mechanoreceptors have encapsulated endings, others have nonencapsulated endings

Nociceptors, thermoreceptors, and some mechanoreceptors have free nerve endings

Pain serves a useful function

Cutaneous receptors are not distributed uniformly

Receptors in Muscles and Joints Detect Muscle Status and Limb Position

Muscle spindles detect muscle length

Golgi tendon organs detect muscle tension

Joints have receptors

Muscle spindles are important proprioceptors

Visceral Structures Contain a Variety of Receptive Endings

Particular Sensations Are Sometimes Related to Particular Receptor Types

PERIPHERAL NERVES CONVEY INFORMATION TO AND FROM THE CNS

Extensions of the Meninges Envelop Peripheral Nerves

The Diameter of a Nerve Fiber Is Correlated With Its Function

191

The ongoing activity and output of the CNS are greatly influenced, and sometimes more or less determined, by incoming sensory information. An example is our constant awareness of the position of our limbs in space and the use of this awareness in guiding movements. The basis of this incoming sensory information is an array of **sensory receptors,*** cells that detect various stimuli and produce **receptor potentials** in response, often with astonishing effectiveness. Rod photoreceptors, for example, can produce measurable responses to single photons (see Chapter 17), and olfactory receptors can respond to single odorant molecules (see Chapter 13). The physiological processes employed by sensory receptors turn out to be gratifyingly similar to those found in synapses.

This chapter considers some general principles of the anatomy and physiology of sensory receptors. The emphasis is on the general receptors of the body—the principal purveyors of sensory information to the spinal cord (see Chapter 10). Specialized receptors, such as those of the eye and the ear, are described in more detail in later chapters.

RECEPTORS ENCODE THE NATURE, INTENSITY, DURATION, AND LOCATION OF STIMULI

There are many types of receptors on and within the human body and several different systems for classifying them. One system subdivides receptors according to the traditional five senses of vision, hearing, touch, smell, and taste. This is too restrictive, however, because it does not recognize sensations such as balance, position, or pain, or sensory information from internal organs that usually does not reach consciousness. Another system distinguishes **interoceptors, proprioceptors,** and **exteroceptors.** Interoceptors monitor events within the body, such as distention of the stomach or changes in the pH of the blood. Proprioceptors respond to changes in the position of the body or its parts; examples are the receptors in muscles and joint capsules. Vestibular receptors of the inner ear are commonly classified as proprioceptors because they signal movement and changes in the orientation of the head in space. Exteroceptors respond to stimuli that arise outside the body, such as the receptors involved in touch, hearing, and vision. Exteroceptors are sometimes subdivided into **teloreceptors** (from the Greek word *tele*, meaning "distant," as in television), which respond to stimuli or objects separated from the body (e.g., visual receptors and auditory receptors), and **contact receptors** (e.g., tactile receptors and pain receptors). Interoceptor-proprioceptor-exteroceptor terminology is not used as commonly as it was in the past, partly because some receptors do not fit neatly and uniquely into one of these categories. For example, heat-sensitive receptors respond to both radiant heat and contact with a warm object, so to classify them as either teloreceptors or contact receptors is somewhat arbitrary. Also, some vestibular receptors respond to gravity, an external force, but are classified as proprioceptors; on the other hand, the visual system is very much involved in our perception of motion and body position, but visual receptors are considered exteroceptors.

Each Sensory Receptor Has an Adequate Stimulus, Allowing It to Encode the Nature of a Stimulus

A more commonly used and straightforward classification system subdivides receptors on the basis of the type of stimulus to which they are most sensitive (called the **adequate stimulus**). **Chemoreceptors** include those for smell, taste, and many internal stimuli such as pH and metabolite concentrations. **Photoreceptors** are the visual receptors of the retina. **Thermoreceptors** respond to temperature and its changes. **Mechanoreceptors,** the most varied group, respond to physical deformation. They include cutaneous receptors for touch, receptors that monitor muscle length and tension, auditory and vestibular receptors, and others. Pain receptors are a bit difficult to classify in this system because different pain receptors have varying degrees of sensitivity to mechanical, thermal, and chemical stimuli. This problem is commonly finessed by classifying pain receptors separately as **nociceptors** (from the Latin word *noci* meaning "hurt," as in noxious or obnoxious).

To a first approximation, the kind of receptors that get stimulated define the nature, or **modality,** of the sensation that is experienced—you experience touch if something actually touches you, or if a peripheral nerve attached to a touch receptor is stimulated electrically. Each sensory modality has a series of submodalities, or **qualities,** associated with it. Stimuli delivered to the skin, for example, can feel like light touch, pressure, a tickle, or vibration. This roughly corresponds to the presence in the skin of multiple receptor types, whose separate outputs the CNS can combine to produce sensations that are richer and more complex, for example, sensations such as the texture of objects.

Many sensory receptors have a receptive field, allowing them to encode the location of a stimulus

Specific wiring patterns in ascending sensory pathways and in the cerebral cortex preserve information about the nature of a stimulus. In some sensory systems, individual receptors convey information not only about the nature of

---

Receptor, like *nucleus*, thus becomes a term with two meanings in neurobiology. A sensory receptor, as described in this chapter, is a specialized cell that conveys to the nervous system information about some stimulus. Neurotransmitter receptors, as described in Chapter 8, are molecules in postsynaptic membranes. To make matters worse, some sensory receptors receive feedback synapses, and so have neurotransmitter receptors in their membranes!

a stimulus, but also about its location. That is, individual receptors not only have adequate stimuli, they also may have **receptive fields,** particular areas in the periphery where application of an adequate stimulus will cause them to respond. For a cutaneous receptor, for example, its receptive field is an area of skin where its receptive endings reside (Figure 9-1). The receptive field of a retinal photoreceptor is some small location in the outside world whose image falls on the particular spot on the retina where that photoreceptor is located. This preservation of spatial information is apparent in the CNS as the common occurrence of systematic maps (see Figure 3-28). Even arrays of receptors with no obvious spatial domain to map may have maps of some other parameter, as in the mapping of sound frequencies in the cochlea and in auditory cortex (see Figure 14-18).

Neurons in successive levels of sensory pathways—second-order neurons, thalamic and cortical neurons—also have receptive fields, although they may be considerably more elaborate than those of the receptors. Neurons in visual cortex, for example, typically respond not to spots of light, but rather to edges with particular orientations.

Receptor Potentials Encode the Intensity and Duration of Stimuli

The nature and location of a stimulus are indicated by the identities of the receptors that respond. To a great extent the intensity and duration of a stimulus are indicated by the size and duration of the receptor potentials produced—more intense stimuli produce larger receptor potentials, and longer stimuli cause longer receptor potentials (Figure 9-2). There is a bit more to the intensity/duration

story than this, however. Some sensory systems include more-sensitive and less-sensitive receptors (as in the rods and cones of the retina), so increasing intensity may be signaled in part by the identities of the active receptors. In addition, as discussed a little later in this chapter, some sensory receptors produce only brief receptor potentials even in response to maintained stimuli.

Sensory receptors utilize stimulus-gated ion channels and G protein–coupled ion channels to produce receptor potentials

Sensory receptors **transduce*** some physical stimulus into an electrical signal, a receptor potential, that the nervous system can understand. Receptor potentials, like other electrical signals across neuronal membranes, are produced by the opening or closing of ion channels. (The only exception known at this point is one kind of taste receptor, as discussed in Chapter 13.) It has become clear in recent years that in many ways most sensory receptors can be thought of as analogous to postsynaptic membranes, and their adequate stimuli as analogous to neurotransmitters (Figure 9-3). Although the transduction mechanism is not understood for all sensory receptors, almost all known mechanisms involve ion channels whose conductance is affected either directly by a stimulus (as in transmitter-gated ion channels), or indirectly by way of a G protein–coupled mechanism. Just as in the case of synapses, some sensory receptors (e.g., somatosensory mechanoreceptors) produce depolarizing receptor potentials when stimulated and oth-

---

*From a Latin word meaning "to lead across."

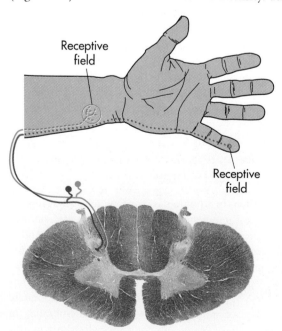

FIGURE 9-1
Receptive fields of two cutaneous receptors.

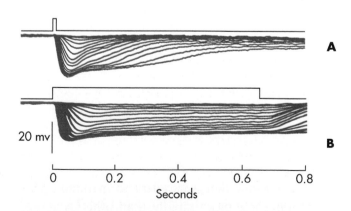

FIGURE 9-2
Intracellular recordings of the receptor potentials produced by a single cone photoreceptor in response to a series of brief (**A**) or longer flashes (**B**), each about twice as bright as the next dimmer. Brief, dim flashes cause brief hyperpolarizations that are graded with light intensity (vertebrate photoreceptors produce hyperpolarizing receptor potentials). Longer flashes produce a sustained receptor potential that lasts as long as the flash. (From Baylor DA, Hodgkin AL, Lamb TD: Reconstruction of the electrical responses of turtle cones to flashes and steps of light, *J Physiol* 242:759, 1974.)

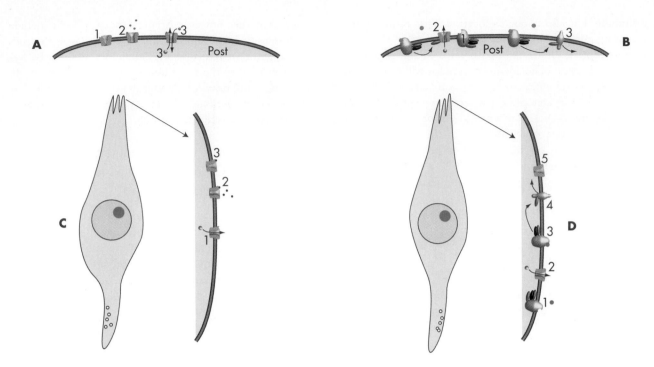

FIGURE 9-3
Similarities between the general mechanisms of postsynaptic potentials and receptor potentials; taste receptor cells (see Chapter 13) are used as examples, but almost all receptors use similar mechanisms. **A,** Rapid synaptic transmission involves ligand-gated ion channels (*I*) that bind neurotransmitter (*2*) and then change permeability (*3*). **C,** Some bitter-sensitive taste receptor cells contain normally-open, ligand-gated K⁺ channels (*I*) that bind bitter substances (*2*) and close (*3*), causing a depolarizing receptor potential. **B,** Slow synaptic transmission involves G protein–coupled receptors (*I*). Dissociation of the G protein in response to neurotransmitter binding may affect ion channels either directly (*2*) or indirectly via enzymatic cascades (*3*). **D,** Sweet-sensitive taste receptor cells contain normally-open K⁺ channels (*2*) and G protein–coupled receptors for sweet substances (*I*). Dissociation of the G protein (*3*) activates an enzyme (*4,* adenyl cyclase), which catalyzes the production of a second messenger (cyclic AMP) that in turn closes K⁺ channels (*5*), causing a depolarizing receptor potential.

ers (e.g., photoreceptors) produce hyperpolarizing receptor potentials. Auditory and vestibular receptors can produce either, depending on the details of the stimulus.

Receptors with directly gated ion channels include most of the somatosensory receptors discussed in this chapter, auditory and vestibular receptors, some taste receptors, and some visceral receptors. Some have channels that are directly sensitive to mechanical distortion and others have channels directly gated by some molecule or ion. Receptors with a G protein–coupled transduction mechanism include photoreceptors, olfactory receptors, some taste receptors, and probably some nociceptors and visceral receptors.

Most sensory receptors adapt to maintained stimuli, some more rapidly than others

Nearly all receptors show some **adaptation,** which means they become less sensitive during the course of a maintained stimulus. Those that adapt relatively little are called **slowly adapting** and are suitable receptors for such things as static position. Those that adapt a great deal are called **rapidly adapting** and can only indicate change and movement of stimuli (Figure 9-4). Adaptation is gen-

erally a property of one or more parts of the receptor's membrane: a maintained stimulus may cause less and less receptor potential with time, or a given value of the receptor potential may generate progressively fewer action potentials. In addition, various accessory structures may modify the physical stimulus before it reaches the sensory ending, as in the case of the pupil constricting in response to bright light and decreasing the amount of light reaching the retina.

Sensory Receptors All Share Some Organizational Features

Although their morphologies vary widely, all receptors seem to have three general parts: a receptive area, an area rich in mitochondria (near the receptive area), and a synaptic area, where the receptor's message is passed toward or into the CNS (Figure 9-5). The receptive area may have specializations suited to the adequate stimulus, as in the case of photoreceptors, which have an elaborately folded array of photopigment-bearing membrane; in other cases, there are no obvious specializations in this area. The area rich in mitochondria is either immediately adjacent to the receptive membrane or nearby and is pre-

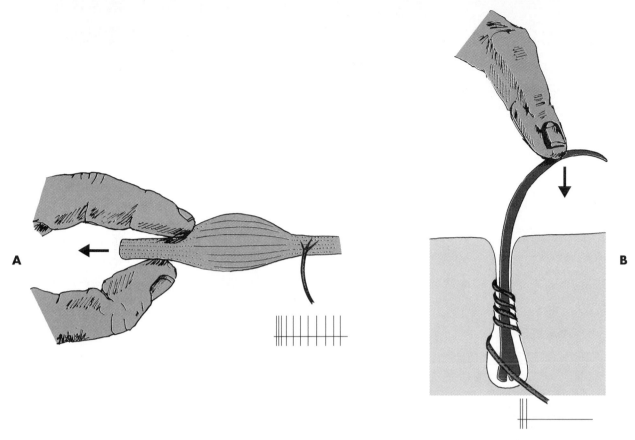

FIGURE 9-4
Slowly adapting versus rapidly adapting receptors. **A,** A tendon receptor (Golgi tendon organ) continues to fire action potentials as long as tension is maintained on the tendon. **B,** Most hair receptors fire a short burst of action potentials and are then silent, even if the bending of the hair is maintained.

sumed to supply the energy needs of the transduction process. In some receptors the synaptic area may be far removed from the other two, as in the case of a cutaneous mechanoreceptor with its receptive endings in the skin and its synaptic terminals in the spinal cord or brainstem.

Some sensory receptors do not produce action potentials

Receptor potentials, like postsynaptic potentials, are focally produced events that spread electrotonically. If a particular sensory receptor is physically small relative to its length constant—that is, if it contacts the next cell in its neuronal pathway close to the site of transduction—then the receptor potential itself can adequately modulate the rate of transmitter release at the synaptic terminal. This in turn will cause a postsynaptic potential, and typically a change in action potential frequency, in the second cell (Figure 9-6, *A*). This is the case for many receptors, prominently including photoreceptors and auditory and vestibular receptors, all of which produce receptor potentials but no action potentials. Some receptors, however,

must convey information over long distances (e.g., from a big toe to the spinal cord), even though the receptor potential dies out within a few millimeters. In such cases, most of the receptor, beginning near the site of transduction, is capable of propagating action potentials. The action potential frequency is then modulated by the receptor potential (Figure 9-6, *B*). Receptor potentials that directly cause changes in action potential frequency are also called **generator potentials.** All somatosensory receptors of the body operate in this manner, as do olfactory receptors and many visceral receptors.

SOMATOSENSORY RECEPTORS DETECT MECHANICAL OR CHEMICAL CHANGES

Somatosensory receptors include an assortment of mechanoreceptors, thermoreceptors, and nociceptors. All are pseudounipolar neurons with cell bodies in a dorsal root ganglion, a central process that terminates in the spinal cord or brainstem, and a peripheral receptive ending in someplace such as skin, a muscle, or a joint (Fig-

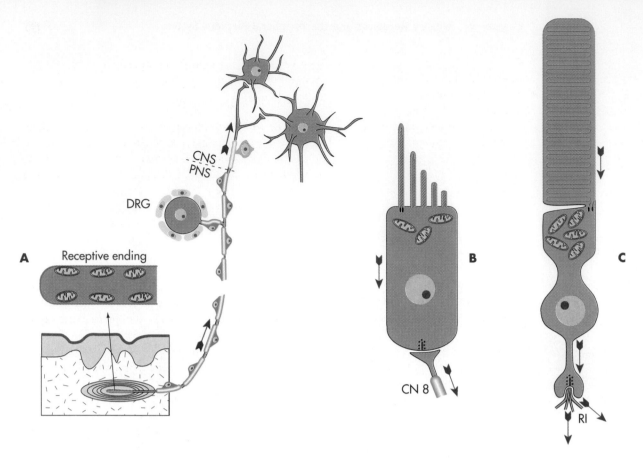

FIGURE 9-5
General organization of sensory receptors, as illustrated by a somatosensory receptor (Pacinian corpuscle, **A**), a hair cell of the inner ear (**B**), and a retinal rod photoreceptor (**C**). Each has a receptive area (*orange*) and mitochondria nearby. The receptive ending of the Pacinian corpuscle has no obvious anatomical specializations, but is surrounded by a layered capsule. The microvillar projections of the hair cell contain mechanosensitive channels (see Chapter 14), and the receptive area of the rod contains a collection of pigment-studded membranous disks (see Chapter 17). Somatosensory receptors make synapses far away in the CNS, whereas hair cells and photoreceptors make synapses nearby on peripheral endings of vestibulocochlear nerve fibers (*CN 8*) or on retinal interneurons (*RI*), respectively.

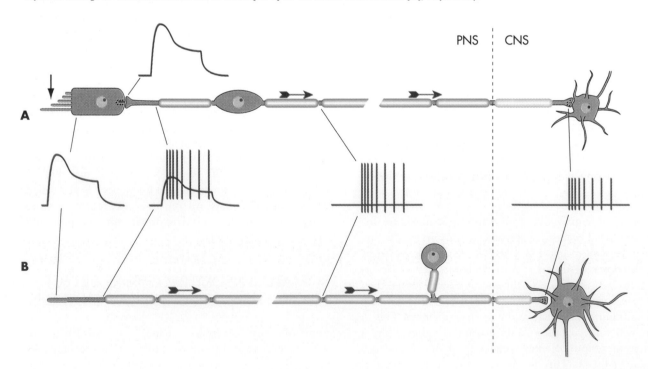

FIGURE 9-6
Short and long receptors, as illustrated by a hair cell of the inner ear (**A**) and a somatosensory ending (**B**). Hair cells produce a depolarizing receptor potential, but no action potentials, in response to deflection in the direction of the longest microvillar process (*arrow*). The receptor potential spreads passively to the synaptic area of the hair cell, where it increases release of neurotransmitter onto the peripheral ending of an eighth nerve fiber. The postsynaptic potential then spreads passively to the trigger zone of the nerve fiber and initiates the firing of action potentials, which are conducted to synaptic terminals in the CNS. Events in the somatosensory receptor are similar, except that no peripheral synapse is involved: the trigger zone of the peripheral nerve fiber is part of the same neuron that contains the receptive ending.

ure 9-1). A great deal is understood about the moment-to-moment responses of many of these receptors, mostly from animal studies but also in large part because it is possible to record from the axons of single receptors of human volunteers, using a process called **microneurography** (Figure 9-12, insets).

Cutaneous Receptors Have Free Nerve Endings or Encapsulated Endings

The skin and adjacent subcutaneous tissues are richly innervated by a wide variety of sensory endings. These endings may be divided conveniently into **encapsulated** and **nonencapsulated** receptors (Table 9-1), depending on whether a capsule surrounds the ending. A bewildering variety of encapsulated receptors have been described in the past, and an equally bewildering variety of mostly eponymous names have been attached to them. These classifications are merely variations on two common themes: receptors with layered capsules and receptors with thin capsules. This chapter describes only the best known of these. The function of the capsule is not known for all encapsulated receptors, but in at least some instances it serves as a mechanical filter, modifying mechanical stimuli before they reach the sensory ending. For example, receptors with layered capsules are rapidly adapting, due in large part to these mechanical properties of the capsules. The capsules also have barrier properties (discussed later in this chapter) that may be important in regulating the composition of the fluid surrounding the sensory endings contained within them.

Nonencapsulated receptors may be divided into two categories: **free nerve endings** and endings with **accessory structures** that do not surround the ending. Free nerve endings, as the name implies, are formed by branching terminations of sensory fibers in the skin, with no obvious specialization around them. Such endings are not restricted to the skin but are found throughout the body. Even though microscopically they look similar to one another, many are known to be nociceptors, others thermoreceptors, and still others mechanoreceptors.

Some cutaneous mechanoreceptors have encapsulated endings, others have nonencapsulated endings

In addition to mechanoreceptive free nerve endings, there are five other prominent types of mechanoreceptors found in the skin and adjacent subcutaneous tissue. Two are nonencapsulated endings with accessory structures, and three are encapsulated.

Endings around hairs vary in their degrees of complexity. Those around the base of a cat's whiskers are very elaborate, but those around most ordinary human body hairs are longitudinal neural processes and spiral endings that wrap around the base of the hair (Figure 9-7). Bending the hair is presumed to deform the sensory ending, distort mechanically sensitive channels, and lead to the production of a generator potential (although the precise molecular events coupling the stimulus at the receptor membrane to the receptor potential are not known for this or for any other somatosensory mechanoreceptor). Most hair receptors are rapidly adapting; they respond well to something brushing across the skin but not to a steady pressure.★

The second type of nonencapsulated receptor is the **Merkel ending,** which is found in both hairy and glabrous skin (Figure 9-7). The ending is a disc-shaped expansion of the terminal of a sensory fiber, which is inserted into the base of a specialized cell called a **Merkel cell.** A single fiber branches to innervate several Merkel cells, which tend to occur in groups. Each Merkel cell is situated in the basal layer of the epidermis and contains dense-cored vesicles in what looks like a synaptic ending onto the sensory terminal. This apparent synapse led naturally to the hypothesis that the Merkel cell is sensitive to deformation and uses this synapse to pass information about mechanical stimuli along to the nerve ending. However, the available evidence on this issue is inconclusive, and the role of the Merkel cell is currently uncertain. Recordings from these sensory fibers have shown that Merkel endings are slowly adapting mechanoreceptors.

★You can easily demonstrate this to yourself; bend a single hair on the back of your hand (or have someone else do it), then hold it in the bent position. You will feel it bending but will almost immediately lose awareness of its new position.

Table 9-1   Principal Types of Cutaneous Receptors

	Accessory structures	Receptors	Modality
Encapsulated	Layered capsule	Pacinian corpuscle	Vibration
		Meissner corpuscle	Touch
	Thin capsule	Ruffini ending	Pressure
Nonencapsulated ending	Present	Endings around hairs	Touch
		Merkel endings	Touch
	Absent	Free nerve ending	Pain, temperature, touch

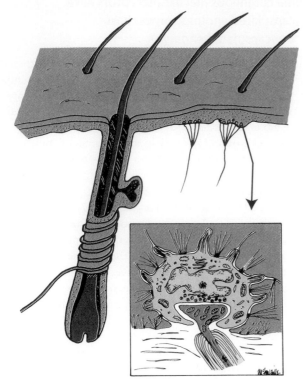

FIGURE 9-7
Two receptor types from hairy skin. Receptor endings wrap around hairs in a variety of configurations; a simple helical winding is shown. The inset is an enlarged drawing of a Merkel ending–Merkel cell complex in the basal layer of the epidermis. (Inset modified from Bannister LH: Sensory terminals of peripheral nerves. In Landon DN, editor: *The peripheral nerve*, London, 1976, Chapman & Hall.)

Meissner corpuscles are elongated, encapsulated endings in the dermal papillae of hairless skin just beneath the epidermis and are oriented with their long axis perpendicular to the surface of the skin (Figure 9-8). The encapsulation consists of a thin outer capsule and a layered stack of epithelial cells within the capsule, each cell oriented perpendicular to the long axis of the capsule. One or more myelinated fibers approach the base of the corpuscle, lose their myelin, and wind back and forth between the stacked cells within the capsule. These are rapidly adapting receptors, and it is assumed that the capsule and the layered epithelial cells within it are important in determining the degree of adaptation. Vertical pressure on a dermal papilla compresses the nerve endings between the stacked capsular cells of a Meissner corpuscle, whereas pressure on a neighboring papilla is not nearly so effective. Meissner corpuscles are quite numerous in the skin of fingertips, and it is thought that they and Merkel endings are largely responsible for our ability to perform fine tactile discriminations with our fingertips (Figures 9-9 and 9-16). Most animals have their own species-specific patterns of distribution of receptors, with specializations in functionally important parts of the body. Rats and cats have elaborate arrays of receptors surrounding their whiskers and large areas of somatosensory cortex devoted

to their whiskers. Elephants mind their trunks. Other animals have other patterns (Box 9-1).

Pacinian corpuscles are almost as widespread as free nerve endings. They are found subcutaneously over the entire body and in numerous other connective tissue sites. They are wrapped in the ultimate expression of a layered capsule and look like an onion in cross section (Figure 9-8). The capsule consists of many concentric layers of very thin epithelial cells, with fluid spaces between adjacent layers. Pacinian corpuscles are also rapidly adapting, and in this case the role of the capsule is understood. Quickly applied forces are transmitted through the interior of the capsule and reach the ending, but maintained forces are not, as a result of the elastic properties of the capsular layers. During maintained pressure, each successive layer is slightly less deformed than its outer neighbor—imagine indenting the outermost of a series of balloons, one inflated inside another—and the ending itself is not deformed at all. These corpuscles are amazingly sensitive: much like the Merkel endings, they can respond to skin indentations as small as 1 μm.

Because Pacinian corpuscles are probably the most rapidly adapting receptors we have, they are poor receptors for pressure but good ones for the rapidly changing mechanical stimulation that we perceive as vibration. That is, a vibratory stimulus causes a steady train of impulses from such an ending, so that in this sense the receptor is "slowly adapting." It is important to understand that slowly adapting receptors, as they are conventionally defined, are simply receptors that respond best to *unchanging* stimuli. Rapidly adapting receptors, on the other hand, respond best to *changing* stimuli, giving a constant output to a stimulus with constant velocity, constant acceleration, or some other temporal property.

The fifth type of cutaneous mechanoreceptor is an encapsulated receptor called a **Ruffini ending,** which is widespread in the dermis and in subcutaneous and other connective tissue sites. It consists of a thin, cigar-shaped capsule traversed longitudinally by strands of collagenous connective tissue. A sensory fiber enters the capsule and branches profusely, so that many small processes are interspersed among the collagenous strands. This is a slowly adapting receptor and is thought to work by the squeezing of sensory terminals between strands of connective tissue when tension is applied to one or both ends of the capsule. Because collagen is not very elastic, the deformation of the endings is maintained as long as the tension is maintained, so adaptation is slow.

Nociceptors, thermoreceptors, and some mechanoreceptors have free nerve endings

Nociceptors, thermoreceptors, and some mechanoreceptors are all free nerve endings; no pronounced morphological differences are seen among them with presently available techniques. Electrophysiological studies, however,

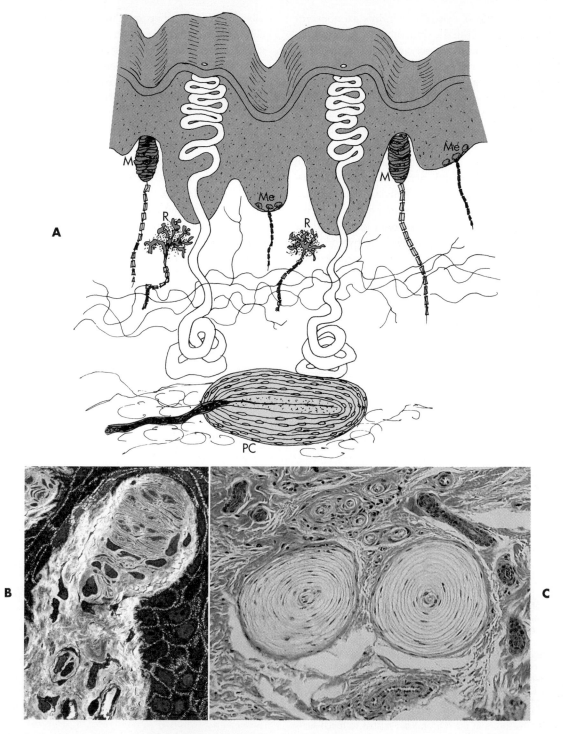

FIGURE 9-8

A, Some of the sensory endings found in glabrous skin. *M*, Meissner corpuscle; *Me*, Merkel cell; *PC*, Pacinian corpuscle; *R*, Ruffini ending. **B** and **C,** Electron micrograph of a Meissner corpuscle sectioned along its long axis and light micrograph of two Pacinian corpuscles sectioned transversely, all from monkey skin. (**B** courtesy Dr. David Moran, University of Colorado Health Sciences Center. **C** courtesy Dr. Nathaniel T. McMullen, Department of Cell Biology and Anatomy, The University of Arizona College of Medicine.)

have clearly shown that all exist. Some individual fibers respond selectively to cooling the skin, others to warming it, and still others to stimuli that are perceived as touch or pain. Many of the latter respond not only to damaging mechanical stimuli but also to heat or a variety of chemicals.

Some free nerve endings have axons that are small and thinly myelinated, whereas others are very small and unmyelinated. Each of these groups of free nerve endings includes some nociceptors. Some thinly myelinated nociceptors respond exclusively to intense mechanical stimuli, others to both mechanical and thermal stimuli. Most unmyelinated nociceptors respond to mechanical, thermal, and chemical stimuli, and for this reason are often referred to as **polymodal nociceptors.** Corresponding to these two different size classes, pain is perceived in two different stages, as most of us can attest to from common experience. If a painful stimulus is applied abruptly—you hit your thumb with a hammer, for example—there is an initial sensation of sharp, pricking, well-localized pain (Ow!). This is followed by an aching, longer-lasting pain (Ohhh!!). The initial sharp pain is carried by the more rapidly conducting, thinly myelinated fibers. For reasons explained later in the chapter, these are classified as Aδ

fibers, so this phase is sometimes referred to as **delta pain.** The aching pain that follows is carried by the more slowly conducting, unmyelinated fibers. This has been verified experimentally on human volunteers because it is possible to block different classes of nerve fibers selectively. Local anesthetics applied to peripheral nerves block unmyelinated fibers before myelinated fibers; during the period when only unmyelinated fibers are blocked, a pinprick is felt only as a sharp, brief pain. Externally applied pressure, however, blocks axons in order of size, so that myelinated fibers can be blocked while unmyelinated fibers continue to conduct. In this situation, most forms of tactile sensation disappear, and a pinprick is felt only as a dull, aching pain that is even more unpleasant than usual. The two forms of pain are processed differently within the CNS, so they may be dissociated at sites other than peripheral nerves. This can be of major clinical importance and is discussed further in subsequent chapters.

Causalgia sometimes follows injury (such as a partial transection) to a peripheral nerve. The patient has episodes of severe burning pain in the area of distribution of the affected nerve. The pain may be triggered by normally trivial stimuli, such as the mere pressure of clothing, or by

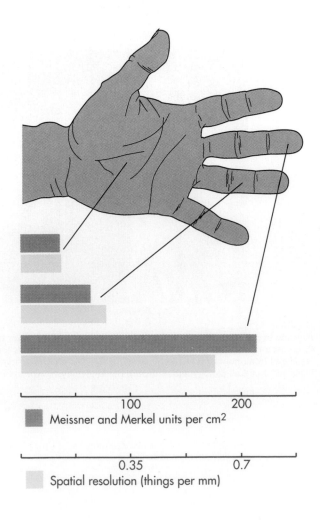

FIGURE 9-9
Correlation of spatial resolution and numbers of cutaneous receptors in different areas of the human hand. Spatial resolution (the reciprocal of the two-point discrimination threshold) was determined in psychophysical experiments, by touching humans with two points and determining the minimum separation needed for them to be recognized as two separate points; this separation is less than 2 mm for fingertips, but more than 8 mm for the palm of the hand. Correspondingly, there are many more Meissner corpuscles and Merkel endings per cm² in the fingertips than in the palm. (Modified from Vallbo ÅB, Johansson RS: Properties of cutaneous mechanoreceptors in the human hand related to touch sensation, *Human Neurobiol* 3:3, 1984.)

100   200
$\blacksquare$ Meissner and Merkel units per cm²

0.35   0.7
Spatial resolution (things per mm)

Box 9-1 A Remarkable Somatosensory Specialization: The Snout of the Star-Nosed Mole

Star-nosed moles (*Condylura cristata*, Figure 9-10, *A*) live beneath the surface of wetlands, burrowing through the mud with large, powerful forelimbs, searching for worms and insects. Vision is not very useful in a dark environment such as this, and these moles have relatively tiny eyes. Instead, they find their prey with the help of one of the most remarkable sets of somatosensory appendages ever described. Each nostril is surrounded by a series of 11 rays (Figure 9-10, *B*) that move backward and forward as rapidly as 10 times a second as the mole searches for food. The surface of each ray is paved with a series of papillae (Figure 9-10, *C* and *D*), each about 40 μm across.

The function of these rays has long been a mystery. One might logically have suspected that they are somehow related to the sense of smell, but recent studies have demonstrated that they are in fact largely or totally devoted to somatic sensation (Figure 9-11). Each ray in cross section (Figure 9-11, *A*) contains a large central nerve from which smaller nerve bundles leave to innervate receptor complexes called *Eimer's organs* that underlie each of the surface papillae. Each Eimer's organ (Figure 9-11, *B-E*) contains an elaborate array of free nerve endings, a Merkel cell-neurite complex, and an associated Pacinian-like corpuscle. The most superficial of the free nerve endings is a mere 5μm from the mole's surface.

The numbers of Eimer's organs and the accompanying innervation density are extraordinary. The 11 rays surrounding each nostril contain a total of about 13,000 Eimer's organs, innervated by more than 50,000 nerve fibers. By comparison, a human hand, with its very highly developed somatosensory capabilities, is innervated by about 17,000 somatosensory nerve fibers. The obvious functional implication is that star-nosed moles are probably capable of amazingly subtle somatosensory discriminations, although this has not yet been tested rigorously. Certainly they devote a large proportion of their cortical processing power to these rays (see Figure 22-12).

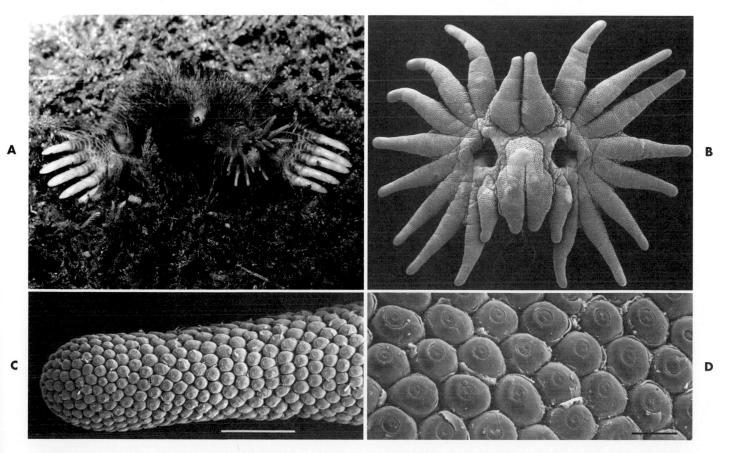

FIGURE 9-10
Surface anatomy of the star-nosed mole. A, A mole peering out from its burrow. **B-D,** Scanning electron micrographs at successively higher magnifications of the rays surrounding the nose. The scale marks in **C** and **D** are 250 μm and 50 μm, respectively. (**A, C,** and **D** courtesy Dr. Kenneth C. Catania, Department of Psychology, Vanderbilt University. **B** from Catania KC: Structure and innervation of the sensory organs on the snout of the star-nosed mole, *J Comp Neurol* 351:536, 1995.)

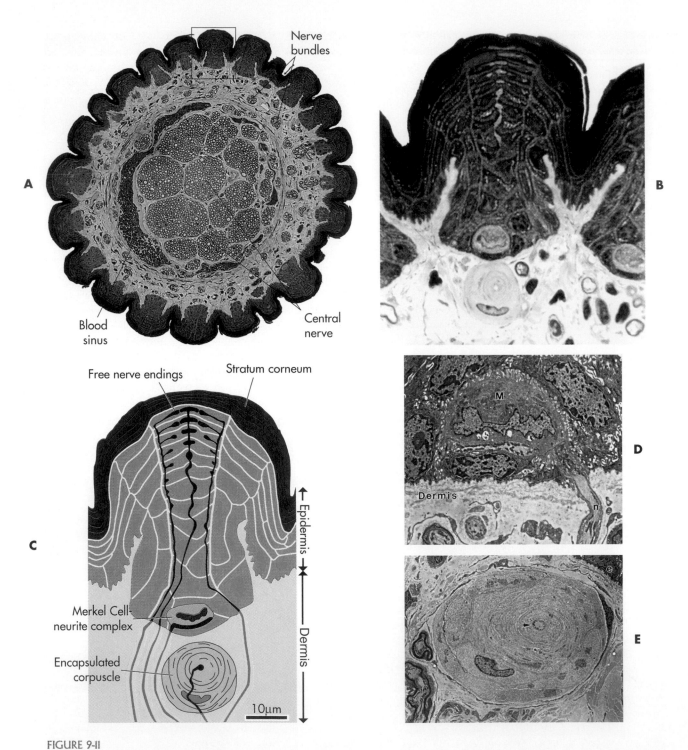

FIGURE 9-11

Microscopic anatomy of Eimer's organs. **A,** Cross section of one ray from a star-nosed mole, showing the large central nerve partially surrounded by a blood sinus. An Eimer's organ such as that outlined in **A** is enlarged in **B** and its components indicated schematically in **C**. **D,** Electron micrograph of an Eimer's organ Merkel cell *(M)* and the neural process *(n)* that innervates it. **E,** Electron micrograph of an Eimer's organ Pacinian-like corpuscle and the neural process *(arrow)* that innervates it; *e,* epidermal cell column at the core of the Eimer's organ. (**A** and **B** from Catania KC: Structure and innervation of the sensory organs on the snout of the star-nosed mole, *J Comp Neurol* 351:536, 1995. **C-E** from Catania KC: Ultrastructure of the Eimer's organ of the star-nosed mole, *J Comp Neurol* 365:343, 1996.)

emotional states. The exact mechanism of causalgia is not known, but it is usually associated with autonomic disturbances in the affected area and is typically relieved by sympathetic blockade. This has led to the conjecture that efferent sympathetic activity somehow stimulates unmyelinated fibers at the site of injury, and the subsequent activity is then perceived as pain. A complementary explanation relies on the phenomenon, noted previously, that activity restricted to unmyelinated fibers (during blockade of the myelinated fibers) causes particularly intense pain. This led some investigators to reason that if myelinated fibers were selectively stimulated in patients with causalgia, then the normal "balance" of activity between large and small fibers would be restored, and the pain would be relieved. Amazingly enough, this works in many patients. Small electrodes placed on the skin over the affected nerve (proximal to the lesion), if adjusted to stimulate only myelinated fibers, can provide dramatic relief from pain. The relief can outlast the electrical stimulus by minutes or even hours.

Pain serves a useful function

Most people think that freedom from pain would be a terrific condition. However, pain has a useful function, which is to warn us of damage; its absence is actually a handicap. Some rare individuals are born without the capability to feel pain. They characteristically have many injuries that heal poorly or remain unhealed. They may fracture bones without realizing it, have mutilated fingers and toes, or incur serious burns. The deficit may involve only the sensa-

tion of pain, but sometimes other forms of sensation are involved as well. The condition takes several different forms. Some patients have a selective loss of unmyelinated sensory fibers in their peripheral nerves; others have apparently normal nerves, so in these cases the disorder is probably within the CNS.

Cutaneous receptors are not distributed uniformly

The skin is often thought of as a uniform sensory surface varying in hairiness but basically uniform in sensitivity. This is far from true, however; some areas (such as the lips and fingertips) are much more densely innervated than other areas (such as the back). More densely innervated areas can subserve subtler tactile discriminations than can less densely innervated areas because of the close packing of receptors. One way this capability can be measured is in terms of **two-point discrimination,** which refers to the minimum distance by which two stimuli can be separated and still be perceived as two stimuli. This minimum distance is only about 2 mm for the fingertips (Figure 9-9) but is several centimeters for the back. Corresponding to this two-point discrimination ability is the capacity to localize single stimuli accurately. We can easily detect the movement of a stimulus from one ridge to the next on a fingertip, but we are not nearly so accurate for stimuli delivered to the back of the thigh. The CNS generally does a very good job of keeping us unaware of this and of many other limitations in our ability to localize stimuli (Box 9-2).

Box 9-2   Perceptual Illusions: Getting Fooled by the Nervous System*

Subjectively, we usually feel as though our sensory receptors in collaboration with our CNS present us with a precisely accurate report of the nature, location, and intensity of stimuli. In fact, however, the nervous system economizes on receptors and neural processing, collecting only the most important subset of the data that would be required to be 100% accurate and then making an "educated guess" about the stimulus. A consequence is that the nervous system can be fooled by stimuli of certain configurations: we may misinterpret the nature, location, or even the existence or nonexistence of a stimulus. One well-known example is our lack of awareness of the blind spot in the visual field of each eye (see Figure 17-10), but illusions occur in all other sensory systems as well.

The sense of taste provides another example. We perceive the taste of something we are eating as localized to that bit of food, although taste actually involves stimulation not only of taste buds, but also of the olfactory epithelium and of somatosensory endings inside the mouth that signal the texture of the food (see Chapter 13). So even though soluble factors

such as salt and sugar get distributed widely to taste buds in various parts of the tongue, and volatile substances from the same food stimulate olfactory receptors high in the nasal cavity, we localize the taste to the site at which the food touches the tongue.

Similarly, although we feel subjectively that we can localize thermal stimuli on the skin accurately, the nervous system actually localizes the touch and uses this information to decide the position of a thermal stimulus. This forms the basis of a striking somatosensory illusion described by Green in 1977†, which you can easily demonstrate to yourself. Take three similar coins, put two of them in a freezer, and leave one at room temperature. After a few minutes, set all three coins in a row on a table with the room-temperature coin in the center. Now touch the two cold coins with your index and ring fingers while simultaneously touching the room-temperature coin with your middle finger. You will experience a very compelling illusion that the room-temperature coin is just as cold as the other two coins.

---

*Modified in part from Bartoshuk LM, Weiffenbach JM: Chemical senses and aging. In Schneider EL, Rowe JW, editors: *Handbook of the biology of aging,* ed 3, San Diego, 1990, Academic Press, Inc.
†Green BG: Localization of thermal sensation: an illusion and synthetic heat, *Perception & Psychophysics* 22:331, 1977.

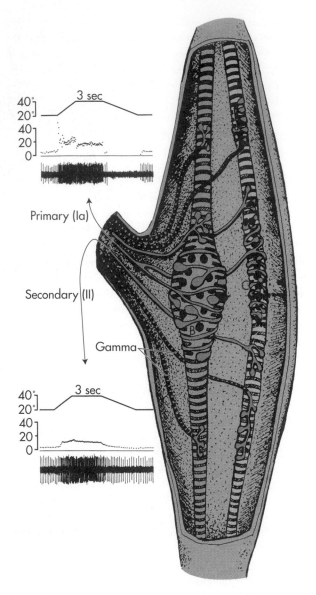

FIGURE 9-12

Simplified diagram of a muscle spindle. A single nuclear bag fiber and a single nuclear chain fiber are shown. A single afferent fiber (group *Ia*) supplies all the intrafusal fibers with primary endings. Several smaller afferents (group *II*) provide secondary endings, mostly to nuclear chain fibers. Small motor axons (of *gamma* motor neurons) of two different types innervate the contractile portions of nuclear bag and nuclear chain fibers. (The Ia-II-gamma terminology is explained later in this chapter.) The upper and lower insets show the response properties of axons from primary and secondary endings in human finger extensors, stretched by passive bending at the metacarpophalangeal joint. For each inset, the upper trace shows the metacarpophalangeal joint angle, the middle trace shows the firing rate of the axon (impulses/sec), and the lower trace shows the actual action potentials recorded. (Drawing modified from Warwick R, Williams PL, editors: *Gray's anatomy*, British ed 35, Philadelphia, 1975, WB Saunders Co. Insets from Edin BB, Vallbo ÅB: Dynamic response of human muscle spindle afferents to stretch, *J Neurophysiol* 63:1297, 1990.)

Granted that acuity is better in some areas than in others, many of us still tend to consider the skin a uniform sensory surface because we think we can detect the occurrence of a stimulus anywhere on it. This too is inaccurate because receptors are discrete entities whose zones of termination in the skin may not overlap each other. For example, temperature sensitivity is distributed like polka dots across the skin (more densely in some areas than in others). A fine, cold probe touched to an appropriate spot on the skin elicits a sensation of coolness. The same probe touched to the skin between cold-sensitive spots may elicit only a sensation of touch. Because the skin is more or less densely innervated everywhere, there are probably no places that are insensitive to all stimuli, but a given small location is likely to be most sensitive to a particular *type* of stimulus. In real life, we are usually not stimulated by fine probes, so we are not aware that sensitivity is distributed across the skin in small, selective spots.

Receptors in Muscles and Joints Detect Muscle Status and Limb Position

Muscle, like other tissues, receives an abundant supply of free nerve endings. The function of these endings is largely unknown, but some are undoubtedly involved in muscle pain, whereas others may be chemoreceptors responsive to changes in extracellular fluid composition during muscle activity. Muscles are also supplied with two important types of encapsulated receptors: the **muscle spindle,** which is unique to muscle, and the **Golgi tendon organ,** which is similar to a Ruffini ending.

Muscle spindles detect muscle length

Scattered throughout virtually every striated muscle in the body are long, thin stretch receptors called *muscle spindles* (Figure 9-12). They are quite simple in principle, consisting of a few small muscle fibers with a capsule surrounding the middle third of the fibers. These fibers are called **intrafusal muscle fibers** (from the Latin words *intra*, meaning "within," and *fusus*, meaning "spindle"), in contrast to the ordinary **extrafusal muscle fibers** (from the Latin word *extra*, meaning "outside"). The ends of the intrafusal fibers are attached to extrafusal fibers, so whenever the muscle is stretched, the intrafusal fibers are also stretched. The central region of each intrafusal fiber has few myofilaments and is noncontractile, but it does have one or more sensory endings applied to it. When the muscle is stretched, the central part of the intrafusal fiber is stretched, presumably distorting mechanically sensitive channels, and each sensory ending fires impulses.

Numerous specializations occur in this simple basic organization, so that in fact the muscle spindle is one of the most complex receptor organs in the body. Only three of these specializations are described here; their overall effect is to make the muscle spindle adjustable and give it a dual function, part of it being particularly sensitive to the length of the muscle in a static sense and part of it being particularly sensitive to the rate at which this length changes.

1. Intrafusal muscle fibers are of two types. All are multinucleated, and the central, noncontractile region contains the nuclei. In one type of intrafusal fiber, the nuclei are lined up single file; these are called **nuclear chain fibers.** In the other type, the nuclear region is broader, and the nuclei are arranged several abreast; these are called **nuclear bag fibers.** There are typically two or three nuclear bag fibers per spindle and about twice that many chain fibers, but these numbers are variable.

2. There are also two types of sensory endings in the muscle spindle. The first type, called the **primary ending,** is formed by a single, very large nerve fiber that enters the capsule and then branches, supplying every intrafusal fiber in a given spindle (although it innervates* the bag fibers more heavily than the chain fibers). Each branch wraps around the central region of an intrafusal fiber, frequently in a spiral fashion, so these are sometimes called **annulospiral endings.** The second type of ending is formed by a few smaller nerve fibers that branch and primarily innervate nuclear chain fibers on both sides of the primary ending. These are the **secondary endings,** which are sometimes referred to as **flower-spray endings** because of their appearance. Primary endings are selectively sensitive to the onset of muscle stretch but discharge at a slower rate while the stretch is maintained (Figure 9-12). Secondary endings are less sensitive to the onset of stretch, but their discharge rate does not decline very much while the stretch is maintained (Figure 9-12).

3. Muscle spindles also receive a motor innervation. The large motor neurons that supply extrafusal muscle fibers are called **alpha motor neurons,** whereas the smaller ones supplying the contractile portions of intrafusal fibers are called **gamma motor neurons** (or **fusimotor neurons**). Intrafusal fibers are too small and too few to contribute to the strength of a muscle, and firing all the gamma motor neurons to a muscle does not generate significant tension. The function of this motor innervation is discussed in conjunction with motor control systems (Chapter 18), but a simple example can indicate one of the possibilities (Figure 9-13). Consider a muscle spindle in the biceps, and suppose that this muscle is contracted. This will relieve most or all of

the tension on the nuclear region of the intrafusal fibers, so the sensory endings will be quite insensitive to muscle stretch that starts from this contracted state. Suppose that, at the same time, the gamma motor neurons to that spindle fire. This will cause the parts of each intrafusal fiber on both sides of the nuclear region to contract. This in turn will generate some tension on the nuclear region and restore its sensitivity. Thus gamma motor neurons can regulate the sensitivity of a muscle spindle so that this sensitivity can be maintained during voluntary contractions. Not surprisingly, there are two types of gamma motor neurons, one of which preferentially ends on bag fibers, the other on chain fibers.

This is just one example of feedback control by the nervous system over its sensory pathways. Such control is very common; sometimes it occurs at the level of the receptor (as in this instance), and sometimes it occurs at relay nuclei, but it seems to occur at one or more locations in every sensory pathway.

Golgi tendon organs detect muscle tension

Spindle-shaped receptors called *Golgi tendon organs* are found at the junctions between muscles and tendons. They are similar to Ruffini endings in their basic organization, consisting of interwoven collagen bundles surrounded by a thin capsule (Figure 9-14). Large sensory fibers enter the capsule and branch into fine processes that are inserted among the collagen bundles. It is thought that tension on the capsule along its long axis squeezes these fine processes, and the resulting distortion stimulates them. As in the case of Ruffini endings, these are slowly adapting receptors, because the collagen is nonelastic and the squeezing action is maintained as long as the tension is maintained.

For many years, Golgi tendon organs were studied physiologically by pulling on a tendon while recording from the sensory axon. When they are stimulated in this way, considerable tension must be applied to the tendon before a response is obtained, and so it was thought that these were high-threshold receptors designed to inform the nervous system when muscle tension was reaching dangerous levels. However, the amount of tension actually applied to a tendon organ by such a stimulus is quite small: the muscle acts something like a rubber band attached to a piece of string, and most of the tension is absorbed by the muscle. However, if tension is generated in a tendon by making its attached muscle contract, the tendon organ is found to be much more sensitive and can actually respond to the contraction of just a few muscle fibers. Thus the Golgi tendon organ very specifically monitors the tension generated by muscle contraction; it is currently considered to play an active role in the process by which the nervous system controls motor activity.

*The word *innervate* means "to supply with nerve endings." The nerve endings can be sensory, as in the case of these stretch-sensitive endings, or motor, as in the endings made by motor neurons on muscle fibers.

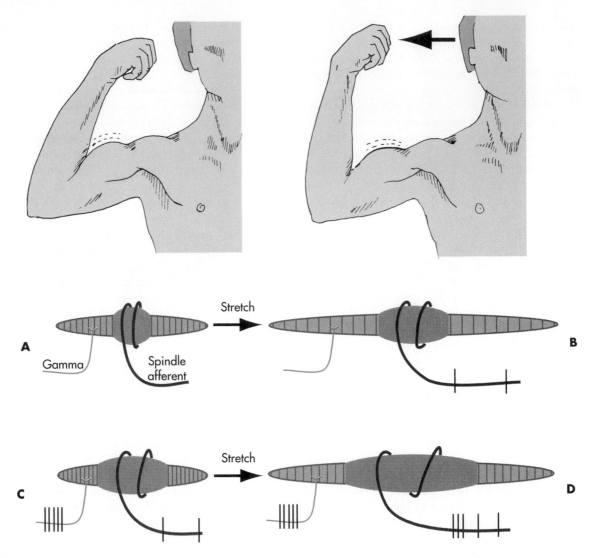

FIGURE 9-13
Mechanism of action of gamma motor neurons. **A,** Muscle spindles in a contracted muscle (in this case the biceps) are unstretched and thus electrically silent. As a result, slight stretching of the muscle causes little or no response (**B**). Activity of gamma motor neurons "prestretches" the central receptive region of the muscle spindle, causing some background activity when the biceps is contracted (**C**) and many more action potentials when it is stretched (**D**).

Thus the mode of action of the Golgi tendon organ is quite different from that of the muscle spindle (Figure 9-15). If a muscle contracts isometrically, tension will be generated across its tendons, and the tendon organs will signal this; however, the muscle spindles will signal nothing because muscle length has not changed (assuming that the activity of the gamma motor neurons remains unchanged). On the other hand, a relaxed muscle can be stretched easily, and the muscle spindles will fire; the tendon organs, in contrast, will experience little tension and will remain silent. A muscle, by virtue of these two types of receptors, can simultaneously monitor its own length and tension.

Joints have receptors

The receptors found in joints and their capsules are similar to some of those found in skin and muscle. In addition

to the usual free nerve endings, there are endings equivalent to Golgi tendon organs in the ligaments and Ruffini endings and a few Pacinian corpuscles in joint capsules (Table 9-2). As might be expected from their morphology, a few joint receptors (presumably the Pacinian corpuscles) are rapidly adapting, but most are slowly adapting and respond to joint position and movement.

Muscle spindles are important proprioceptors

The identity of the receptors involved in position sense and kinesthesia (conscious awareness of movement) has long been a topic of debate. It was generally assumed in the past that joint receptors are primarily responsible, and that the output of muscle spindles and Golgi tendon organs does not reach consciousness, being utilized in subconscious motor feedback circuits and in reflexes. This

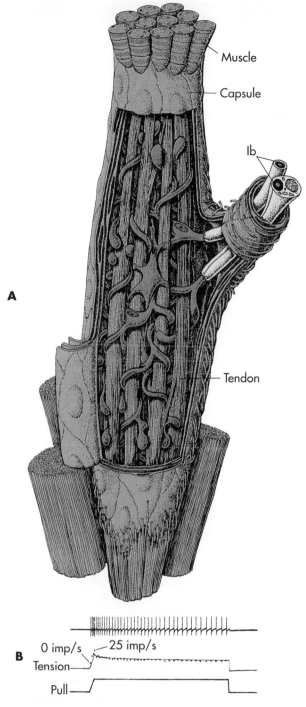

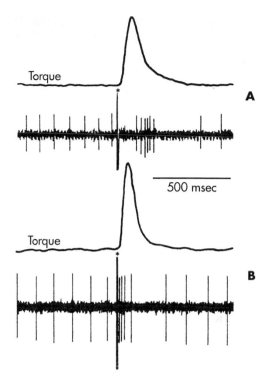

FIGURE 9-15

Responses of single afferents from a muscle spindle (**A**) and a Golgi tendon organ (**B**) in a human finger extensor in response to an electrically elicited twitch of the muscle. The spindle afferent stops firing as the muscle contracts and shortens, then fires a burst of action potentials as the muscle relaxes and lengthens. In contrast, the tendon organ afferent fires faster as the muscle contracts and increases tension on the tendon, then falls silent as the muscle relaxes and tension diminishes. (From Edin BB, Vallbo ÅB: Twitch contraction for identification of human muscle afferents, *Acta Physiol Scand* 131:129, 1987.)

FIGURE 9-14

A, Golgi tendon organ. One or more large-diameter afferent fibers enter a capsule around part of the myotendinous junction and then break up into many branches that interweave with bundles of collagen. **B,** Responses of a single afferent fiber from a Golgi tendon organ to a pull on the tendon that stretched it by 50 μm. The firing rate of the afferent, indicated by dots in the middle trace, closely tracks the tension developed in the tendon. (**A** from Krstić RV: *General histology of the mammal*, Berlin, 1985, Springer-Verlag. **B** from Fukami Y, Wilkinson RS: Responses of isolated Golgi tendon organs of the cat, *J Physiol* 265:673, 1977.)

never fit very well with the observation that individuals who have had joint-replacement surgery retain position sense at that joint despite the loss of receptors. This, together with more recent experimental work, has led to a reversal in thinking about proprioception. Although the relative importance of different receptor types varies at different joints, muscle receptors usually play a major role, and joint and cutaneous receptors are of more limited importance. If a local anesthetic is injected into the knee joint capsule of a human volunteer or into the skin of the knee, there is no loss of position sense or kinesthesia. However, if tendons of human volunteers are vibrated (through the skin), illusions of movement and altered perceptions of position are experienced at the joints where the muscles of these tendons act. A vibrating stimulus of moderate intensity should be ineffective at activating Golgi tendon organs, but it should activate muscle spindles. In particular, it should excite the primary endings because these are especially sensitive to changing stimuli. Hence it is thought that the muscle spindles but not the tendon organs are involved in these illusions and in our sense of limb position and movement. However, the tendon organs appear to contribute to our sense of the force exerted during a movement.

Table 9-2   Principal Types of Somatosensory Receptors Found in Various Tissues*

	Free nerve endings with accessory structures	Receptors with layered capsules	Receptors with thin capsules
Hairy skin	Endings around hairs (R); Merkel endings	Pacinian corpuscles (R)	Ruffini endings
Glabrous skin	Merkel endings	Pacinian corpuscles (R) Meissner corpuscles (R)	Ruffini endings
Muscle/tendon			Muscle spindles; Golgi tendon organs
Joints		Pacinian corpuscles (R)	Ruffini endings; Golgi endings

*Free nerve endings are not included because they are ubiquitous. *R*, Receptor adapts rapidly to a maintained stimulus.

Visceral Structures Contain a Variety of Receptive Endings

Much less is known about visceral receptors than about the other types discussed in this chapter; they have been studied mostly in terms of their physiology and reflex effects. Visceral receptors tend to be supplied by thinly myelinated and unmyelinated fibers that terminate as free nerve endings, sometimes with complex branching patterns. Functionally, most of these receptors act at a subconscious level through visceral reflexes. They include (1) mechanoreceptors in the walls of hollow organs (such as the endings in the aortic arch and carotid sinus, which, when stimulated by increased arterial pressure, cause reflex vasodilation and decreased heart rate), (2) chemoreceptors (such as those of the carotid body, which, when stimulated by changes in blood gases or pH, cause compensating cardiovascular and respiratory changes), and (3) nociceptors (which can cause severe pain when stimulated, as by distention of an organ or its capsule). In some instances a single visceral receptor may be able to serve as a mechanoreceptor at low discharge frequencies and a nociceptor at higher frequencies.

Particular Sensations Are Sometimes Related to Particular Receptor Types

Because we have a variety of morphologically distinct types of receptors, it was widely assumed in the past that different types are uniquely responsible for particular sensations. Certainly, the photoreceptor cells of the retina and the hair cells of the cochlea unequivocally form the basis of vision and hearing. This kind of association is true in a very general way for somatic sensation, which has perhaps been shown most elegantly in microneurography experiments on human volunteers. By recording from single nerve fibers innervating Meissner corpuscles of the fin-

gertip, it has been found that a tiny mechanical indentation of a few micrometers, just enough to cause a single action potential in one nerve fiber, can give rise to perception of the touch. Conversely, stimulation of a fiber electrically, without touching the fingertip, also gives rise to the perception of touch. Because Meissner corpuscles are rapidly adapting, a continuous train of impulses would be expected to signify repeated touches—and subjects do in fact report a sensation of repeated, gentle tapping. In contrast, stimulation of a fiber associated with a slowly adapting Merkel ending gives rise to a sensation of maintained pressure. A train of impulses in the axon from a Pacinian corpuscle, which is very rapidly adapting, is interpreted as vibration. Some receptor types are well suited for detecting fine spatial details of tactile stimuli, whereas others are not (Figure 9-16).

However, thinking of somatic sensation in terms of a unique, one-to-one pairing of specific receptor types and specific sensations is an oversimplification. First, there are counterexamples in which a single receptor type signals different types of stimulation, depending on the location of the receptor. For example, Ruffini endings in the skin are activated by touch, but morphologically similar receptors in joint capsules are activated by changes in limb position. Another example involves free nerve endings. As noted previously, some of these respond best to temperature changes, others to mechanical stimuli, and still others to intense, tissue-damaging stimuli. Second, few situations dealing with mechanical stimuli such as touch and movement involve only one receptor type. The microneurography experiments just cited were performed under carefully controlled laboratory conditions, and it seems likely that under ordinary circumstances the overall pattern of activity in an array of receptors is important in determining the resulting sensation. Here again, Ruffini endings provide an instructive example. Whereas touching the skin

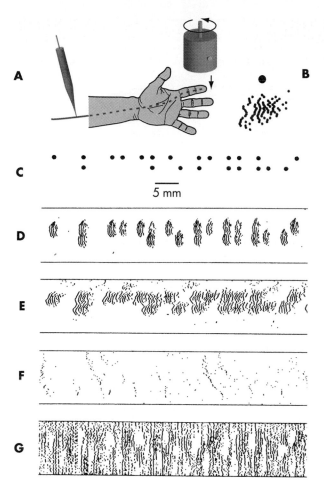

FIGURE 9-16
Responses of receptors in human fingertips to Braille characters.
A, Recordings were made from single axons in the median nerve as a rotating drum swept embossed Braille characters across a fingertip. After each revolution the drum was advanced 200 μm, thereby slowly moving the Braille characters through the receptive field of the receptor whose responses were being recorded. **B,** Sample records from the fiber also shown in **E.** The upper dot indicates the size of one Braille dot relative to the size of the receptive field. Each dot in the lower swarm corresponds to a single action potential, and each horizontal row corresponds to a single revolution of the drum. **C,** An array of Braille characters swept across a fingertip while recording from an axon innervating a probable Merkel ending **(D),** Meissner corpuscle **(E),** Ruffini ending **(F),** and Pacinian corpuscle **(G).** Meissner corpuscles and especially Merkel endings are able to encode the spatial properties of the Braille characters, but Ruffini endings and Pacinian corpuscles are not. [**B-G** from Phillips JR, Johansson RS, Johnson KO: Representation of braille characters in human nerve fibres, *Exp Brain Res* 81:589, 1990.]

overlying a Ruffini ending causes its axon to discharge, stimulating the same axon selectively in microneurography experiments causes no sensation at all. Presumably, because any naturally occurring touch stimulates many afferents in addition to the Ruffini ending, the CNS is unable to interpret isolated activity in the latter. Similarly, causing unmyelinated nociceptors to fire in response to chemical irritants produces a sensation of pain; causing the same firing rate with mechanical stimuli (and simultaneously exciting myelinated mechanoreceptor fibers) may produce only a sensation of firm pressure. The CNS thus

seems to survey all the information coming in from a given area of the body before deciding about the nature of a stimulus.

PERIPHERAL NERVES CONVEY INFORMATION TO AND FROM THE CNS

The nerve fibers innervating the receptors described thus far have their cell bodies in dorsal root ganglia adjacent to the spinal cord or, in the case of those serving the head, in various cranial nerve ganglia near the brainstem. The central process of each of these ganglion cells enters the CNS. Each peripheral process joins motor axons emerging from the spinal cord (or brainstem) to form spinal nerves (or cranial nerves). The formal boundary between the central and peripheral nervous systems occurs between the sensory ganglia and the spinal cord/brainstem, at the point where the myelinating cells change from oligodendrocytes to Schwann cells. However, it is more convenient in the present discussion to consider only those portions peripheral to the sensory ganglia (i.e., the wrappings and contents of spinal and cranial nerves). Aspects of the sensory ganglia and of the sensory and motor roots of the spinal and cranial nerves are discussed in subsequent chapters.

Extensions of the Meninges Envelop Peripheral Nerves

Extensions of the meninges invest peripheral nerves with three connective tissue coverings (Figure 9-17), each with a different function. From the outside layer in, these are the **epineurium,** the **perineurium,** and the **endoneurium** (Figure 9-18).

The epineurium is a loose connective tissue sheath surrounding each peripheral nerve. Composed mainly of collagen and fibroblasts, it forms a substantial covering over nerve trunks, then thins to an incomplete layer around smaller branches near their terminations. The abundant longitudinally and spirally arranged collagen fibers of the epineurium are largely responsible for the considerable tensile strength of peripheral nerves. The epineurium is continuous centrally with the dura mater. Peripherally, it usually ends near the termination of a nerve fiber, but it may continue as the capsule of Meissner corpuscles and a few other encapsulated endings.

The perineurium, lying within the epineurium, is a layer of thin, concentrically arranged cells with interspersed collagen. Adjacent perineurial cells are connected to one another by tight junctions that effectively isolate the epineurial spaces from the endoneurial spaces around peripheral nerve fibers. In addition, the endothelial cells of capillaries within the perineurium are connected to one another by tight junctions. Thus functional equivalents of the arachnoid barrier and the blood-brain barrier persist in the PNS as a **blood-nerve barrier.** The perineurium

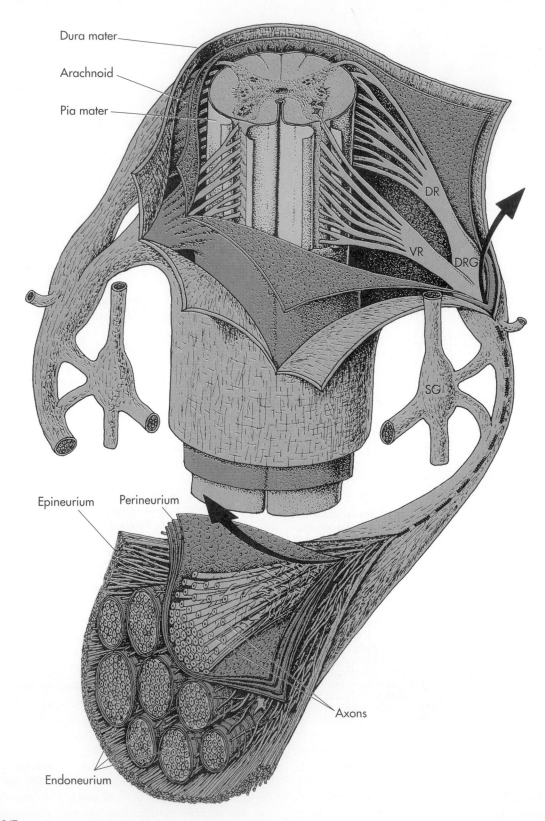

Dura mater

Arachnoid

Pia mater

DR

VR

DRG

SG

Epineurium   Perineurium

Axons

Endoneurium

FIGURE 9-17
Continuity of spinal meninges and the sheaths of peripheral nerves. The continuity between spinal subarachnoid space and extracellular space within nerve fascicles is indicated by the arrow emerging from both the cut end of the nerve and the vicinity of a dorsal root ganglion (DRG). DR, Dorsal root; SG, sympathetic ganglion; VR, ventral root. The pia mater is reflected from the exit zone of the ventral rootlets for clarity. [From Krstić RV: General histology of the mammal, Berlin, 1985, Springer-Verlag.]

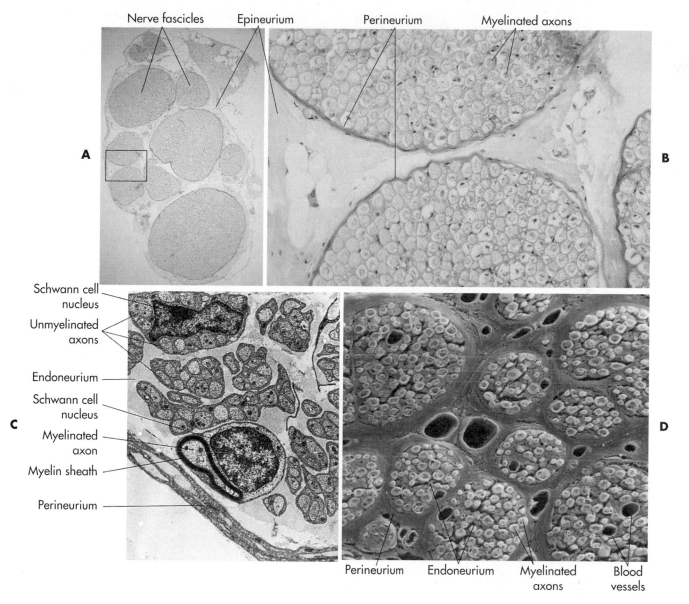

FIGURE 9-18

Wrappings of peripheral nerves. **A,** Light micrograph of a peripheral nerve, showing its several bundles (fascicles) of nerve fibers and its en-sheathment by epineurium. The outlined area is enlarged in **B,** showing the perineurial sheath around nerve fascicles and the extension of epineurium between fascicles. **C,** Electron micrograph of part of one fascicle from another nerve, showing part of the perineurium surrounding myelinated and unmyelinated axons, and endoneurium between nerve fibers. **D,** Scanning electron micrograph of a freeze-fractured preparation of peripheral nerve. (**A** and **B** courtesy Dr. Nathaniel T. McMullen, Department of Cell Biology and Anatomy, The University of Arizona College of Medicine. **C** from Moran DT, Rowley JC III: *Visual histology,* Philadelphia, 1988, Lea & Febiger. **D** from Kessel RG, Kardon RH: *Tissues and organs: a text-atlas of scanning electron microscopy,* San Francisco, WH Freeman and Company, © 1979.)

continues as the capsule of some endings, such as Pacinian corpuscles, muscle spindles, and Golgi tendon organs. However, at other places, such as near neuromuscular junctions, the perineurium is open-ended, allowing the endoneurial space around nerve fibers to communicate with the general extracellular space of the body. This is of clinical importance because certain toxins and viruses gain access to the nervous system at these sites.

The endoneurium is the loose connective tissue within the perineurium that continues into nerve fascicles and surrounds individual fibers. In at least some species, these

individual endoneurial sheaths are compact enough that they may help to direct the regrowth of nerve fibers after injury.

The Diameter of a Nerve Fiber Is Correlated With Its Function

Peripheral nerve fibers come in a wide range of diameters; some are myelinated, others are not. There is some correlation between the size of a fiber and its function, so it has proven useful to subdivide them. Unfortunately, there are

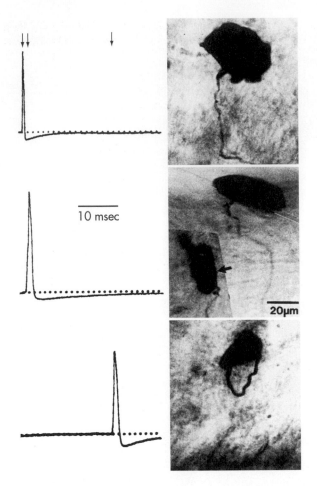

FIGURE 9-19
Action potentials recorded from dorsal root ganglion cells after stimulation of the sciatic nerve (at the beginning of each electrical record on the left). The size of a dorsal root ganglion cell is correlated with the diameter of its axon, so larger cells typically have axons that conduct more rapidly; the peak of the action potentials of these three neurons are indicated by *arrows*. The upper neuron was about 38 μm in diameter and had an axon in the Aβ range. The middle neuron (the one *not* indicated by the arrow) was about 24 μm in diameter and had an axon in the Aδ range. The lower neuron was about 17 μm in diameter and had an unmyelinated (C) axon. (From Villière V, McLachlan EM: Electrophysiological properties of neurons in intact rat dorsal root ganglia classified by conduction velocity and action potential duration, *J Neurophysiol* 76:1924, 1996.)

two major classification systems, and neither is used universally for all fibers.

The first system is based on conduction velocity. Larger fibers conduct action potentials faster than do smaller fibers (Figure 9-19). If the compound action potential of a peripheral nerve is recorded at some distance from the site at which the nerve was stimulated electrically, the fast impulses will reach the recording electrode before the slower ones. Conduction velocities (and axonal diameters)

are not distributed in a bell-shaped curve but rather in a curve with several peaks. Therefore the remotely recorded compound action potential will have several peaks corresponding to these favored conduction velocities. Three deflections can be easily demonstrated; they are named **A, B,** and **C.** The fibers responsible for the A deflection (the A fibers) are the myelinated sensory and motor fibers. B fibers are myelinated visceral fibers, both preganglionic autonomic fibers and some visceral afferents. C fibers are unmyelinated. The A deflection is complex and was subdivided into α, β, γ, and δ peaks (α being the fastest). Although the β and γ peaks as originally described were probably recording artifacts, the terminology has become established in the literature and is still commonly used. Thus Aα fibers are the largest and most rapidly conducting myelinated fibers, and Aδ are the smallest and slowest of the A group.

The second classification system is based on direct microscopic measurement of axonal diameters. In this system myelinated fibers are placed into group **I, II,** or **III** in order of decreasing size. Unmyelinated fibers are group **IV.**

Portions of both systems are still used. Most commonly the letter system is used for myelinated efferent fibers and the roman numeral system for myelinated afferents. Unmyelinated fibers are usually referred to as *C fibers* but may be called *group IV.* The sizes, conduction velocities, and functional correlates involved in both systems are listed in Table 9-3 for reference purposes.

The commonly used terminology for efferent fibers is fairly simple. The large axons innervating the extrafusal fibers of skeletal muscle are in the Aα category, and the smaller axons innervating intrafusal muscle fibers are in the Aγ category. The "A" is commonly dropped, and these are simply called α and γ motor neurons. Preganglionic autonomic axons are usually called just that, but may also be referred to as *B fibers.*

Myelinated afferents are slightly more complicated. The largest fibers, group I, are found only in muscle nerves; some form the primary endings of muscle spindles and others innervate Golgi tendon organs. To distinguish between them, spindle primary fibers are called **Ia** and tendon organ fibers are called **Ib.** Group II, corresponding to Aβ fibers, is quite diverse and includes the fibers that form the secondary endings of muscle spindles and those that form all the encapsulated receptors of skin and joints. Group III consists of small myelinated afferents that form free nerve endings and includes mechanoreceptors, cold-sensitive thermoreceptors, and the nociceptors responsible for fast pain. Group III corresponds to Aδ, and so these fibers are sometimes referred to as δ fibers.

Table 9-3 Classification of Peripheral Nerve Fibers

Roman numeral classification	Diameter	Letter classification	Conduction velocity	Myelinated	Types of structures innervated
1a★	12-20 μm	—	70-120 m/sec	Yes	Muscle spindle primary endings
1b★	12-20 μm	—	70-120 m/sec	Yes	Golgi tendon organs
—	12-20 μm	α	70-120 m/sec	Yes	Efferents to extrafusal muscle fibers
II	6-12 + μm	Aβ†	30-70 m/sec	Yes	Other encapsulated endings and endings with accessory structures: Meissner corpuscles, Merkel endings, muscle spindle secondary endings, etc.
—	2-10 μm	γ	10-50 m/sec	Yes	Efferents to intrafusal muscle fibers
III	1-6 μm	Aδ	5-30 m/sec	Yes	Some nociceptors (sharp pain) Cold receptors Most hair receptors Some visceral receptors
—	<3 μm	B	3-15 m/sec	Yes	Preganglionic autonomic efferents
IV	<1.5 μm	C	0.5-2 m/sec	No	Most nociceptors (dull, aching pain) Some visceral receptors Warmth receptors Few mechanoreceptors Postganglionic autonomic efferents

★Data from carefully studied peripheral nerves of cats. Muscle afferents in primates, including humans, probably conduct more slowly, up to only about 80 m/sec.

†Some afferents in nonmuscle nerves, particularly joint afferents, range up to 17 μm in diameter. Some investigators refer to these larger fibers, in the 12-17 μm range, as Aα and call those in the 6-12 μm range Aβ. Others refer to all nonmuscle afferents larger than 6 μm as Aβ.

SUGGESTED READINGS

Bannister LH: Sensory terminals of peripheral nerves. In Landon DN, editor: *The peripheral nerve*, London, 1976, Chapman & Hall. *A well-written overview of the anatomy and physiology of somatic, olfactory, and gustatory receptors.*

Belmonte C, Cervero F, editors: *Neurobiology of nociceptors*, New York, 1996, Oxford University Press.

Block SM: Biophysical principles of sensory transduction. In Corey DP, Roper SD, editors: *Sensory transduction*, New York, 1992, The Rockefeller University Press. *An interesting discussion of the physical limits on the transduction process in sensory receptors.*

Burgess PR et al: Signaling of kinesthetic information by peripheral sensory receptors, *Ann Rev Neurosci* 5:171, 1982.

Caterina MJ et al: The capsaicin receptor: a heat-activated ion channel in the pain pathway, *Nature* 389:816, 1997. *Homing in on the molecular basis of nociception.*

Cervero F: Sensory innervation of the viscera: peripheral basis of visceral pain, *Physiol Rev* 74:95, 1994.

Chambers MR et al: The structure and function of the slowly adapting type II mechanoreceptor in hairy skin, *Quart J Exp Physiol* 57:417, 1972. *The anatomy and physiology of the Ruffini ending of the cat.*

Dow RR, Shinn SL, Ovalle WK Jr: Ultrastructural study of a blood-muscle spindle barrier after systematic administration of horseradish peroxidase, *Am J Anat* 157:375, 1980.

Dyson C, Brindley GS: Strength-duration curves for the production of cutaneous pain by electrical stimuli, *Clin Sci* 30:237, 1966. *Direct production of both sharp, pricking pain and slow, burning pain by small electrical stimuli.*

Gandevia SC, McCloskey DI: Joint sense, muscle sense, and their combination as position sense, measured at the distal interphalangeal joint of the middle finger, *J Physiol* 260:387, 1976. *Clever experiments taking advantage of an anatomical quirk of the middle finger. This finger can be positioned in such a way that muscles and their receptors are functionally disengaged from its terminal phalanx, so the position sense of the distal interphalangeal joint can be measured both with and without a contribution from muscle receptors.*

Ghabriel MN, Jennings KH, Allt G: Diffusion barrier properties of the perineurium: an in vivo ionic lanthanum tracer study, *Anat Embryol* 180:237, 1989.

Goodwin GM, McCloskey DI, Matthews PBC: The contribution of muscle afferents to kinaesthesia shown by vibration induced illusions of movement and by the effects of paralysing joint afferents, *Brain* 95:705, 1972. *The paper that sparked the reinvestigation of the role of muscle spindles in our sense of position and movement. It contains a skeptical review of the earlier literature on this topic, as well as several simple but interesting experiments.*

Hallin RG, Torebjörk HE: Studies on cutaneous A and C fiber afferents, skin nerve blocks and perception. In Zotterman Y, editor: *Sensory functions of the skin of primates*, Elmsford, NY, 1976, Pergamon Press. *A description of experiments involving recording from the radial nerve; the experimenter notes afferent fiber activity in response to stimulation, and the experimentee reports his sensations, all during selective block of A fibers by pressure or of C fibers by a local anesthetic.*

Hensel H: Cutaneous thermoreceptors. In Iggo A, editor: *Handbook of sensory physiology.* Vol. II, *Somatosensory system*, New York, 1973, Springer-Verlag.

Houk J, Henneman E: Responses of Golgi tendon organs to active contraction of the soleus muscle of the cat, *J Neurophysiol* 30:466, 1967. *Experiments demonstrating that tendon organs are really highly sensitive receptors when responding to muscle contraction.*

Hunt CC: Mammalian muscle spindle: peripheral mechanisms, *Physiol Rev* 70:643, 1990.

Iggo A: Sensory receptors in the skin of mammals and their sensory functions, *Rev Neurol* 141:599, 1985.

Iggo A, Muir AR: The structure and function of a slowly adapting touch corpuscle in hairy skin, *J Physiol* 200:763, 1969. *The slowly adapting receptor of this paper is the Merkel ending of the cat.*

Jami L: Golgi tendon organs in mammalian skeletal muscle: functional properties and central actions, *Physiol Rev* 72:623, 1992.

Jänig W, Koltzenburg M: On the function of spinal primary afferent fibres supplying colon and urinary bladder, *J Autonom Nerv Sys* 30:S89, 1990. *Single receptors in cats that apparently can signal both normal fullness and painful distention.*

Kenshalo DR, Gallegos ES: Multiple temperature-sensitive spots innervated by single nerve fibers, *Science* 158:1064, 1967.

Kruger L, Perl ER, Sedivic MJ: Fine structure of myelinated mechanical nociceptor endings in cat hairy skin, *J Comp Neurol* 198:137, 1981.

Landau W, Bishop GH: Pain from dermal, periosteal, and fascial endings and from inflammation: electrophysiological study employing differential nerve block, *Arch Neurol Psychiatr* 69:490, 1953. *The volunteers in this case were the authors themselves who, with admirable fortitude, studied the effects of pressure blocks and local anesthetics on the pain caused by needles, bee stings, and other methods.*

Low FN: The perineurium and connective tissue of peripheral nerve. In Landon DN, editor: *The peripheral nerve*, London, 1976, Chapman & Hall.

Macefield G, Gandevia SC, Burke D: Conduction velocities of muscle and cutaneous afferents in the upper and lower limbs of human subjects, *Brain* 112:1519, 1989. *Evidence that human muscle afferents may not conduct as rapidly as those of cats and other experimental animals, and that they may be no faster than large-diameter cutaneous afferents.*

Matthews PBC: *Mammalian muscle receptors and their central actions*, London, 1973, Edward Arnold.

Matthews PBC: Where does Sherrington's "muscular sense" originate? Muscles, joints, corollary discharges? *Ann Rev Neurosci* 5:189, 1982.

McCloskey DI et al: Sensory effects of pulling or vibrating exposed tendons in man, *Brain* 106:21, 1983. *Heroic experiments in which one of the investigators had the tendon of his own extensor hallucis longus transected and then pulled on.*

McMahon SB, Koltzenburg M: Itching for an explanation, *Trends Neurosci* 15:497, 1992. *Itch is conveyed by fibers the same size as those that convey pain, but the mechanism remains a mystery.*

Meyer GA, Fields HL: Causalgia treated by selective large fibre stimulation of peripheral nerve, *Brain* 95:163, 1972.

Meyer RA, Campbell JN, Raja SN: Peripheral neural mechanisms of nociception. In Wall PD, Melzack R, editors: *Textbook of pain*, ed 3, Edinburgh, 1994, Churchill Livingstone.

Munger BL et al: A re-evaluation of the cytology of cat Pacinian corpuscles. I. The inner core and clefts, *Cell Tissue Res* 253:83, 1988.

Ochoa J, Torebjörk E: Sensations evoked by intraneural microstimulation of single mechanoreceptor units innervating the human hand, *J Physiol* 342:633, 1983.

Sato J, Perl ER: Adrenergic excitation of cutaneous pain receptors induced by peripheral nerve injury, *Science* 251:1608, 1991. *Recent evidence indicating that partial nerve injury may make the sensory terminals of C fibers sensitive to sympathetic stimulation, thus leading or contributing to causalgia.*

Schmelz M et al: Specific C-receptors for itch in human skin, *J Neurosci* 17:8003, 1997.

Schoultz TW, Swett JE: The fine structure of the Golgi tendon organ, *J Neurocytol* 1:1, 1972.

Shanthaveerappa TR, Bourne GH: Perineural epithelium: a new concept of its role in the integrity of the peripheral nervous system, *Science* 154:1464, 1966.

Sinclair D: *Mechanisms of cutaneous sensation*, New York, 1981, Oxford University Press.

Thrush DC: Congenital insensitivity to pain: a clinical genetic and neurophysiological study of four children from the same family, *Brain* 96:369, 1973.

Torre V et al: Transduction and adaptation in sensory receptor cells, *J Neurosci* 15:7757, 1995. *A nice discussion of unifying themes in the transduction mechanisms used by different kinds of receptors.*

Vallbo ÅB, Johansson RS: Properties of cutaneous mechanoreceptor in the human hand related to touch sensation, *Hum Neurobiol* 3:3, 1984. *Good review of the properties of skin receptors, as determined by recording from individual sensory axons of human volunteers.*

Vallbo ÅB et al: Somatosensory, proprioceptive, and sympathetic activity in human peripheral nerves, *Physiol Rev* 59:919, 1979.

Vallbo Å et al: A system of unmyelinated afferents for innocuous mechanoreception in the human skin, *Brain Res* 628:301, 1993.

Van Hees J, Gybels J: C nociceptor activity in human nerve during painful and nonpainful skin stimulation, *J Neurol Neurosurg Psych* 44:600, 1981. *Direct demonstration that a given level of activity in the axon of a nociceptor can be interpreted as pain in some situations but not in others.*

Winkelmann RK, Lambert EH, Hayles AB: Congenital absence of pain, *Arch Derm* 85:325, 1962.

Zelená J: *Nerves and mechanoreceptors*, London, 1994, Chapman and Hall.

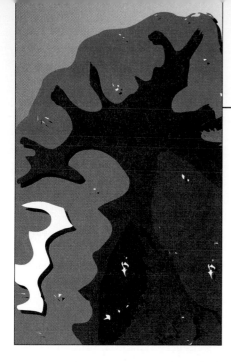

SPINAL CORD

The spinal cord is the traditional starting point for a detailed consideration of the CNS. It is a uniformly organized part of the CNS and also one of the simplest (in a relative sense), but many principles of cord function apply to other levels of the nervous system. At the same time, the spinal cord is extraordinarily important in the day-to-day activities we tend not to think about. In it reside all the motor neurons supplying the muscles we use to move our bodies around, as well as most autonomic efferents. It also receives all the sensory input from the body and some from the head and performs the initial processing operations on most of this input.

THE SPINAL CORD IS SEGMENTED

An adult human spinal cord appears surprisingly small on first inspection, being only about 42 to 45 cm long and about 1 cm in diameter at its widest point. It weighs about 35 g, so one could be mailed for just two stamps. It is anatomically segmented—not obviously, like an earthworm, but in terms of the nerve roots attached to it (Figure 10-1). A continuous series of dorsal (i.e., posterior) rootlets enters the cord in a shallow longitudinal groove (the **posterolateral sulcus**) on its posterolateral surface, and a continuous series of ventral (i.e., anterior) rootlets leaves from the poorly defined **anterolateral sulcus.** The dorsal and ventral rootlets from discrete sections of the cord coalesce to form **dorsal** and **ventral roots,** which in turn join to form **spinal nerves** (Figure 10-2, *A*). Each dorsal root bears a **dorsal root ganglion** just proximal to the junction between dorsal and ventral roots; it contains the cell bodies of the primary sensory neurons whose processes travel through that particular spinal nerve. A portion of the cord that gives rise to a spinal nerve constitutes a **segment.** There are 31 segments in the human spinal cord: 8 **cervical,** 12 **thoracic,** 5 **lumbar,** 5 **sacral,** and 1 **coccygeal.**

The spinal cord itself, stripped of its dorsal and ventral rootlets, gives no obvious sign of segmentation. Rather, it is a continuous column with two enlargements that ends caudally in the pointed **conus medullaris** (Figure 10-2, *B-D*). The two enlargements occur in those regions of the cord that supply the upper and lower extremities and therefore contain increased numbers of motor neurons and interneurons. The limits of the enlargements are not distinct, but the **cervical enlargement,** which supplies the upper extremities, is conventionally considered to extend from the fifth cervical to the first thoracic segment (C5 to T1), inclusive. The **lumbar** (or **lumbosacral**) **enlargement,** which supplies the lower extremities, extends from the second lumbar to the third sacral segment (L2 to S3).

Each Spinal Cord Segment Innervates a Dermatome

As the neural tube closes, adjacent mesoderm also segments, here into a series of somites (see Figure 2-3) that will go on to give rise to skin, muscle, and bone. Each spinal nerve retains its relationship with a somite during development, with the result that spinal segments are related systematically to areas of skin, to muscles, and in some instances to bones (e.g., vertebrae). Hence, each spinal nerve (except C1, which typically lacks a dorsal root) comes to innervate a single **dermatome** (Figure 10-3). This dermatomal arrangement is particularly apparent in the trunk, where pairs of dermatomes form bands that encircle the chest and abdomen; outgrowth of limb buds during development makes the dermatomal arrangement somewhat more complex in the upper and lower extremities.★ Similarly, the innervation of skeletal muscles is related systematically to spinal segments (Table 10-1).

Knowledge of the segmental innervation of muscles and cutaneous areas (Table 10-2) can be extremely help-

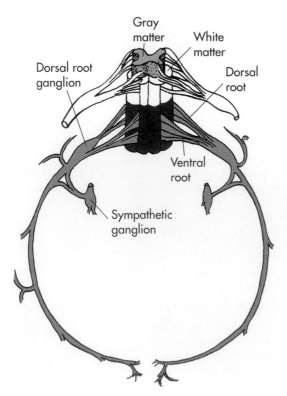

FIGURE 10-1

Segmentation of the spinal cord. The portion in color, giving rise to a single spinal nerve on each side, represents a single segment. (From Mettler FA: *Neuroanatomy,* ed 2, St. Louis, 1948, Mosby.)

★Dermatomes are generally not demarcated from each other as abruptly as Figure 10-3 indicates. When neighboring areas of skin are innervated by consecutive spinal segments (e.g., T6 and T7), the territories innervated by the two segments overlap considerably. On the other hand, when neighboring areas of skin are innervated by *non*consecutive segments (e.g., the C4 and T2 dermatomes), the overlap between the two territories is limited.

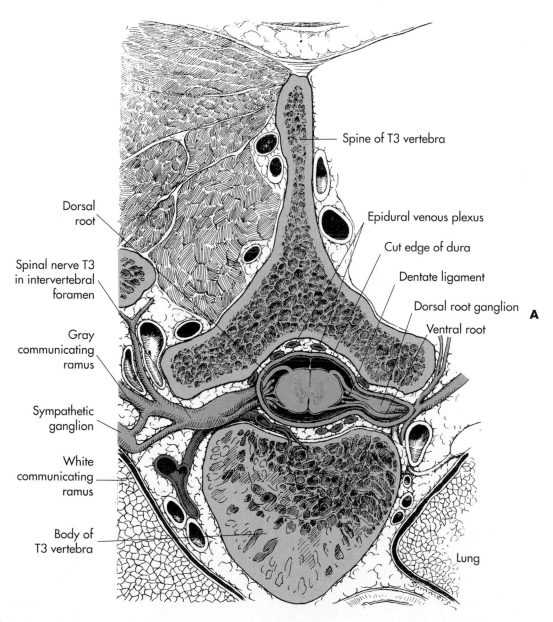

FIGURE 10-2
Relationships between spinal cord, vertebrae, and vertebral column. **A,** Section through the third thoracic vertebra and the spinal cord at that level. (From Mettler FA: *Neuroanatomy,* ed 2, St. Louis, 1948, Mosby.)

Continued

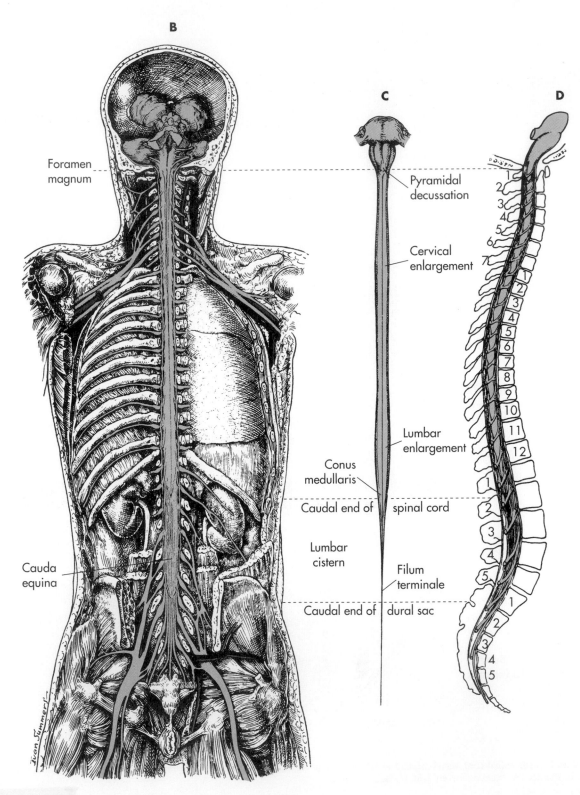

B

Foramen
magnum

Cauda
equina

C

Pyramidal
decussation

Cervical
enlargement

Lumbar
enlargement

Conus
medullaris

Caudal end of   spinal cord

Lumbar
cistern

Filum
terminale

Caudal end of   dural sac

D

FIGURE 10-2, cont'd
B, Posterior surface of a spinal cord within a vertebral canal dissected from the back. **C,** How the anterior surface of the same spinal cord would look after removal of dura, arachnoid, and spinal nerves. **D,** Spinal cord exposed from the lateral direction, showing the way in which the cord ends at about the L1-L2 level and spinal nerves travel progressively longer distances in the cauda equina to reach their exits from the vertebral canal.

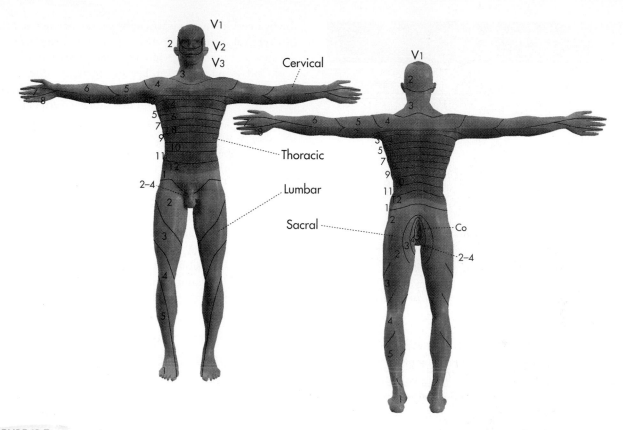

FIGURE 10-3

Cutaneous territories innervated by spinal nerves (dermatomes) and the trigeminal nerve *(VI, V2, V3)*. Co, Coccygeal segment. (Based on Bonica JJ: Applied anatomy relevant to pain. In Bonica JJ, editor: *The management of pain*, ed 2, Philadelphia, 1990, Lea & Febiger.)

Table 10-1   Innervation of Major Muscles

Movement	Peripheral nerve (muscle)	Cord segment(s)*	Movement	Peripheral nerve (muscle)	Cord segment(s)*
ARM			**HIP**		
Abduction	Suprascapular (supraspinatus)	**C5**, C6	Flexion	Lumbar spinal nerves, femoral (iliopsoas)	L1, **L2**, L3
	Axillary (deltoid)	**C5**, C6	Extension	Inferior gluteal (gluteus maximus)	L5, **S1**, S2
ELBOW			**KNEE**		
Flexion	Musculocutaneous (brachialis, biceps)	C5, **C6**	Flexion	Sciatic (hamstrings)	**L5, S1**, S2
	Radial (brachioradialis)	C5, **C6**	Extension	Femoral (quadriceps)	L2, **L3, L4**
Extension	Radial (triceps)	C6, **C7, C8**			
WRIST			**ANKLE**		
Flexion	Median, ulnar	C6, **C7**, C8	Dorsiflexion	Sciatic→peroneal (tibialis anterior)	**L4**, L5
Extension	Radial	C5, **C6, C7**, C8	Plantar flexion	Sciatic→tibial (gastrocnemius)	**S1**, S2
HAND					
Finger movements	Median, radial, ulnar	C7, **C8**, T1			
Thumb movements	Median, radial, ulnar	C7, **C8**, T1			

*Major segments indicated in **bold**.

Neurological Exams also test muscles

Table 10-2   Dermatomal Levels of Clinical Importance*

Cutaneous area	Cord segment
Upper arm (lateral surface)	C5
Thumb and lateral forearm	C6
Middle finger	C7
Little finger	C8
Nipple	T4
Umbilicus	T10
Big toe	L5
Heel	S1
Back of the thigh	S2

*See Figure 10-3 for additional details.

ful in diagnosing the site of damage in or near the spinal cord. For example, compression of a dorsal root can cause pain in its dermatome, allowing pain caused by root compression to be differentiated from pain caused by peripheral nerve damage. In addition, the highest level of a sensory or motor deficit may allow deductions about the segmental level of a suspected spinal cord lesion (Figure 10-29).

The Spinal Cord Is Shorter Than the Vertebral Canal

The spinal cord approaches its adult length long before the vertebral canal does. Until the third month of fetal life, both grow at about the same rate, and the cord fills the canal. Thereafter the body and the vertebral column grow faster than the spinal cord does, so that at the time of birth the spinal cord ends at the third lumbar vertebra. A small additional amount of differential growth in the vertebral column occurs subsequent to this, and by a few months of age the cord ends at about the level of the disk between the first and second lumbar vertebrae. However, the spinal nerves still exit through the same intervertebral foramina as they did early in development, and each dorsal root ganglion remains at the level of the appropriate foramen. Proceeding from cervical to sacral levels, the dorsal and ventral roots become progressively longer because they have longer and longer distances to travel before reaching their sites of exit from the vertebral canal (Figure 10-2, *B*). The **lumbar cistern,** from the end of the spinal cord at vertebral level L1 to L2 to the end of the dural sheath at vertebral level S2, is filled with this collection of dorsal and ventral roots, collectively referred to as the **cauda equina** (Latin for "horse's tail"; Figure 10-4, *E*). Hence a needle carefully inserted into the lumbar cistern will pass harmlessly among nerve roots, allowing safe sampling of CSF.

Each of the first seven cervical nerves leaves the vertebral canal *above* the corresponding vertebra; for instance, the first cervical nerve leaves between the occiput and the first cervical vertebra (the atlas), the second leaves between the first and second cervical vertebrae (the atlas and the axis), and so on. However, because there are only seven cervical vertebrae, the eighth cervical nerve leaves between the seventh cervical and first thoracic vertebrae, and each of the subsequent nerves leaves *below* the corresponding vertebra.

The meningeal coverings of the spinal cord were described in Chapter 4 (see Figure 4-13) and Figure 10-2, *A*. The cord is suspended within an arachnoid-lined dural tube by the dentate ligaments, which are extensions of the pia-arachnoid, similar to but more substantial than arachnoid trabeculae. In addition, the caudal end of the cord is anchored to the end of the dural tube by the **filum terminale,** an extension of the pial covering of the conus medullaris. The filum terminale then acquires a dural outer layer and in turn is anchored to the coccyx.

ALL LEVELS OF THE SPINAL CORD HAVE A SIMILAR CROSS-SECTIONAL STRUCTURE

In cross section the spinal cord consists of a roughly H-shaped area of gray matter that floats like a butterfly in a surround of white matter. The gray matter can be divided into **horns** and the white matter into **funiculi** (from the Latin *funiculus,* meaning "string") (Figure 10-5). Keep in mind that the spinal cord is, to a great extent, a longitudinally organized structure, even though it is most conveniently studied in cross section. For example, the posterior gray horns are continuous cell columns rather than a series of discrete nuclei, and at any given level the posterior horn cells interact with cells from many other levels.

In addition to the posterolateral and anterolateral sulci, several other longitudinal grooves indent the cross-sectional outline of the cord (Figure 10-5). The deep **anterior median fissure** extends almost to the center of the cord; at the apex of this fissure, only a thin zone of white matter (the **anterior white commissure**) and a thin zone of gray matter separate the central canal from the subarachnoid space. The **posterior median sulcus** is much less distinct, but a glial septum extends from it all the way to the gray matter surrounding the central canal. Therefore the two sides of the spinal cord can communicate with each other through only a narrow band of neural tissue near the central canal. Because the fibers of many ascending pathways cross the midline in the spinal cord, this small area where crossing occurs can become important clinically in diseases affecting the center of the cord (Figure 10-30). Finally, at cervical and upper thoracic levels, a **posterior intermediate sulcus** is found. Another glial septum projects from this sulcus, partially subdividing each posterior funiculus.

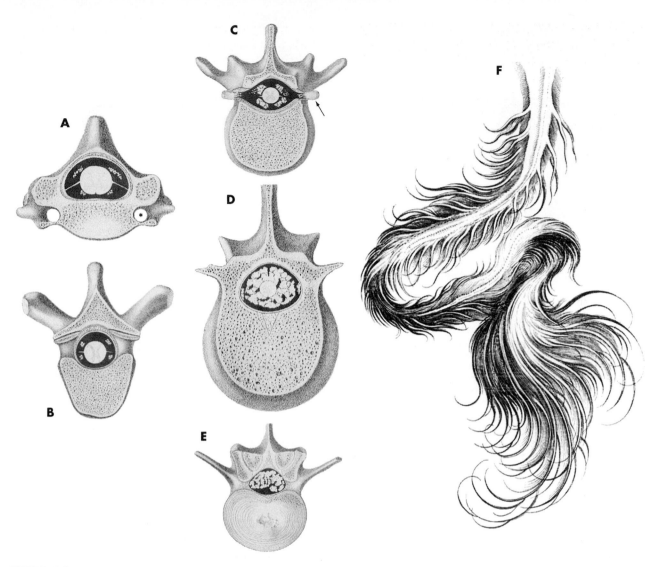

FIGURE 10-4

Formation of the cauda equina. **A-E** show cross sections from progressively more caudal levels of a vertebral column in which the subarachnoid space had been filled with dyed gelatin (C3, T3, L1, L2, and L3 vertebrae, respectively). The C3 and T3 vertebrae encase spinal cord segments C4 and T4/5, each adjacent to the dorsal and ventral roots of these segments and suspended by dentate ligaments. The L1 and L2 vertebrae encase the sacral spinal cord together with a collection of dorsal and ventral roots from lumbar and sacral segments. By the level of the L3 vertebra the spinal cord has ended and only the cauda equina remains. **F**, A depiction of the cauda equina from *Historia Anatomica Humani Corporis* by Andreas Laurentius (Frankfurt, 1600, Becker), who was apparently the first to name and illustrate this structure. The dissection from which this illustration was made was "obtained by immersion in water, suggesting a horse's tail." *, Foramen for the vertebral artery; *arrow*, spinal nerve emerging from intervertebral foramen. (**A-E** from Key A, Retzius G: *Studien in der anatomie des nervensystems und des bindegewebes*, vol I, Stockholm, 1875, Norstad. **F**, my thanks to Dr. Francis Schiller, University of California, San Francisco, for calling attention to this illustration [*Neurol* 38:161, 1988]).

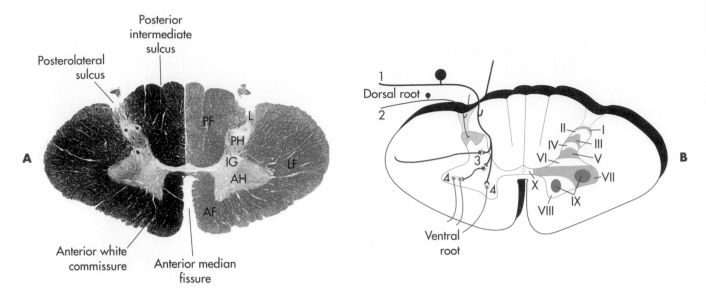

FIGURE 10-5

General cross-sectional anatomy of the spinal cord, represented in this case by the eighth cervical segment. **A,** A cross section of C8. **B,** Laminae of Rexed are indicated on the right, and the general kinds of cells and connections in these different areas are indicated on the left. Large-diameter, heavily myelinated afferents *(I)* enter medially through the posterior funiculus, whereas small-diameter afferents *(2)* enter laterally near the substantia gelatinosa. This corresponds to the way in which tactile and proprioceptive information is processed, relative to pain and temperature information. These afferents then contact interneurons *(3)*, and in some cases contact motor neurons *(4)* directly. *AF,* Anterior funiculus; *AH,* anterior horn; *IG,* intermediate gray matter; *L,* Lissauer's tract; *LF,* lateral funiculus; *PF,* posterior funiculus; *PH,* posterior horn; *asterisks* indicate the substantia gelatinosa.

THE SPINAL CORD IS INVOLVED IN SENSORY PROCESSING, MOTOR OUTFLOW, AND REFLEXES

Afferent fibers enter the cord via the dorsal roots* and then end almost exclusively on the ipsilateral side of the CNS. They may reach their site of termination either by ascending directly and uncrossed to relay nuclei in the medulla or by synapsing on neurons in the ipsilateral gray matter of the spinal cord. The relay cells in the spinal gray matter or the medulla then project their axons through defined sensory pathways to more rostral structures. In subsequent discussions of these sensory pathways, it may sometimes sound as if a particular primary afferent synapses on only one relay cell and sends its information into one and only one pathway. However, it is important to realize that each primary afferent fiber gives rise to many branches and feeds into more than one ascending sensory pathway as well as into local reflex circuits (see Figure 3-25). It is estimated, for example, that a single Ia afferent from a muscle spindle may give rise to 500 or more branches within the spinal cord.

The motor neurons that innervate skeletal muscle are located in the anterior horns, and many preganglionic autonomic neurons are located in the intermediate gray matter of appropriate segments. The axons of these motor neurons leave the cord in the ventral roots. Activity in these neurons is modulated by local reflex circuits and by pathways that descend through the spinal white matter from the cerebral cortex and from various brainstem structures.

Certain specified afferent inputs cause stereotyped motor outputs, called **reflexes,** as in the familiar knee jerk reflex. Many of these involve neural circuitry that is wholly contained within the spinal cord; several examples are discussed in this chapter.

SPINAL GRAY MATTER IS REGIONALLY SPECIALIZED

The Posterior Horn Contains Sensory Interneurons

The posterior horn consists mainly of interneurons whose processes remain within the spinal cord and of projection neurons whose axons collect into long, ascending sensory pathways. This area of gray matter contains two prominent parts, the **substantia gelatinosa** and the **body** of the posterior horn, both present at all spinal levels.

The substantia gelatinosa is a distinctive region of gray matter that caps the posterior horn (Figure 10-6). In

---

*The Bell-Magendie law, a long-standing neuroanatomical tenet, states that the dorsal root contains only primary afferent fibers and the ventral root only efferent fibers of various sorts. However, it now appears that a small percentage of ventral root fibers are finely myelinated or unmyelinated primary afferents. Ventral root afferents may be at least partially responsible for the persistence or the return of pain after the dorsal roots have been sectioned.

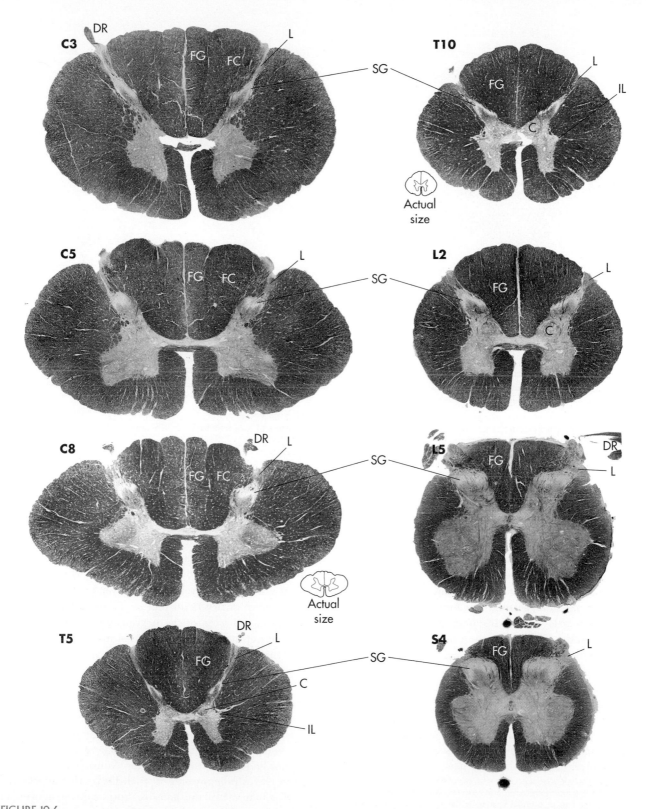

FIGURE 10-6

Cross sections of the spinal cord at various levels; note the large lateral extensions of the anterior horns in C5, C8, and L5. *C,* Clarke's nucleus; *DR,* dorsal root; *FC,* fasciculus cuneatus; *FG,* fasciculus gracilis; *IL,* intermediolateral cell column; *L,* Lissauer's tract; *SG,* substantia gelatinosa.

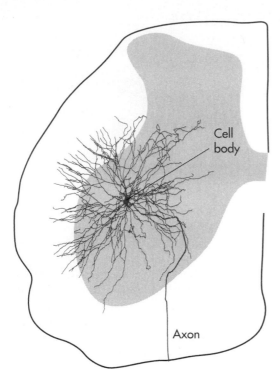

FIGURE 10-7
A single motor neuron from the lumbar spinal cord of an adult cat. A marker substance (horseradish peroxidase) was injected from the intracellular tip of a microelectrode, and the neuron was subsequently reconstructed from a series of sections. The extent and complexity of the dendritic trees of real neurons are obviously different from those of the "cartoon" neurons in most of the diagrams in this book. (Modified from Ulfhake B et al: *J Comp Neurol* 278:69, 1988.)

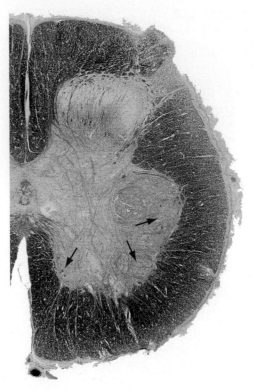

FIGURE 10-8
Clusters of motor neurons in the anterior horn at S4.

myelin-stained preparations this region looks pale compared with the rest of the gray matter because it deals mostly with finely myelinated and unmyelinated sensory fibers that carry pain and temperature information. Between the substantia gelatinosa and the surface of the cord is a relatively pale-staining area of white matter called **Lissauer's tract.** ★ This tract stains more lightly than the rest of the white matter because it contains the finely myelinated and unmyelinated fibers with which the substantia gelatinosa deals.

The body of the posterior horn consists mainly of interneurons and projection neurons that transmit many types of somatic and visceral sensory information. In this respect it functionally overlaps parts of the intermediate gray matter.

The Anterior Horn Contains Motor Neurons

The anterior horn contains the cell bodies of the large motor neurons that supply skeletal muscle (Figure 10-7). These alpha motor neurons, also referred to as **lower motor neurons,** ★ are the only means by which the nervous system can exercise control over body movements, whether voluntary or involuntary; a number of different pathways and parts of the nervous system can influence these lower motor neurons, but they alone can effect muscle contraction. Destruction of the lower motor neurons supplying a muscle or interruption of their axons therefore causes complete paralysis of that muscle. Lower motor neuron lesions cause paralysis of a type called **flaccid paralysis,** indicating that the muscle is limp and uncontracted. Reflex contractions can no longer be elicited, and the muscle slowly atrophies (for lack of trophic factors normally delivered to it by motor axons). This occurs, for example, in poliomyelitis (a viral disease that attacks the motor neurons of the anterior horn) and in injuries in which ventral roots are damaged.

Alpha motor neurons occur in groups (Figure 10-8), separated from one another by areas of interneurons; the groups that innervate axial muscles are medial to those

---

★Lissauer's tract is an unusual case in which an eponym is becoming more commonly used rather than fading away. For many years Lissauer's tract was also known by the descriptive term *dorsolateral fasciculus*. However, as described elsewhere in this chapter, the dorsal part of the lateral funiculus is now known to contain some distinctively important ascending and descending pathways. As a result, many now refer to the latter area of spinal white matter as the *dorsolateral fasciculus* or *funiculus*. To avoid ambiguity, Lissauer's tract is probably best referred to by its eponymous name.

★They are also referred to simply as *anterior horn cells*, even though other cell types also live in the anterior horn.

Table 10-3   Important Subdivisions of Spinal Cord Gray Matter

Nucleus	Levels	Lamina	Function
Marginal zone	All	I	Some spinothalamic tract cells
Substantia gelatinosa	All	II	Modulate pain and temperature
Body of posterior horn	All	III-VI	Sensory processing
Clarke's nucleus	T1–L2	VII	Posterior spinocerebellar tract cells
Intermediolateral column	T1–L3	VII	Preganglionic sympathetics *Autonomic*
Sacral parasympathetic nucleus	S2–S4	VII	Preganglionic parasympathetics→pelvic viscera
Accessory nucleus	Medulla–C5	IX	Motor neurons→trapezius and sternocleidomastoid
Phrenic nucleus	C3–C5	IX	Motor neurons→diaphragm

that innervate limb muscles. In the cervical and lumbar enlargements, which innervate the limbs, the anterior horns are enlarged laterally to accommodate the additional motor neurons (Figure 10-6). Smaller gamma motor neurons are interspersed with alpha motor neurons in all such groups. They innervate the intrafusal muscle fibers of muscle spindles, and so they are also referred to as **fusimotor neurons.**

Two columns of motor neurons in the anterior horn of the cervical cord are recognized as separate entities. The **spinal accessory nucleus** extends from the caudal medulla to about C5. The axons of these motor neurons emerge from the lateral surface of the spinal cord just posterior to the dentate ligament as a separate series of rootlets that form the accessory nerve (see Figure 3-15). The **phrenic nucleus,** containing the motor neurons that innervate the diaphragm, is located in the medial portion of the anterior horn in segments C3 to C5. This makes injuries to the upper cervical spinal cord a matter of grave concern because destruction of the descending pathways that control the phrenic nucleus and other respiratory motor neurons renders a patient unable to breathe.

The Intermediate Gray Matter Contains Autonomic Neurons

The gray matter that is intermediate to the anterior and posterior horns has some characteristics of both and also contains the spinal preganglionic autonomic neurons. In addition, at some levels it includes a distinctive region called **Clarke's nucleus.**

The preganglionic sympathetic neurons for the entire body lie between segments T1 and L3, most of them located in a column of cells called the **intermediolateral cell column,** which forms a pointy lateral horn on the spinal gray matter (Figure 10-6). Their axons leave through the ventral roots. Cells in a corresponding location in segments S2 to S4 form the **sacral parasympathetic nucleus** but do not form a distinct lateral horn. Their axons leave through the ventral roots and synapse on the postganglionic parasympathetic neurons for the pelvic viscera.

Clarke's nucleus (or **nucleus dorsalis**) is a rounded collection of large cells located on the medial surface of the base of the posterior horn from about T1 to L2. It is particularly prominent at lower thoracic levels (Figure 10-6). This is an important relay nucleus for the transmission of information to the cerebellum and may also play a role in forwarding proprioceptive information from the leg to the thalamus. Because of its prominent role in sensory processing, it is considered by many to be part of the posterior horn.

The remainder of the intermediate gray matter is a collection of various projection neurons, sensory interneurons, and interneurons that synapse on motor neurons.

Spinal Cord Gray Matter Is Arranged in Layers

In 1952 Rexed devised a system for subdividing the gray matter of the cat's spinal cord into layers, or laminae. The same system has since been applied to the cords of other mammals, including humans (Figure 10-5, *B*). **Lamina I** (also called the **marginal zone**) is a thin layer of gray matter that covers the substantia gelatinosa, **lamina II** is the substantia gelatinosa, and **laminae III** through **VI** are the body of the posterior horn; **lamina VII** roughly corresponds to the intermediate gray matter but also includes Clarke's nucleus and large extensions into the anterior horn; **lamina VIII** comprises some of the interneuronal zones of the anterior horn, whereas **lamina IX** is the clusters of motor neurons embedded in the anterior horn; **lamina X** is the zone of gray matter surrounding the central canal.

This terminology has proved useful for experimental anatomists and physiologists because the histological differences between the laminae correspond to functional differences (Table 10-3). For example, the functional dichotomy between large- and small-diameter peripheral nerve fibers is maintained to a great extent in the patterns of termination of these fibers in the spinal gray matter: there are prominent (though not exclusive) terminations of pain and temperature afferents in laminae I and II, tactile afferents from cutaneous nerves in lamina III, and Ia muscle spindle afferents in laminae VI, VII, and IX.

REFLEX CIRCUITRY IS BUILT INTO THE SPINAL CORD

A reflex is an involuntary, stereotyped response to a sensory input. All reflex pathways therefore must involve at least a receptor structure and associated afferent neuron (with its cell body in a dorsal root ganglion or some other sensory ganglion) and an efferent neuron (with its cell body within the CNS). With the exception of the **stretch reflex,** all reflexes involve one or more interneurons as well.

Reflexes range from the very simple ones described in this chapter (which serve as a useful introduction to neural integration and are the basis for common clinical tests) to neural subroutines so complex that calling them "reflexes" seems an oversimplification. For example, a cat with its spinal cord transected at thoracic levels can, under certain conditions, perform coordinated walking movements with its hind limbs. If its hind feet are placed on a moving treadmill, the gait changes in a predictable fashion with the speed of the treadmill, from alternating stepping movements at low speeds to galloping movements (in which both legs move together in phase) at higher speeds.

Muscle Stretch Leads to Excitation of Motor Neurons

All skeletal muscles have a tendency, more pronounced in some than others, to contract in response to being stretched. The reflex arc responsible for this contraction is the simplest possible because it involves only two neurons and a single intervening synapse. It is therefore sometimes referred to as the **monosynaptic reflex** or the **myotatic reflex** (from two Greek words meaning "muscle stretch"). The afferent limb of the arc is a Ia afferent with its associated muscle spindle primary ending. Central processes of the Ia afferent synapse within the spinal cord directly on the alpha motor neurons that innervate the muscle containing the stimulated spindle (Figure 10-9).

The stretch reflex is commonly used for clinical testing purposes. Tapping the patellar tendon, as in the familiar **knee jerk reflex,** stretches the quadriceps slightly. Ia endings in quadriceps muscle spindles are excited and in turn excite quadriceps alpha motor neurons; these cause the quadriceps to contract, completing the reflex. Similarly, tapping the Achilles tendon stretches the gastrocnemius slightly, thereby causing a reflex contraction. Testing a variety of stretch reflexes can provide valuable clinical information about the integrity not only of peripheral nerves, but also of predictable spinal cord segments (Table 10-4). Because stretch reflexes are usually elicited by tapping a tendon, they are often referred to as **deep tendon reflexes** (sometimes abbreviated as **DTRs**). One should remember that even though the reflex is studied in this manner, the responsible receptors are actually in the muscles attached to the tapped tendons.

Table 10-4 Deep Tendon Reflexes Commonly Tested Clinically			
Reflex	Muscle(s) involved	Principal cord segment	Peripheral nerve
Biceps	Biceps brachii	C5	Musculocutaneous
Brachioradialis	Brachioradialis	C6	Radial
Triceps	Triceps brachii	C7	Radial
Knee-jerk (patellar)	Quadriceps femoris	L4	Femoral
Ankle-jerk (Achilles)	Gastrocnemius, soleus	S1	Tibial

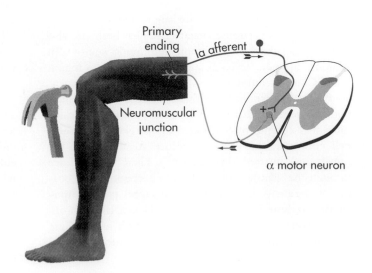

FIGURE 10-9

Stretch reflex. Striking the patellar tendon activates muscle spindle primary endings, which then monosynaptically excite alpha motor neurons that innervate the stretched muscle.

Stretch reflexes are thought to be important for the constant automatic corrections we perform during movements and postures (although other reflexes may in fact be even more important for this function). As an example, when we stand still and upright, we actually sway to and fro a bit. Each time we sway in one direction, some muscles are stretched and the resulting reflex contraction helps return us toward the desired position.

Muscle Tension Can Lead to Inhibition of Motor Neurons

Stimulation of a Ib fiber from a Golgi tendon organ has an effect that varies depending on the position and activity of the limb at the time of stimulation. It sometimes has an effect opposite to that of stimulating a Ia fiber: the alpha motor neurons that innervate the muscle connected to that tendon organ are inhibited. This effect is termed **autogenic inhibition** and involves an inhibitory interneuron between the afferent and efferent fibers (Figure 10-10). Under other circumstances (e.g., stimulating a tendon organ attached to a weight-supporting muscle), excitation of the motor neurons can result (again, through an interneuron).

The normal role of reflexes mediated by Golgi tendon organs is not yet completely understood. It was thought for a time that autogenic inhibition is protective in nature, preventing muscles from developing excess tension. However, in view of the great sensitivity of tendon organs to actively generated tension, it is clear that this reflex would be activated long before hazardous levels are reached. Therefore it now seems likely that Golgi tendon organs contribute to fine adjustments in the force of muscle contraction during ordinary motor activities.

Clinically, autogenic inhibition may be manifested in a phenomenon called the **clasp-knife response.** In certain pathological conditions that follow damage to descending motor pathways, the resistance of muscles to manipulation is greatly increased. Thus one would have considerable

difficulty flexing the leg of an individual with such a condition. If sufficient force is applied, however, the leg slowly flexes until at some point all resistance suddenly disappears and the leg collapses in flexion, like a clasp knife snapping shut. This collapse of resistance is commonly attributed to autogenic inhibition initiated by Golgi tendon organs, although other receptors are probably also involved.

Painful Stimuli Elicit Coordinated Withdrawal Reflexes

Whereas stretch reflexes and autogenic inhibition are initiated by muscle or tendon receptors and primarily involve the muscle stretched or tensed, the **flexor reflex** is initiated by cutaneous receptors and involves a whole limb. A familiar example is withdrawal from a painful stimulus; after accidentally touching something painfully hot, we automatically remove the offended hand from that vicinity by flexing the arm to which it is attached.

The flexor reflex pathways in the spinal cord are normally held in a somewhat inhibited state by descending influences from the brainstem, so that only noxious stimuli result in a strong reflex. If these descending influences are removed, either surgically in experimental animals or as a result of certain pathological conditions, reflex flexion can result from harmless tactile stimulation. This indicates that most or all cutaneous receptors feed into the pathway, but ordinarily only nociceptors have a powerful enough influence to cause a reflex withdrawal.

Because the flexor reflex involves an entire limb, its pathway must spread over several spinal segments to include the motor neurons innervating all the various flexor muscles of that limb. This spreading occurs in two ways. First, all primary afferent fibers bifurcate on entering the spinal cord, and their processes then extend one or more segments in both rostral and caudal directions. Second, the flexor pathway includes at least one interneuron, which itself may have processes extending over several segments (Figure 10-11).

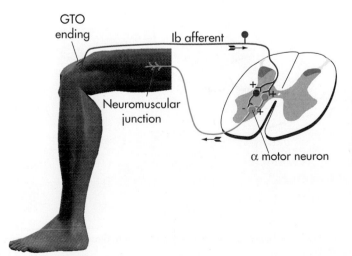

FIGURE 10-10
Reflex connections of Golgi tendon organs. Contraction of a muscle activates the Golgi tendon organs in its attached tendon. Under some conditions, the Ib afferents then activate inhibitory interneurons that inhibit the motor neurons to that muscle (autogenic inhibition). Under other conditions, the opposite effect is noted, mediated by excitatory interneurons.

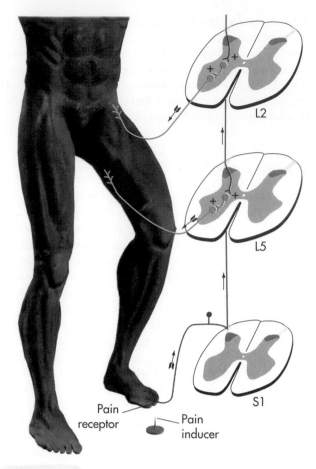

Flexor reflex. This reflex involves several segments, and all connections are polysynaptic. In the example shown, a nociceptive fiber from the foot enters the spinal cord at SI and activates (through at least one interneuron) motor neurons to iliopsoas and hamstring muscles.

Although this reflex is usually called the **flexor reflex,** the term **withdrawal reflex** is also used and is perhaps more appropriate. The reflex is not an all-or-none phenomenon for a given limb but rather shows different patterns depending on which portion of the limb is stimulated (the pattern being appropriate to withdraw the stimulated area). It would be imprudent to flex a lower extremity when a painful stimulus was applied to the anterior surface of the thigh because this would drive the thigh into the stimulus. In such a situation, it would make much more sense to activate the extensors, which is in fact what happens. Modification of the reflex response so that it reflects the area being stimulated is called **local sign.**

Reflexes Are Accompanied by Reciprocal and Crossed Effects

So far, we have given a simplified description of reflex circuits, including only the most direct and dominant motor effects. However, these reflexes also include weaker influences on other muscles of the same limb and even of contralateral limbs.

It would clearly be easier to shorten a stretched muscle if the motor neurons to its synergists were excited and those to its antagonists inhibited. This actually does occur and is a general principle in all reflexes: reflex activity in a given muscle produces similar activity in its ipsilateral synergists and the opposite activity in its ipsilateral antagonists (Figure 10-12). Thus the standard tap on the patellar tendon causes not only excitation of quadriceps motor neurons but also inhibition (through an interneuron) of motor neurons to the hamstring muscles. If one extensor muscle of the thigh were selectively stretched, its motor

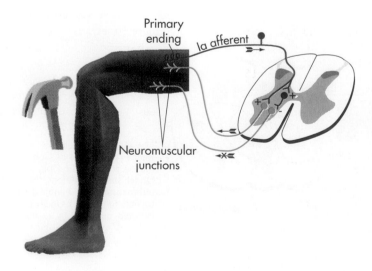

Reciprocal inhibition. Striking the patellar tendon initiates a stretch reflex, as in Figure 10-9. It also causes inhibition, through an interneuron, of the motor neurons to the antagonist hamstring muscles.

neurons would be monosynaptically excited, as would those of all the other thigh extensors. After stimulation of a Golgi tendon organ the pattern may be just the reverse. If tension is applied to the patellar tendon during certain phases of a movement, the quadriceps is inhibited and the hamstring muscles are excited, both actions occurring through interneurons. Finally, the flexor reflex is accompanied by inhibition of the extensors of that limb.

The crossed effects in reflex actions are most easily understood with reference to the flexor reflex (Figure 10-13). If the only effect of stepping on a tack with the left foot were withdrawal of the left leg, the maladaptive behavior of falling over and possibly landing on the tack might follow. This is avoided by a simultaneous and opposite pattern of activity in the contralateral limb; as the left leg flexes and withdraws, the right leg extends and is thus better able to support the body. Similar observations have been made after stimulation of muscle spindles and

Golgi tendon organs, although the effects on contralateral antagonists are not pronounced.

These crossed effects may be the basic building blocks for more complex subroutines, such as those for the coordinated stepping movements referred to earlier. Individual interneurons receive multiple inputs and can participate in tendon organ-mediated reflexes, withdrawal reflexes, and more complex movements.

Reflexes Are Modifiable

The preceding discussion makes it sound as though reflexes are fixed and unchangeable, a function only of the type and magnitude of the stimulus. This is largely an illusion created by the way in which reflexes are tested, with relaxed patients in static postures; the sensitivity of reflex arcs in fact varies substantially, depending on the functional requirements of the nervous system at any given time. The stretch reflex, for example, must be variable or we would be unable to sit: sitting should stretch the quadriceps just as tapping the patellar tendon does, in which case reflex contraction of the quadriceps would then be expected to make us stand up again! Part of the answer to this apparent dilemma lies in the gamma motor neurons. During the act of sitting, the gamma motor neurons to quadriceps muscle spindles decrease their firing rate. This decreases the excitability of the quadriceps spindles just enough that they do not respond to the stretch imposed by sitting. The activities of the alpha and gamma motor neuron populations are coordinated generally during movements; this is discussed in more detail in Chapter 18.

In addition to generally suppressing or enhancing reflexes during different behavioral states, the CNS also adjusts the sensitivity of individual reflex arcs from moment to moment in response to different postures or during different parts of a task. For example, during normal walking each leg alternates between a stance phase in which it supports the body and then pushes off, and a swing phase in which the foot is lifted off the ground and moved forward. The foot is dorsiflexed during the swing phase, keeping the toes clear of the ground. This dorsiflexion stretches the soleus. The monosynaptic stretch reflex involving the soleus is almost completely suppressed specifically during this phase of the step cycle, preventing it from contracting, extending the foot, and possibly causing the toes to contact the ground. Reflex responses to something touching the sole of the foot can actually reverse direction, depending on the phase of the step cycle during which the touch occurs (Figure 10-14, *A*). Similarly, the withdrawal reflex in response to a painful stimulus can be enhanced or suppressed, depending on the postural-support role being played by that limb at the moment of the stimulus (Figure 10-14, *B*). Some of these adjustments to reflex sensitivity are accomplished by circuitry built into the spinal cord, others depend on pathways descending from the brainstem.

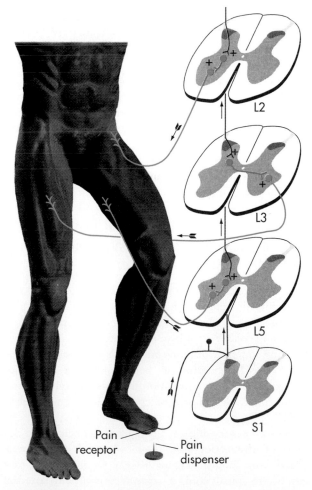

FIGURE 10-13
Crossed extension. Stepping on a tack initiates a flexor reflex, as in Figure 10-11. It also causes excitation, through an interneuron, of the contralateral antagonist muscles. In this case contraction of the contralateral quadriceps helps the leg with the nonpunctured foot to support the body.

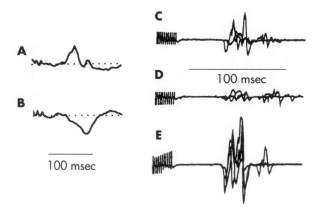

FIGURE 10-14

Moment-to-moment changes in the sensitivity of reflexes. **A-E** show the mass electrical activity (electromyogram) of a foot flexor (tibialis anterior) recorded from the skin surface. **A** and **B** show average responses to 20 or more stimuli; **C-E** each shows three superimposed single responses. Innocuous electrical stimuli delivered to the ipsilateral posterior tibial nerve as a subject walked on a treadmill caused somatic sensations in the sole of the foot and reflex changes in the electrical activity of the muscle. A stimulus delivered during the swing phase caused increased activity of the muscle (**A**), but a stimulus delivered as the heel touched down caused decreased activity (**B**). A painful electrical stimulus delivered to the sole of one foot caused some ipsilateral contraction and foot flexion when the subject stood on both legs (**C**), much less when standing on the leg whose foot was stimulated (**D**), and much more when standing on the other leg (**E**). [**A** and **B** from De Serres SJ, Yang JF, Patrick SK: Mechanism for reflex reversal during walking in human tibialis anterior muscle revealed by single motor unit recording, *J Physiol* 488:249, 1995. **C-E** from Rossi A, Decchi B: Flexibility of lower limb reflex responses to painful cutaneous stimulation in standing humans: evidence of load-dependent modulation, *J Physiol* 481:521, 1994.]

ASCENDING AND DESCENDING PATHWAYS HAVE DEFINED LOCATIONS IN THE SPINAL WHITE MATTER

The nerve fibers in the white matter of the spinal cord are of three general types:

1. Long, ascending fibers projecting to the thalamus, the cerebellum, or various brainstem nuclei
2. Long, descending fibers projecting from the cerebral cortex or from various brainstem nuclei to the spinal gray matter
3. Shorter **propriospinal** fibers interconnecting various spinal cord levels, such as the fibers responsible for the coordination of flexor reflexes.

Fibers having similar connections tend to travel together, forming the various tracts of the spinal cord. Propriospinal fibers mostly remain in a thin shell surrounding the gray matter called the **propriospinal tract** or **fasciculus proprius** (the Latin word *fasciculus* means "little bundle"); descending tracts are found primarily in the lateral and anterior funiculi; ascending tracts are found in all funiculi.

A great many ascending and descending tracts have been described, largely on the basis of their origins and terminations; the function of some is unknown. In this chapter we describe the largest and best-known tracts descending from the cerebral cortex or ascending to the cerebellum or the thalamus. Consideration of several other tracts is deferred until the structures where they arise or terminate are discussed.

As mentioned previously, there is a tendency to think of individual primary afferents as performing a single function (e.g., either participating in a particular reflex arc or transmitting information to a single ascending tract). Single fibers are drawn that way in textbooks for convenience and clarity, but in fact each primary afferent probably participates in one or more reflex arcs and also in one or more ascending tracts. In a similar way, there is a tendency to think of particular sensory functions as uniquely associated with particular tracts (e.g., pain with one tract and touch with another), so that damage to an ascending tract should result in total loss of some sensory function. This is not actually the case, and most kinds of sensory information reach the thalamus and the cerebellum by more than one route. Why this is so and the consequences in an intact nervous system are not understood, but one result is that the loss of a single tract can often be compensated for, to a surprising extent, by the remaining tracts.

The following section describes the principal pathways by which somatic sensory information reaches the thalamus and the cerebellum. Information that reaches the thalamus is relayed to the cerebral cortex and perceived consciously. Information that reaches the cerebellum is used in the regulation of motor patterns; we are not consciously aware of cerebellar activity.

The Posterior Column–Medial Lemniscus System Conveys Information About Touch and Limb Position

The term *posterior column* refers to the entire contents of a posterior funiculus, exclusive of its share of the propriospinal tract. The posterior columns consist mainly of ascending collaterals of large myelinated primary afferents carrying impulses from various kinds of mechanoreceptors.* This has traditionally been considered the major pathway by which information from low-threshold cutaneous, joint, and muscle receptors reaches the cerebral cortex.

Spinal primary afferent fibers of all diameters and degrees of myelination have their cell bodies in ipsilateral dorsal root ganglia (Figure 10-15). As the dorsal root enters the spinal cord, it segregates itself into **medial**

---

*Significant numbers of unmyelinated fibers have also been noted in the posterior columns, but at this point little is known of their significance. Some are branches of primary visceral afferents.

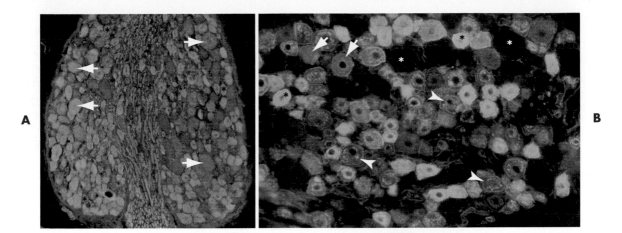

FIGURE 10-15

Heterogeneity of dorsal root ganglion cells. **A,** A low-power view of a single dorsal root ganglion double-labeled with fluorescent antibodies. Green and yellow-green fluorescence *(arrows)* is seen primarily in large neurons, and indicates a neurofilament protein concentrated in myelinated axons and their parent cell bodies. Orange fluorescence *(asterisks)* is seen primarily in small neurons and indicates an intermediate filament protein concentrated in unmyelinated axons and their parent cell bodies. Similarly labeled nerve fibers run vertically through the ganglion on their way out. **B,** Higher-power view of a dorsal root ganglion double-labeled with fluorescent antibodies. Orange fluorescence indicates the presence of a membrane receptor (for nerve growth factor) characteristic of nociceptors, green fluorescence indicates the presence of another cell surface molecule characteristic of neurons with unmyelinated axons, and yellow fluorescence indicates the presence of both markers. Hence in this image orange neurons *(arrows)* presumably give rise to thinly myelinated nociceptive fibers, yellow neurons *(asterisks)* to unmyelinated nociceptive fibers, and green neurons *(arrowheads)* to unmyelinated thermoreceptive or mechanoreceptive fibers. Unlabeled areas *(white asterisks)* are large cell bodies that give rise to heavily myelinated axons that end peripherally in skin, muscle, and joints. (From Molliver DC et al: Presence or absence of TrkA protein distinguishes subsets of small sensory neurons with unique cytochemical characteristics and dorsal horn projections, *J Comp Neurol* 361:404, 1995.)

and **lateral divisions** (Figure 10-16). The medial division contains large, myelinated afferents, whereas the lateral division contains small, finely myelinated or unmyelinated afferents. Fibers of the medial division enter the posterior column. Most of them give off numbers of collaterals to deeper laminae of the spinal gray matter and finally terminate at some spinal level, but some reach the caudal medulla and synapse there. Caudal to T6, each posterior column is an undivided bundle called the **fasciculus gracilis** (the Latin word *gracilis* means "slender"). Rostral to T6, fibers may leave the fasciculus gracilis, but few if any are added. Afferents entering rostral to T6 accumulate in a second bundle, roughly triangular in shape and lateral to the fasciculus gracilis, called the **fasciculus cuneatus** (the Latin word *cuneus* means "wedge"). A glial partition (the **posterior intermediate septum**) extends inward to partially separate the two.

At each successive spinal level, fibers entering the posterior columns add on laterally to those already present (Figure 10-17). A lamination results, with layers of fibers from sacral levels most medial and layers from cervical levels most lateral. This sort of arrangement, in which particular portions of the body are represented in particular regions of a pathway or nucleus, is called **somatotopic** organization and is characteristic of most sensory and motor pathways.

Those posterior column fibers that reach the brainstem synapse in the **nucleus gracilis** or the **nucleus cunea-**

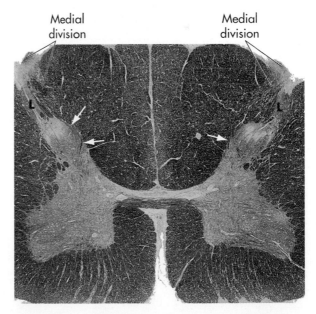

FIGURE 10-16

Dorsal root entry zone, using C5 as an example. Small-diameter fibers enter the cord laterally and join Lissauer's tract *(L)* before terminating in superficial laminae of the posterior horn. Large-diameter fibers enter the spinal cord through the medial division and join the posterior columns. Collaterals of many of these fibers sweep over the medial surface of the posterior horn *(arrows)* to reach deeper laminae.

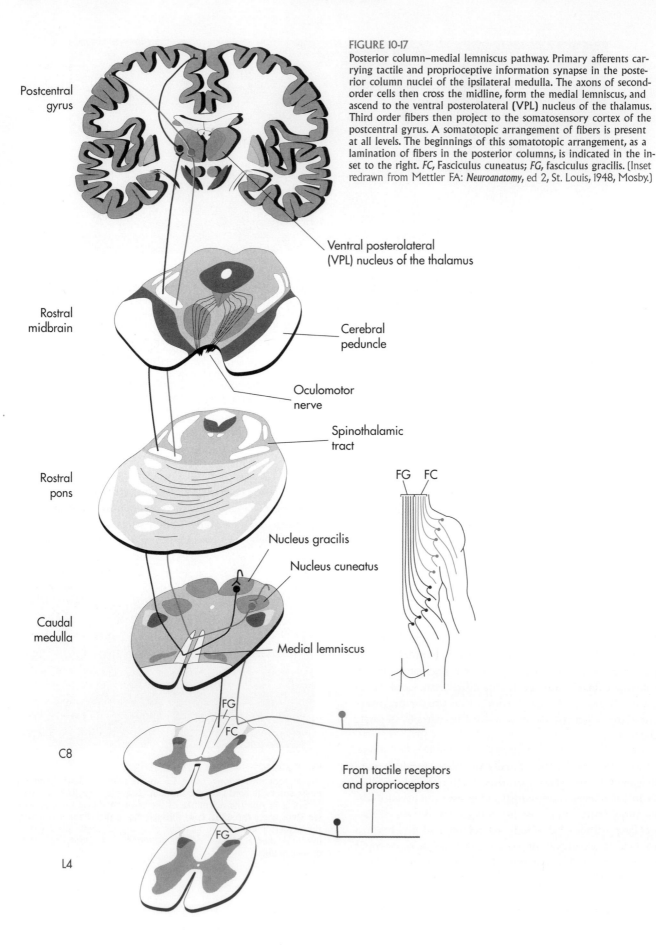

Postcentral
gyrus

Ventral posterolateral
(VPL) nucleus of the thalamus

Rostral
midbrain

Cerebral
peduncle

Oculomotor
nerve

Spinothalamic
tract

FG   FC

Rostral
pons

Nucleus gracilis

Nucleus cuneatus

Caudal
medulla

Medial lemniscus

FG

FC

C8

From tactile receptors
and proprioceptors

FG

L4

FIGURE 10-17

Posterior column–medial lemniscus pathway. Primary afferents carrying tactile and proprioceptive information synapse in the posterior column nuclei of the ipsilateral medulla. The axons of second-order cells then cross the midline, form the medial lemniscus, and ascend to the ventral posterolateral (VPL) nucleus of the thalamus. Third order fibers then project to the somatosensory cortex of the postcentral gyrus. A somatotopic arrangement of fibers is present at all levels. The beginnings of this somatotopic arrangement, as a lamination of fibers in the posterior columns, is indicated in the inset to the right. *FC*, Fasciculus cuneatus; *FG*, fasciculus gracilis. (Inset redrawn from Mettler FA: *Neuroanatomy*, ed 2, St. Louis, 1948, Mosby.)

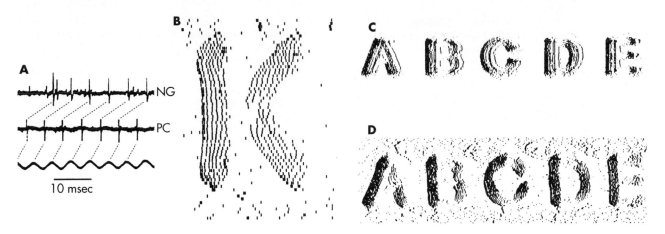

FIGURE 10-18
Preservation of spatial information in the posterior column–medial lemniscus pathway. **A,** One-to-one transmission from the posterior columns to the posterior column nuclei. A small probe vibrating at 200 Hz *(lower trace)* and moving less than 2 μm was applied to the skin of a cat's hindlimb while simultaneous recordings were made from a Pacinian corpuscle *(PC)* afferent in fasciculus gracilis and from a neuron on which it synapsed in nucleus gracilis *(NG)*. Each oscillation caused a spike in the primary afferent. The first of these caused a pair of spikes in the postsynaptic neuron, after which there was a faithful one-to-one coupling between spikes in the primary afferent and the postsynaptic neuron. **B-D,** Responses of a probable Merkel afferent **(C)** and a neuron in somatosensory cortex **(B, D)** as a rotating drum swept embossed letters across a monkey's fingertip. After each revolution the drum was advanced 200 μm, thereby slowly moving the letters through the receptive field of the receptor whose responses were being recorded. One part of such a record, obtained as the letter K was swept across the fingertip, is shown enlarged in **B,** in which each small tick mark corresponds to the occurrence of a single action potential; for additional details on this technique see Figure 9-16. (**A** from Ferrington DG, Rowe MJ, Tarvin RPC: Actions of single sensory fibres on cat dorsal column nuclei neurones: vibratory signalling in a one-to-one linkage, *J Physiol* 386:293, 1987. **B** from Phillips JR, Johnson KO, Hsaio SS: Spatial pattern representation and transformation in monkey somatosensory cortex, *Proc Nat Acad Sci* 85:1317, 1988.)

tus (the **posterior column nuclei**) in the caudal medulla. Second-order fibers arising in these nuclei cross the midline and form the **medial lemniscus** (the Greek word *lemniskos* means "ribbon"), a flattened, ribbon-shaped bundle of fibers that proceeds rostrally through the brainstem and terminates in the thalamus (Figure 10-17). Third-order fibers arising in the thalamus (specifically in the **ventral posterolateral nucleus** of the thalamus, or **VPL**) ascend through the internal capsule to synapse mainly in the cortex of the postcentral gyrus, the primary somatosensory cortex.

Information about the location and nature of a stimulus is preserved in the posterior column–medial lemniscus system

When the primary afferents of the posterior columns terminate in the posterior column nuclei, they maintain their somatotopic organization. Fibers from sacral levels terminate in the most medial portions of the nucleus gracilis, and fibers from cervical levels terminate in the most lateral portions of the nucleus cuneatus. A somatotopic arrangement is found throughout the rest of this pathway, so that information from sacral segments travels through a particular part of the medial lemniscus, projects to a particular portion of VPL, and proceeds to a particular region of the postcentral gyrus. This does not mean that the sacral-to-cervical sequence remains along a medial-to-lateral line throughout the pathway, but rather that sacral information remains segregated from cervical information

at all points along the way to somatosensory cortex. You may find it easier to keep track of the somatotopic arrangement of the pathway at different levels if you envision it as an actual map of the body (a **homunculus,** from the Latin word meaning "little person"), with sacral and lumbar levels corresponding to the legs, thoracic to the trunk, and cervical to the arms and neck. Viewed in this way, the homunculus is lying down, with its feet toward the midline, up to the level of the posterior column nuclei. Its subsequent gyrations are described in the next chapter.

Details about the nature and time course of a stimulus are also preserved in this pathway. Some individual neurons of the posterior column nuclei receive sufficiently powerful excitatory input from individual posterior column fibers that information is transmitted faithfully to the medial lemniscus (Figure 10-18, *A*). Similar subsequent transmission at thalamic and cortical levels results in a remarkably precise representation of certain peripheral stimuli in somatosensory cortex (Figure 10-18, *B-D*).

Damage to the posterior column–medial lemniscus system causes impairment of proprioception and discriminative tactile functions

As might be expected from the types of afferents contained in the posterior columns, this pathway carries information relevant to the conscious appreciation of touch, pressure, and vibration and of joint position and movement. However, because input from cutaneous receptors also reaches the cortex by other routes, damage to the posterior columns causes impairment, but not abolition, of tactile sensibility. Complex discrimination tasks are more severely affected than is simple detection of stimuli.* Other functions, such as proprioception and kinesthesia, are classically considered to be totally lost after posterior column destruction. The result is a distinctive type of **ataxia** (incoordination of muscular activity); the brain is unable to direct motor activity properly without sensory feedback as to the current position of parts of the body (see Figure 18-8). This ataxia is particularly pronounced when the patient's eyes are closed, so that visual compensation is not possible.

The posterior columns actually provide a particularly instructive example of the notion that sensory information travels in multiple pathways, so that damage to a single pathway seldom causes total loss of a function. Classical views of the posterior columns as the pathway responsible for fine tactile discrimination and kinesthesia were based mostly on clinical observations. However, selective lesions of the posterior columns are rare. For example, any process impinging on the posterior columns, such as a tumor, would probably also affect the adjacent posterior horns and dorsal roots, as well as ascending pathways in the posterior part of the lateral funiculus. Tabes dorsalis, a disease process seen in the late stages of neurosyphilis, was traditionally regarded as typifying posterior column damage. Tabetic patients show all the symptoms one would expect if the classical view were correct: their two-point discrimination and vibratory sense are impaired; their senses of movement and position are impaired, and they have great difficulty walking unless they can watch their limbs; and if they try to stand erect with their eyes closed and their feet together, they tend to sway and fall **(Romberg's sign).** Consistent with this, there is pronounced degeneration in the posterior columns. However, there is also degeneration of dorsal root fibers, particularly the heavily myelinated fibers of the medial division, so mechanoreceptive input to all spinal pathways is affected to some extent.

If the posterior columns of a monkey are selectively transected surgically, there is severe impairment initially. The animal has great difficulty coordinating the affected limbs and tends to neglect and not use them. Over a period of months, a remarkable recovery ensues, particularly if the animal is encouraged to use those limbs. After this recovery process, movement and coordination appear nearly normal, tactile threshold is normal, and two-point discrimination and position sense are only slightly impaired. What remains permanently impaired is the ability to use somatosensory information for more complex

tasks, for example, judging the shape of an object pressed against the skin **(stereognosis)** or the direction or speed of a stimulus moving across the skin.

The Spinothalamic Tract Conveys Information About Pain and Temperature

Pain is a complex sensation, in that a noxious stimulus leads not only to a perception of where it occurred, but also to things such as a rapid increase in level of attention, emotional reactions, autonomic responses, and a tendency to remember the event and its circumstances. Corresponding to this complexity, multiple pathways convey nociceptive information rostrally from the spinal cord. One of them (the **spinothalamic tract**) is analogous to the posterior column–medial lemniscus pathway. It reaches the VPL nucleus of the thalamus and is involved in the localization of painful stimuli. The others convey nociceptive information to a variety of other sites in the thalamus, reticular formation, and limbic system that subserve the other aspects of pain. These tracts (including the spinothalamic tract) travel together in the spinal cord and are referred to collectively as the **anterolateral pathway,** reflecting their location in the anterior part of the lateral funiculus.

Collaterals of the nociceptive, thermoreceptive, and some mechanoreceptive fibers of the lateral division of the dorsal root enter the posterior horn and synapse in its superficial laminae (Figure 10-19, *A*), on neurons of lamina I, on neurons of deeper laminae whose dendrites project dorsally into the substantia gelatinosa (Figure 10-19, *B*), and on the small interneurons of the substantia gelatinosa, which in turn convey this information to neurons in other laminae. These second- and third-order cells of the pain and temperature pathways then send their axons across the midline with a slight rostral inclination to form the anterolateral pathway (Figure 10-20). The tract occupies most of the anterior half of the lateral funiculus. New fibers join the anterolateral pathway at its anteromedial edge, so that this system, like the posterior columns, is somatotopically organized. Fibers from the most caudal segments occupy its most posterolateral portion, and those from more rostral segments occupy more anteromedial portions.

As mentioned previously, the anterolateral pathway can be subdivided on the basis of the origin, destination, and probable function of the fibers. One subset of spinothalamic fibers arises from laminae I and V and projects directly to its own part of the VPL and adjoining nuclei of the thalamus in a somatotopic pattern similar to that of the medial lemniscus. It is thought to have a special role in the appreciation of sharp, pricking, well-localized pain (related to that mediated by Aδ fibers), and is also one alternate pathway by which mechanoreceptive input reaches the thalamus and cerebral cortex. A second subset of spinothalamic fibers, aris-

---

*For this reason, whereas posterior column function is commonly tested clinically by touching a vibrating tuning fork to the surface of the body, a more effective test is having a patient try to identify a pattern drawn on the skin.

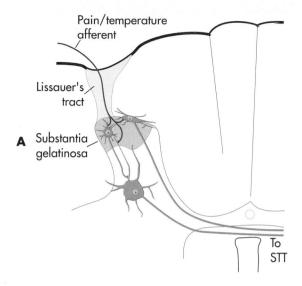

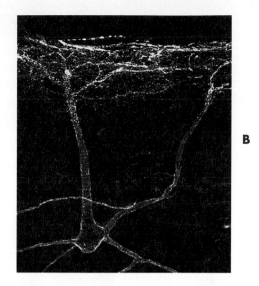

FIGURE 10-19

A, Origin of the spinothalamic tract from the posterior horn, both from neurons on the surface of the substantia gelatinosa (lamina I) and from deeper neurons. Transmission to these deeper tract cells is modulated by small neurons of the substantia gelatinosa, reflecting inputs from large-diameter afferents and from descending pain-control pathways (discussed in Chapter 11). The details of the mechanisms involved in these interactions are not fully understood; other parts of the posterior horn are also involved. **B,** A single spinothalamic tract neuron from the spinal cord of a rat, demonstrated by staining substance P receptors using a fluorescent antibody technique. The cell body of the neuron is located in lamina III, but its dendrites extend into more superficial layers where nociceptive fibers terminate. (**B** from Mantyh PW et al: Receptor endocytosis and dendritic reshaping in spinal neurons after somatosensory stimulation, *Science* 268:1629, 1995.)

ing mainly from the intermediate gray and parts of the anterior horn, projects to different parts of the thalamus (intralaminar and other nuclei) without a somatotopic arrangement. Many of the latter projections are indirect, following a polysynaptic course through the reticular formation, which makes up much of the core of the brainstem (see Chapter 11), and so they are more properly called **spinoreticular** fibers. There is some evidence that these direct and indirect projections to other thalamic nuclei have a special role in the sensation of dull, aching, poorly localized pain related to that mediated by C fibers. Finally, a collection of **spinomesencephalic fibers,** also arising mainly from laminae I and V, probably plays an important role in pain control (discussed in Chapter 11). All these spinothalamic, spinoreticular, and spinomesencephalic fibers are intermingled or adjacent to one another in the spinal cord.

The role of the substantia gelatinosa in the transmission of pain information is still not completely understood. Anatomically it consists of large numbers of small cells among which many unmyelinated afferents terminate. Several populations of these small neurons have been identified based on their neurotransmitter content, but very few from any category give rise to long ascending axons. Rather, they appear to be involved in multiple ways in regulating the access of pain and temperature information to the projection neurons of the anterolateral pathway, either by conveying such information or by participating in pain-suppression processes (discussed in Chapter 11).

Damage to the anterolateral system causes diminution of pain and temperature sensations

Although the spinothalamic tract carries some tactile and pressure information, a great deal also travels in the posterior column system, so destruction of the spinothalamic tract causes no significant tactile deficit. There are, however, several types of sensation (in addition to pain and temperature) subserved more or less predominantly by the spinothalamic tract. These are itch (and probably tickle) sensations, pressure sensations from bladder and bowel, and sexual sensations. However, with the exception of itch (and possibly tickle), this information is carried bilaterally, so unilateral damage generally results in little dysfunction. This may be considered a particularly elegant example of the providence of nature.

The spinothalamic tract is, however, the principal pathway for somatic pain sensations, and its destruction produces contralateral analgesia. An operation to destroy the tract (called **cordotomy**) is sometimes performed on patients suffering from intractable pain. This operation consists of cutting the lateral funiculus from the dentate ligament to the line of ventral rootlets. The cut is usually made several segments rostral to the highest dermatomal level of pain, for two reasons (Figure 10-20). First, collaterals of primary afferents may ascend one or more segments in Lissauer's tract before synapsing, so input from these is spared if the cut is made at the highest dermatomal level of pain. Second, the axons that form the spinothalamic tract cross the midline with a rostral inclination, so a cut at any given level spares fibers that arise

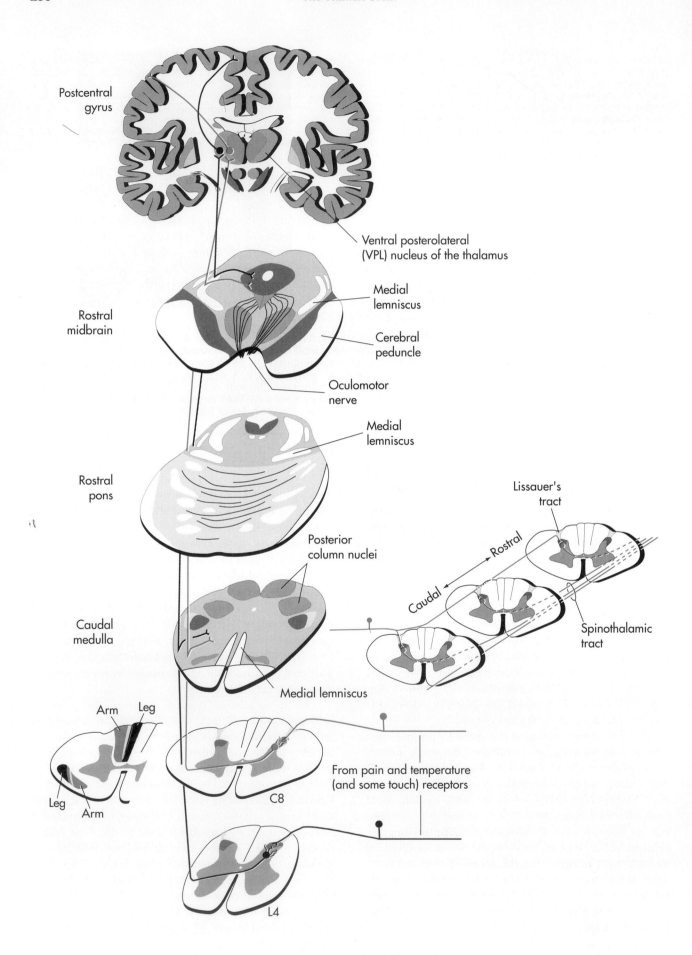

Postcentral
gyrus

Ventral posterolateral
(VPL) nucleus of the thalamus

Rostral
midbrain

Medial
lemniscus

Cerebral
peduncle

Oculomotor
nerve

Medial
lemniscus

Rostral
pons

Lissauer's
tract

Rostral

Caudal

Posterior
column nuclei

Spinothalamic
tract

Caudal
medulla

Medial lemniscus

Arm   Leg

From pain and temperature
(and some touch) receptors

Leg   Arm

C8

L4

FIGURE 10-20

Spinothalamic tract. Pain, temperature, and some touch and pressure afferents end in the posterior horn. Second- or higher-order fibers cross the midline, form the spinothalamic tract, and ascend to the ventral posterolateral (VPL) nucleus of the thalamus (and also to other thalamic nuclei not indicated in this figure). Thalamic cells then project to the somatosensory cortex of the postcentral gyrus. Along their course through the brainstem, spinothalamic fibers give off many collaterals to the reticular formation. The inset to the left shows the lamination of fibers in the posterior columns and the spinothalamic tract, in a leg–lower trunk–upper trunk–arm sequence. The inset to the right shows the longitudinal formation of the spinothalamic tract. Primary afferents ascend several segments in Lissauer's tract before all their branches terminate; fibers crossing to join the spinothalamic tract do so with a rostral inclination. As a result, a cordotomy incision at any given level will spare most of the information entering the contralateral side of the spinal cord at that level, and to be effective the incision must be made several segments rostral to the highest dermatomal level of pain.

---

contralaterally at that level because they join the tract rostral to the cut.

Cordotomy provides prompt contralateral analgesia, but surprisingly the analgesia is usually not permanent. After a varying interval (generally several months), the patient's pain frequently returns. The reason is not known but may be the increasing efficacy of a few uncrossed fibers in the contralateral spinothalamic tract, of additional spinothalamic fibers located more dorsally in the lateral funiculus, or of a limited number of pain fibers in other pathways. Visceral pain is much less affected by cordotomy; recent evidence indicates that much of this information may be conveyed instead in the posterior columns, in the most medial part of fasciculus gracilis.

Additional Pathways Convey Somatosensory Information to the Thalamus

Additional routes for the transmission of tactile and proprioceptive (and to a lesser extent, pain) information have also been described. One such route consists of nonprimary afferents, fibers with their cell bodies in the posterior horn, that nevertheless project to the posterior column nuclei. Some of these travel within the posterior columns, but others travel in the posterior part of the lateral funiculus. The latter route seems to be particularly important for conveying proprioceptive information from the leg to the nucleus gracilis.

Another alternate route is the **spinocervical tract.** Primary afferents conveying information from hair receptors, some other tactile receptors, and some nociceptors synapse on projection neurons in the body of the posterior horn. These projection neurons send their axons ipsilaterally through the posterior part of the lateral funiculus as the spinocervical tract. The spinocervical tract then terminates in the small **lateral cervical nucleus,** which is embedded in the lateral funiculus of the first two cervical segments. The axons of neurons in the lateral cervical nucleus then cross the midline, join the medial lemniscus as it forms in the caudal medulla, and ascend to the VPL.

The size and importance of these alternate pathways in the lateral funiculus are not known for humans, although both are known to exist in monkeys. The acute and chronic effects of posterior column damage, for example, leave little doubt that the posterior columns are ordinarily involved in a major way in kinesthesia and tactile sensation. On the other hand, the degree of recovery that occurs also leaves little doubt that much of this information reaches the thalamus by additional routes. One of these additional routes is undoubtedly the ascending fibers in the posterior part of the lateral funiculus, bound for the posterior column nuclei or the lateral cervical nucleus. These fibers lie near the surface of the cord and can be transected without damaging the lateral corticospinal tract. Such a lesion by itself has no particular effects, but when added to a posterior column lesion, it makes the effects of the latter much more severe and prolonged.

Spinal Information Reaches the Cerebellum Both Directly and Indirectly

The spinal cord is an important source of information used by the cerebellum in the coordination of movement (discussed in greater detail in Chapter 20). This information reaches the cerebellar cortex and nuclei both directly, by way of **spinocerebellar tracts,** and indirectly, by way of relays in brainstem nuclei described further in Chapters 11 and 20. A number of spinocerebellar tracts have been described, some representing the upper extremity and others the lower extremity. Only three have been well characterized (Table 10-5, Figure 10-21).

The posterior spinocerebellar tract and cuneocerebellar tract convey proprioceptive information

Collaterals of posterior column fibers conveying tactile, pressure, and proprioceptive information (mainly the latter, from muscle spindles and Golgi tendon organs) synapse on neurons of Clarke's nucleus. These then send their axons into the lateral funiculus of the same side, forming the **posterior (dorsal) spinocerebellar tract** (Figure 10-21). This tract, a curved band of fibers extending from the dorsal root entry zone to the dentate ligament, lies at the surface of the spinal cord. Fibers in the tract project ipsilaterally to medial zones of the cerebellum (the vermis and adjoining areas) through the **inferior cerebellar peduncle.** Collaterals of some of these fibers end in the nucleus gracilis, providing an important route by which nonprimary afferents transmit proprioceptive

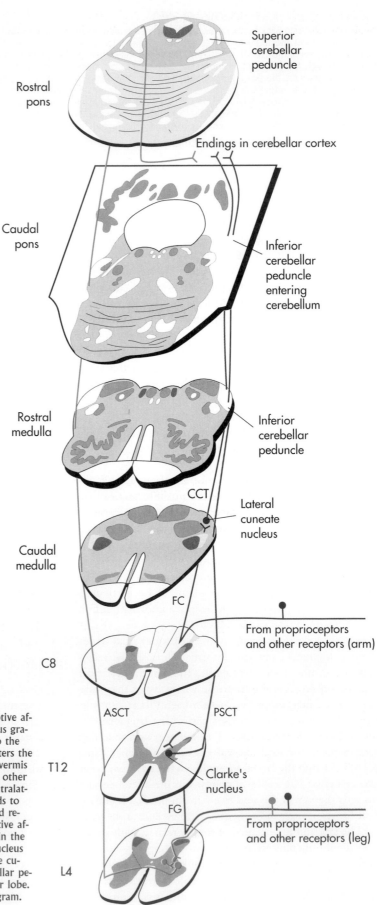

Rostral
pons

Superior
cerebellar
peduncle

Endings in cerebellar cortex

Caudal
pons

Inferior
cerebellar
peduncle
entering
cerebellum

Rostral
medulla

Inferior
cerebellar
peduncle

CCT

Lateral
cuneate
nucleus

Caudal
medulla

FC

From proprioceptors
and other receptors (arm)

C8

ASCT   PSCT

T12   Clarke's
                                       nucleus

FG

From proprioceptors
and other receptors (leg)

L4

FIGURE 10-21

Spinocerebellar and cuneocerebellar tracts. Mechanoreceptive afferents from the lower extremity ascend through fasciculus gracilis *(FG)* to reach Clarke's nucleus, whose cells give rise to the
ipsilateral posterior spinocerebellar tract *(PSCT)*, which enters the
inferior cerebellar peduncle and ends ipsilaterally in the vermis
of the anterior lobe. A larger variety of afferents end on other
cells of the spinal gray matter, whose axons form the contralateral anterior spinocerebellar tract *(ASCT)*; this tract ascends to
the pons, loops over the superior cerebellar peduncle, and recrosses in the vermis of the anterior lobe. Mechanoreceptive afferents from the upper extremity ascend to the medulla in the
fasciculus cuneatus *(FC)* and end in the lateral cuneate nucleus
(analogous to Clarke's nucleus); these cells give rise to the cuneocerebellar tract *(CCT)*, which enters the inferior cerebellar peduncle and ends ipsilaterally in the vermis of the anterior lobe.
The rostral spinocerebellar tract is not shown in this diagram.

Table 10-5	Major Spinocerebellar Tracts		
	Posterior spinocerebellar tract	Anterior spinocerebellar tract	Cuneocerebellar tract
Origin	Clarke's nucleus, T1–L2/3	Spinal border cells, T12–L5	Lateral cuneate nucleus (medulla)
Body part represented	Trunk, lower extremity	Trunk, lower extremity	Trunk, upper extremity
Major inputs	Mechanoreceptors in muscle, joints, skin	Mechanoreceptors, movement-related interneurons	Mechanoreceptors in muscle, joints, skin
Midline crossing	None	Once in cord, again in cerebellum	None
Peduncle used to enter cerebellum	Inferior	Superior	Inferior

information from the leg to the posterior column–medial lemniscus system. Because Clarke's nucleus does not exist caudal to about L2, neither does the posterior spinocerebellar tract. However, afferents from segments caudal to L2 ascend to that level in the fasciculus gracilis to synapse in Clarke's nucleus. This probably explains why Clarke's nucleus is so large at upper lumbar and lower thoracic levels (Figure 10-6), because at these levels it has a substantial backlog of afferent input to process.

The posterior spinocerebellar tract is principally concerned with the ipsilateral leg. Most spinocerebellar-type afferents that enter in cervical and upper thoracic segments, for example, those representing the arm, do not project to Clarke's nucleus. Rather, they travel in the fasciculus cuneatus to a nucleus in the medulla analogous to Clarke's nucleus called the **lateral** (or **external**) **cuneate nucleus** because it is located just lateral to the nucleus cuneatus (see Figures 11-8 and 11-9). Axons of these cells form the **cuneocerebellar tract,** which also projects ipsilaterally to the vermis of the cerebellum through the inferior cerebellar peduncle.

The anterior spinocerebellar tract conveys more complex information

Cells on the lateral surface of the lumbar anterior horn (called *spinal border cells*) give rise to the **anterior (ventral) spinocerebellar tract.** Although this tract is also concerned primarily with the leg, it differs from the posterior spinocerebellar tract in three important respects. First, inputs to these projection neurons are more complex. They come not only from group I muscle afferents (mainly Golgi tendon organs) but also from a wide variety of cutaneous receptors, from spinal interneurons, and from fibers of descending tracts. As a result, activity in anterior spinocerebellar tract neurons is related more to attempted movement than simply to sensory signals. Second, the tract is crossed at the level of the spinal cord, in contrast to the posterior spinocerebellar tract, which ascends uncrossed to an ipsilateral termination in the cere-

bellum. Finally, the anterior spinocerebellar tract takes a roundabout route to the cerebellum (Figure 10-21). It ascends as far as the rostral pons, then turns caudally and enters the cerebellum via the **superior cerebellar peduncle.** There, most of its fibers recross the midline before ending in the vermis of the anterior lobe, so they too ultimately end in the cerebellum on the side ipsilateral to their origin.

A presumed forelimb equivalent of the anterior spinocerebellar tract, called the **rostral spinocerebellar tract,** originates from the posterior horn of lower cervical segments, ascends uncrossed, and enters the cerebellum via both inferior and superior cerebellar peduncles. Little is known of its properties, and it is mentioned here mainly for reasons of symmetry.

Clinically detectable deficits that can be attributed with confidence to damage to the spinocerebellar tracts are rare, partially because the spinocerebellar tracts are rarely if ever affected in isolation. Even in the family of inherited diseases referred to as the *spinocerebellar atrophies,* other areas of the cord are always affected as well. For example, the most common type of spinocerebellar atrophy is Friedreich's ataxia. This disorder is characterized by loss of coordination, which is consistent with cerebellar damage, but also by other impairments not consistent with cerebellar damage, such as disturbed tactile sensation and proprioception and loss of reflexes. Correspondingly, widespread damage is found in and around the spinal cord, affecting not only the posterior spinocerebellar tracts but also the posterior columns and some dorsal root fibers. If the spinocerebellar tracts were selectively affected, one would not expect any sensory changes at all because the cerebellum and its connections have nothing directly to do with sensation.

Descending Pathways Influence the Activity of Lower Motor Neurons

The alpha and gamma motor neurons of the anterior horn are regulated in a variety of ways by supraspinal centers.

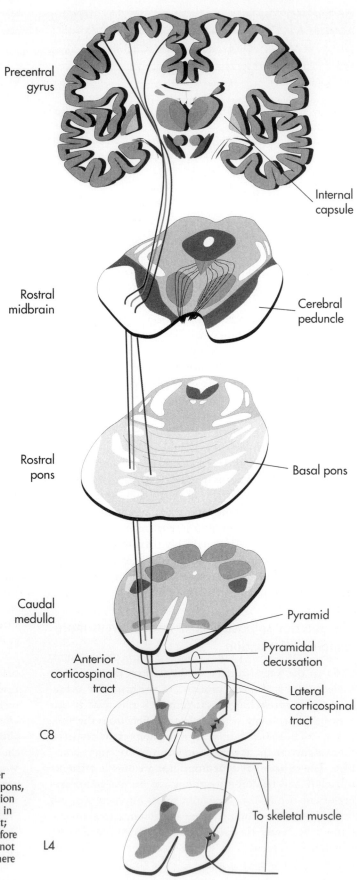

Precentral gyrus

Internal capsule

Rostral midbrain

Cerebral peduncle

Rostral pons

Basal pons

Caudal medulla

Pyramid

Pyramidal decussation

Anterior corticospinal tract

Lateral corticospinal tract

C8

L4

To skeletal muscle

FIGURE 10-22
Corticospinal tracts. Fibers from the precentral gyrus and other
nearby cortical areas descend through the cerebral peduncles, pons,
and medullary pyramids; most cross in the pyramidal decussation
to form the lateral corticospinal tract. Those that do not cross in
the pyramidal decussation form the anterior corticospinal tract;
most of these fibers cross in the anterior white commissure before
ending in the spinal gray matter. Most corticospinal fibers do not
synapse directly on motor neurons; they are drawn that way here
for simplicity.

Table 10-6	Effects of Upper (UMN) and Lower (LMN) Motor Neuron Damage	
	LMN damage	UMN damage
Strength	Decreased	Decreased
Muscle tone	Decreased	Increased
Deep tendon reflexes	Decreased	Increased
Atrophy	Severe	Mild
Other signs	Fasciculations Fibrillations	Clonus Pathological reflexes (e.g., Babinski's sign)

Some of these centers are located in the brainstem and are discussed in later chapters. The major descending outflow is from the cerebral cortex, particularly the precentral gyrus. This **corticospinal** system is dealt with at greater length in Chapter 18, but a few basic concepts are introduced here.

The corticospinal tracts mediate voluntary movement

The **lateral corticospinal tract** (Figure 10-22) is a large, crossed, descending tract that contains the approximately 85% of fibers from the contralateral pyramid that cross in the pyramidal decussation. It is also known as the **pyramidal tract** (because of its course through the pyramid) and occupies the posterior portion of the lateral funiculus, medial to the posterior spinocerebellar tract. Its fibers originate in the cerebral cortex (in the precentral gyrus and nearby areas); descend through the cerebral peduncle, basal pons, and medullary pyramid; decussate; and end in the anterior horn or intermediate gray matter. They terminate on the motor neurons of the anterior horn or, more often, on smaller interneurons that in turn synapse on these motor neurons. Surprisingly, and in contrast to sensory tracts, no anatomical evidence has yet been found for a somatotopic arrangement of the fibers in this tract.*

Fibers of the pyramidal tract and motor axons of the ventral root have distinctly different, though obviously interrelated, roles in the generation of movement. Alpha motor neurons (and the ventral root fibers to which these neurons give rise) contact striated muscle directly and are called **lower motor neurons.** They are also sometimes called the "final common pathway" of the motor system

because, as noted earlier, they are the only means by which the nervous system can exercise control over body movements. Interruption of the lower motor neurons supplying a muscle causes flaccid paralysis and, eventually, atrophy of the muscle.

Neurons with axons that descend from the cerebral cortex or brainstem and end on lower motor neurons, either directly or by way of an interneuron, are called **upper motor neurons.★** An upper motor neuron lesion caused by corticospinal damage has very different effects from those of a lower motor neuron lesion (Table 10-6). Characteristically, the muscles involved show hyperactive reflexes. Their resting tension is increased (i.e., they are **hypertonic**), and there is paralysis or weakness **(paresis),** particularly of fine voluntary movements. This complex of symptoms is referred to as **spastic paralysis.** A number of pathological reflexes are associated with upper motor neuron lesions. The best known is Babinski's sign—dorsiflexion of the big toe and fanning of the others in response to firmly stroking the sole of the foot.†

The 15% or so of the fibers in each pyramid that do not cross in the pyramidal decussation continue into the anterior funiculus (located adjacent to the anterior median fissure) as the **anterior corticospinal tract** (Figure 10-22). These fibers terminate on motor neurons or interneurons in medial portions of the anterior horn or intermediate gray matter, so they preferentially affect the activity of motor neurons for axial muscles. Many of them cross in the anterior white commissure before synapsing, but some do not. Most anterior corticospinal tract fibers end in cervical and thoracic segments, so they may have a special role in the control of neck and shoulder muscles. However, damage to this tract typically does not result in obvious weakness, perhaps partly because of bilateral distribution of fibers from the contralateral tract. Strictly speaking, the term "pyramidal tract" refers to the combination of lateral and anterior corticospinal tracts.

THE AUTONOMIC NERVOUS SYSTEM MONITORS AND CONTROLS VISCERAL ACTIVITY

The goings on of our cardiac and smooth muscles and our glands proceed, for the most part, without conscious supervision—indeed, in spite of attempts at conscious supervision. For instance, we automatically digest our food, regulate our heartbeat, sweat when appropriate, and divert blood to active muscles. Because of the relative automaticity of such functions, the afferents and efferents that

*Nevertheless, damage arising in the center of the cervical spinal cord is often associated with bilateral weakness that is more pronounced in the arms than in the legs. This has led to long-standing clinical teaching that lateral corticospinal fibers are arranged somatotopically, with those destined for more caudal cord levels located more laterally. It has been suggested that this apparent discrepancy may simply reflect the greater importance of this tract for arm movement than for leg movement.

*Some use this term in a more restricted sense to refer only to corticospinal neurons.
†Babinski's sign is either present or not present; it is not "positive" or "negative."

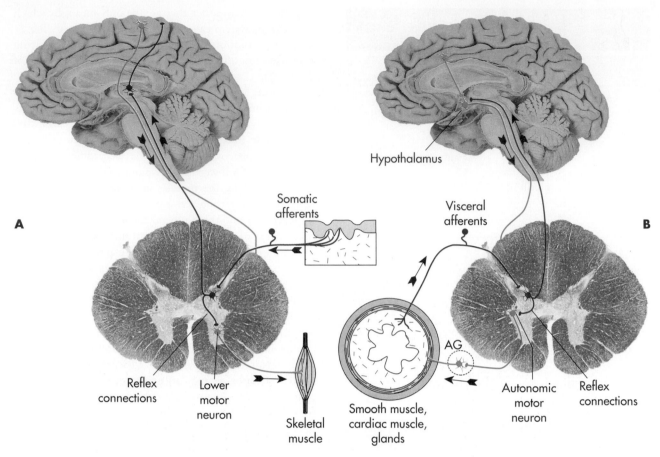

FIGURE 10-23

Parallels between somatic and autonomic parts of the nervous system. Both involve specialized afferents and efferents, reflex connections, and ascending and descending pathways to and from higher levels of the CNS. In the case of the sympathetic and parasympathetic systems, however, the hypothalamus rather than the thalamus receives much of the ascending information, and the hypothalamus rather than the cerebral cortex is a major source of descending pathways. In addition, sympathetic and parasympathetic transmission to the periphery involves an intermediate synapse in an autonomic ganglion *(AG)*.

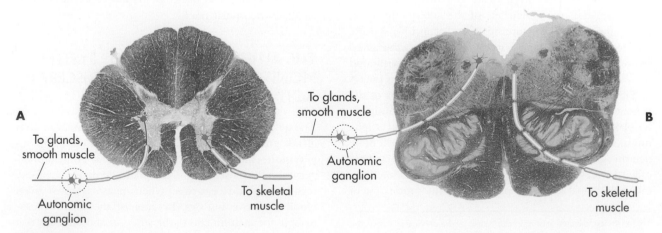

FIGURE 10-24

One major difference between somatic and autonomic efferents. The myelinated axons of lower motor neurons leave the spinal cord (**A**) through ventral roots (or leave the brainstem through cranial nerves, **B**) and reach skeletal muscle directly. The autonomic system, in contrast, uses a two-neuron path. The thinly myelinated axons of preganglionic neurons leave through ventral roots or cranial nerves and end on postganglionic neurons in autonomic ganglia outside the CNS. Unmyelinated axons of postganglionic neurons then innervate smooth muscle, cardiac muscle, and glands.

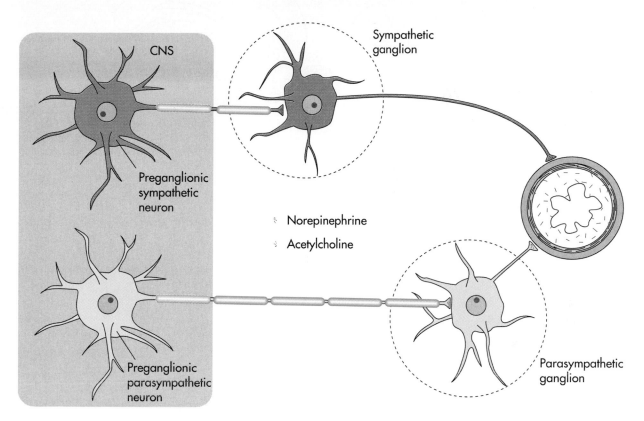

FIGURE 10-25
Major differences between the sympathetic and parasympathetic systems. The axons of preganglionic sympathetic neurons end in ganglia near the spinal cord, whereas those of preganglionic parasympathetic neurons travel a longer distance and reach ganglia near the innervated organ. The preganglionic neurons of both systems use acetylcholine as a neurotransmitter, but at the synapses of postganglionic neurons the parasympathetic system uses acetylcholine and the sympathetic system typically uses norepinephrine.

innervate these organs are referred to as the **autonomic nervous system.**★

The autonomic nervous system has three subdivisions: the **sympathetic, parasympathetic,** and **enteric nervous systems.** Although less well known than the other two, the enteric nervous system perhaps best exemplifies the concept of automatic, self-regulating function. It consists of two interconnected plexuses (the **myenteric plexus** [of Auerbach] and the **submucous plexus** [of Meissner]), including sensory neurons, interneurons, and visceral motor neurons, in the walls of the alimentary canal; all of these neurons and their processes lie entirely outside the CNS. The plexuses are quite extensive. It has been estimated that they contain 10^8 neurons, a number comparable to the number of neurons in the entire spinal cord! The enteric nervous system accounts for the observation that near-normal, coordinated gut motility persists even in the total absence of connections between the gut and the CNS. The normally present sympathetic and parasympathetic connections between the gut and the CNS allow for modulation of this motility.

The sympathetic and parasympathetic divisions of the autonomic nervous system, on the other hand, have a more familiar organization. Similar to the somatic portions of the nervous system considered thus far, there are visceral sensory fibers, ascending visceral sensory pathways, visceral reflex arcs, and descending pathways that control the activity of visceral motor neurons (Figure 10-23). One fundamental difference is that sympathetic and parasympathetic efferents originating in the CNS do not reach their targets directly; rather, a two-neuron chain is involved (Figure 10-24). The first neuron, referred to as a **preganglionic neuron,** has its cell body in the CNS. Its axon terminates in a peripheral ganglion on the second neuron, termed a **postganglionic neuron.** Preganglionic fibers are thinly myelinated (group B), whereas postganglionic fibers are unmyelinated. Sympathetic ganglia are located near the CNS; parasympathetic ganglia are located near the organs they innervate (Figure 10-25). The sympathetic and parasympathetic nervous systems also differ in the neurotransmitter used by their postganglionic neurons (Figure 10-25). The preganglionic neurons of both systems liberate acetylcholine onto the postganglionic neurons. Postganglionic parasympathetic neurons also release acetylcholine onto their targets. Most postganglionic sympathetic neurons, in contrast, release

---

★The autonomic nervous system as originally defined consists only of visceral efferents. However, most now use the term to refer to afferents as well.

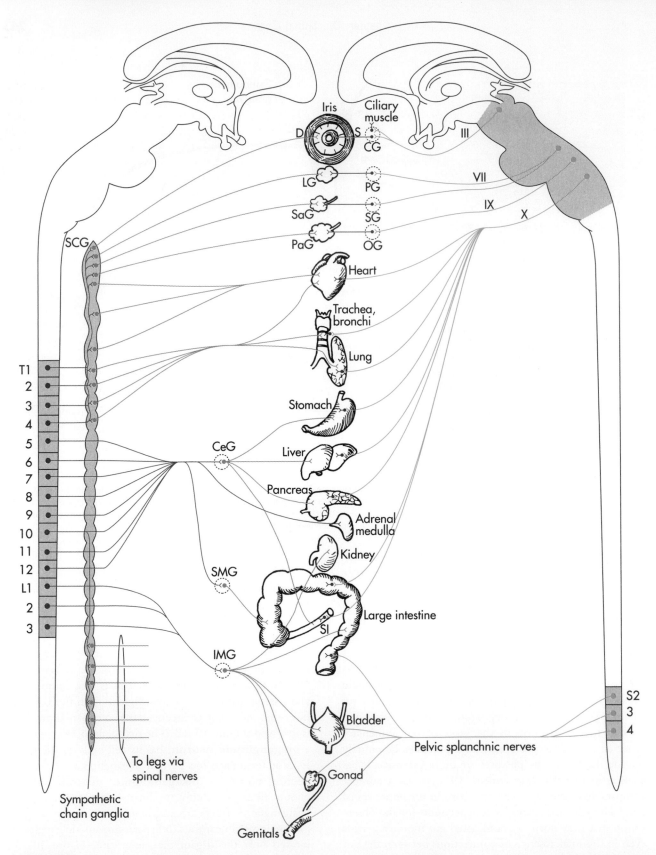

FIGURE 10-26
Origin and distribution of sympathetic *(left)* and parasympathetic *(right)* efferents. Postganglionic neurons that live in sympathetic chain ganglia and project to the body wall and upper extremity are omitted from the diagram to avoid excessive complexity; their axons travel in spinal nerves in a way analogous to that indicated for the lower extremity supply. Although the cranial nerves have distinct and separate parasympathetic contents, there is substantial overlap in the contents of ventral roots S2 to S4. *CG,* Ciliary ganglion; *CeG,* celiac ganglion; *D,* pupillary dilator; *IMG,* inferior mesenteric ganglion; *LG,* lacrimal gland; *OG,* otic ganglion; *PaG,* parotid gland; *PG,* pterygopalatine ganglion; *S,* pupillary sphincter; *SaG,* submandibular and sublingual salivary glands; *SCG,* superior cervical ganglion; *SG,* submandibular ganglion; *SMG,* superior mesenteric ganglion. [Modified from Mettler FA: *Neuroanatomy,* ed 2, St. Louis, 1948, Mosby.)

norepinephrine (a prominent exception is the sympathetic innervation of sweat glands, which is cholinergic). Other differences between the sympathetic and parasympathetic systems are reviewed briefly in the following sections.

Preganglionic Parasympathetic Neurons Are Located in the Brainstem and Sacral Spinal Cord

Preganglionic parasympathetic fibers originate from neurons in two widely separated parts of the CNS, the brainstem and the sacral spinal cord (Figure 10-26). They travel in sacral spinal nerves or in certain cranial nerves (III, VII, IX, and most important, X, as discussed further in Chapter 12) to ganglia in or near their targets. Postganglionic neurons in these peripheral parasympathetic ganglia then innervate the target organ. Relative to the case in sympathetic ganglia, there is little divergence in parasympathetic ganglia. This, together with the location of parasympathetic ganglia in individual organs, makes it possible for the parasympathetic system to exert restricted, localized control. Sympathetic activation, in contrast, tends to be more widespread.

The parasympathetic (or **craniosacral**) outflow goes almost exclusively to thoracic, abdominal, and pelvic viscera (Figure 10-26). There are, for example, no parasympathetic fibers to the limbs. (One clinically important exception is the pupillary sphincter of the eye; the parasympathetic fibers included in the oculomotor nerve serve as the efferent limb of the pupillary light reflex [Figure 17-36].) In a general sense, the parasympathetic system enhances energy storage. Activation of parasympathetic nerves causes decreased cardiac output and blood pressure, increased peristalsis in the gut and salivation, as well as pupillary constriction and bladder contraction. Visceral afferents traveling with sacral spinal nerves and with cranial nerves IX and X are appropriate for these functions, carrying information about things such as blood pressure and chemistry and fullness of the bladder and gastrointestinal tract. Cranial nerves VII, IX, and X also carry information from taste buds, obviously relevant to energy intake.

Preganglionic Sympathetic Neurons Are Located in Thoracic and Lumbar Spinal Segments

Preganglionic sympathetic fibers originate from neurons in the thoracic and upper two or three lumbar segments (Figure 10-26). This division of the autonomic nervous system therefore is also referred to as the **thoracolumbar outflow.** The preganglionic fibers travel in spinal nerves to ganglia relatively close to the spinal cord. Some of these ganglia form an interconnected **sympathetic chain** adjacent to the spinal cord (Figures 10-1 and 10-2), whereas others, referred to as **prevertebral ganglia,** are a little

farther away. The major exception is the adrenal medulla, which is directly innervated by preganglionic sympathetic fibers. The adrenal medulla develops from the neural crest and, similar to postganglionic sympathetic neurons, its cells secrete norepinephrine; it can therefore be thought of as a displaced sympathetic ganglion.

Sympathetic fibers are more widely distributed than parasympathetic fibers, reaching all parts of the body. Preganglionic fibers exit the spinal cord in thoracic and lumbar nerves and then travel from the spinal nerves to the sympathetic chain via **white communicating rami,** so called because the preganglionic fibers are myelinated and hence white (Figure 10-2, *A*). Some end in sympathetic chain ganglia, from which unmyelinated postganglionic fibers rejoin spinal nerves via **gray communicating rami.** Others continue through the chain without synapsing and reach prevertebral ganglia. Postganglionic fibers destined for the head, thorax, and limbs originate in sympathetic chain ganglia, whereas those destined for abdominal and pelvic viscera originate in prevertebral ganglia.

Generally, the sympathetic system prepares us for situations in which energy needs to be expended. Activation of sympathetic fibers increases heart rate, decreases peristalsis, and diverts blood from the gut to skeletal muscles. Because there is a great deal of divergence in sympathetic ganglia and because sympathetic stimulation causes the adrenal medulla to secrete norepinephrine and epinephrine into the circulation, sympathetic activation tends to produce widespread and relatively long-lasting effects.

Although in some instances, such as effects on gut motility and heart rate, the sympathetic and parasympathetic systems have opposite effects, in other instances one or the other is unopposed or both act cooperatively (Table 10-7). For example, sweat glands and limb vasculature receive only sympathetic innervation, but the parasympathetic system is the dominant influence in control of the pupil and the bladder. The two systems cooperate in male sexual function in which erection is mediated primarily by parasympathetic fibers and ejaculation by sympathetic fibers.

Visceral Distortion or Damage Causes Pain That Is Referred to Predictable Dermatomes

Visceral afferent fibers, with their cell bodies in T1 to L2 or L3 dorsal root ganglia, accompany sympathetic efferents in spinal nerves. Similarly, visceral afferents with cell bodies in S2 to S4 dorsal root ganglia or certain cranial nerve ganglia accompany parasympathetic efferents. Most of these afferents carry information that subserves visceral reflexes and does not reach consciousness, such as data about vascular tone. Others, primarily in sympathetic nerves, carry messages about distortion or inflammation of visceral organs, which are interpreted as pain. Visceral pain

Table 10-7   Principal Physiological Effects of Autonomic Activity

Structure or system	PSN	Sympathetic effect	PPN*	Parasympathetic effect
HEAD				
Pupillary sphincter			E-W	Contracts (miosis)
Pupillary dilator	T1–T3	Contracts (mydriasis)		
Superior tarsal muscle	T1–T3	Contracts (lid elevation)		
Ciliary muscle			E-W	Contracts (accommodation)
Lacrimal gland	T1–T3	↓Secretion	SSN	↑Secretion
Salivary glands	T1–T3	↓Secretion, ↑Viscosity	ISN, SSN	↑Secretion, ↓Viscosity
RESPIRATORY SYSTEM				
Bronchial muscles	T1–T5	Relax	DMN X	Contract
CARDIOVASCULAR SYSTEM				
Heart rate and output	T1–T5	↑	NA	↓
Arteries (skeletal muscle)	T1–L3	Dilate or constrict†		
Arteries (skin)	T1–L3	Constrict		
Arteries (viscera)	T1–L3	Constrict	DMN X	Dilate
GASTROINTESTINAL SYSTEM				
Motility	T6–L3	↓	DMN X‡	↑
Sphincters	T6–L3	Contract	DMN X‡	Relax
Secretion	T6–L3	↓	DMN X‡	↑
Gallbladder	T6–T9	Relax	DMN X	Contract
UROGENITAL SYSTEM				
Bladder detrusor	T12–L2	Relax	S2–S4	Contract
Bladder sphincter	T12–L2	Contract	S2–S4	Relax
Seminal vesicles, vas deferens	T10–L1	Contract (during ejaculation)		
Penile/clitoral arteries	T10–L1	Dilate or constrict§	S2–S4	Dilate (erection)
SKIN				
Sweat glands	T1–L3	↑Secretion‖		
Piloerector muscles	T1–L3	Contract (goose bumps)		
ADRENAL MEDULLA	T8–L1	↑Secretion		

DMN X, Dorsal motor nucleus of the vagus (in the medulla); *E-W*, Edinger-Westphal nucleus (in the midbrain); *ISN*, inferior salivary nucleus (in the medulla); *NA*, nucleus ambiguus (in the medulla); *PPN*, location of preganglionic parasympathetic neurons; *PSN*, location of preganglionic sympathetic neurons; *SSN*, superior salivary nucleus (in the pons).

*Brainstem sites containing preganglionic parasympathetic neurons are discussed in Chapter 12.

†Effect depends on conditions of stimulation. Most postganglionic sympathetic fibers to skeletal muscle arteries cause constriction, but there are some cholinergic vasodilator fibers. In addition, sympathetic activation of the adrenal medulla causes skeletal muscle vasodilation in response to circulating catecholamines.

‡Spinal segments S2-S4 provide the preganglionic parasympathetic neurons for the digestive tract below the left colic flexure.

§Depends on conditions of stimulation. Sympathetic fibers have been implicated both in psychogenic erection and in detumescence.

‖Most postganglionic sympathetic fibers to sweat glands are atypical in that they are cholinergic.

Table 10-8 Typical Patterns of Referred Pain

Organ damaged	Dermatomes in which pain may be felt
Diaphragm	C3–C4
Heart	T1–T4 (mainly left)
Stomach	T6–T9 (mainly left)
Gallbladder	T7–T8 (right)
Duodenum	T9–T10
Appendix	T10 (right)
Reproductive organs	T10–T12
Kidney, ureter	L1–L2

is different from somatic pain in that it is poorly localized to the diseased organ and commonly is **referred** to an area of the body surface. The area to which the pain is referred corresponds to the dermatome innervated by the spinal segment to which the visceral afferents project. Thus the heart is supplied by visceral afferents that enter the cord in upper thoracic segments, and coronary artery disease is associated with pain referred to the left side of the chest and part of the left arm (angina pectoris). The most satisfactory explanation available for referred pain at present is that visceral and somatic pain fibers at a given level of the spinal cord converge on the same spinothalamic tract cells, and the brain interprets spinothalamic tract impulses as pain in the somatic region. The functional utility of such an arrangement is not clear, but knowledge of typical patterns of referred pain is important clinically (Table 10-8).

A LONGITUDINAL NETWORK OF ARTERIES SUPPLIES THE SPINAL CORD

The arterial supply of the spinal cord is by way of the vertebral arteries and of branches, ultimately from the thoracic and abdominal aorta, called **radicular arteries.** Each vertebral artery gives rise to an **anterior spinal artery;** the two anterior spinal arteries fuse to form a single midline vessel that courses along the anterior median fissure of the spinal cord (Figure 10-27). The vertebral or posterior inferior cerebellar artery of each side also gives rise to a **posterior spinal artery,** which proceeds along the line of attachment of the dorsal roots. The posterior spinal arteries and the midline anterior spinal artery supply upper cervical levels with blood from the vertebral arteries. Below this, all three spinal arteries form a more or less continuous series of anastomoses with radicular arteries for the length of the cord. The spinal arteries are rather small; beginning with lower cervical segments, the spinal cord depends on these radicular arteries for its survival.

One particular radicular artery, present at about spinal cord level T12 in most individuals, is called the **great radicular artery** (or **artery of Adamkiewicz**) and may provide the entire arterial supply for the lumbosacral spinal cord.

The very long anterior spinal artery, which is usually a continuous vessel for the length of the spinal cord, gives rise to a series of hundreds of central and circumferential branches (Figure 10-27) that supply the anterior two thirds of the spinal cord, including the base of the posterior horn and a variable portion of the lateral corticospinal tract (Figure 10-28). The posterior spinal arteries may subdivide into longitudinal branches medial and lateral to the dorsal roots (Figure 10-27) and are really more of a plexiform network of small arteries. Collectively they supply the posterior columns, substantia gelatinosa, dorsal root entry zone, and a variable portion of the lateral corticospinal tract.

Venous drainage is by a series of six irregular, plexiform channels: one each along the anterior and posterior midlines and one along the line of attachment of the dorsal and ventral roots of each side. These are drained by **radicular veins,** which in turn empty into the **epidural venous plexus.**

SPINAL CORD DAMAGE CAUSES PREDICTABLE DEFICITS

Long-Term Effects of Spinal Cord Damage Are Preceded by a Period of Spinal Shock

If the spinal cord of a cat is transected at a midcervical level, you might expect, among other things, a spastic (upper motor neuron) paralysis of its whole body. This does happen eventually, but first there is a period, lasting for a few days, of more or less completely flaccid paralysis and areflexia. Deep tendon reflexes then begin to return and finally become hyperactive. The areflexic period is called **spinal shock.** The mechanism of spinal shock is incompletely understood, but the whole sequence of events is thought to be a consequence of interruption of fibers from the brainstem and cerebrum descending to spinal cord motor neurons and interneurons. In addition to corticospinal tracts, there are a number of other descending influences, some facilitatory and some inhibitory. Spinal shock would thus be caused by sudden loss of a collection of descending influences whose net effect is facilitatory. The mechanism by which this period of spinal shock resolves into spasticity is not fully understood. It may be the result, at least in part, of the formation of new synaptic connections. The degeneration of the endings of descending fibers would leave vacant synaptic sites at various places on motor neurons and interneurons, adjacent to intact reflex connections. Multiplication of these reflex connections to fill up the vacated sites would be expected to

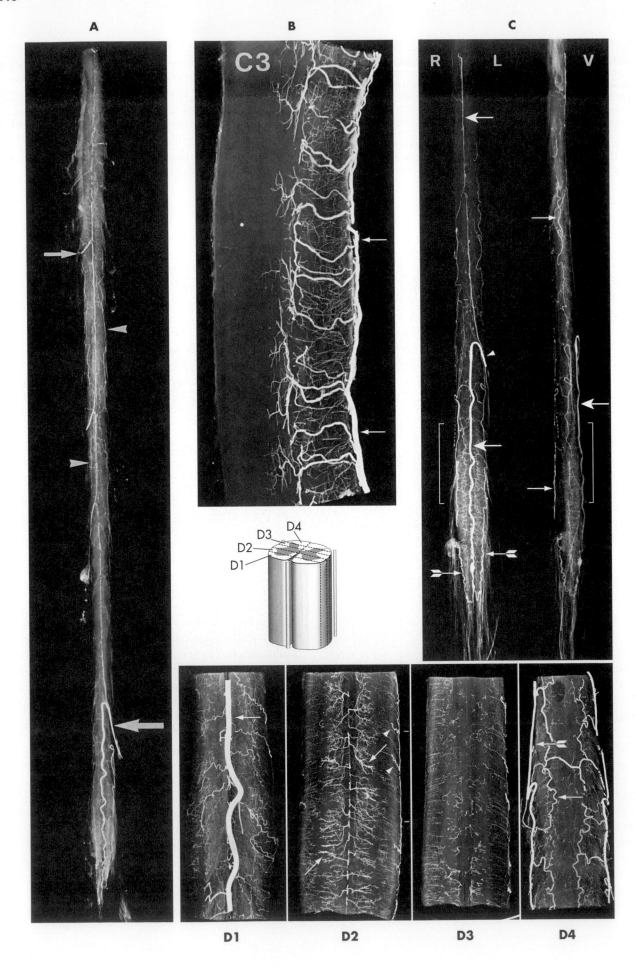

A

B

C3

C

R L V

D4
D3
D2
D1

D1   **D2**   **D3**   **D4**

FIGURE 10-27

Arterial supply of the spinal cord, demonstrated in a beautiful series of angiograms obtained after postmortem injection of barium sulfate and gelatin. **A,** An anterior view, showing the anterior spinal artery joined by a large radicular artery at C7 *(small arrow)* and by the great radicular artery of Adamkiewicz *(large arrow)* at T11. Parts of posterior spinal arteries *(arrowheads)* can also be seen. **B,** Midsagittal view at C3 showing the anterior spinal artery *(arrows)*, giving rise to many branches that run posteriorly through the anterior median fissure to reach central regions of the cord. **C,** Anterior and lateral (*V,* ventral) views of the thoracic and lumbosacral portions of a spinal cord, showing the anterior *(large arrows)* and posterior *(small arrows)* spinal arteries and the artery of Adamkiewicz *(arrowhead).* Near the cauda equina, anastomoses *(tailed arrows)* typically interconnect the anterior and posterior spinal arteries in a kind of miniature circle of Willis. **D,** Vertical slices of the bracketed region in **C,** showing the anterior spinal artery *(arrow,* **D1**), its branches to central regions of the cord *(arrows,* **D2**), branches from circumferential anterior-posterior arterial interconnections that feed parts of the cord closer to the surface (**D3** and *arrowheads,* **D2**) and posterior spinal arteries medial and lateral to the dorsal root entry zone *(arrow* and *tailed arrow,* **D4**). [From Thron AK: *Vascular anatomy of the spinal cord,* Vienna, 1988, Springer-Verlag.]

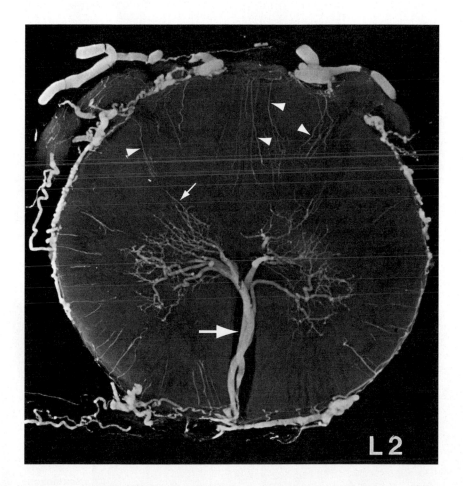

FIGURE 10-28

Microangiogram of a cross section at L2. Branches *(large arrow)* of the anterior spinal artery run posteriorly through the anterior median fissure to reach central regions of the cord. Branches of circumferential connections between the anterior and posterior spinal arteries supply parts of the cord closer to the surface. Branches *(arrowheads)* of the posterior spinal artery supply the posterior columns and share with anterior spinal branches *(small arrow)* in the supply of the posterior horn. [From Thron AK: *Vascular anatomy of the spinal cord,* Vienna, 1988, Springer-Verlag.]

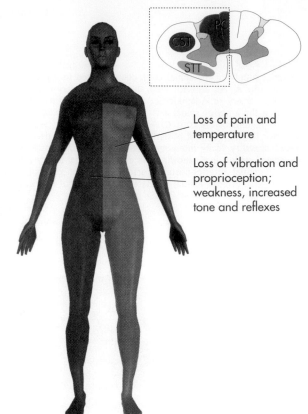

FIGURE 10-29
Brown-Séquard syndrome. Damage to the outlined area of the spinal cord (in this example at C8) would affect the indicated tracts, causing *ipsi*lateral spastic paralysis and loss of fine touch and proprioception, and *contra*lateral loss of pain and temperature beginning one or more segments below the level of damage.

Loss of pain and temperature

Loss of vibration and proprioception; weakness, increased tone and reflexes

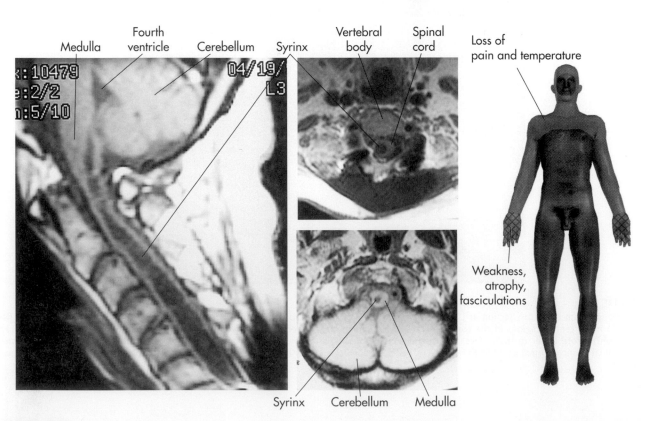

Medulla   Fourth ventricle   Cerebellum   Syrinx   Vertebral body   Spinal cord

Loss of pain and temperature

Weakness, atrophy, fasciculations

Syrinx   Cerebellum   Medulla

FIGURE 10-30
Syringomyelia. A 39-year-old man was thrown from the bed of a pickup truck in a motor vehicle accident, sustaining vertebral fractures at T5-6 and C4-5. About 2 years later, he began to notice progressive weakness and atrophy of his hand muscles. MRI revealed a central cavity in his spinal cord (syringomyelia), extending into the caudal medulla. The cavity is somewhat irregular in shape, and damage is more extensive at some levels than others. Typical findings in such a case would be a band of bilateral loss of pain and temperature sensation (extending into the distribution of the trigeminal nerve, in a pattern explained in Chapter 12), and weakness and atrophy at levels where the damage extended into the anterior horns (in this case at lower cervical levels). [MRIs courtesy Dr. Raymond F. Carmody, Department of Radiology, The University of Arizona College of Medicine.]

increase the sensitivity and intensity of reflexes. Other mechanisms, such as increased sensitivity to the transmitter substances released at remaining synapses, may also be involved.

Spinal shock occurs in humans as well, even in cases of contusion of the spinal cord, in which total or near-total recovery can be expected. It may last for weeks or even months in cases of complete transection. A complicating factor in spinal shock is the complete loss of bladder function (and loss of a sensation of distention) that accompanies it. Early catheterization is called for to minimize bladder distention and consequent damage. With proper care, even in cases of complete cord transection, a state of automatic or reflex emptying of the bladder develops.

The Side and Distribution of Deficits Reflect the Location of Spinal Cord Damage

Partial lesions of the spinal cord are (fortunately) much more common than complete transections. Complete transection of one side of the cord (hemisection), although rare, results in an instructive complex of symptoms called the **Brown-Séquard syndrome** (Figure 10-29). After a period of spinal shock (particularly prominent in those areas subserved by the damaged portion of the cord), a spastic paralysis develops below the level of the lesion and ipsilateral to it because of interruption of the lateral corticospinal tract. Tactile, vibratory, and position senses are disturbed ipsilaterally below the level of the lesion because of interruption of the posterior column. There is loss of pain and temperature sensation *contralateral* to the lesion, beginning one or two segments caudal to the level of the lesion, as a result of interruption of the spinothalamic tract. This is one of many examples of **crossed findings,** that is, some symptoms referable to one side of the head or body and others to the other side, which may seem strange and inexplicable unless one understands the anatomical sites at which different pathways cross the midline.

Syringomyelia (the Greek word *syrinx* means "tube," as in syringe) is a disease of the central part of the spinal cord in which a tubelike enlargement of the central canal develops, typically at lower cervical or upper thoracic levels (Figure 10-30). As the syrinx enlarges, surrounding neural tissue is destroyed. The first damage is to fibers crossing through the limited available area around the central canal (Figure 10-5, *A*). The next area damaged is usually the anterior horn. The result is a distinctive combination of loss of pain and temperature sensation bilaterally over the arms and shoulders (as a result of the damage to crossing fibers) and weakness and atrophy of the muscles of the hands (as a result of anterior horn damage). Of course, if the syrinx occurred at a different spinal level, the symptoms would be referred to a correspondingly different part of the body.

SUGGESTED READINGS

Andersson K-E, Wagner G: Physiology of penile erection, *Physiol Rev* 75:191, 1995.

Apkarian AV, Hodge CJ: Primate spinothalamic pathways. I. A quantitative study of the cells of origin of the spinothalamic pathway, *J Comp Neurol* 288:447, 1989.

Appel NM, Elde RP: The intermediolateral cell column of the thoracic spinal cord is comprised of target-specific subnuclei: evidence from retrograde transport studies and immunohistochemistry, *J Neurosci* 8:1767, 1988.

Appenzeller O: *The autonomic nervous system: an introduction to basic and clinical concepts,* ed 4, Amsterdam, 1990, Elsevier.

Applebaum ML et al: Organization and receptive fields of primate spinothalamic tract neurons, *J Neurophysiol* 38:572, 1975.

Basbaum AI: Conduction of the effects of noxious stimulation by short-fiber multisynaptic systems of the spinal cord in the rat, *Exp Neurol* 40:699, 1973. *A series of experiments showing that rats can learn to avoid painful stimuli even after hemisection of both sides of the spinal cord, which should transect the long ascending fibers of both sides.*

Batzdorf U, editor: *Syringomyelia: current concepts in diagnosis and treatment,* Baltimore, 1991, Williams & Wilkins.

Besson JM, Chaouch A: Peripheral and spinal mechanisms of nociception, *Physiol Rev* 67:67, 1987.

Briner RP et al: Evidence for unmyelinated sensory fibers in the posterior columns in man, *Brain* 111:999, 1988.

Brown AG: The spinocervical tract, *Prog Neurobiol* 17:59, 1981.

Bryan RN, Coulter JD, Willis WD: Cells of origin of the spinocervical tract in the monkey, *Exp Neurol* 42:574, 1974.

Calne DB, Pallis CA: Vibratory sense: a critical review, *Brain* 89:723, 1966. *Interesting reading, with a review of old clinical observations.*

Cervero F, Iggo A: The substantia gelatinosa of the spinal cord: a critical review, *Brain* 103:717, 1980.

Cervero F, Morrison JFB, editors: *Visceral sensation,* vol 67, *Prog Brain Res,* Amsterdam, 1986, Elsevier.

Cervero F, Sharkey KA: More than just gut feelings about visceral sensation, *Trends Neurosci* 8:188, 1985. *A brief review of a neglected topic—the pathways and mechanisms used by visceral afferents.*

Chung K, Coggeshall RE: Unmyelinated primary afferent fibers in dorsal funiculi of cat sacral spinal cord, *J Comp Neurol* 238:365, 1985.

Coggeshall RE: Law of separation of function of the spinal roots, *Physiol Rev* 60:716, 1980.

Collins WF, Nulsen FE, Randt CT: Relation of peripheral nerve fiber size and sensation in man, *Arch Neurol* 3:381, 1960. *Postcordotomy abolition of the painful consequences of controlled electrical stimulation of the sural nerve.*

Craig AD, Serrano LP: Effects of systemic morphine on lamina I spinothalamic tract neurons in the cat, *Brain Res* 636:233, 1994.

Creed RS et al: *Reflex activity of the spinal cord,* reprinted with annotations by DPC Lloyd, New York, 1972, Oxford University Press.

Critchley E, Eisen A, editors: *Spinal cord disease: basic science, diagnosis and management,* London, 1997, Springer-Verlag.

Crock HV, Yoshizawa H: *The blood supply of the vertebral column and spinal cord in man,* New York, 1977, Springer-Verlag.

Davidoff RA: The dorsal columns, *Neurol* 39:1377, 1989. *A good recent review of the complications lurking in this seemingly simple pathway.*

deGroat WC et al: Mechanisms underlying the recovery of urinary bladder function following spinal cord injury, *J Autonom Nerv Sys* 30:S71, 1990.

Furness JB, Costa M: *The enteric nervous system,* Edinburgh, 1987, Churchill Livingstone.

Gillilan LA: The arterial blood supply of the human spinal cord, *J Comp Neurol* 110:75, 1958.

Gillilan LA: Veins of the spinal cord, *Neurol* 20:860, 1970.

Glees P, Soler J: Fibre content of the posterior column and synaptic connections of nucleus gracilis, *Z Zellforsch* 36:381, 1951. *Documents the fact that, at least in the cat, only about 25% of the fibers that enter the posterior columns actually reach the posterior column nuclei; the rest end within the spinal cord.*

Goyal RK, Hirano I: The enteric nervous system, *New Engl J Med* 334:1106, 1996.

Grillner A: Locomotion in the spinal cat. In Stein RB et al, editors: *Control of posture and locomotion: advances in behavioral biology,* vol 7, New York, 1973, Plenum Press. *Walking with the hind limbs by cats whose spinal cords had been transected at low thoracic levels.*

Ha H: Cervicothalamic tract in the rhesus monkey, *Exp Neurol* 33:205, 1971.

Hirshberg RM et al: Is there a pathway in the posterior funiculus that signals visceral pain? *Pain* 67:291, 1996. *Evidence from human neurosurgical procedures that second-order fibers specifically conveying visceral pain information travel near the midline in the posterior funiculus.*

Hosobuchi Y: The majority of unmyelinated afferent axons in human ventral roots probably conduct pain, *Pain* 8:167, 1980.

Jenny A, Smith J, Decker J: Motor organization of the spinal accessory nerve in the monkey, *Brain Res* 441:352, 1988.

Keswani NH, Hollinshead WH: Localization of the phrenic nucleus in the spinal cord of man, *Anat Rec* 125:683, 1956.

Kuhn RA: Functional capacity of the isolated human spinal cord, *Brain* 73:1, 1950. *A careful study of the course of events after complete transection of the spinal cord, particularly spinal shock and its gradual fading.*

Kuo DC, DeGroat WC: Primary afferent projections of the major splanchnic nerve to the spinal cord and gracile nucleus of the cat, *J Comp Neurol* 231:421, 1985.

Levi ADO, Tator CH, Bunge RP: Clinical syndromes associated with disproportionate weakness of the upper versus the lower extremities after spinal cord injury, *Neurosurg* 38:179, 1996. *A review of the evidence that the corticospinal tract, surprisingly, is not somatotopically organized in the lower brainstem and the spinal cord.*

Liddell EGT, Sherrington C: Reflexes in response to stretch (myotatic reflexes), *Proc R Soc Lond,* series B, 96:212, 1924.

Matthews PBC: The 1989 James A.F. Stevenson memorial lecture. The knee jerk: still an enigma, *Can J Physiol Pharmacol* 68:347, 1990.

Melzack R, Wall PD: Pain mechanisms: a new theory, *Science* 150:971, 1965. *A seminal paper, in which the modulating effect of the substantia gelatinosa on pain transmission was proposed in a scheme called the "gate control theory" of pain. Although apparently wrong in some of its details, the gate control theory has nevertheless been very influential on pain research since 1965.*

Mense S: Structure-function relationships in identified afferent neurones, *Anat Embryol* 181:1, 1990. *A review of elegant demonstrations of how single primary afferents with known functions end in precisely defined patterns in the spinal cord.*

Miller S, van der Meché FGA: Coordinated stepping of all four limbs in the high spinal cat, *Brain Res* 109:395, 1976.

Morin F: A new spinal pathway for cutaneous impulses, *Am J Physiol* 183:245, 1955. *The original physiological description of the spinocervical tract.*

Nathan PW, Smith MC: The location of descending fibres to sympathetic preganglionic vasomotor and sudomotor neurons in man, *J Neurol Neurosurg Psychiatry* 50:1253, 1987.

Nathan PW, Smith MC, Cook AW: Sensory effects in man of lesions of the posterior columns and of some other afferent pathways, *Brain* 109:1003, 1986. *"The total evidence from all the relevant cases shows that the major pathway subserving every kind of mechanoreception is in the posterior third of the cord."*

Nathan PW, Smith MC, Deacon P: The corticospinal tracts in man: course and location of fibres at different segmental levels, *Brain* 113:303, 1990.

Norrsell U: Behavioral studies of the somatosensory system, *Physiol Rev* 60:327, 1980.

Nudo RJ, Masterton RB: Descending pathways to the spinal cord: a comparative study of 22 mammals, *J Comp Neurol* 277:53, 1988.

Oscarsson O: Functional organization of spinocerebellar paths. In Iggo A, editor: *Handbook of sensory physiology, vol. II, Somatosensory system,* New York, 1973, Springer-Verlag.

Perl ER: Effects of muscle stretch on excitability of contralateral motoneurones, *J Physiol* 145:193, 1959.

Petras JM: Spinocerebellar tract neurons in the rhesus monkey, *Brain Res* 130:146, 1977.

Pratt CA: Evidence of positive force feedback among hindlimb extensors in the intact standing cat, *J Neurophysiol* 73:2578, 1995. *Conditions under which Golgi tendon organs cause excitatory reflex effects.*

Rexed B: The cytoarchitectonic organization of the spinal cord in the cat, *J Comp Neurol* 96:415, 1952.

Rossi A, Decchi B: Flexibility of lower limb reflex responses to painful cutaneous stimulation in standing humans: evidence of load-dependent modulation, *J Physiol* 481:521, 1994.

Rustioni A, Hayes NL, O'Neill SO: Dorsal column nuclei and ascending afferents in macaques, *Brain* 102:95, 1979. *An account of the nonprimary afferents ascending to nuclei gracilis and cuneatus in the posterior columns and the posterior part of the lateral funiculus.*

Rymer WZ, Houk JC, Craggo PE: Mechanisms of the clasp-knife reflex studied in an animal model, *Exp Brain Res* 37:93, 1979. *Physiological experiments suggesting that Golgi tendon organs cannot entirely account for the clasp-knife reflex and that group III and IV muscle afferents may be involved.*

Shealy CN, Mortimer JT, Hagfors NR: Dorsal column electroanalgesia, *J Neurosurg* 32:560, 1970. *Another example of treating pain by shifting the balance of activity toward large-fiber afferent systems, this time by stimulating the posterior columns.*

Smith MC, Deacon P: Topographical anatomy of the posterior columns of the spinal cord in man: the long ascending fibers, *Brain* 107:671, 1984.

Snyder R: The organization of the dorsal root entry zone in cats and monkeys, *J Comp Neurol* 174:47, 1977.

Stein RB, Capaday C: The modulation of human reflexes during functional motor tasks, *Trends Neurosci* 11:328, 1988.

Takahashi Y, Takahashi K, Moriya H: Mapping of dermatomes of the lower extremities based on an animal model, *J Neurosurg* 82:1030, 1995.

Thron AK: *Vascular anatomy of the spinal cord: neuroradiological investigations and clinical syndromes*, Vienna, 1988, Springer-Verlag.

Truex RC et al: The lateral cervical nucleus of cat, dog and man, *J Comp Neurol* 139:93, 1970.

Uddenberg N: Functional organization of long second-order afferents in the dorsal funiculus, *Exp Brain Res* 4:377, 1968. *Physiological description of the minority of fibers in the posterior column that are not primary afferents.*

Vierck CJ Jr: Alterations of spatio-tactile discrimination after lesions of primate spinal cord, *Brain Res* 58:69, 1973. *Some speculations on how primates compensate for loss of a posterior column, plus experiments to show the much greater deficits caused by damage to both a posterior column and the posterior part of the ipsilateral lateral funiculus.*

Vierck CJ Jr, Luck MM: Loss and recovery of reactivity to noxious stimuli in monkeys with primary spinothalamic cordotomies, followed by secondary and tertiary lesions of other cord sectors, *Brain* 102:233, 1979.

Wall PD, Noordenbos W: Sensory functions which remain in man after complete transection of dorsal columns, *Brain* 100:641, 1977. *A description of the surprising sensory capabilities left in two unfortunate patients after transection of all but one anterior quadrant of the cord. "We conclude that patients with dorsal column lesions do not lose one or more of the classical primary modalities of sensation but lose an ability to carry out tasks where they must simultaneously analyze spatial and temporal characteristics of the stimulus."*

Weaver TA, Walker AE: Topical arrangement within the spinothalamic tract of the monkey, *Arch Neurol Psychiatry* 46:877, 1941.

White JC, Sweet WH: *Pain and the neurosurgeon: a forty year experience*, Springfield, Ill, 1969, Charles C Thomas.

Willis WD, Coggeshall RE: *Sensory mechanisms of the spinal cord*, ed 2, New York, 1991, Plenum Press. *A well-written, thoroughly documented review of the literature.*

Willis WD, Kenshalo DR Jr, Leonard RB: The cells of origin of the primate spinothalamic tract, *J Comp Neurol* 188:543, 1979.

Wilson DA, Prince JR: MR imaging determination of the location of the normal conus medullaris throughout childhood, *Am J Roentgenol* 152:1029, 1989.

Yang JF, Stein RB: Phase-dependent reflex reversal in human leg muscles during walking, *J Neurophysiol* 63:1109, 1990.

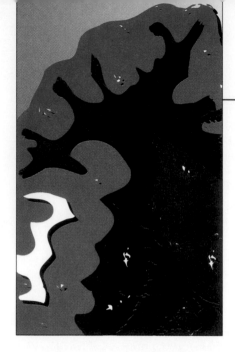

ORGANIZATION OF THE BRAINSTEM

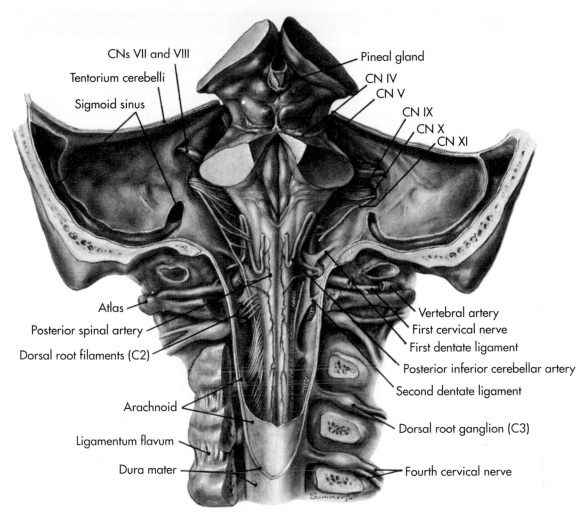

FIGURE 11-1
Posterior aspect of the brainstem and upper spinal cord. The cerebellum and cerebral hemispheres have been removed. (From Mettler FA: *Neuroanatomy*, ed 2, St. Louis, 1948, Mosby.)

The spinal cord continues rostrally into the brainstem (Figure 11-1), which performs spinal cord–like functions for the head. It contains the lower motor neurons for the muscles of the head and does the initial processing of general afferent information concerning the head. However, the brainstem does much more than this, reflecting in large part the additional functions of the cranial nerves attached to it, as well as some distinctive built-in brainstem functions.

THE BRAINSTEM HAS CONDUIT, CRANIAL NERVE, AND INTEGRATIVE FUNCTIONS

Brainstem activities may be divided (not very cleanly) into three general types: **conduit functions, cranial nerve functions,** and **integrative functions.**

The need for conduit functions is apparent; the only way for ascending tracts to reach the thalamus or cerebel-

lum, or for descending tracts to reach the spinal cord, is through the brainstem. Many of these tracts, however, are not straight-through affairs, and identifiable relay nuclei in the brainstem are frequently involved.

The cranial nerves contain not only the head's equivalent of spinal nerve fibers but also those involved in the special senses of olfaction, sight, hearing, equilibrium, and gustation, or taste (Table 11-1). The olfactory and optic nerves project directly to the telencephalon and diencephalon, respectively, but the others project to or emerge from the brainstem. Thus a wide assortment of sensory and motor nuclei related to cranial nerve function can be found at various brainstem levels.

A number of integrative functions are organized at the level of the brainstem, such as complex motor patterns, aspects of respiratory and cardiovascular activity, and even some regulation of the level of consciousness itself. Much of this is accomplished by the **reticular formation,** which forms the central core of the brainstem.

Table 11-1	Highly Simplified Overview of Cranial Nerve Functions*	
Cranial nerve	Main sensory function	Main motor function
I. Olfactory	Smell	—
II. Optic	Sight	—
III. Oculomotor	—	Eye movements, pupil and lens function
IV. Trochlear	—	Eye movements
V. Trigeminal	Facial sensation	Chewing
VI. Abducens	—	Eye movements
VII. Facial	Taste	Facial expression
VIII. Vestibulocochlear	Hearing, equilibrium	—
IX. Glossopharyngeal	Taste	Swallowing
X. Vagus	Thoracic and abdominal viscera	Speech, swallowing; thoracic and abdominal viscera
XI. Accessory	—	Head and shoulder movements
XII. Hypoglossal	—	Tongue movements

*For more details, see Table 12-2 and Chapters 12-14.

It is clear that these three general types of activity are far from mutually exclusive. For example, ascending pathways to the thalamus arise not only in the spinal cord, but also from cranial nerve nuclei; the latter therefore have a hybrid conduit and cranial nerve function. However, this parcelization does provide a useful framework on which to organize a treatment of the brainstem. It is difficult to learn about this portion of the nervous system all at once, so it is presented here in several parts. This chapter describes the overall anatomy of the brainstem and presents a series of sections showing the locations of some prominent nuclei and of major ascending and descending tracts. The next three chapters describe the central connections of cranial nerves III to XII, and Chapter 15 is a similar series of sections, labeled in more detail, with summary descriptions of the contents of various tracts and nuclei.

THE MEDULLA, PONS, AND MIDBRAIN HAVE CHARACTERISTIC GROSS ANATOMICAL FEATURES

Each of the three major subdivisions of the brainstem—the medulla, pons, and midbrain (Figure 11-2)—has a characteristic set of surface features. As will be explained in subsequent sections, knowledge of these surface features can help make sense of the internal organization of the brainstem.

The Medulla Includes Pyramids, Olives, and Part of the Fourth Ventricle

The medulla is vaguely scoop shaped (Figure 11-2). The "handle" corresponds to the **caudal** or **closed** portion, containing a central canal continuous with that of the spinal cord. The open portion of the scoop corresponds to the **rostral** or **open medulla,** in which the central canal expands as the fourth ventricle. The apex of the V-shaped caudal fourth ventricle, where it narrows into the central canal, is called the **obex** (Figure 11-3, *A*).

The longitudinal grooves of the surface of the spinal cord continue into the medulla. They divide the surface of the caudal medulla and part of the rostral medulla into a series of columns that completely encircle it (Figure 11-3). The anterior median fissure is briefly interrupted by the pyramidal decussation at the junction between spinal cord and brainstem, but then continues rostrally to the edge of the pons, separating the two pyramids (Figure 11-3, *B*). Proceeding around in a posterior direction, the anterolateral sulcus marks the other side of the pyramid. The rootlets of the hypoglossal nerve (XII) emerge from this sulcus, mainly in the rostral medulla. In the rostral medulla, the column dorsal to the hypoglossal rootlets is enlarged to form an oval swelling called the **olive.** The rootlets of the glossopharyngeal (IX) and vagus (X)* nerves emerge from a shallow lateral groove dorsal to the olive. The posterolateral sulcus also continues into the medulla; the area between it and the line of rootlets of IX and X (which in the spinal cord would overlie Lissauer's tract and the posterior horn) overlies the **spinal tract of the trigeminal nerve.** As explained in the next chapter, the spinal tract of the trigeminal nerve is the head's equivalent of Lissauer's tract. Finally, the posterior columns continue into the medulla. The fasciculus cuneatus, adjacent

---

*The most caudal vagal filaments join the accessory nerve briefly while passing through the jugular foramen, and so for a long time were spoken of as the **cranial part of the accessory nerve.** However, in most other aspects of their origin, course, and termination these caudal filaments resemble vagal fibers (see Chapter 12). Hence most now include all of these filaments as part of the vagus, and consider the fibers emerging from the lateral surface of the upper cervical cord as the definitive accessory nerve.

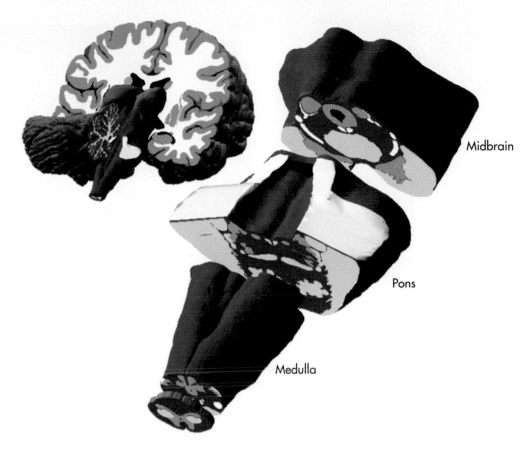

FIGURE II-2
The three major subdivisions of the brainstem.

to the posterolateral sulcus, extends rostrally to a small swelling called the **cuneate tubercle,** which marks the site of the nucleus cuneatus. The fasciculus gracilis, adjacent to the midline, extends rostrally to a similar small swelling called the **gracile tubercle,** which marks the site of the nucleus gracilis.

If the cerebellum is removed (as it has been in Figure 11-3), one can peer down on the floor of the fourth ventricle. Here, too, various grooves and elevations signify the presence of underlying nuclei. The sulcus limitans can often be followed rostrally along the floor of the ventricle into the pons (Figure 11-3, *A*). As in the embryonic spinal cord, it is a line of separation between motor nuclei (now medial to it) and sensory nuclei (now lateral to it; see Figures 2-9 and 12-1). The portion of the medulla and pons immediately beneath the floor of the ventricle, lateral to the sulcus limitans, is mostly occupied by vestibular nuclei and is referred to as the **vestibular area.** The area medial to the sulcus limitans overlies a series of motor nuclei, three of which make visible elevations. In the medulla, the hypoglossal nucleus and the dorsal motor nucleus of the vagus make small triangular swellings, appropriately called the **hypoglossal** and **vagal trigones.** Farther rostrally, in the pons, is another elevation called the **facial colliculus.** This elevation is not caused by an underlying motor nucleus of the facial nerve, as one might surmise from its

name. Rather, it is the location of the abducens nucleus; fibers destined for the facial nerve loop over it at this location on their way out of the brainstem (see Figures 12-5 and 12-6).

The Pons Includes the Basal Pons, Middle Cerebellar Peduncles, and Part of the Fourth Ventricle

The pons is dominated by the massive, transversely oriented structure on its ventral surface from which it derives its name (Figures 11-3 and 11-4). *Pons* is the Latin word for "bridge," and this portion of it (called the **basal pons**) looks like a bridge interconnecting the two cerebellar hemispheres. It is not, however, a direct interconnection. Rather, many of the fibers descending in a cerebral peduncle synapse in scattered nuclei of the ipsilateral half of the basal pons. These nuclei in turn project their fibers across the midline, after which they funnel into the **middle cerebellar peduncle (brachium pontis★)** and finally enter the cerebellum.

★*Brachium* is the Latin word for "arm" and is used neuroanatomically to refer to some prominent bands of white matter extending from or to an area of gray matter. In this case the brachium pontis—literally "the arm of the pons"—extends dorsally from the pons to reach the cerebellum.

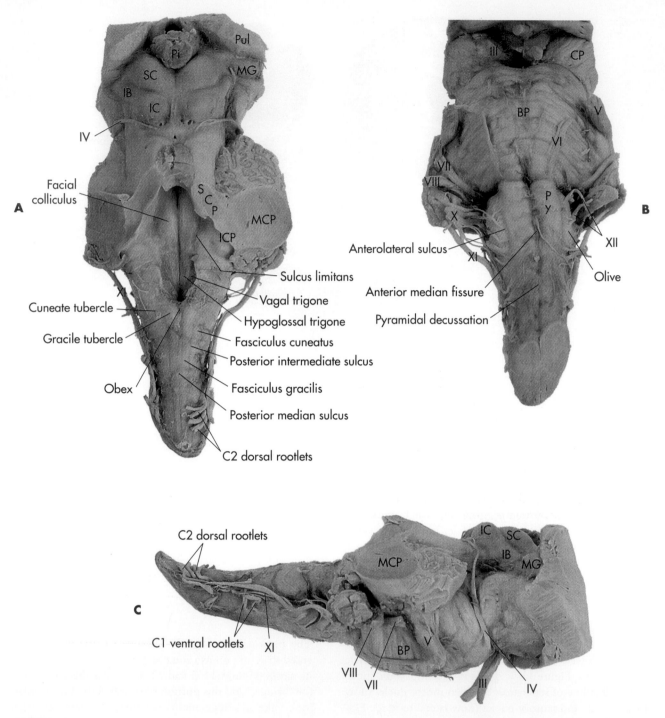

FIGURE 11-3

Posterior (A), anterior (B), and lateral (C) aspects of the brainstem, after the cerebellum and cerebrum were removed. Actual length is 8 cm. Cranial nerves indicated by Roman numerals. *BP*, Basal pons; *CP*, cerebral peduncle; *IB*, brachium of the inferior colliculus; *IC*, inferior colliculus; *ICP*, inferior cerebellar peduncle; *MCP*, middle cerebellar peduncle; *MG*, medial geniculate nucleus; *Pi*, pineal gland; *Pul*, pulvinar; *Py*, pyramid; *SC*, superior colliculus; *SCP*, superior cerebellar peduncle. [From Nolte J, Angevine JB Jr: *The human brain in photographs and diagrams*, St. Louis, 1995, Mosby.]

The trigeminal nerve (V) enters the brainstem at the midpons, and three others enter (or leave) along the groove between the basal pons and the medulla (Figure 11-3). The abducens nerve (VI) is the smallest and most medially located of these three, exiting where the pyramid emerges from the basal pons. The facial nerve (VII) is farther lateral and consists of two parts: a larger and more medial motor root and a smaller sensory root (sometimes referred to as the **intermediate nerve** [see Figure 3-15, *B*]). The vestibulocochlear nerve (VIII) is slightly lateral

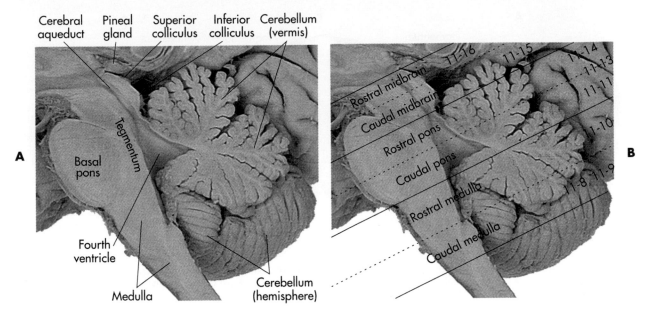

Cerebral aqueduct   Pineal gland   Superior colliculus   Inferior colliculus   Cerebellum (vermis)

Tegmentum

Basal pons

A

Fourth ventricle

Medulla

Cerebellum (hemisphere)

Rostral midbrain
Caudal midbrain
Rostral pons
Caudal pons
Rostral medulla
Caudal medulla

11-16   11-15   11-14   11-13   11-11   11-10   11-8, 11-9

B

FIGURE 11-4
Medial surface of the right half of a hemisected brain, showing major features of the brainstem and cerebellum **(A). B,** Transverse planes defining the subdivisions of the brainstem and the planes of sections shown elsewhere in this chapter. (Modified from Nolte J, Angevine JB Jr: *The human brain in photographs and diagrams,* St. Louis, 1995, Mosby.)

to the facial nerve and also has two parts: a vestibular division and a more lateral cochlear division.

The superior cerebellar peduncle **(brachium conjunctivum*)** forms much of the roof of the fourth ventricle in the pons. It emerges from the cerebellum, moves toward the midline and the brainstem, and enters the latter near the junction between the pons and midbrain. At this same junction, the trochlear nerve (IV) emerges from the dorsal surface of the brainstem. The superior cerebellar peduncle is covered in the rostral pons by a flattened band of fibers called the **lateral lemniscus,** which forms part of the ascending auditory system and terminates in the inferior colliculus.

The Midbrain Includes the Superior and Inferior Colliculi, the Cerebral Peduncles, and the Cerebral Aqueduct

The midbrain is characterized by four bumps (the paired superior and inferior colliculi) on its posterior surface and by the large cerebral peduncles on its anterior surface. The oculomotor nerve (III) emerges from the interpeduncular fossa between the peduncles.

The broad, low ridge extending rostrally from the inferior colliculus is the **brachium of the inferior colliculus** (usually shortened to **inferior brachium**). This is a continuation of the ascending auditory pathway, projecting from the inferior colliculus to the thalamic relay nucleus for hearing (the **medial geniculate nucleus**).

---

*Latin for "joined-together arm," named for the path taken by the two peduncles as they enter the brainstem and decussate (see Figure 20-20, *A*).

THE INTERNAL STRUCTURE OF THE BRAINSTEM REFLECTS SURFACE FEATURES AND THE POSITION OF LONG TRACTS

At any given brainstem level rostral to the obex, three general areas can be identified in cross section (Figure 11-5). These are (1) the area posterior to the ventricular space, (2) the area anterior to the ventricular space, and (3) large structures "appended" to the anterior surface of the brainstem. (In the caudal medulla the central canal is surrounded by structures, including some that will be anterior to the ventricular space at more rostral levels).

The only place where the portion posterior to the ventricular space contains a substantial amount of neural tissue is the midbrain. Here this region is called the **tectum** (Latin for "roof") and consists of the superior and inferior colliculi. In the pons and rostral medulla, the fourth ventricle is covered posteriorly by the superior and inferior medullary vela (and, of course, the cerebellum).

The area anterior to the ventricular space is called the **tegmentum** (Latin for "covering") as a general term. The tegmentum contains most of the structures to be described in this and the next three chapters: the reticular formation, cranial nerve nuclei and tracts, ascending pathways from the spinal cord, and some descending pathways.

The structures appended to the anterior surface of the brainstem contain fibers descending from the cerebral cortex to the spinal cord, to certain cranial nerve nuclei, or to pontine nuclei (which in turn project to the cerebellum). These appended structures primarily include the

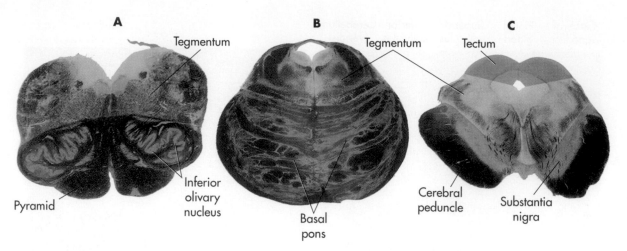

FIGURE 11-5

General areas in cross sections of the brainstem, as seen in the rostral medulla (**A**), pons (**B**), and midbrain (**C**). The tegmentum is prominent at all levels, the tectum only in the midbrain. Anteriorly appended structures include the pyramids and inferior olivary nuclei of the rostral medulla, the basal pons, and the cerebral peduncles and substantia nigra of the rostral midbrain.

large fiber bundles of the cerebral peduncles, the basal pons, and the pyramids of the medulla.

Although the brainstem is derived embryologically from a serial array of vesicles, in the adult it no longer possesses an organization quite so neat (Figure 11-4). For example, the basal pons usually extends rostrally to a point ventral to the tectum of the midbrain; the pineal gland and part of the thalamus extend caudally to a point dorsal to the tectum of the midbrain. Because the most instructive way to study the brainstem is to consider a series of parallel sections through it (all perpendicular to its long axis), I have ignored minor inconveniences such as the intrusion of the basal pons under the midbrain and have used, for the purposes of the following discussion, reference transverse planes (Figure 11-4, *B*) that subdivide the brainstem into six parts: caudal and rostral medulla, caudal and rostral pons, and caudal and rostral midbrain.

The following discussion points out major brainstem structures at these levels and the locations of tracts that begin or end in the spinal cord. The next three chapters deal with the cranial nerves and their tracts and nuclei. Finally, as noted previously, the material of all four chapters is integrated in a series of extensively labeled sections that form Chapter 15.

The Corticospinal and Spinothalamic Tracts Have Consistent Locations Throughout the Brainstem*

The three major longitudinal pathways (corticospinal tract, posterior columns, and spinothalamic tract) that were followed through the spinal cord in Chapter 10 can be followed systematically through the brainstem, as indicated in Figure 11-6. Two of the three stay in more or less

*This discussion was modified from Nolte J, Angevine JB Jr: *The human brain in photographs and diagrams*, St. Louis, 1995, Mosby.

the same location throughout the brainstem. Corticospinal fibers travel in the most ventral part of the brainstem, traversing the cerebral peduncle, basal pons, and medullary pyramid. At the spinomedullary junction, most of the fibers in the pyramids decussate and form the lateral corticospinal tracts. The spinothalamic tract at all levels of the brainstem is in or near the ventrolateral corner of the tegmentum, similar to its position in the spinal cord. The posterior columns terminate in the posterior column nuclei (nucleus gracilis and nucleus cuneatus) of the medulla. Efferent fibers from these nuclei decussate in the medulla to form the medial lemniscus, which reaches the thalamus. The medial lemniscus starts out near the midline and then moves progressively more laterally as it proceeds through the brainstem.

The Medial Lemniscus Forms in the Caudal Medulla

The caudal (closed) medulla extends from the caudal edge of the pyramidal decussation (where the medulla becomes continuous with the spinal cord) to the obex, which marks the caudal end of the fourth ventricle.

The caudal medulla (Figures 11-7 and 11-8) looks somewhat like the spinal cord. Part of the anterior horn is still present caudally (Figure 11-7), as are structures similar to Lissauer's tract and part of the posterior horn. The latter two are actually the **spinal tract** and **spinal nucleus of the trigeminal nerve.** These are the head's equivalent of Lissauer's tract and the substantia gelatinosa (i.e., they deal with pain, temperature, and some tactile information).

The fasciculi gracilis and cuneatus continue into the caudal medulla but are gradually replaced by the posterior column nuclei (nucleus gracilis and nucleus cuneatus). The nucleus cuneatus begins and ends a bit rostral to the nucleus gracilis, so even in Figure 11-8 part of the fasci-

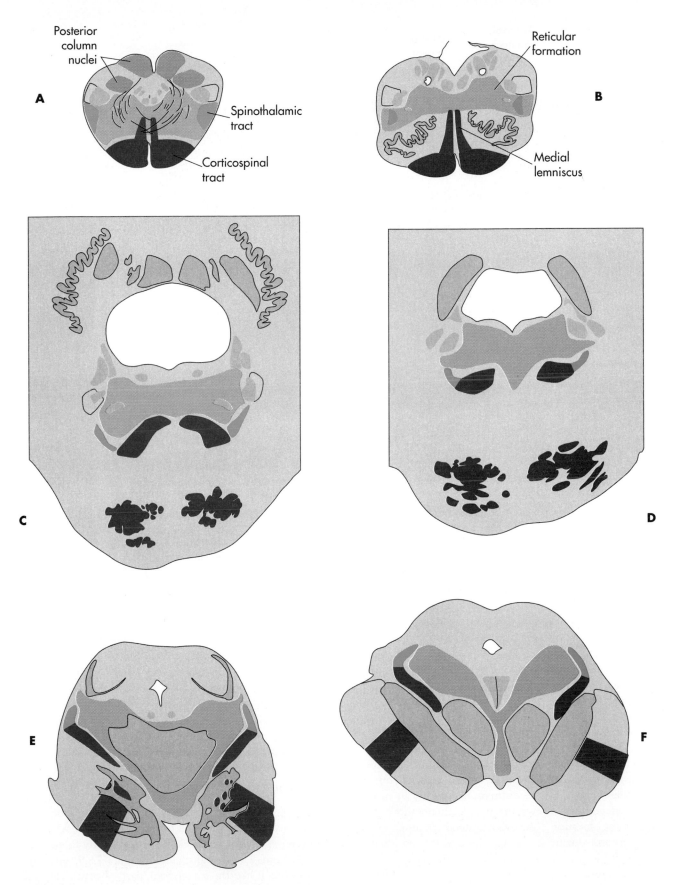

FIGURE 11-6
Locations of the corticospinal tract, medial lemniscus, spinothalamic tract, and reticular formation in the caudal and rostral medulla (**A, B**), pons (**C, D**) and midbrain (**E, F**). (Modified from Nolte J, Angevine JB Jr: *The human brain in photographs and diagrams*, St. Louis, 1995, Mosby.)

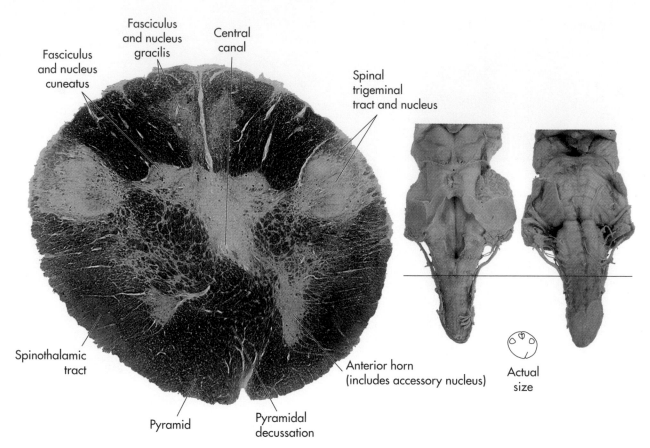

FIGURE 11-7
Caudal medulla near the spinomedullary junction at the level of the pyramidal decussation.

culus cuneatus is still present. Postsynaptic fibers leave these two nuclei in a ventral direction and arch across the midline to form the contralateral medial lemniscus, a vertically oriented band of fibers (Figure 11-8). These decussating fibers are part of the collection of **internal arcuate fibers** and are sometimes called the **sensory decussation.** Throughout the medulla, the medial lemniscus is organized so that fibers representing cervical segments are most posterior (i.e., as though the homunculus were standing upright).

Adjacent to the nucleus cuneatus and embedded in the fasciculus cuneatus is the **lateral** (or **external**) **cuneate nucleus** (Figure 11-8). This is the forelimb equivalent of Clarke's nucleus, and the axons of these cells join the posterior spinocerebellar tract in the inferior cerebellar peduncle at a slightly more rostral level.

The spinothalamic tract is one of several that are not so compact or heavily myelinated as the medial lemniscus and therefore cannot be distinguished clearly in myelin-stained sections. However, this tract maintains more or less the same location (the ventrolateral portion of the tegmentum) during its passage through the brainstem, at least until it reaches the rostral midbrain.

The prominent pyramids (Figure 11-8) and their decussation (Figure 11-7) are located most anteriorly in the caudal medulla. Each pyramid consists of corticospinal

fibers that originated in ipsilateral cerebral cortex and are (mostly) bound for the contralateral anterior horn.

Most of the area traversed by internal arcuate fibers in Figure 11-8 is **reticular formation.** A casual observer, looking at this region in photographs such as these, will not see much. This is, to a first approximation, what distinguishes the reticular formation from the rest of the brainstem; the posterior column nuclei, for example, *look* like nuclei, whereas the reticular formation just looks like the uniform neural tissue filling the gaps between identifiable structures, forming a central core throughout the brainstem tegmentum (Figure 11-6). In fact, however, the reticular formation is organized—but on a microscopic level, as discussed briefly later in this chapter.

The Rostral Medulla Contains the Inferior Olivary Nucleus and Part of the Fourth Ventricle

The rostral (open) medulla, as defined here, extends from the obex to the rostral wall of the lateral recess, where the inferior cerebellar peduncle turns posteriorly to enter the cerebellum. The rostral medulla (Figure 11-9) no longer looks much like the spinal cord, partly because the walls of the embryonic neural tube have been pushed outward to form the floor of the fourth ventricle (see Figure 2-9).

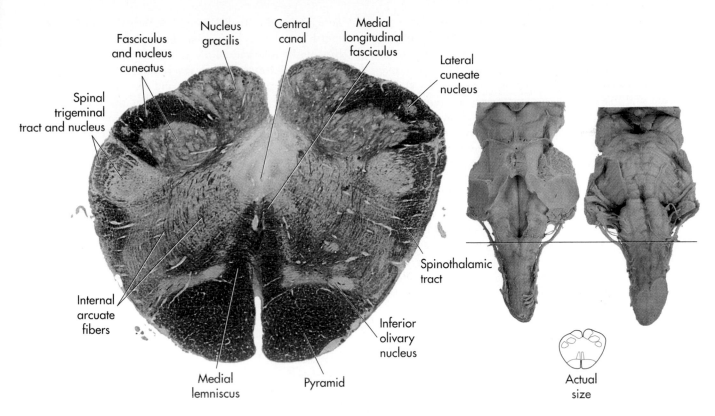

FIGURE 11-8
Caudal medulla just caudal to the obex. A small portion of the inferior olivary nucleus, a landmark of the rostral medulla, extends into the caudal medulla.

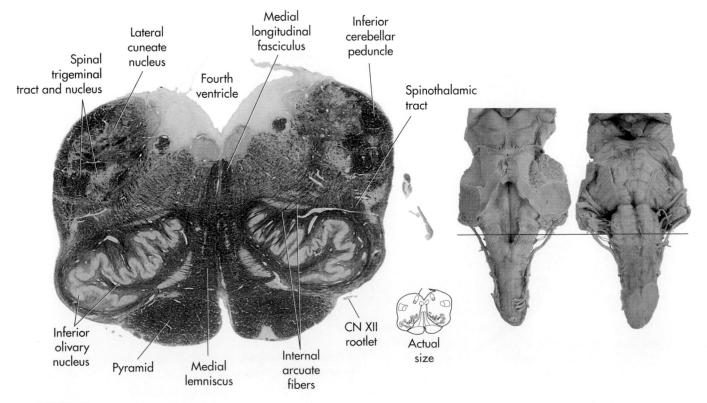

FIGURE 11-9
Rostral medulla just rostral to the obex.

The caudal boundary (the obex) is approximately co-incident with the caudal edge of the **inferior olivary nucleus,** a prominent structure that is responsible for the surface swelling called the **olive** (Figure 11-3). The inferior cerebellar peduncle is located dorsolaterally at these levels and grows progressively larger as it continues rostrally. Fibers can be seen leaving the medially facing mouth (or **hilus**) of the inferior olivary nucleus, arching across the midline, and joining the contralateral inferior cerebellar peduncle. These too are internal arcuate fibers. More and more are added at progressively more rostral levels of the medulla, increasing the size of the peduncle.

Medial to the inferior olivary nucleus is the medial lemniscus, which still has the shape of a flattened band with a dorsal-ventral axis. Anterior to the medial lemniscus is the pyramid. Fascicles of the hypoglossal (XII) nerve (Figures 11-3 and 11-9) emerge lateral to the pyramid in the groove between it and the inferior olivary nucleus.

Posterior to the medial lemniscus, near the floor of the fourth ventricle, is a small but distinctive bundle of fibers that can be followed all the way to the midbrain. This is the **medial longitudinal fasciculus (MLF),** which is involved in vestibular functions and eye movements.

The spinothalamic tract remains in the ventrolateral portion of the tegmentum, just above the inferior olivary nucleus, as does the anterior spinocerebellar tract. The posterior spinocerebellar tract moves posteriorly and joins the inferior cerebellar peduncle.

The Caudal Pons Is Attached to the Cerebellum by the Middle Cerebellar Peduncle

The caudal pons (Figure 11-10), as defined here, extends from the rostral wall of the lateral recess of the fourth ventricle to the rostral edge of the middle cerebellar pedun-

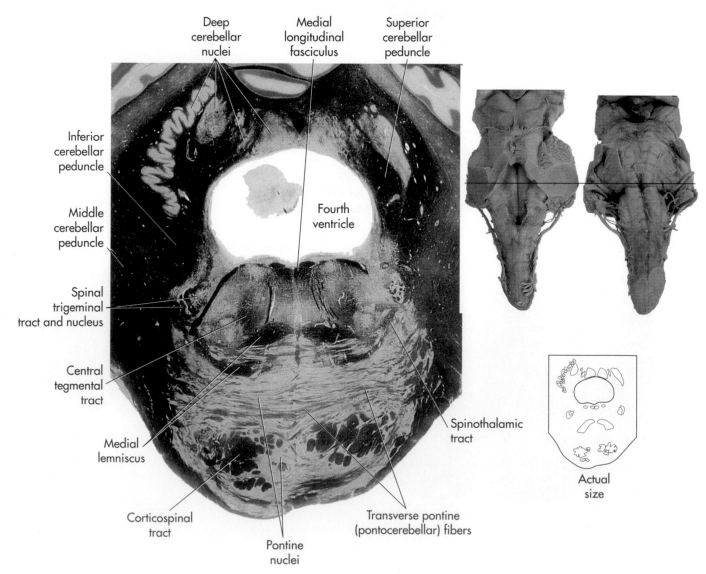

FIGURE 11-10
Caudal pons at the level of the facial colliculus.

cle. In the caudal pons the inferior olivary nucleus ends, and the inferior cerebellar peduncle bends posteriorly and enters the cerebellum (see Figure 20-6, *A*). The MLF is in the same relative position as it was previously, adjacent to the midline and the floor of the fourth ventricle.

As the inferior olivary nucleus ends, the medial lemniscus assumes a more oval shape, as though it had previously been held upright against the midline. Now the homunculus is allowed to slump down slowly into a horizontal position, with its feet directed laterally.

The pyramidal tract becomes dispersed in the basal pons, which contains bundles of longitudinally oriented fibers, bundles of transversely oriented fibers, and **pontine nuclei** scattered among these bundles. Some of the longitudinally oriented fibers are those of the pyramidal tract. Most of the others are **corticopontine fibers;** these fibers originate in many areas of the cerebral cortex and terminate in ipsilateral pontine nuclei (see Figure 20-18). Fibers arising in the pontine nuclei cross the midline and form the massive middle cerebellar peduncle (brachium pontis).

The spinothalamic tract and the anterior spinocerebellar tract remain in the ventrolateral portion of the tegmen-

tum. Spinoreticular fibers related to the spinothalamic system terminate medial to the direct spinothalamic fibers in the reticular formation throughout the brainstem, as do collaterals of direct spinothalamic fibers.

The Superior Cerebellar Peduncle Joins the Brainstem in the Rostral Pons

The rostral pons extends from the rostral edge of the middle cerebellar peduncle to the beginning of the cerebral aqueduct. The trigeminal nerve (V) is attached to the brainstem at a midpontine level (Figure 11-11), and the trochlear nerve (IV) emerges at the pons-midbrain junction (Figure 11-3). The MLF is visible throughout the rostral pons, as is the basal pons (Figure 11-12). The fourth ventricle narrows as the cerebral aqueduct is approached, and the superior cerebellar peduncle (brachium conjunctivum) becomes apparent in the wall of the ventricle. This is the major outflow from the cerebellum, projecting to the thalamus and to other structures (see Figure 20-20).

The medial lemniscus gradually takes on a more flattened profile, now with a medial-lateral axis, and assumes a trans-

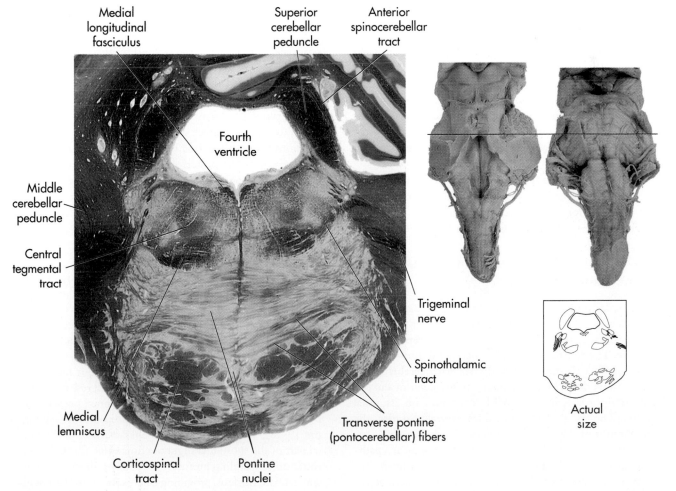

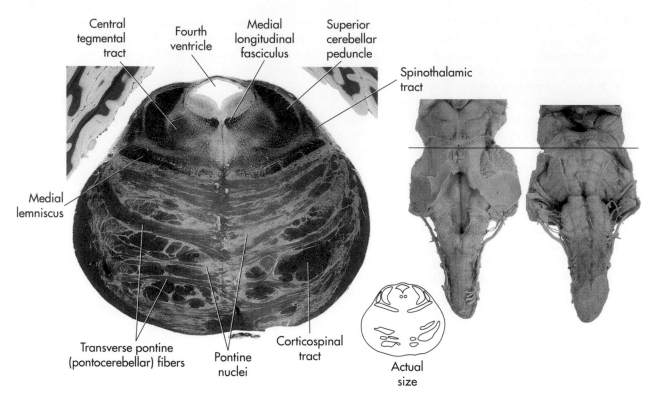

Central tegmental tract Fourth ventricle Medial longitudinal fasciculus Superior cerebellar peduncle

Spinothalamic tract

Medial lemniscus

Transverse pontine (pontocerebellar) fibers Pontine nuclei Corticospinal tract

Actual size

FIGURE 11-12
Rostral pons near the pons–midbrain junction.

verse orientation at the junction between the basal pons and the pontine tegmentum. As in the caudal pons, the homunculus is arranged so that its feet are most lateral. As the medial lemniscus moves laterally, it approaches the spinothalamic tract; from here through the midbrain, the two are adjacent. The corticospinal tract travels through the rostral pons as a series of longitudinally oriented bundles of fibers, accompanied by more numerous corticopontine bundles.

The anterior spinocerebellar tract moves posteriorly onto the surface of the superior cerebellar peduncle (Figure 11-11). From here it turns caudally and enters the cerebellum, traveling "backwards" along the peduncle.

The Superior Cerebellar Peduncles Decussate in the Caudal Midbrain

The caudal midbrain is essentially the part that contains the inferior colliculi. It extends from the point of emergence of the trochlear nerve to the **intercollicular groove.** The fourth ventricle has narrowed into the cerebral aqueduct (Figure 11-13), the superior cerebellar peduncles sink deeper into the midbrain tegmentum and begin to decussate, and the MLF continues on its usual course. The basal pons protrudes rostrally under the tegmentum of the caudal midbrain. The inferior colliculus, a major component of the ascending auditory pathway discussed in Chapter 14, is (literally) a prominent nuclear mass. Ventromedial to it, encircling the aqueduct, is a particularly pale-staining region of gray matter called, ap-

propriately enough, the **periaqueductal gray.** The periaqueductal gray is part of an important descending pain-control system discussed a little later in this chapter.

The medial lemniscus is still a flattened band of fibers, now curving a bit dorsally, and the spinothalamic tract is dorsal to it at the surface of the brainstem. These adjacent locations position the two tracts to terminate in overlapping regions of the posterior thalamus. In the caudal midbrain, the basal pons gives way to a **cerebral peduncle** on each side, through which the corticospinal tract travels.

The Rostral Midbrain Contains the Red Nucleus and Substantia Nigra

The rostral midbrain contains the superior colliculi (Figure 11-14). It extends from the intercollicular groove to the **posterior commissure.** At this level the MLF is ending, decussation of the superior cerebellar peduncles is complete, and in their place the large **red nucleus** becomes visible on each side. Some fibers from the contralateral half of the cerebellum end here, but most continue on to the thalamus. Anterior to the red nucleus is the **substantia nigra** (pale in myelin-stained preparations but dark in unstained or cell-stained preparations; see Figure 19-18). The pigmented cells characteristic of the dorsal part of the substantia nigra use dopamine for their neurotransmitter, ending profusely on neurons of the putamen and caudate nucleus, providing one example of the chemically coded systems discussed later in this chapter. Mal-

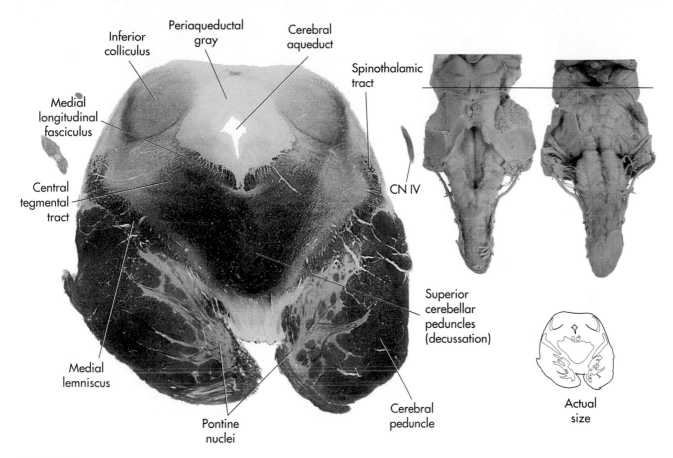

FIGURE 11-13

Caudal midbrain at the level of the inferior colliculus.

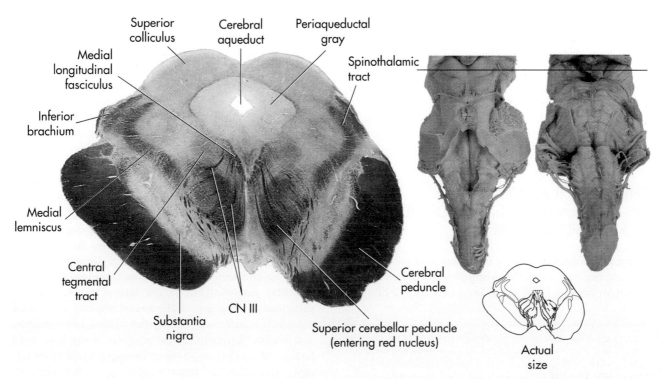

FIGURE 11-14

Rostral midbrain at the level of the superior colliculus.

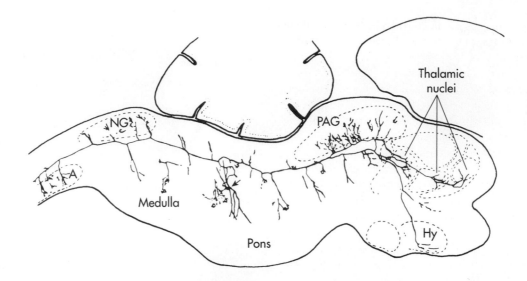

FIGURE 11-15
Drawing of a Golgi-stained parasagittal section from the brain of a young rat. The single stained cell (arrow) in the pontine reticular formation has an axon that bifurcates and ends in wide areas of the CNS, reaching the anterior horn of the spinal cord (A), nucleus gracilis (NG), periaqueductal gray (PAG), hypothalamus (Hy), thalamus, and multiple levels of the reticular formation. If one cell has projections this extensive, imagine the complexity of the reticular formation as a whole. [From Scheibel ME, Scheibel AB: Structural substrates for integrative patterns in the brainstem reticular core. In Jasper HH et al, editors: *Reticular formation of the brain*, Boston, 1958, Little, Brown & Co.)

function of this particular dopamine system results in Parkinson's disease (see Chapter 19).

Ventral to the substantia nigra is a massive bundle of fibers commonly referred to as the **cerebral peduncle.*** This bundle consists principally of descending corticopontine and corticospinal fibers. The oculomotor nerve (III) emerges into the space between the cerebral peduncles (the interpeduncular fossa). Several parts of the diencephalon (the pineal gland and some thalamic nuclei) hang back over and alongside the rostral midbrain.

At rostral midbrain levels, the medial lemniscus and the spinothalamic tract form a continuous curved band of fibers. Spinomesencephalic fibers (sometimes referred to as the **spinotectal tract**) that have accompanied the spinothalamic tract through the brainstem terminate in the periaqueductal gray, adjacent regions of the reticular formation, and certain portions of the superior colliculus.

THE RETICULAR CORE OF THE BRAINSTEM IS INVOLVED IN MULTIPLE FUNCTIONS

The reticular formation is an apparently (but not actually) diffusely organized area that forms the central core of the brainstem (Figure 11-6). It has been likened to a hot dog

surrounded by a bun of discrete tracts and nuclei.* The reason it appears to be diffusely organized is twofold.

1. Its pattern of connectivity is characterized by a great deal of convergence and divergence, so that a single cell may respond to several different sensory modalities or to stimuli applied practically anywhere on the body.

2. Although it is involved in several quite separate functions, the areas involved in these functions overlap considerably, almost as though several nuclei had been scrambled together and dispersed along the brainstem, while their constituent cells retained their original connections.

At most levels of the brainstem, the reticular formation can be divided into three longitudinal zones arranged in a medial-to-lateral sequence. The **raphe nuclei** (from the Greek word *rhaphe* meaning "seam," referring to the midline seam of the brainstem) are thin plates of cells in and immediately adjacent to the sagittal plane. The **medial zone,** alongside the midline raphe nuclei, contains a mixture of large and small neurons and is the source of most of the long ascending and descending projections from the reticular formation. Some of the neurons in the medial zone of the rostral medullary reticular formation are so large that this area is referred to as the **gigantocellular reticular nucleus.** Finally, the **lateral zone,** which is particularly prominent in the rostral medulla and caudal pons, is primarily concerned with cranial nerve reflexes and visceral functions. These reticular zones have been further subdivided into a series of nuclei based on histology, connections, and function, although such nuclei can-

---

*Strictly speaking, the term *cerebral peduncle* refers to all of the midbrain anterior to the superior colliculus, and the term **basis pedunculi** (or **crus cerebri**) refers to the massive fiber bundle in the anterior part of the peduncle. However, in common usage, *basis pedunculi* and *cerebral peduncle* have become more or less interchangeable, both referring to the fiber bundle.

---

*Earnest, Michael: Personal communication, 1974.

not be distinguished easily in conventionally prepared sections such as those shown in this chapter.

Many reticular neurons have extensive and complex axonal projections. They may innervate multiple levels of the spinal cord, send numerous collaterals to the brainstem and diencephalon, or even have bifurcating axons that give rise to both ascending and descending connections (Figure 11-15). Some reticular neurons with distinctive neurochemical characteristics (described later in this chapter) project directly to the cerebral cortex; these are an exception to the usual pattern of transmission through the thalamus on the way to the cortex. Reticular neurons also have large fields of dendrites, sometimes spreading out in a plane perpendicular to the long axis of the brainstem, that allow them to receive synaptic inputs from ascending sensory pathways, descending cortical axons, and a variety of other sources. A look at the processes of a single reticular cell in a single plane (Figure 11-15) should demonstrate why the reticular formation has been a tremendously difficult area of the brain to study; still, some progress has been made.

The Reticular Formation Participates in the Control of Movement Through Connections With Both the Spinal Cord and the Cerebellum

Two **reticulospinal tracts** arise from the medial zone of the pontine and the rostral medullary reticular formation. Fibers from the pons descend with the ipsilateral MLF and travel through the anterior funiculus in the spinal cord (Figure 11-16). Those from the medulla descend bilaterally, but mostly uncrossed, in the anterior part of the lateral funiculus. The reticulospinal tracts are a major alternate route (to the pyramidal tract) by which spinal motor neurons are controlled, both influencing motor neurons directly and regulating the sensitivity of spinal reflex arcs. For example, tonic inhibition of flexor reflexes originates in the reticular formation, with the result that only noxious stimuli can normally evoke such a reflex. Reticulospinal neurons receive projections from many areas, including the basal ganglia, vestibular nuclei, and substantia nigra. Input from widespread areas of the cerebral cortex, particularly the somatosensory and motor cortex, is especially important. Most of these descending fibers travel to their reticular terminations in the **central tegmental tract** (Figures 11-10 through 11-14). This is a complex tract containing afferents to, and efferents from, the reticular formation and descending projections from the red nucleus to the inferior olivary nucleus.

The reticulospinal tracts also carry descending motor commands generated within the reticular formation itself. Just as the spinal cord contains the basic neural machinery for simple (and some not-so-simple) reflexes, so the reticular formation contains the neural machinery for considerably more complex patterns of movement. A cat whose

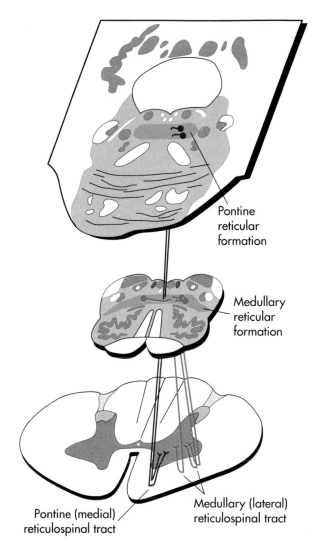

Pontine
reticular
formation

Medullary
reticular
formation

Pontine (medial)
reticulospinal tract

Medullary (lateral)
reticulospinal tract

FIGURE 11-16
Medullary and pontine reticulospinal tracts.

brainstem has been surgically separated from its diencephalon can, after a recovery period, walk and run spontaneously, properly right itself if tipped over, and assume a variety of complex postures. There have been cases of human infants born without cerebral hemispheres who were nevertheless capable of apparently normal yawning, stretching, suckling, and orienting behavior. It is assumed that their reticular formations formed the basis for these activities.

Finally, certain reticular regions are closely related to the cerebellum and its motor control functions. A fairly discrete collection of cells in the medullary reticular formation called the **lateral reticular nucleus** can often be resolved adjacent to the spinothalamic tract in conventionally prepared brainstem sections. It extends rostrally to midolivary levels and caudally into the caudal medulla, receiving direct spinoreticular fibers and collaterals of spinothalamic fibers and projecting to the cerebellum. It also receives input from the red nucleus, so it is more than a straightforward somatosensory relay to the cerebellum. Collections of reticular neurons near the medullary midline, collectively called the **paramedian reticular nucleus,** also project to the cerebellum. Afferents to the paramedian nucleus arise in the cerebellum and in other locations, including the cerebral cortex. Finally, the **reticular tegmental nucleus,** located between the medial lemnisci in the rostral pons, receives inputs from the cerebral cortex and other sites and projects to the cerebellum.

The Reticular Formation Modulates the Transmission of Information in Pain Pathways

It is a common experience that we are able to focus attention on particular sensory modalities at some times and to ignore them (with varying success) at others. This is particularly evident in the case of noxious stimuli, which are experienced as more painful or less painful depending on an individual's circumstances. The classic example of this is soldiers wounded in battle who nevertheless continue to function and are not nearly as distressed as one would expect. The nervous system has several pain-control pathways available, and the reticular formation plays a prominent role in one of them.

Electrical stimulation (through implanted electrodes) of the periaqueductal gray of the midbrain of rats causes an analgesia so profound that major surgery can then be performed without the aid of an anesthetic. Similar stimulation of the periaqueductal gray of humans can ameliorate intractable pain. This effect is a selective stimulation-produced analgesia, diminishing pain without substantially affecting other somatosensory modalities such as touch. The periaqueductal gray receives information about the level of noxious stimulation through spinomesencephalic fibers; it also receives inputs from the hypothalamus and several cortical areas, presumably related to behavioral state and relevant to decisions about whether to activate this pain-control system. Efferents from the periaqueductal gray then project to one of the raphe nuclei (**nucleus raphe magnus**) of the rostral medulla and caudal pons, and to adjacent areas of the medullary reticular formation. These areas in turn project to superficial laminae of the posterior horn via a pathway that travels through the posterior part of the lateral funiculus (Figure 11-17), suppressing the transmission of pain information by spinothalamic neurons.

Opium and its derivatives, especially morphine, have long been used for pain control, and one way they work is by activating the periaqueductal gray–raphe nucleus pain-control system at multiple levels. Opiate receptors are found in abundance in the periaqueductal gray, nucleus raphe magnus, and superficial laminae of the posterior horn. Microinjection of opiates at any of these three sites causes analgesia, and the analgesia induced by stimulation of the periaqueductal gray is blocked by opiate antago-

nists. (Opiate receptors are also found at a number of other sites in the CNS, presumably accounting for some of the other effects of morphine and related drugs.) The endogenous ligands for opiate receptors are various opi-oid peptides, in this pathway **enkephalin** and **dynorphin.** Small enkephalin-containing inhibitory interneurons are involved in suppressing transmission by spinothalamic tract neurons (Figure 11-17), but many of the details of the pain-control circuitry described here are still unknown.

The Reticular Formation Contains Autonomic Reflex Circuitry

A great deal of visceral information reaches the reticular formation, which programs appropriate responses to environmental changes and projects to the autonomic nuclei of the brainstem and spinal cord. Centers controlling inspiration, expiration, and the normal rhythm of breathing have been identified physiologically in the medulla and pons. Other centers controlling heart rate and blood pressure have been identified in the medullary reticular formation. These are in many ways comparable to the previously mentioned pattern generators in the reticular formation for various kinds of complex movements.

The hypothalamus also gives rise to numerous fibers concerned with autonomic regulation. Many of those involved in sympathetic control traverse the brainstem near the spinothalamic tract and reach the intermediolateral cell column of the spinal cord (mostly uncrossed). The numbers and types of synapses in the pathway are not completely understood, but at least some of the fibers reach the spinal cord directly from the hypothalamus. Interruption of the descending sympathetic pathway causes ipsilateral **Horner's syndrome,** which refers to a combination of miosis (small pupil), ptosis (drooping eyelid), and enophthalmos (recession of the eyeball; this is more apparent than real). Horner's syndrome may be accompanied by flushing and lack of sweating in ipsilateral skin of the face and part of the body.

The Reticular Formation Is Involved in the Control of Arousal and Consciousness

Ascending projections from the reticular formation terminate in the thalamus, subthalamus, hypothalamus, and basal ganglia. The functions of most of these are poorly understood, but those to the thalamus seem to be particularly important. Neurons in the reticular formation of the midbrain and rostral pons collect information about multiple sensory modalities, for example, information about pain via spinoreticular fibers and project to the intralaminar nuclei of the thalamus. The intralaminar nuclei in turn project to widespread areas of the cortex, causing heightened arousal in response to sensory stimuli or attention-demanding tasks (Figure 11-18). This pathway

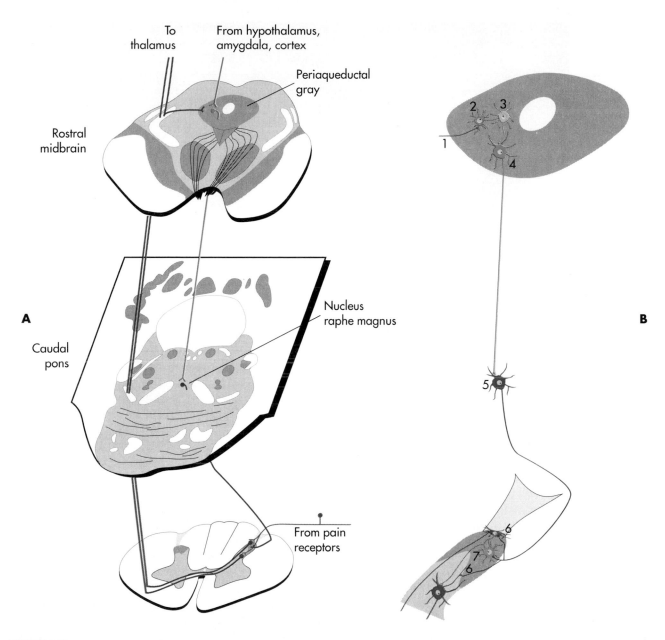

FIGURE 11-17

A, The periaqueductal gray–raphe nuclei pathway, one of several descending and ascending pain-control systems. Although the details of the neural circuitry are not completely known, the fact that microinjection of opiates into either the periaqueductal gray or the posterior horn of the spinal cord elicits analgesia suggests that elements such as those in **B** are involved. Serotonin-containing neurons of nucleus raphe magnus *(5)*, when stimulated by projection neurons of the periaqueductal gray *(4)*, inhibit spinothalamic tract neurons either directly *(6)* or by making excitatory synapses on inhibitory, enkephalin-containing interneurons *(7)* in the substantia gelatinosa. The system can be activated by spinomesencephalic and other inputs *(1)* that stimulate periaqueductal, enkephalin-containing inhibitory interneurons *(2)*. These in turn inhibit inhibitory interneurons *(3)* that ordinarily suppress this pain-control pathway.

collaborates with monoamine-containing reticular projections (described in the next section) in modulating the activity of the cerebral cortex. The reticulothalamic and monoamine projections are essential for the maintenance of a normal state of consciousness, and bilateral damage to neurons of the midbrain reticular formation and fibers passing through it results in prolonged coma. This is an astounding notion: a normal, intact cerebrum is incapable of functioning in a conscious manner by itself; sustaining input from the brainstem reticular formation is required. The portion of the reticular formation that provides this input is known as the **ascending reticular activating system** (ARAS). It is important to understand that the ARAS is defined by physiological criteria; it is not synonymous with the anatomically defined reticular formation but rather is a portion of it. Modulation of the ARAS has a basic role in the sleep-wakefulness cycle, as discussed in Chapter 22.

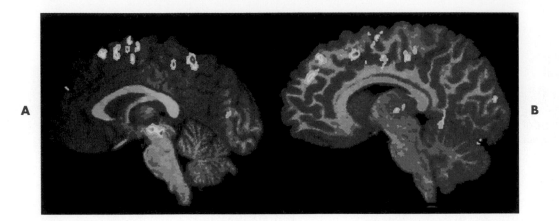

FIGURE 11-18
PET images in parasagittal planes, demonstrating increased blood flow in the midbrain reticular formation (**A**) and intralaminar nuclei of the thalamus (**B**) as a subject engages in an attention-demanding task (pressing a key as quickly as possible after a visual or somatosensory stimulus). The plane in **A** is about 2 mm from the midline, that in **B** is about 9 mm from the midline, and areas of increased blood flow are indicated in red and yellow. [From Kinomura S et al: Activation by attention of the human reticular formation and thalamic intralaminar nuclei, *Science* 271:512, 1996.]

SOME BRAINSTEM NUCLEI HAVE DISTINCTIVE NEUROCHEMICAL SIGNATURES

Most of the connections discussed thus far in this book are quite precise, obviously designed to convey a particular type of information from one part of the nervous system to another. Some neurons of the reticular formation are an exception, projecting to multiple areas in a way consistent with a general alerting function (Figure 11-15). An extreme example of such widely distributed connections is provided by brainstem neurons that contain monoamine neurotransmitters (norepinephrine, dopamine, and serotonin). Similarly configured neurons that contain acetylcholine are found primarily in the telencephalon, although some are also present in the reticular formation.

Neurons of the Locus Ceruleus Contain Norepinephrine

CNS neurons containing norepinephrine (called **noradrenergic** neurons* from the synonym **noradrenaline** for norepinephrine) are found only in the pons and medulla. Most are located in the **locus ceruleus** (Latin for "blue spot"), a collection of pigmented cells located near the floor of the fourth ventricle (Figure 11-19). The pigmented neurons contain neuromelanin, accounting for the blue-black appearance of the locus ceruleus in unstained brain tissue. The remainder of the noradrenergic neurons are located in lateral parts of the medullary reticular formation, in some nuclei associated with cranial

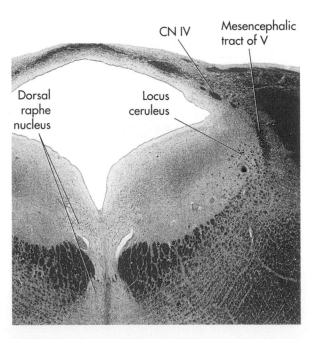

FIGURE 11-19
Section through the rostral pons showing the locus ceruleus. One of the serotonin-containing raphe nuclei can also be seen. (The mesencephalic tract of the trigeminal nerve is discussed in Chapter 12.) This figure is an enlargement of part of the section shown in Figure 11-12.

nerves (the solitary nucleus and the dorsal motor nucleus of the vagus; see Chapter 12), and in a few other sites (Figure 11-20). Collectively, these noradrenergic neurons innervate virtually the entire CNS. Ascending fibers, many of which travel through the central tegmental tract, reach the thalamus, hypothalamus, limbic forebrain structures, and the cerebral cortex. All areas of the cerebral cortex appear to receive some noradrenergic innervation, but that to somatosensory cortex is particularly dense. Descending fibers project to other parts of the brainstem and

*The relatively small number of neurons that use epinephrine as a neurotransmitter, together with noradrenergic neurons, are referred to collectively as **adrenergic** neurons.

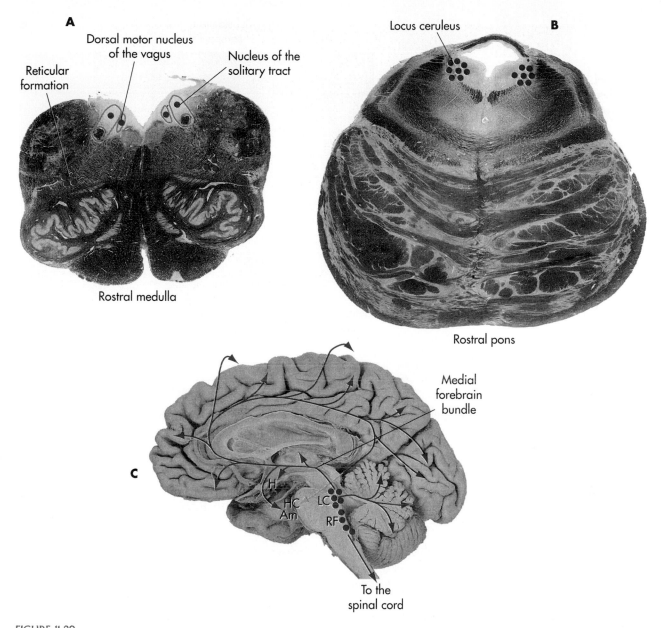

A
Reticular formation
Dorsal motor nucleus of the vagus
Nucleus of the solitary tract
Rostral medulla

B
Locus ceruleus
Rostral pons

C
Medial forebrain bundle
H
HC
Am
LC
RF
To the spinal cord

FIGURE 11-20
Locations of noradrenergic neurons in the medulla **(A)** and pons **(B)**, and a schematic indication of their widespread CNS projections **(C)**. *Am,* Amygdala; *H,* hypothalamus; *HC,* hippocampus; *LC,* locus ceruleus; *RF,* reticular formation. (Modified from Nolte J, Angevine JB Jr: *The human brain in photographs and diagrams,* St. Louis, 1995, Mosby.)

to all spinal levels, and some travel through the superior cerebellar peduncle to reach the cerebellum. Despite the diverse nature of these projections, there is some anatomical specificity in their pattern. For example, the locus ceruleus provides most of the output to the cerebral cortex, whereas the lateral reticular formation provides most of the output to the spinal cord.

As might be expected from the extensive pattern of these terminations, activation of noradrenergic neurons and pathways results in widespread effects in other areas of the CNS. Some hints about possible functions of this system are provided by the response patterns of neurons in the locus ceruleus. These cells are nearly silent electrically

during sleep, become somewhat active during wakefulness, and are most active in situations that are startling or call for watchfulness. Hence the locus ceruleus and other noradrenergic neurons may play a role in maintaining attention and vigilance.

Neurons of the Substantia Nigra and Ventral Tegmental Area Contain Dopamine

Most **dopaminergic** neurons are mesencephalic, located in dorsal portions of the substantia nigra (the **compact part** of the substantia nigra) and in the medially adjacent **ventral tegmental area** (Figure 11-21), and project ros-

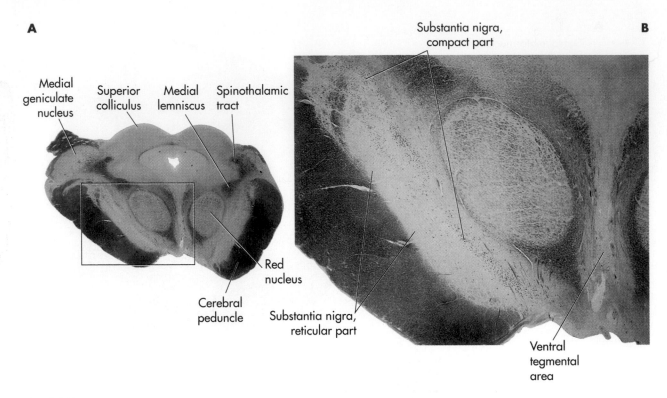

A

Medial geniculate nucleus

Superior colliculus

Medial lemniscus

Spinothalamic tract

Red nucleus

Cerebral peduncle

Substantia nigra, reticular part

B

Substantia nigra, compact part

Ventral tegmental area

FIGURE 11-21
Section through the rostral midbrain showing the locations of dopaminergic neurons. The area outlined in **A** is enlarged in **B**.

trally in three partially overlapping streams of fibers. The first, a massive projection from the substantia nigra to the caudate nucleus and putamen, is discussed in Chapter 19. These fibers are referred to as **nigrostriatal,** because the caudate and putamen together constitute the **striatum,** or as **mesostriatal,** reflecting their origin in the midbrain. **Mesolimbic** and **mesocortical** fibers originate primarily in the ventral tegmental area and travel to a variety of forebrain destinations, including the cerebral cortex and limbic structures such as the amygdala (Figure 11-22). As in the case of the locus ceruleus, the cortical projections are extensive but nonuniform; in this instance motor and limbic areas are emphasized. The nigrostriatal projection and the mesocortical projection to motor cortex are both consistent with the idea that the dopaminergic system is involved in the initiation of movement, and that its disruption is instrumental in the movement deficits seen in Parkinson's disease. However, the extensive dopaminergic projections to limbic structures and other cortical areas suggest that this system is also involved in motivation and cognition. Consistent with this, there is evidence that imbalances in the dopamine system may play a role in certain forms of mental illness. Interestingly, many drugs of abuse directly or indirectly cause dopamine release in limbic forebrain structures, suggesting that the mesolimbic projection may be involved in whatever it is that makes some things pleasurable.

Additional dopaminergic neurons are found in the retina (see Figure 1-6, *D*), the olfactory bulb, and the hy-

pothalamus (where dopamine participates in the control of prolactin secretion).

Neurons of the Raphe Nuclei Contain Serotonin

Serotonergic neurons are found at most levels of the brainstem, concentrated in the **raphe nuclei** (Figure 11-19). Like the noradrenergic neurons described above, they innervate virtually all parts of the CNS (Figure 11-23); the serotonergic innervation is in fact even more extensive and profuse. Projections from the rostral raphe nuclei reach the forebrain, providing a cortical innervation that is most dense in sensory and limbic areas. Caudal raphe nuclei provide most of the projection to the brainstem and spinal cord.

The firing rates of both serotonergic and noradrenergic neurons fluctuate with sleep and wakefulness, suggesting that both play a role in modulating the general activity levels of the CNS. However, there are differences in the cortical layers and areas emphasized by these two transmitters, indicating that their roles are at least somewhat different. For example, it has been proposed that the serotonin system is more important for determining the overall level of arousal, and the norepinephrine system more important for phasic changes in level of attention. In addition, it seems clear that the serotonin system has at least one other important role, as part of the descending pain-control system described earlier.

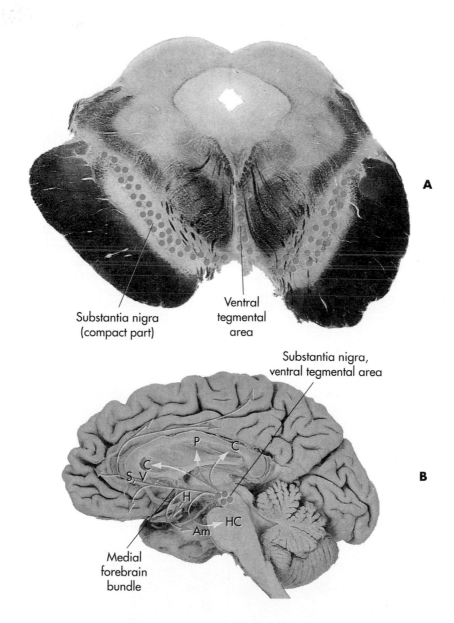

FIGURE II-22
Locations of dopaminergic neurons in the midbrain (**A**), and a schematic indication of their widespread CNS projections (**B**). *Am*, Amygdala; *C*, caudate nucleus; *H*, hypothalamus; *HC*, hippocampus; *P*, putamen; *S*, septal nuclei (see Chapter 23); *V*, ventral striatum (the area of fusion between the putamen and caudate nucleus; see Chapter 19). [Modified from Nolte J, Angevine JB Jr: *The human brain in photographs and diagrams*, St. Louis, 1995, Mosby.]

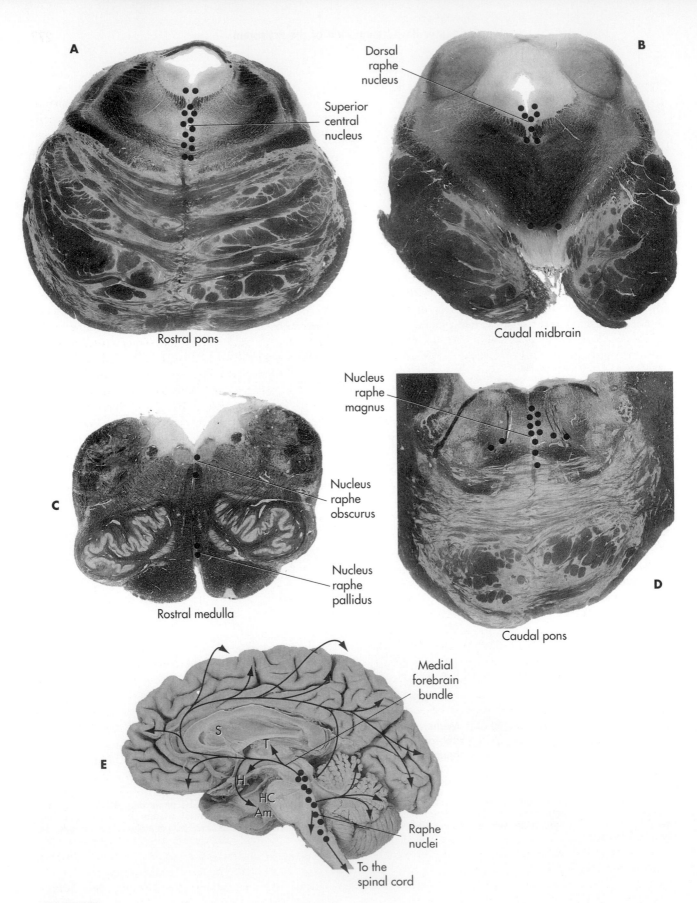

A Rostral pons

Superior central nucleus

B Dorsal raphe nucleus

Caudal midbrain

C Rostral medulla

Nucleus raphe obscurus

Nucleus raphe pallidus

D Caudal pons

Nucleus raphe magnus

E Medial forebrain bundle

S

T

H

HC

Am

Raphe nuclei

To the spinal cord

FIGURE 11-23

Locations of serotonergic neurons and nuclei in the brainstem **(A-D)**, and a schematic indication of their widespread CNS projections **(E)**. Names of individual raphe nuclei are indicated for reference purposes. *Am,* Amygdala; *H,* hypothalamus; *HC,* hippocampus; *T,* thalamus; *S,* septal nuclei (see Chapter 23). [Modified from Nolte J, Angevine JB Jr: *The human brain in photographs and diagrams,* St. Louis, 1995, Mosby.]

Neurons of the Basal Forebrain Contain Acetylcholine

Acetylcholine plays an especially prominent role in the PNS as the transmitter released by alpha and gamma motor neurons, preganglionic autonomic neurons, and postganglionic parasympathetic neurons. It was thought for a time that acetylcholine might be similarly widespread in the CNS, but we know now that its distribution there is more restricted. **Cholinergic** neurons (Figure 11-24) are concentrated in parts of the reticular formation and in the **basal forebrain,** and are also found in the caudate nucleus and putamen, where they account for some large interneurons. The physiological action of acetylcholine is different at central and peripheral endings. As discussed in Chapter 8, nicotinic receptors mediate brief and spatially precise excitatory events in the periphery, whereas muscarinic receptors in the CNS have slower and more diffuse effects.

Basal forebrain is a loosely used term that refers approximately to the area at and near the inferior surface of the telencephalon, between the hypothalamus and the orbital cortex. The basal forebrain reaches the surface of the brain in the anterior perforated substance and extends superiorly into limbic regions near the rostrum of the corpus callosum. The connections and function of this portion of the telencephalon have been notoriously difficult to unravel; partly as a result of this difficulty, the area beneath the anterior commissure has long been referred to somewhat oxymoronically as the **substantia innominata** (literally, the "stuff with no name"). Recent work has demonstrated that a prominent component of the substantia innominata, the **nucleus basalis** (or **basal nucleus of Meynert**) is the major collection of forebrain cholinergic neurons. Neurons of the nucleus basalis, together with some from related nearby nuclei, blanket the cerebral cortex, hippocampal formation, and amygdala with cholinergic endings. These widespread projections suggest that the nucleus basalis is also involved in general regulation of the level of forebrain activity, and there is considerable evidence that these cholinergic neurons (together with cholinergic projections from the reticular formation to the thalamus) play a critical role in the sleep-wakefulness cycle.

Neurochemical Imbalances May Be Involved in Certain Forms of Mental Illness

Many of the drugs used to treat neurological and psychiatric disorders are known to have effects at synapses involving particular neurotransmitters. For example, phenothiazine derivatives (e.g., Thorazine) and related drugs used as antipsychotics in the treatment of schizophrenia block dopamine receptors, suggesting that the mesolimbic and mesocortical projections may be involved in this disorder. Similarly, drugs commonly used as antidepressants

enhance the effectiveness of transmission at norepinephrine and serotonin synapses. Observations like these, coupled with our recent ability to map out the cells, axons, and synaptic endings that use a neurotransmitter, have raised hopes of being able to better understand these disorders and to develop more effective drugs for their treatment. Although there are few disorders in which malfunction of a single neurotransmitter system accounts for all findings, there is a growing number of examples in which one transmitter plays a major role.

Alzheimer's disease is a devastating and sadly common illness characterized by extensive neuronal atrophy (particularly in the cerebral cortex and hippocampus), memory loss, personality change, and, ultimately, profound dementia. There is a dramatic loss of acetylcholine in the cortex and hippocampus of Alzheimer's patients, and a corresponding loss of neurons in the basal nucleus and nearby cholinergic cell groups. This finding led to the hope that an acetylcholine replacement therapy (analogous to the use of L-dopa in Parkinson's disease; see Chapter 19) might help Alzheimer's patients. Unfortunately such attempts have been unsuccessful, and it has since been found that multiple transmitter systems are affected in Alzheimer's disease. For example, cortical somatostatin-containing interneurons are affected as much as cholinergic neurons. Although acetylcholine deficiency is still thought to be important in the pathogenesis of Alzheimer's disease, the fundamental basis of the neuronal degeneration is still unknown.

THE BRAINSTEM IS SUPPLIED BY THE VERTEBRAL-BASILAR SYSTEM

The brainstem depends almost entirely on the vertebral-basilar system for its blood supply (Figures 11-25 and 11-26). The caudal medulla has a supply much like that of the spinal cord. Anterior and lateral portions are supplied by the anterior spinal artery and/or small branches of the vertebral artery. Posterior portions are supplied by the posterior spinal artery and/or small branches of the posterior inferior cerebellar artery (PICA). The rostral medulla receives a varying supply. Anterior and medial structures, such as the pyramid and the medial lemniscus, depend on some combination of vertebral branches and the anterior spinal artery. Lateral and posterior structures, such as the spinothalamic tract and the inferior cerebellar peduncle, depend on the branches of the vertebral artery, PICA, and, to a lesser extent, the posterior spinal artery.

Most of the pons is supplied by unnamed **paramedian** and **circumferential** branches of the basilar artery. The anterior inferior cerebellar artery (AICA) and the superior cerebellar artery contribute branches to the middle and superior cerebellar peduncles and to dorsal and lateral portions of the pontine tegmentum.

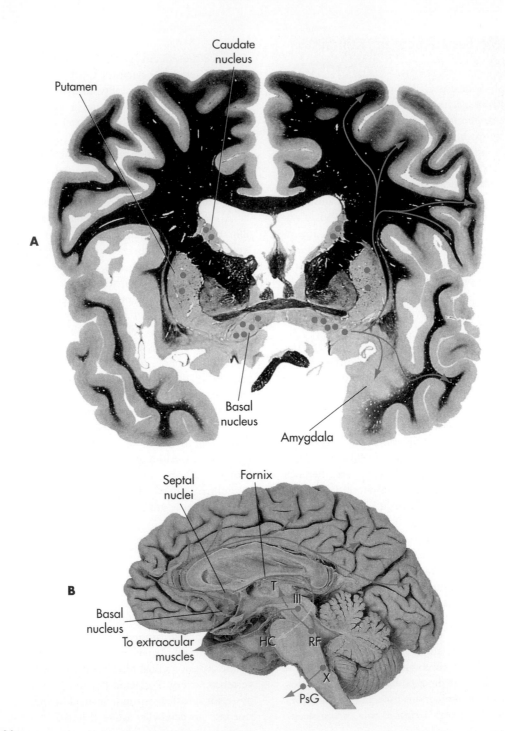

FIGURE 11-24
Locations of cholinergic neurons in the forebrain (**A**), and a schematic indication of their widespread CNS projections and of the locations of other cholinergic neurons (**B**). *III*, Oculomotor nucleus (representing motor neurons in general); *X*, dorsal motor nucleus of the vagus (representing preganglionic autonomic neurons in general); *HC*, hippocampus; *PsG*, parasympathetic ganglion cell; *RF*, reticular formation; *T*, thalamus. (Modified from Nolte J, Angevine JB Jr: *The human brain in photographs and diagrams*, St. Louis, 1995, Mosby.)

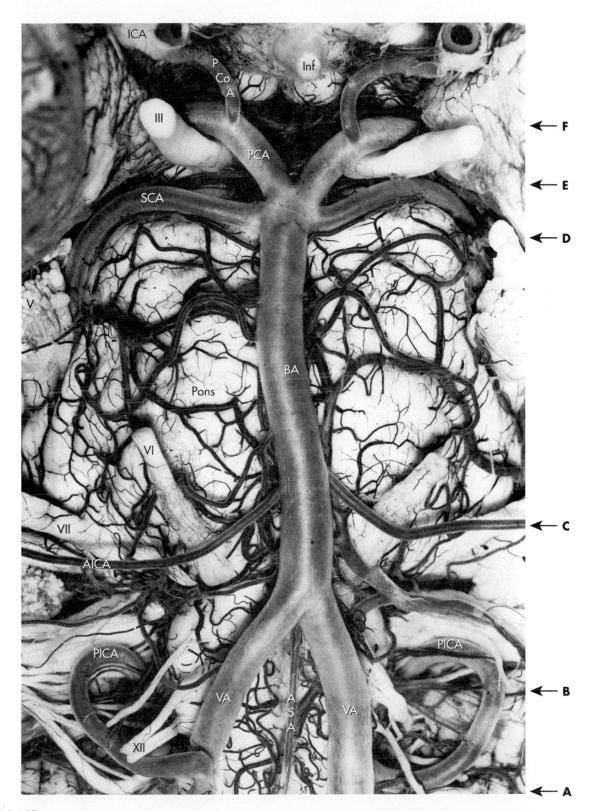

FIGURE 11-25

The anterior surface of a human brainstem, after its arteries had been injected with a mixture of gelatin and India ink. Arteries of the vertebral-basilar systems can be seen clearly, overlying the various divisions of the brainstem. By considering where different vessels and branches leave the vertebral-basilar system, one can imagine the vascular supply of each brainstem level; the arrows on the right indicate the levels for which vascular territories are charted in Figure 11-26. *AICA,* Anterior inferior cerebellar artery; *ASA,* anterior spinal artery; *BA,* basilar artery; *ICA,* internal carotid artery; *Inf,* infundibular stalk; *PCA,* posterior cerebral artery; *PCoA,* posterior communicating artery; *PICA,* posterior inferior cerebellar artery; *SCA,* superior cerebellar artery; *VA,* vertebral artery; cranial nerves indicated by Roman numerals. [From Duvernoy HM: *Human brainstem vessels,* New York, 1978, Springer-Verlag.]

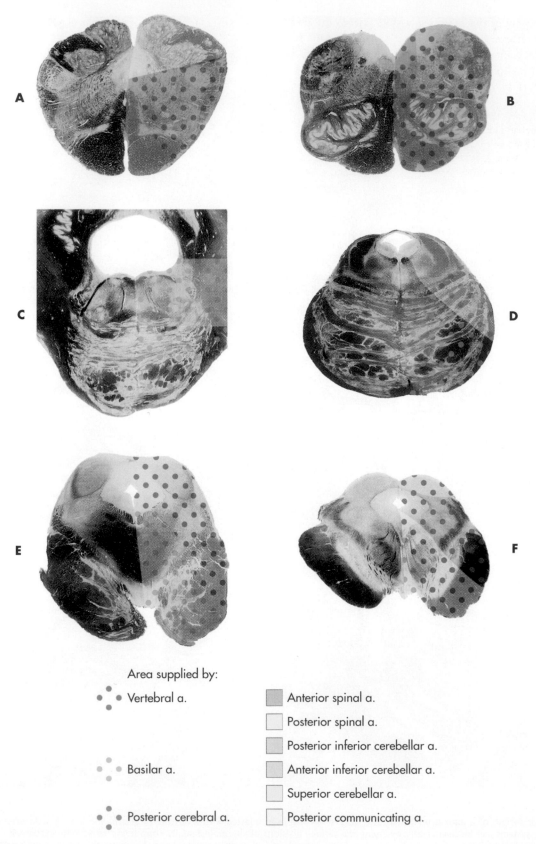

Area supplied by:

Vertebral a.

Basilar a.

Posterior cerebral a.

Anterior spinal a.

Posterior spinal a.

Posterior inferior cerebellar a.

Anterior inferior cerebellar a.

Superior cerebellar a.

Posterior communicating a.

FIGURE II-26

Approximate arterial supply of various brainstem levels; corresponding levels of an intact brainstem are indicated in Figure II-25. Although there is variability from one individual to another, different vertebral-basilar branches, or combinations of these branches, typically supply wedge-shaped areas at each brainstem level. The zones of damage in brainstem strokes frequently correspond to these wedge-shaped areas.

The supply of the midbrain is chiefly from the posterior cerebral artery, with some contribution from the basilar and superior cerebellar arteries caudally. In addition, the anterior choroidal artery and the posterior communicating artery may send branches to the cerebral peduncle.

SUGGESTED READINGS

Baker KG et al: The human locus coeruleus complex: an immunohistochemical and three-dimensional reconstruction study, *Exp Brain Res* 77:257, 1989.

Bandler R, Shipley MT: Columnar organization in the midbrain periaqueductal gray: modules for emotional expression? *Trends Neurosci* 17:379, 1994.

Beecher HR: Pain in men wounded in battle, *Ann Surg* 123:96, 1946. *A fascinating paper showing that wounds we would expect to be terribly painful may not be, depending in part on the circumstances surrounding the incurrence of the injury.*

Behbehani MM: Functional characteristics of the midbrain periaqueductal gray, *Prog Neurobiol* 46:575, 1995. *It's involved in a lot more than modulation of pain pathways.*

Brozoski TJ et al: Cognitive deficit caused by regional depletion of dopamine in prefrontal cortex of rhesus monkey, *Science* 205:929, 1979.

Caplan LR: *Posterior circulation disease: clinical findings, diagnosis, and management,* Cambridge, 1996, Blackwell Science, Inc. *An extensive review of the vascular anatomy and symptoms involved in brainstem strokes.*

Carlsson A, Falck B, Hillarp N-Å: Cellular localization of brain monoamines, *Acta Physiol Scand* 56 (Suppl):196, 1962. *The first systematic mapping of monoamine-containing neurons in the CNS, using a histochemical technique that makes them fluorescent.*

Cohen MI: Neurogenesis of respiratory rhythm in the mammal, *Physiol Rev* 59:1105, 1979.

Cooper JR, Bloom FE, Roth RH: *The biochemical basis of neuropharmacology,* ed 7, New York, 1996, Oxford University Press.

Duvernoy HM: *Human brainstem vessels,* New York, 1978, Springer-Verlag.

Duvernoy HM: *The human brain stem and cerebellum: surface structure, vascularization, and three-dimensional sectional anatomy with magnetic resonance imaging,* Vienna, 1995, Springer-Verlag.

Engberg I, Lundberg A, Ryall RW: Reticulospinal inhibition of transmission in reflex pathways, *J Physiol* 194:201, 1968.

Fibiger HC: Cholinergic mechanisms in learning, memory and dementia: a review of recent evidence, *Trends Neurosci* 14:220, 1991.

Fields HL, Basbaum AI: Central nervous system mechanisms of pain modulation. In Wall PD, Melzack R: *Textbook of pain,* ed 3, Edinburgh, 1994, Churchill Livingstone.

Fillenz M: *Noradrenergic neurons,* New York, 1990, Cambridge University Press.

Foote SL, Bloom FE, Aston-Jones G: Nucleus locus ceruleus: new evidence of anatomical and physiological specificity, *Physiol Rev* 63:844, 1983.

Foote SL, Morrison JH: Extrathalamic modulation of cortical function, *Ann Rev Neurosci* 10:67, 1987. *A review of direct cortical input from fiber systems containing norepinephrine, dopamine, serotonin, and acetylcholine.*

Gaspar P et al: Catecholamine innervation of the human cerebral cortex as revealed by comparative immunohistochem-

istry of tyrosine hydroxylase and dopamine-beta-hydroxylase, *J Comp Neurol* 279:249, 1989.

Grant SJ, Aston-Jones G, Redmond DE Jr: Responses of primate locus coeruleus neurons to simple and complex sensory stimuli, *Brain Res Bull* 21:401, 1988.

Hobson JA, Brazier MAB, editors: *The reticular formation revisited: specifying function for a nonspecific system,* International Brain Research Organization monograph series, vol 6, New York, 1980, Raven Press.

Hosobuchi Y, Adams JE, Linchitz R: Pain relief by electrical stimulation of the central gray matter in humans and its reversal by naloxone, *Science* 197:183, 1977. *Evidence that the analgesia caused by stimulation of the periaqueductal gray has properties in common with morphine analgesia.*

Huang X-F, Paxinos G: Human intermediate reticular zone: a cyto- and chemoarchitectonic study, *J Comp Neurol* 360:571, 1995. *The anatomy of the part of the reticular formation most closely related to autonomic control mechanisms.*

Hughes J: Isolation of an endogenous compound from the brain with pharmacological properties similar to morphine, *Brain Res* 88:295, 1975. *The original discovery of enkephalins.*

Jacobs BL: Single-unit activity of locus ceruleus neurons in behaving animals, *Prog Neurobiol* 27:183, 1986.

Jacobs BL, Azmitia EC: Structure and function of the brain serotonin system, *Physiol Rev* 72:165, 1992.

Kinomura S et al: Activation by attention of the human reticular formation and thalamic intralaminar nuclei, *Science* 271:512, 1996.

Koob GF: Drugs of abuse: anatomy, pharmacology and function of reward pathways, *Trends Pharmacol Sci* 13:177, 1992.

Kuhar MJ, Pert CB, Snyder SH: Regional distribution of opiate receptor binding in monkey and human brain, *Nature* 245:447, 1973.

Le Moal M, Simon H: Mesocorticolimbic dopaminergic network: functional and regulatory roles, *Physiol Rev* 71:155, 1991.

Loewy AD, Araujo JC, Kerr FWL: Pupillodilator pathways in the brain stem of the cat: anatomical and electrophysiological identification of a central autonomic pathway, *Brain Res* 60:65, 1973.

Luiten PGM et al: The course of paraventricular hypothalamic efferents to autonomic structures in medulla and spinal cord, *Brain Res* 329:374, 1985.

Mayer DJ, Price DD, Rafii A: Antagonism of acupuncture analgesia in man by the narcotic antagonist naloxone, *Brain Res* 121:368, 1977. *A provocative paper providing initial evidence that acupuncture works by somehow causing the release of enkephalins.*

Mesulam M-M, Geula C: Nucleus basalis (Ch 4) and cortical cholinergic innervation in the human brain: observations based on the distribution of acetylcholinesterase and choline acetyltransferase, *J Comp Neurol* 275:216, 1988.

Mesulam M-M et al: Human reticular formation: cholinergic neurons of the pedunculopontine and laterodorsal tegmental nuclei and some cytochemical comparisons to forebrain cholinergic neurons, *J Comp Neurol* 281:611, 1989.

Mitani A et al: Descending projections from the gigantocellular tegmental field in the cat: cells of origin and their brainstem and spinal cord trajectories, *J Comp Neurol* 268:546, 1988.

Newman DB, Ginsberg CY: Brainstem reticular nuclei that project to the thalamus in rats: a retrograde tracer study, *Brain Behav Evol* 44:1, 1994.

Nieuwenhuys R: *Chemoarchitecture of the brain,* Berlin, 1985, Springer-Verlag.

Nygren L-G, Olson L: A new major projection from locus coeruleus: the main source of noradrenergic nerve terminals in the ventral and dorsal columns of the spinal cord, *Brain Res* 132:85, 1977.

Olszewski J, Baxter D: *Cytoarchitecture of the human brainstem,* Philadelphia, 1954, JB Lippincott.

Paxinos G: *The human nervous system,* San Diego, 1990, Academic Press.

Paxinos G, Huang X-F: *Atlas of the human brainstem,* San Diego, 1995, Academic Press, Inc.

Pearson J et al: Human brainstem catecholamine neuronal anatomy as indicated by immunocytochemistry with antibodies to tyrosine hydroxylase, *Neurosci* 8:3, 1983.

Peterson BW: The reticulospinal system and its role in the control of movement. In Barnes CD, editor: *Brainstem control of spinal cord function,* Orlando, Fla, 1984, Academic Press.

Reynolds DV: Surgery in the rat during electrical analgesia induced by focal brain stimulation, *Science* 164:444, 1969. *The original demonstration of stimulation-induced analgesia.*

Saper CB et al: Direct hypothalamo-autonomic connections, *Brain Res* 117:305, 1976.

Saper CB, Chelimsky TC: A cytoarchitectonic and histochemical study of nucleus basalis and associated cell groups in the normal human brain, *Neurosci* 13:1023, 1984.

Savoiardo M et al: The vascular territories in the cerebellum and brainstem: CT and MR study, *AJNR* 8:199, 1987.

Schwartz J-C et al: Histaminergic transmission in the mammalian brain, *Physiol Rev* 71:1, 1991. *One more amine neurotransmitter, this one prominent in hypothalamic neurons.*

Steriade M, McCarley RW: *Brainstem control of wakefulness and sleep,* New York, 1990, Plenum Press. *A recent, extensive review of the structure, connections, and electrophysiology of the reticular formation.*

Torack RM, Morris JC: The association of ventral tegmental area histopathology with adult dementia, *Arch Neurol* 45:497, 1988.

Tracey DJ, Stone J, Paxinos G, editors: Neurotransmitters in the human brain. In *Advances in behavioral biology,* vol 43, New York, 1995, Plenum Press.

Whitehouse PJ et al: Alzheimer's disease and senile dementia: loss of neurons in the basal forebrain, *Science* 215:1237, 1982.

Willis WD, Haber LH, Martin RF: Inhibition of spinothalamic tract cells and interneurons by brain stem stimulation in the monkey, *J Neurophysiol* 40:968, 1977.

Willner P, Scheel-Kruger J: *The mesolimbic dopamine system: from motivation to action,* New York, 1991, John Wiley and Sons.

Woolf NJ: Cholinergic systems in mammalian brain and spinal cord, *Prog Neurobiol* 37:475, 1991.

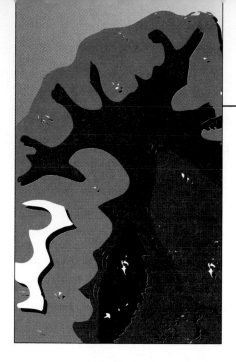

CRANIAL NERVES AND THEIR NUCLEI

The caudal medulla looks somewhat similar to the spinal cord, but this similarity seems to disappear at more rostral levels of the brainstem. One of the complicating factors is the arrangement of the tracts and nuclei associated with cranial nerves III to XII. These tracts and nuclei appear discouragingly intricate on first inspection, but there is a common way of systematizing the cranial nerves so that their central connections make sense. This involves categorizing the tracts and nuclei according to the kinds of afferent and efferent fibers contained within each nerve (often referred to as the **functional components** of each nerve).

CRANIAL NERVE NUCLEI HAVE A GENERALLY PREDICTABLE ARRANGEMENT

Spinal nerves contain sensory and motor fibers. Some of each kind are related to visceral structures and some to somatic structures. A given spinal nerve fiber can therefore be placed in one of the following four categories:

1. **Somatic sensory** fibers are related to receptors for pain, temperature, and mechanical stimuli in somatic structures such as skin, muscles, and joints.

2. **Visceral sensory** fibers are related to receptors in visceral structures such as the walls of blood vessels or of the digestive tract.

3. **Visceral motor** fibers are preganglionic autonomic axons.

4. **Somatic motor** fibers innervate skeletal muscle (i.e., they are the axons of alpha and gamma motor neurons).

By and large the cell bodies on which spinal afferents synapse and the cell bodies of spinal efferent fibers are located in portions of the spinal gray matter predictable from its embryological development (Figure 12-1, A). The sulcus limitans separates the alar plate (which develops into the posterior horn) from the basal plate (which develops into the anterior horn). Within both the alar and the basal plates, cells concerned with visceral function tend to be located nearer the sulcus limitans. This is shown most clearly in the adult by the location of the cell bodies of visceral motor fibers in the intermediolateral cell column. Thus for each of the four spinal axon categories there is a corresponding column of cells in the spinal gray matter. The somatic sensory and motor columns extend the length of the cord; the visceral sensory and motor columns are found at spinal levels T1 to L2 or L3 and S2 to S4.

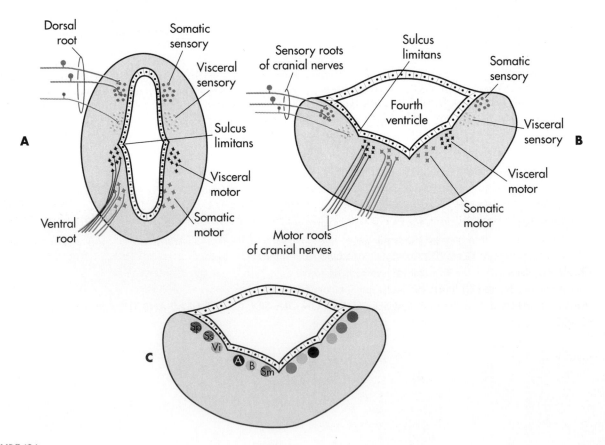

FIGURE 12-1

Arrangement of cranial nerve nuclei in the brainstem. **A,** Arrangement of the general afferent and efferent cell columns in the embryonic spinal cord. **B,** Movement of these columns to the floor of the fourth ventricle in the embryonic rhombencephalon. **C,** Further subdivision of these cell columns, showing the "ideal" locations of the cranial nerve nuclei, corresponding to the six functional categories of cranial nerve fibers. A, Preganglionic autonomic (visceral motor); B, branchial motor; Sm, somatic motor; Ss, somatic sensory; Sp, special sensory; Vi, visceral sensory.

The Sulcus Limitans Intervenes Between Motor and Sensory Nuclei of Cranial Nerves

Axons from all four of the categories found in spinal nerves are also found in various cranial nerves, where they subserve the same functions for the head. However, some cranial nerves contain axons from additional categories, reflecting specialized structures and functions associated with the head. Thus there are **special sensory** fibers that, in the case of the cranial nerves attached to the brainstem, are related to the special senses of hearing and equilibrium.★ In addition, motor axons in certain cranial nerves innervate striated muscles with a special embryological origin, referred to as the **branchiomeric muscles.** Structures that develop into the gill arches (or branchial arches) in fish develop instead into various structures in and near the head and neck in humans and other mammals. Branchiomeric muscles (notably the muscles of the larynx, pharynx, jaw, and face) are associated with these branchial arch structures. Functionally and histologically, branchiomeric muscles are identical to ordinary skeletal muscle, but the motor neurons for branchiomeric muscles have a distinctive location in the brainstem, different from that of ordinary somatic motor neurons. In recognition of their special development and location they are classified as a separate category, here called **branchial motor**

neurons.★ Hence there are six different categories of nerve fibers in the cranial nerves attached to the brainstem (Table 12-1).

As in the case of the spinal cord, the locations of the cell bodies where cranial nerve afferents terminate or cranial nerve efferents originate can be predicted, to some extent, from the embryology of the brainstem. The walls of the neural tube spread apart in the medulla and pons to form the floor of the fourth ventricle (see Figure 2-9). The sulcus limitans runs longitudinally along the floor of the adult ventricle (see Figure 11-3, *A*), still separating sensory alar plate derivatives (now lateral) from motor basal plate derivatives (now medial) (Figure 12-1, *B*). As in the case of the spinal cord, cells concerned with visceral function tend to be located nearer the sulcus limitans.

Ideally the cell columns subserving the special components of the cranial nerves would be located adjacent to those for the corresponding general components, as indicated in Figure 12-1, *C*. The actual arrangement in the adult brainstem is not quite as simple as in this idealized diagram, for two principal reasons. First, the cell columns of the brainstem are not continuous as are those of the spinal cord; rather, they are interrupted and form a series of nuclei so that all components may not be present in a given transverse plane (Figure 12-2, *A;* see also Figure 15-2). Second, in a few instances, portions of a cell column migrate away from their expected locations

---

★The cranial nerve fibers conveying information from taste buds are often considered special afferents as well—**special visceral afferents**—but, as discussed in this and the next chapter, they have connections similar in many ways to those of other visceral afferents. Hence in this account all visceral afferents are treated as one category.

★Because branchiomeric muscles tend to be concentrated around the mouth at a junction between visceral and somatic areas, the motor fibers that innervate them are often referred to as **special visceral efferent** fibers. This classification is somewhat confusing (particularly because the sensory fibers from these muscles are called *somatic afferent fibers*), but it is a tradition of long standing.

Table 12-1   Categories of Nerve Fibers in Cranial Nerves of the Brainstem★

	Structures innervated	Principal nerve(s)†
SENSORY TYPE		
Somatic	Skin, muscles, joints of head	V
Visceral	Cranial, thoracic, abdominal viscera	X
	Taste buds	VII, IX
Special	Inner ear	VIII
MOTOR TYPE		
Somatic	Extraocular muscles, tongue muscles	III, IV, VI, XII
Visceral	Parasympathetic ganglia for cranial, thoracic, abdominal smooth muscle and glands	X
Branchial	Muscles of jaw, face, larynx, and pharynx	V, VII, X
	Middle ear muscles	V, VII
	Sternocleidomastoid, trapezius	XI

★Does not include the efferents in cranial nerve VIII (described in Chapter 14) that innervate the receptor cells of the inner ear, which do not fit comfortably into any of these categories.
†Smaller contributions that may nevertheless be clinically important (e.g., parasympathetics for the pupil in CN III) not included.

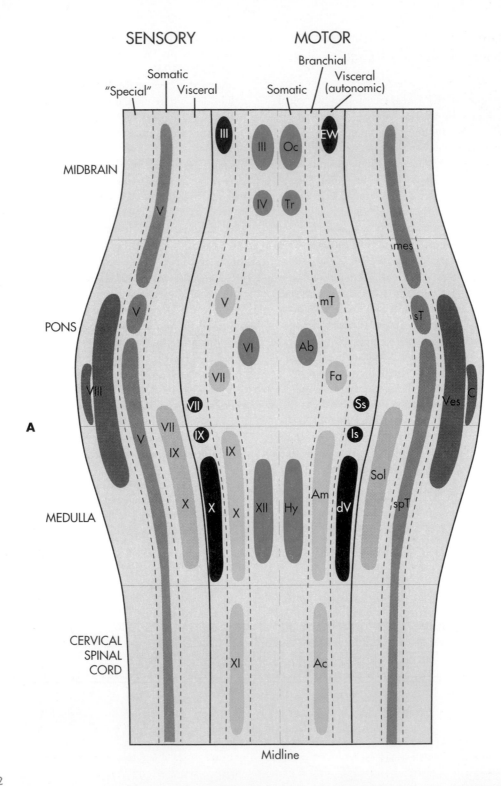

FIGURE 12-2

A, The longitudinal arrangement of functional types of cranial nerve nuclei in the brainstem, indicating their derivation from cell columns. Names of nuclei are indicated on the right and the principal cranial nerves associated with each nucleus are indicated on the left by Roman numerals. This diagram summarizes the way in which, to a first approximation, the medial-lateral location of a nucleus suggests its function, and its location along the longitudinal extent of the brainstem suggests the cranial nerve with which it is associated. *Ab,* Abducens nucleus; *Ac,* accessory nucleus; *Am,* nucleus ambiguus; *C,* cochlear nuclei; *dV,* dorsal motor nucleus of the vagus; *EW,* Edinger-Westphal nucleus (a subdivision of the oculomotor nucleus); *Fa,* facial motor nucleus; *Hy,* hypoglossal nucleus; *Is,* inferior salivatory nucleus; *mes,* mesencephalic nucleus of the trigeminal; *mT,* trigeminal motor nucleus; *Oc,* oculomotor nucleus; *Sol,* nucleus of the solitary tract; *Ss,* superior salivatory nucleus; *sT,* trigeminal main sensory nucleus; *spT,* spinal trigeminal nucleus; *Tr,* trochlear nucleus; *Ves,* vestibular nuclei. (**A** modified from Nieuwenhuys R et al: *The human central nervous system: a synopsis and atlas,* ed 3, New York, 1988, Springer-Verlag.)

Continued

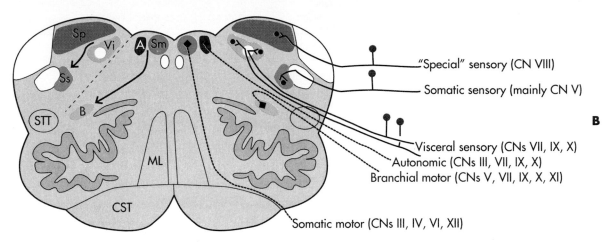

"Special" sensory (CN VIII)

Somatic sensory (mainly CN V)

B

Visceral sensory (CNs VII, IX, X)
Autonomic (CNs III, VII, IX, X)
Branchial motor (CNs V, VII IX, X, XI)

Somatic motor (CNs III, IV, VI, XII)

FIGURE 12-2, cont'd
B, Drawing of an actual section through the rostral medulla of an adult brain. On the left the nuclei corresponding to the six functional categories are indicated. On the right the cranial nerves containing each of these fiber types are indicated; cranial nerves I and II are not included nor are some minor components such as the few somatic sensory fibers in cranial nerve VII. Not all the nerves listed actually emerge at this brainstem level; they are included here for summary purposes. *A,* Preganglionic autonomic (visceral motor); *B,* branchial motor; *CST,* costicospinal tract; *ML,* medial lemniscus; *Sm,* somatic motor; *Ss,* somatic sensory; *Sp,* special sensory; *STT,* spinothalamic tract; *Vi,* visceral sensory.

(Figure 12-2, *B*). For example, most branchial motor neurons are located in the ventrolateral part of the tegmentum rather than in the floor of the ventricle adjacent to other efferent neurons. The actual locations of cranial nerve nuclei in the rostral medulla are shown in Figure 12-2, *B*; also indicated are the functional types of fibers in each of the cranial nerves of the brainstem. However, this is only meant to be a convenient summary; not all cranial nerves project to or originate from the rostral medulla.

It can be seen from Figure 12-2, *B* that no cranial nerve contains axons from all six categories. If the compositions of all the nerves are tabulated (as in Table 12-2), it becomes apparent that there are three types of cranial nerves. Some nerves (III, IV, VI, and XII) contain motor axons for ordinary skeletal muscle and little or nothing else, so they may be referred to as **somatic motor nerves.** Others (I, II, and VIII) contain special sensory fibers and little or nothing else. The remaining nerves (V, VII, IX, X, and XI) are somewhat more complex and typically contain several components; all innervate branchial arch musculature, so they are called **branchiomeric nerves.**

Presenting the cranial nerves requires dealing with a considerable amount of material, which is therefore spread out over several chapters. The remainder of this chapter is divided into two more or less distinct sections, discussing first the somatic motor nerves and then most components of the branchiomeric nerves. Chapter 13 discusses the chemical senses of taste and smell subserved by some brainstem cranial nerves and the olfactory nerve. Chapter 14 deals with the eighth nerve, the special sensory nerve subserving hearing and equilibrium. (The remaining special sensory nerve, the optic nerve, is an outgrowth of the diencephalon and is really a tract of the CNS. It is considered separately in Chapter 17.) Finally, as mentioned previously, Chapter 15 contains a series of brainstem sections with labels and summary descriptions indicating the locations and contents of cranial nerve nuclei and other important brainstem structures.

CRANIAL NERVES III, IV, VI, AND XII CONTAIN SOMATIC MOTOR FIBERS

The somatic motor nerves are the simplest of the cranial nerves because each contains fibers of only one category (except for cranial nerve III, which has a small but important complement of preganglionic parasympathetic fibers).* The nuclei of origin of all these nerves are located adjacent to the midline near the aqueduct or the floor of the fourth ventricle, as would be expected from their embryological origins.

The Oculomotor Nerve (III) Innervates Four of the Six Extraocular Muscles

Cranial nerve III supplies the levator palpebrae superioris and all the internal and external muscles of the ipsilateral eye except the lateral rectus, superior oblique, and pupillary dilator. The fibers originate in the wedge-shaped **ocu-**

*The course of proprioceptive fibers (e.g., from stretch receptors) from extraocular muscles and muscles of the tongue has long been a matter of contention. The hypoglossal nerve almost certainly contains lingual proprioceptive fibers for part or all of its course. Those from the extraocular muscles travel in cranial nerves III, IV, and VI within the orbit, then join the ophthalmic division of the trigeminal nerve for the rest of their course to the brainstem. Eye muscle proprioceptors may play a role in depth perception or its development, but the function of lingual proprioceptors is largely unknown.

Table 12-2 Contents of the Cranial Nerves

Nerve	Axon categories	CNS origin or termination	Peripheral ending
I (Olfactory)	Sp	Olfactory bulb	Originates in olfactory epithelium
II (Optic)	Sp	Lateral geniculate nucleus, superior colliculus	Originates in retinal ganglion cells
III (Oculomotor)	Sm	Oculomotor nucleus	Superior, inferior, and medial recti; inferior oblique; levator palpebrae superioris
	A	Edinger–Westphal nucleus (part of the oculomotor nucleus)	Pupillary sphincter, ciliary muscle★
IV (Trochlear)	Sm	Trochlear nucleus	Superior oblique
V (Trigeminal)	Ss	Spinal and main sensory nuclei	Skin, deep tissues, and dura mater of head
		Mesencephalic nucleus	Muscle spindles and other mechanoreceptors
	B	Trigeminal motor nucleus	Muscles of mastication, tensor tympani, and a few others
VI (Abducens)	Sm	Abducens nucleus	Lateral rectus
VII (Facial)	Ss	Spinal trigeminal nucleus	Outer ear
	Vi	Nucleus of the solitary tract	Taste buds of palate and anterior two thirds of tongue; some mucous membranes of nasopharynx
	A	Superior salivatory nucleus	Submandibular, sublingual salivary glands, nasal and palatine glands, lacrimal gland★
	B	Facial motor nucleus	Muscles of facial expression, stapedius
VIII (Vestibulocochlear)	Sp	Cochlear and vestibular nuclei	Organ of Corti, cristae of semicircular ducts, maculae of utricle and saccule
IX (Glossopharyngeal)	Ss	Spinal trigeminal nucleus	Outer ear
	Vi	Nucleus of the solitary tract	Taste buds, posterior third of tongue; carotid body and sinus
		Nucleus of the solitary tract, spinal trigeminal nucleus	Mucous membranes of posterior third of tongue, nasal and oral pharynx, middle ear
	A	Inferior salivatory nucleus	Parotid gland★
	B	Nucleus ambiguus	Pharynx (stylopharyngeus)
X (Vagus)	Ss	Spinal trigeminal nucleus	Outer ear
	Vi	Nucleus of the solitary tract	Taste buds of epiglottis
		Nucleus of the solitary tract, spinal trigeminal nucleus	Thoracic and abdominal viscera; mucous membranes of larynx and laryngeal pharynx
	A	Dorsal motor nucleus, nucleus ambiguus	Thoracic and abdominal viscera★
	B	Nucleus ambiguus	Larynx and pharynx
XI (Accessory)	B	Accessory nucleus (cervical cord)	Sternocleidomastoid, trapezius
XII (Hypoglossal)	Sm	Hypoglossal nucleus	Muscles of tongue

A, Autonomic (visceral motor); *B*, branchial motor; *Sm*, somatic motor; *Sp*, special sensory; *Ss*, somatic sensory; *Vi*, visceral sensory.
★Final destination after synapse in a parasympathetic ganglion.

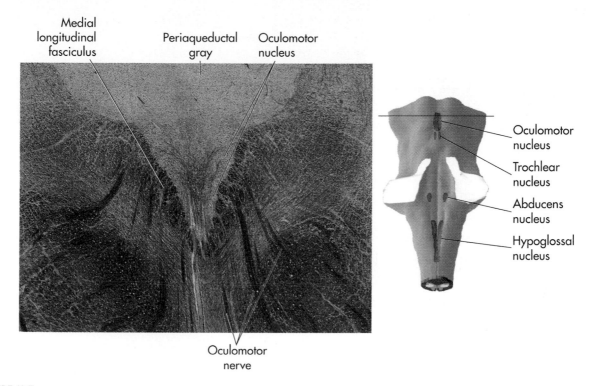

Medial longitudinal fasciculus

Periaqueductal gray

Oculomotor nucleus

Oculomotor nucleus

Trochlear nucleus

Abducens nucleus

Hypoglossal nucleus

Oculomotor nerve

FIGURE 12-3
Section through the rostral midbrain showing the oculomotor nucleus. This figure is an enlargement of part of the section shown in Figure 11-14. The oculomotor nucleus is actually a tight cluster of subnuclei, each of which innervates a different muscle.

lomotor nucleus, which is located at the ventral edge of the periaqueductal gray in the rostral midbrain (Figure 12-3). They then proceed ventrally and arch through the midbrain tegmentum in several separate bundles that join to form the nerve just as they emerge into the interpeduncular fossa.

The oculomotor nucleus actually consists of a series of longitudinal cell columns, or subnuclei. The column supplying the levator palpebrae superioris is located in the midline and innervates this muscle on both sides. The column supplying the superior rectus projects to the contralateral eye. The columns supplying the medial rectus, inferior oblique, and inferior rectus all project to the ipsilateral eye. Finally, a column including preganglionic parasympathetic neurons, which straddles the midline and is known by the tenacious eponym **Edinger-Westphal nucleus,** projects to the ipsilateral ciliary ganglion. The ciliary ganglion in turn innervates the pupillary sphincter and the ciliary muscle.

The partly crossed–partly uncrossed nature of the oculomotor nerve is a curious fact but one of limited clinical significance. This is because the oculomotor nuclei of the two sides are so close to one another that a central lesion in this vicinity is likely to damage both nuclei. On the other hand, once a given oculomotor nerve emerges from the brainstem, it supplies only ipsilateral muscles, so a lesion of the third nerve, or of fibers curving through the midbrain tegmentum on their way to the third nerve, affects only one eye. Therefore the dissociated finding of

paralysis of the superior rectus on one side and of other extraocular muscles on the opposite side is rarely encountered (although there are occasional cases of unilateral nuclear damage in which these deficits are found).

Damage to one oculomotor nerve causes a series of deficits (Figure 12-26, C). The eye ipsilateral to the lesion deviates laterally because the medial rectus is now paralyzed and the lateral rectus is unopposed. This is called **lateral strabismus,** indicating that the eyes are misaligned because one of them deviates laterally from midposition. As a result, the patient complains of **diplopia** (double vision) and is unable to move the affected eye vertically or medially. The ipsilateral levator palpebrae superioris is paralyzed, so **ptosis** occurs. In addition, the pupillary sphincter and ciliary muscle are nonfunctional. The pupil on the affected side is dilated **(mydriasis)** as a result of the now-unopposed pupillary dilator, and does not constrict in response to light★ ; the lens cannot be focused on near objects.

Along the course of the oculomotor nerve from brainstem to orbit, the preganglionic parasympathetic fibers from the Edinger-Westphal nucleus travel in a superficial location and are therefore especially susceptible to external pressures. A dilated pupil, unresponsive to light, may be the first clinically detectable sign of something pressing on the third nerve.

★Both pupils normally constrict when light is shone into either eye. This is the pupillary light reflex, which is discussed further in Chapter 17.

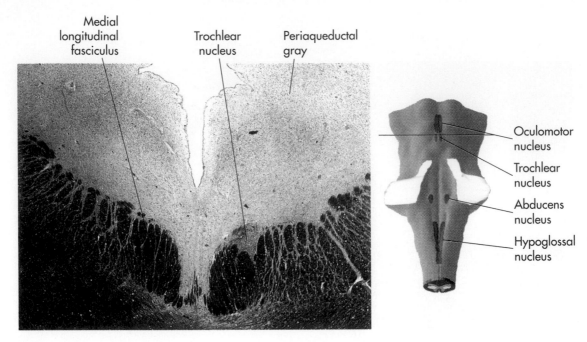

FIGURE 12-4
Section through the caudal midbrain showing the trochlear nucleus. This figure is an enlargement of part of the section shown in Figure 11-13.

Because ptosis and pupils of unequal size accompany Horner's syndrome, one might think this syndrome could be confused with third nerve damage. However, in Horner's syndrome the ptosis is on the same side as a nonfunctional pupillary dilator, hence on the same side as the *smaller* pupil. On the other hand, the ptosis caused by third nerve damage is on the same side as a nonfunctional pupillary sphincter, hence on the same side as the *larger* pupil. Also, the ptosis caused by third nerve damage is more pronounced and is usually accompanied, of course, by defective eye movements and lateral strabismus.

The Trochlear Nerve (IV) Innervates the Superior Oblique Muscle

Cranial nerve IV, the trochlear nerve, supplies the superior oblique muscle and is named for the loop of connective tissue (the *trochlea*—Latin for "pulley") through which the tendon of the superior oblique passes (see Figure 21-1). Its cell bodies of origin are located in the contralateral **trochlear nucleus.** This is a small nucleus (because it has only one small muscle to supply) located at the level of the inferior colliculus, where it indents the medial longitudinal fasciculus (MLF) (Figure 12-4). Fibers leaving the nucleus turn caudally in the periaqueductal gray, then arch dorsally to decussate and leave the brainstem at the pons-midbrain junction. The trochlear nerve is thus unique in two respects: it is the only cranial nerve attached to the dorsal surface of

the brainstem and the only one to originate entirely from a contralateral nucleus.★

Damage to the trochlear nerve results in much less drastic and noticeable deficits than does damage to either the oculomotor or the abducens nerve. The superior oblique muscle helps to move the eye downward and laterally, so attempted movement in these directions (typically in reading or in descending stairs) may cause diplopia.

The Abducens Nerve (VI) Innervates the Lateral Rectus Muscle

Cranial nerve VI, the abducens nerve, supplies the lateral rectus muscle, which abducts the eye (hence the name of the nerve). The fibers originate from the ipsilateral **abducens nucleus,** which is located in the caudal pons beneath the floor of the fourth ventricle (Figure 12-5). Medial to this nucleus are two bundles of fibers. The more medial of the two is the MLF. Between the MLF and the

---

★This probably reflects an adaptation to maintain certain relationships between head movements and eye movements. Eye movements are discussed in more detail in Chapter 21, but consider the following example. Tilting your head toward your left shoulder evokes a reflex counterrotation of your eyes. The principal muscles that need to contract in this counterrotation are the left superior oblique and superior rectus, and the right inferior oblique and inferior rectus. Because fibers to the superior oblique and superior rectus cross before leaving the brainstem, all the lower motor neurons needed for this counterrotation are located on the right side of the brainstem.

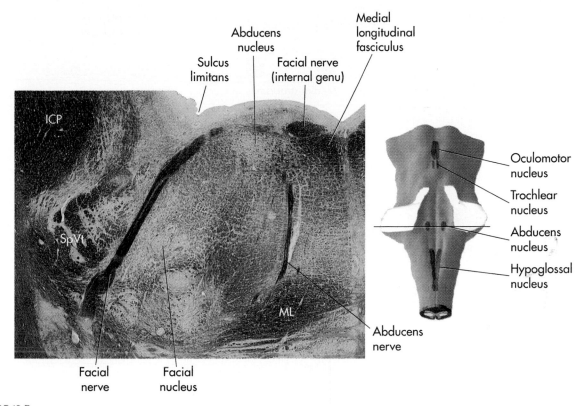

FIGURE 12-5
Section through the caudal pons showing the abducens nucleus and fibers of the facial nerve cut at different points along their course. The rounded elevation in the floor of the fourth ventricle between the midline and the sulcus limitans is the facial colliculus (see Figure 11-3, *A*). This figure is an enlargement of part of the section shown in Figure 11-10. ICP, Inferior cerebellar peduncle; *ML*, medial lemniscus; *SpVt*, spinal trigeminal tract.

abducens nucleus are motor fibers of the facial nerve, which take an unusual course in leaving the brainstem. They originate in the facial nucleus (Figures 12-5 and 12-21), which is located in the ventrolateral part of the pontine tegmentum at about the same level as the abducens nucleus. The facial fibers project dorsomedially, wrap around the abducens nucleus, and turn back ventrally to exit from the brainstem (Figure 12-6). The place where these fibers wrap around the abducens nucleus is called the **internal genu of the facial nerve.** The abducens nucleus, together with the internal genu, is responsible for the facial colliculus in the floor of the fourth ventricle (see Figure 11-3, *A*).

The abducens nucleus also contains interneurons that project to the contralateral oculomotor nucleus

Damage to the abducens nerve causes a **medial strabismus** (i.e., the affected eye deviates medially) as a result of the action of the now-unopposed medial rectus muscle. The individual may be able to move the affected eye from the adducted position to midposition (but not past it) by relaxing its medial rectus muscle (Figure 12-7, *A*). Damage to the abducens nucleus causes the same deficit but with a significant addition. In this case, not only can the

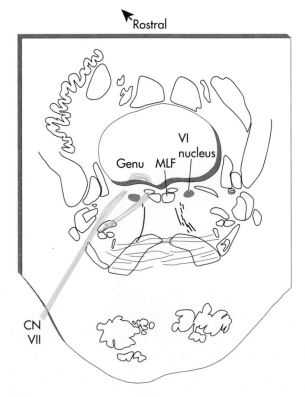

FIGURE 12-6
Course of facial nerve fibers through the internal genu.

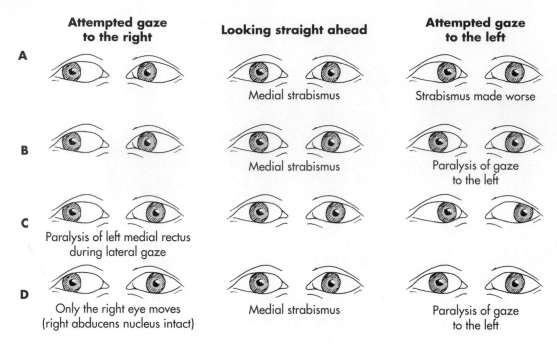

FIGURE 12-7
Deficits of horizontal gaze following damage to the abducens/MLF system as indicated in Figure 12-8. **A,** Abducens palsy resulting from damage to the left abducens nerve. **B,** Lateral gaze paralysis resulting from damage to the left abducens nucleus. **C,** Internuclear ophthalmoplegia resulting from damage to the left MLF. **D,** A "one-and-a-half" (combination of **B** and **C**) resulting from damage to the left abducens nucleus and MLF. In all of these situations, convergence, which does not depend on abducens-oculomotor interconnections, is preserved.

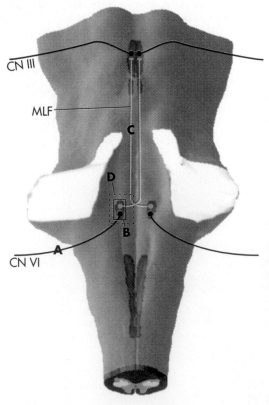

FIGURE 12-8
Connections between abducens and oculomotor nuclei involved in lateral gaze. Lesions labeled **A, B, C,** and **D** would cause the eye movement deficits indicated in Figure 12-7, A–D.

individual not move the ipsilateral eye laterally, but it is also impossible to move the contralateral eye medially when trying to look toward the side of the lesion (Figures 12-7, *B* and 12-9, *A*). This is called **lateral gaze paralysis** and occurs because the abducens nucleus contains not only lateral rectus motor neurons but also an approximately equal number of **internuclear neurons.** The axons of these internuclear neurons project through the MLF to the motor neurons controlling the contralateral medial rectus muscle (Figure 12-8).

The function of the MLF in lateral gaze may be understood by considering that both eyes normally work together. For example, when we look to one side, one lateral rectus muscle contracts, and the contralateral medial rectus muscle also contracts. The pathway that interconnects the abducens, trochlear, and oculomotor nuclei to make these sorts of movements possible is the MLF. Vertical movements and the higher centers that direct coordinated eye movements are discussed in Chapter 21, but for purely horizontal movements the crucial interconnecting fibers are those that arise from the internuclear neurons in the abducens nucleus (Figure 12-8). These cells send their axons across the midline at the level of the abducens nucleus to join the contralateral MLF. These axons then ascend to the oculomotor nucleus, where they make excitatory synapses on medial rectus motor neurons. Simultaneous firing of abducens motor neurons and internuclear neurons thus results in coordinated lateral gaze.

Damage to one MLF removes this excitatory influence from medial rectus motor neurons, so the eye ipsilateral to

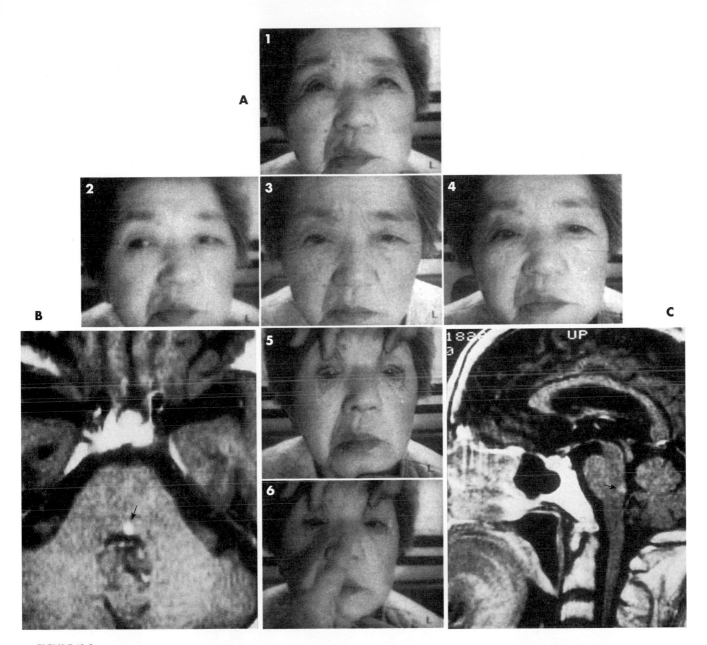

FIGURE 12-9

Horizontal gaze palsy resulting from damage to one abducens nucleus. In this case "an 80-year-old woman was admitted to the hospital with a 1-day history of dizziness, double vision, and facial asymmetry. One day prior to admission she awoke with diplopia and drooping of the left side of her mouth. She could not close her left eye or gargle with water." Examination of her eye movements (A) revealed a slight medial strabismus when she looked straight ahead (A3), preserved upward (A1) and downward (A5) gaze and convergence (A6), and inability of either eye to move past midposition during attempted gaze to the left (A4). Gaze to the right was at least partially preserved (A2) (although adduction of the left eye was reported to be incomplete, indicating some damage to the left MLF). Contrast-enhanced MRI scans in horizontal (B) and parasagittal planes (C) revealed a small ischemic infarct at precisely the location of the abducens nucleus. Flattening of the patient's left nasolabial fold and the left side of her forehead (A), together with inability to close her left eye, is consistent with damage to fibers of the facial nerve as they loop around the abducens nucleus. Her eye movements and facial strength recovered slowly over the next several months. [From Hirose G et al: Unilateral conjugate gaze palsy due to a lesion of the abducens nucleus: clinical and neuroradiological correlations, *J Clin Neuro–ophthalmol* 13:54, 1993.]

the lesion fails to move medially past midposition during attempted horizontal gaze (Figure 12-7, *C*). Because both abducens nuclei are intact, full lateral movements of both eyes are still possible. In addition, although the affected medial rectus fails to contract during attempted horizontal gaze, it still functions normally when used without the opposite lateral rectus (i.e., during convergence). This

condition has the ponderous name **internuclear ophthalmoplegia**★ (often abbreviated as *INO*).

Another eye movement disorder, clinically called a **one-and-a-half,** is rarely seen but is nevertheless instructive. It is caused by damage in the vicinity of the abducens

---

★Literally, "paralysis of the eye caused by damage between the nuclei."

nucleus and is characterized by the patient's inability to move either eye toward the side of the lesion in lateral gaze, or to move the eye on the side of the lesion in gaze toward the opposite side (Figures 12-7, *D* and 12-9). Thus of the two directions of horizontal gaze (right and left), the patient has only half of one intact. This is caused by destruction of one abducens nucleus plus destruction of fibers from the contralateral internuclear neurons as they join the MLF on the side of the lesion.

The Hypoglossal Nerve (XII) Innervates Tongue Muscles

Cranial nerve XII enters the tongue from below and supplies its intrinsic muscles and most of its extrinsic muscles (*hypoglossal* is Greek for "under the tongue"). The fibers originate in the ipsilateral **hypoglossal nucleus,** which extends from the caudal medulla through most of the rostral medulla (Figure 12-10). This nucleus is situated adjacent to the midline just beneath the floor of the fourth ventricle and forms an elevation there called the **hypoglossal trigone** or **triangle.** Hypoglossal axons proceed ventrally and emerge as a series of rootlets in the groove between the pyramid and the olive (see Figure 11-3).

Damage to the hypoglossal nerve causes weakness of one side of the tongue and, because this would be a lower motor neuron lesion, atrophy of that side of the tongue as well. This weakness is most easily demonstrated by asking the patient to protrude his or her tongue; the tongue deviates toward the side of the lesion (i.e., toward the weak side). Bilateral hypoglossal lesions may cause difficulties in both speaking and eating.

BRANCHIOMERIC NERVES CONTAIN AXONS FROM MULTIPLE CATEGORIES

The branchiomeric nerves all innervate striated muscle of branchial arch origin (i.e., they all contain branchial motor fibers). With the possible exception of cranial nerve XI, they all contain other components as well. In spite of this, each has one function with which it is principally associated: the trigeminal nerve (V) is the major general sensory nerve for the head; the facial nerve (VII) is the motor nerve for facial expression; the glossopharyngeal nerve (IX) is the most important conveyor of taste and pharyngeal sensations; the vagus nerve (X) carries the parasympathetic outflow to the thoracic and abdominal viscera; and the accessory nerve (XI) is

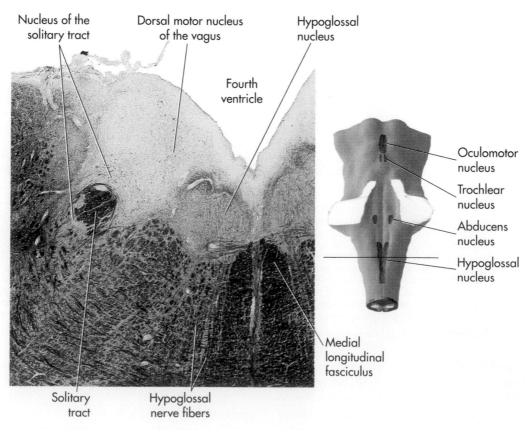

FIGURE 12-10
Section through the rostral medulla showing the hypoglossal nucleus and other cranial nerve nuclei. This figure is an enlargement of part of the section shown in Figure 11-9.

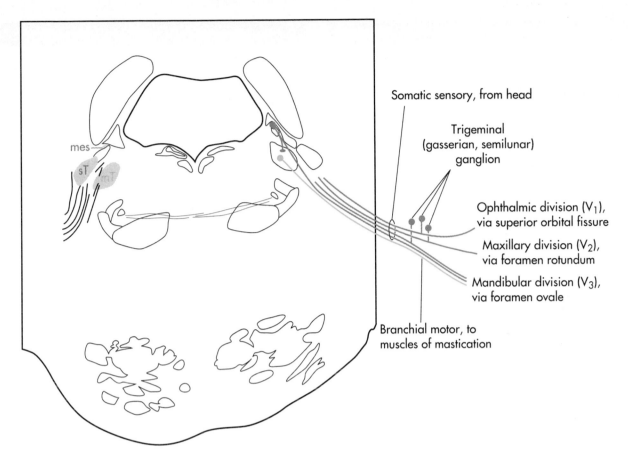

FIGURE 12-11

Fiber types in the trigeminal nerve and their peripheral destinations. *mes*, Mesencephalic nucleus of the trigeminal; *mT*, trigeminal motor nucleus; *sT*, trigeminal main sensory nucleus.

the motor nerve for the sternocleidomastoid and trapezius muscles.

The Trigeminal Nerve (V) Is the General Sensory Nerve for the Head

With respect to somatic sensory innervation, cranial nerve V (Figure 12-11) and its connections are to the head what the dorsal roots and spinal cord are to the body. That is, the trigeminal system is ultimately responsible for the transmission of tactile, proprioceptive, and pain and temperature information from the head to the cerebral cortex, cerebellum, and reticular formation. The primary afferent fibers are distributed peripherally in the three divisions for which the trigeminal nerve was named (*trigeminal* is Latin for "born three at a time"), the **ophthalmic (V₁), maxillary (V₂), and mandibular (V₃)** divisions, in the pattern shown in Figure 12-12.

Three sensory nuclei are associated with trigeminal afferents, connected in ways homologous to spinal cord systems (Table 12-3). They form a long, almost continuous column of cells that extends from the rostral midbrain to the upper cervical spinal cord. The **main sensory nucleus** (Figure 12-13) forms an enlargement in this column in the midpons, slightly lateral to the

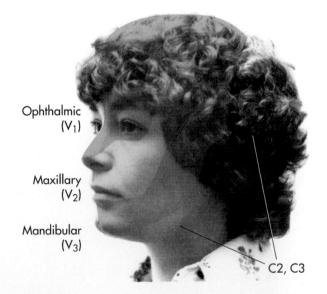

FIGURE 12-12

Peripheral distribution of the ophthalmic, maxillary, and mandibular branches of the trigeminal nerve. Not indicated is the innervation of the outer ear, at the junction between V₃ and C2/C3 territory, by cranial nerves VII, IX, and X.

Table 12-3   Homologous Structures in Spinal and Trigeminal Systems

	Spinal cord	Trigeminal system
TOUCH, PROPRIOCEPTION		
Primary afferents (cell bodies)	Dorsal root ganglia	Trigeminal ganglion, mesencephalic nucleus
Primary afferents (central processes)	Posterior columns	Entering trigeminal fibers
Second-order neurons	Posterior column nuclei	Main sensory nucleus
Ascending pathway	Medial lemniscus	Medial lemniscus, dorsal trigeminal tract
Destination	VPL	VPM
PAIN, TEMPERATURE		
Primary afferents (cell bodies)	Dorsal root ganglia	Trigeminal ganglion
Primary afferents (central processes)	Lissauer's tract	Spinal tract
Second-order neurons	Posterior horn	Spinal nucleus (caudal nucleus)
Ascending pathway	Spinothalamic tract	Spinothalamic tract
Destination	VPL	VPM
PATHWAYS TO CEREBELLUM		
Second-order neurons	Intermediate gray	Spinal nucleus (interpolar and oral nuclei)
REFLEXES		
Stretch reflex components	Dorsal root ganglion cells, anterior horn motor neurons	Mesencephalic nucleus cells, trigeminal motor neurons
Withdrawal reflex interneurons	Intermediate gray	Blink reflex: spinal nucleus (interpolar and oral nuclei)

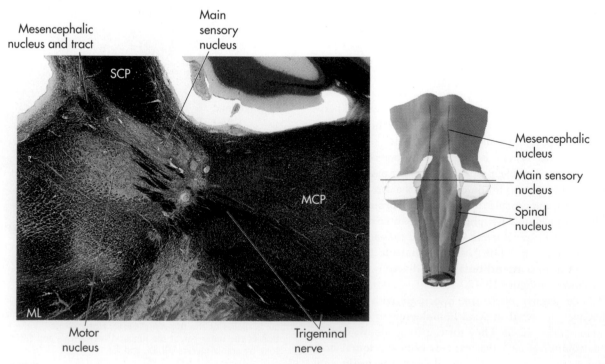

FIGURE 12-13

Section through the midpons showing the trigeminal motor and main sensory nuclei. This figure is an enlargement of the section shown in Figure 11-11. *MCP*, Middle cerebellar peduncle; *ML*, medial lemniscus; *SCP*, superior cerebellar peduncle.

trigeminal motor nucleus. The **spinal nucleus** extends caudally from this level, and the very slender **mesencephalic nucleus** extends rostrally (all the way into the midbrain, as its name implies). The main sensory and spinal nuclei are involved in processing somatosensory information. The mesencephalic nucleus, in contrast, is notable primarily as an anatomical aberration, as it is essentially a bit of the **trigeminal ganglion** located within the CNS rather than in the periphery. The cells of the mesencephalic nucleus are pseudounipolar (homologous to dorsal root ganglion cells), and their myelinated processes collect in a bundle, called the **mesencephalic trigeminal tract,** adjacent to the nucleus (Figure 12-13). The peripheral processes of these fibers are distributed through the trigeminal nerve to muscle spindles in the muscles of mastication and some mechanoreceptors of the gums, teeth, and hard palate. The central processes have connections similar to those of more conventional large-diameter trigeminal afferents with cell bodies in the trigeminal ganglion.

The main sensory nucleus receives information about touch and jaw position

The main sensory nucleus of the trigeminal nerve (Figure 12-13), located near the motor nucleus, is the trigeminal homologue of the posterior column nuclei. Thus it is primarily concerned with discriminative tactile and proprioceptive sensations, and receives large-diameter, heavily myelinated tactile afferents. Unlike the situation in the spinal cord, however, it gives rise to two ascending pathways to the thalamus. One is the expected collection of fibers that cross the midline, join the medial lemniscus adjacent to the representation of cervical dermatomes, and terminate in the **ventral posteromedial (VPM) nucleus** of the thalamus, adjacent to VPL (Figures 12-14 and 12-19). The other is an ipsilateral projection from the dorsomedial portion of the main sensory nucleus (an area that does not project through the medial lemniscus). This is called the **dorsal trigeminal tract;** it travels through the dorsomedial part of the brainstem tegmentum and ends in its own separate portion of VPM. The significance of this tract being uncrossed—indeed, its functional significance in general—is unclear. However, it does end alongside the ascending taste pathway (see Chapter 13), which is also uncrossed; hence intraoral sensations from one side of the mouth are processed in adjacent areas of the thalamus.

The spinal trigeminal nucleus receives information about pain and temperature

Primary afferent fibers reach the spinal trigeminal nucleus by turning caudally as they enter the pons and joining the **spinal trigeminal tract,** which is just lateral to the nucleus. Both nucleus and tract extend caudally to about the

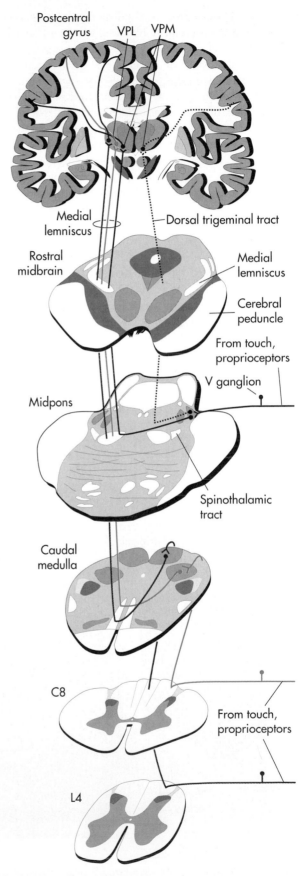

FIGURE 12-14
Ascending trigeminal pathways from the main sensory nucleus.

third cervical segment of the spinal cord (hence their name), the nucleus gradually blending with the posterior horn and the tract gradually blending with Lissauer's tract.

The spinal trigeminal nucleus has been subdivided into three regions on the basis of its histology. The most caudal part, extending from the spinal cord to the obex, is the **caudal nucleus.** The most rostral part, extending from the main sensory nucleus to about the pontomedullary junction, is the **oral nucleus.** Between these two is the **interpolar nucleus** in the rostral medulla. Differences exist among these nuclei in terms of the types of afferents that terminate at each level and the types of secondary connections made from each level. The functional correlates of these differences are incompletely understood for the oral and interpolar nuclei, but the caudal nucleus is known to be particularly important for the processing of pain and temperature information from the head.★ This fits nicely with its appearance (Figure 12-15): the caudal nucleus looks much like the posterior horn of the spinal cord, with a cap of cells resembling the substantia gelatinosa.

Small-diameter trigeminal afferents conveying pain and temperature information descend through the spinal trigeminal tract and synapse in the caudal nucleus. Sec-

ond-order neurons of the caudal nucleus, homologous to spinothalamic tract neurons, give rise to a crossed ascending pain pathway that joins the spinothalamic tract in the rostral medulla or caudal pons★ and terminates in VPM (Figure 12-16). Hence the principal difference between spinal and trigeminal somatosensory projections to the thalamus lies in the position of the second-order neurons (Figure 12-17). Trigeminal pain information also reaches the thalamus indirectly (via relays in the reticular formation) in a manner thought to be similar to spinoreticulothalamic projections. It is often assumed that this similarity holds in a functional sense as well (i.e., that trigeminal contributions to the spinothalamic tract are responsible for sharp, well-localized pain, whereas indirect trigeminal projections through the reticular formation are responsible for dull, aching pain). However, clinical evidence for such a functional similarity seems to be relatively scanty.

Different parts of the ipsilateral half of the face are represented systematically in different parts of a given spinal trigeminal nucleus (Figure 12-18). At all levels of

---

★The only exception is pain in the teeth and other intraoral structures, which is processed partly in more rostral portions of the spinal trigeminal nucleus—the interpolar nucleus and possibly the oral nucleus as well.

★The exact position of this ascending trigeminal pain and temperature projection is not known with certainty for all levels of the human brainstem. It is often said to travel with the medial lemniscus, but clinical evidence indicates it travels adjacent to the representation of cervical dermatomes in the spinothalamic tract (i.e., where it might be expected somatotopically).

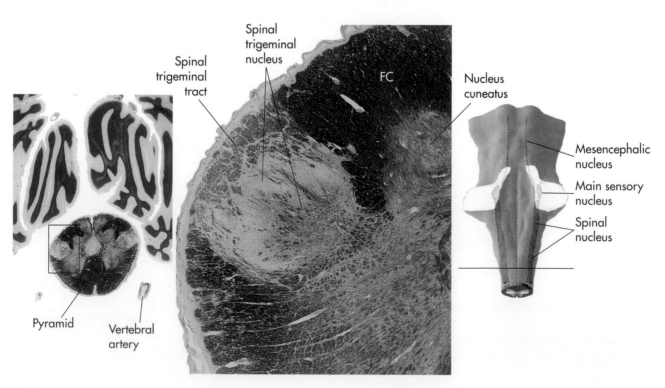

FIGURE 12-15

Section through the caudal medulla where the spinal trigeminal tract and nucleus have an appearance much like that of Lissauer's tract and the posterior horn in the spinal cord. At levels rostral to the obex (e.g., Figures 11-9 and 11-10), the spinal trigeminal tract and nucleus do not have this appearance.

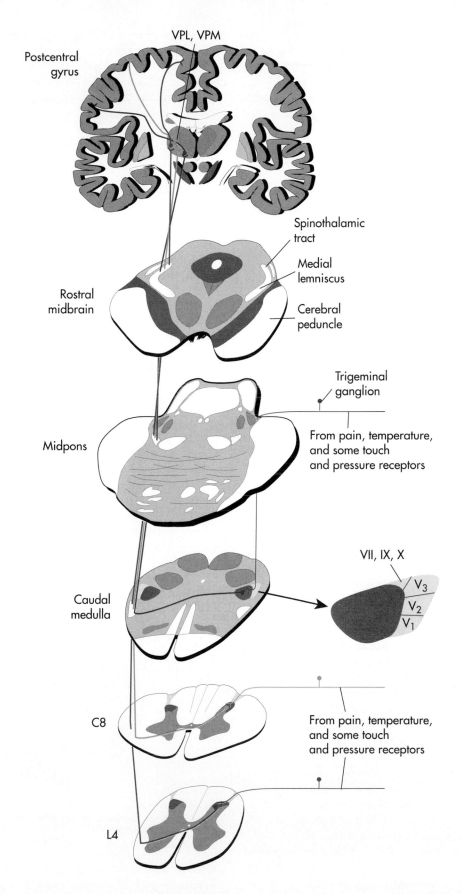

FIGURE 12-16

Ascending trigeminal pathways from the spinal nucleus. The inset near the caudal medulla section indicates the arrangement within the spinal trigeminal tract of fibers from the three subdivisions of the trigeminal nerve, as well as those from cranial nerves VII, IX, and X that innervate the outer ear.

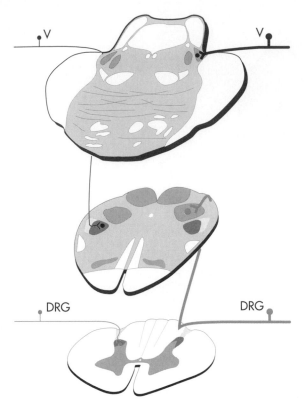

FIGURE 12-17
Locations of second-order neurons for touch/proprioceptive pathways and for pain/temperature pathways. *V*, Trigeminal ganglion; *DRG*, dorsal root ganglion.

the spinal tract mandibular division fibers are most dorsal, ophthalmic division fibers most ventral, and maxillary division fibers in between. The primary afferents retain this arrangement as they terminate in the medially adjacent spinal nucleus, so that neurons in ventral parts of the caudal nucleus, for example, respond to areas of the face in the ophthalmic distribution. Some pain fibers from all three divisions of the trigeminal nerve reach the upper cervical spinal cord, but most end at various levels in the caudal medulla. There is a somatotopic arrangement in this rostral–caudal distribution of endings as well, so that in each trigeminal division pain fibers representing areas near the center of the face end near the obex, whereas fibers representing areas toward the back of the head end in the upper cervical cord. This apparently peculiar arrangement makes sense because it allows for a smooth transition from spinal levels processing cutaneous information from the back of the head to brainstem levels processing similar cutaneous information from the face. That is, the trigeminal fibers ending in the cervical cord are thereby overlapping spinal fibers that represent adjacent areas of skin (Figure 12-12). This gives rise to a characteristic pattern of sensory loss, sometimes referred to clinically as an **onion-skin distribution,** when the spinal trigeminal tract is damaged; the farther caudally a lesion is located, the larger the area surrounding the mouth that is spared from sensory loss. Conversely, de-

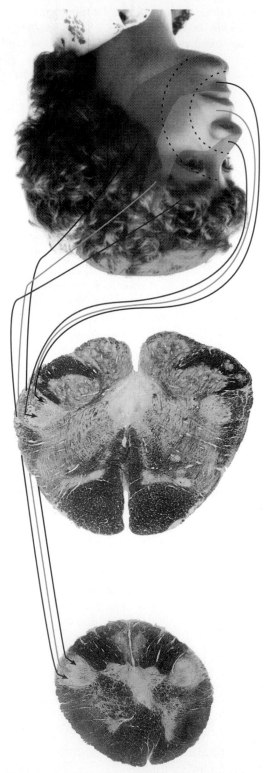

FIGURE 12-18
Somatotopic arrangement of afferents and their endings in the spinal trigeminal system.

structive lesions ascending from the spinal cord into the brainstem (such as a syrinx expanding upward from the cervical spinal cord) can cause sensory loss that starts at the back of the head and converges on the mouth (see Figure 10-30).

Abnormalities in the trigeminal system manifest themselves clinically in a number of syndromes involving head pain. **Trigeminal neuralgia** (also called **tic douloureux**) is a prominent example. This condition is characterized by brief attacks of excruciating pain, usually less than a minute in duration, in the distribution of one (or sometimes more than one) division of the trigeminal nerve. Between attacks, no significant sensory abnormalities can be found. There is frequently a "trigger zone" in the involved area, where tactile stimulation may precipitate an attack. The mechanism is unknown and could be peripheral (e.g., in the trigeminal ganglion) or central (e.g., in the spinal trigeminal nucleus). Most cases can be treated pharmacologically, but a number of surgical treatments are available if absolutely necessary. These include sectioning the involved nerve root and destroying or mechanically disturbing the trigeminal ganglion. The destructive procedures have a serious disadvantage in that the patient loses all tactile sensibility, in addition to pain, in the area. A more complex and rarely performed operation (but one that avoids this problem) is to section the spinal trigeminal tract slightly caudal to the obex, thus removing the afferent input to the caudal nucleus. Tactile sensibility remains intact, and the corneal blink reflex is usually preserved. The fact that this operation abolishes pain sensation over one entire half of the face is a major piece of evidence that the caudal part of the spinal trigeminal nucleus deals with pain and that afferents from all three divisions of the trigeminal extend at least into the caudal medulla.

Remaining parts of the spinal trigeminal nucleus (the interpolar and oral nuclei) are heavily involved in other functions homologous to somatic functions of the spinal cord. Some fibers project to the cerebellum (through the inferior cerebellar peduncle), and some fibers carrying tactile information reach the contralateral VPM. These are presumably similar to spinocerebellar fibers and to the tactile component of the spinothalamic tract, respectively. There are also reflex connections within the brainstem involving the reticular formation and other cranial nerve nuclei. One of these, the corneal reflex, is of considerable clinical importance and is discussed in conjunction with the facial nerve (Figure 12-22). The relative contributions of the three portions of the spinal nucleus to these various functions are not completely understood.

The trigeminal motor nucleus innervates muscles of mastication

There is also a branchial motor nucleus, the **trigeminal motor nucleus,** associated with cranial nerve V. It innervates the muscles of the first branchial arch, which consist mainly of the muscles of mastication. They also include the tensor tympani (discussed in Chapter 14) and several other small muscles. The nucleus is located in the midpons at the level of attachment of the trigeminal nerve to the brainstem (Figure 12-13). Fibers arising in the trigem-

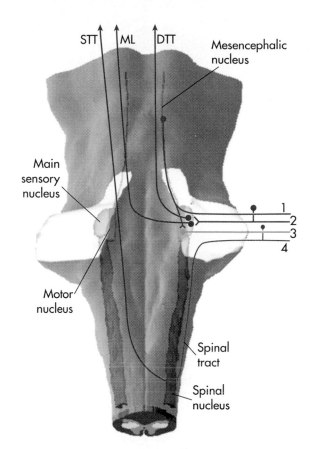

FIGURE 12-19

Major connections of the trigeminal nerve. *1,* Peripheral branches of mesencephalic trigeminal neurons, on their way to innervate things such as masseter muscle spindles; *2,* tactile afferents; *3,* axons of trigeminal motor neurons, on their way to muscles of mastication; *4,* pain/temperature afferents; *DTT,* dorsal trigeminal tract; *ML,* medial lemniscus; *STT,* spinothalamic tract.

inal motor nucleus emerge as a separate motor root and are then distributed peripherally with the mandibular division.

Trigeminal motor neurons form the efferent limb of the **jaw jerk reflex.** Stretching the masseter, typically by a downward tap on the chin, causes it to contract (bilaterally) in a reflex fashion. This is a monosynaptic reflex basically similar to spinal stretch reflexes. The afferent limb is a mesencephalic trigeminal neuron whose peripheral process innervates a masseter muscle spindle and whose central process synapses on a trigeminal motor neuron (Figure 12-19).

The Facial (VII), Glossopharyngeal (IX), and Vagus (X) Nerves All Contain Somatic and Visceral Sensory, Visceral Motor, and Branchial Motor Fibers

Cranial nerves VII, IX, and X all contain fibers belonging to several different categories (Figure 12-20), with the relative importance of each category varying. All three play a comparatively minor role in somatic sensation, whereas the vagus nerve is very important for visceral sensory

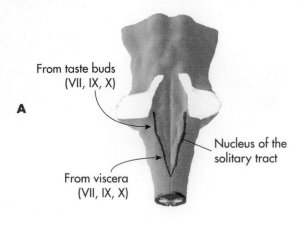

From taste buds
(VII, IX, X)

A

Nucleus of the
solitary tract

From viscera
(VII, IX, X)

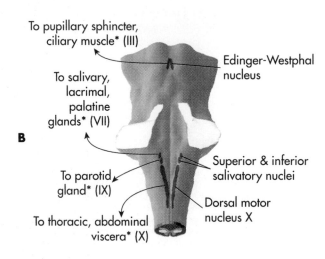

To pupillary sphincter,
ciliary muscle* (III)

Edinger-Westphal
nucleus

To salivary,
lacrimal,
palatine
glands* (VII)

B

To parotid
gland* (IX)

Superior & inferior
salivatory nuclei

To thoracic, abdominal
viscera* (X)

Dorsal motor
nucleus X

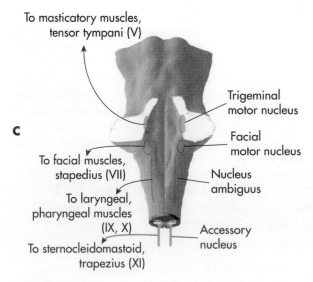

To masticatory muscles,
tensor tympani (V)

Trigeminal
motor nucleus

C

Facial
motor nucleus

To facial muscles,
stapedius (VII)

Nucleus
ambiguus

To laryngeal,
pharyngeal muscles
(IX, X)

Accessory
nucleus

To sternocleidomastoid,
trapezius (XI)

FIGURE 12-20

Visceral afferent (**A**), autonomic (**B**), and branchial motor (**C**) components of cranial nerves VII, IX, X, and XI. *, Final destination after a synapse in a parasympathetic ganglion.

and motor functions, and both the facial and vagus nerves contain large numbers of branchial motor fibers.

All three nerves contain somatic sensory fibers from the skin of the outer ear and its immediate vicinity. The exact distribution and the division of these fibers among the three nerves varies somewhat from one individual to another. These somatic afferent fibers of nerves VII, IX, and X all enter the spinal trigeminal tract and thereafter behave exactly like trigeminal afferents. They are the most dorsomedial fibers in the spinal tract and occupy a position adjacent to those from the mandibular division of nerve V (Figure 12-16).

Nerves VII, IX, and X also contain visceral sensory fibers, some from visceral structures and some from taste buds. The visceral sensory fibers from all three nerves enter a discrete bundle called the **solitary tract** (Figure 12-10). This bundle received its name as a result of its unusual appearance: it is a collection of afferents surrounded by the nucleus of termination of these afferents (the **nucleus of the solitary tract,** or the **solitary nucleus**) and looks isolated in cross sections. Both tract and nucleus extend throughout the rostral medulla and into the caudal medulla and caudal pons. The nucleus of the solitary tract is the principal visceral sensory nucleus of the brainstem. Its further connections related to autonomic control and to conveying taste information to places like the cerebral cortex are discussed in Chapters 23 and 13, respectively.

The Facial Nerve (VII) Innervates Muscles of Facial Expression

Most of the fibers of the facial nerve (Figure 12-21) are branchial motor, innervating muscles derived from the second branchial arch. These are the muscles of facial expression and the stapedius, a small muscle in the middle ear. The large nucleus of origin of all these fibers, the **facial motor nucleus,** is located in the ventrolateral tegmentum of the caudal pons (Figure 12-5). The peculiar course of these fibers, through the internal genu of the facial nerve, was described earlier (Figure 12-6).

The facial motor nucleus is involved in a reflex of considerable functional and clinical importance, the **corneal blink reflex** (Figure 12-22). If either cornea is touched by a foreign object (in testing situations, typically a wisp of cotton), both eyes automatically blink. Sensory innervation of the cornea is by way of the ophthalmic division of the trigeminal nerve, so this is the afferent limb of the reflex. The afferents enter the spinal trigeminal tract and synapse on interneurons in the spinal trigeminal nucleus, mostly rostral to the obex. The spinal trigeminal interneurons then project bilaterally via relays in the reticular formation to motor neurons of the facial motor nucleus, which form the efferent limb. (Some corneal afferents also project to the main sensory nucleus, which then projects to the ipsilateral facial nucleus. This uncrossed component of the blink reflex is brief and relatively small, but it can be

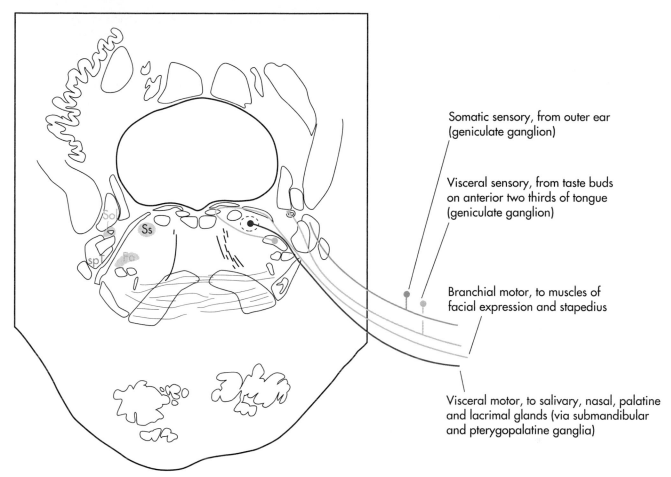

FIGURE 12-21
Fiber types in the facial nerve and their peripheral destinations. *Fa,* Facial motor nucleus; *Sol,* nucleus of the solitary tract; *spT,* spinal trigeminal tract; *Ss,* superior salivatory nucleus.

recorded electrically [Figure 12-22, *B*].) Thus by touching each of an individual's corneas in turn and observing the resulting blinks, it is possible to test, in a crude fashion, the integrity of both trigeminal nerves, both facial nerves, and some of their central connections.

Other components of the facial nerve are somatic sensory fibers from the skin of the outer ear; a small collection of visceral sensory fibers that innervate parts of the nasal cavity and soft palate; visceral afferents from taste buds (see Chapter 13); and preganglionic parasympathetic fibers for the submandibular and sublingual salivary glands, nasal and palatine glands, and the lacrimal gland. The parasympathetic fibers originate from a scattered group of cells called the **superior salivatory nucleus,** located in the reticular formation near the internal genu of the facial nerve.

Upper motor neuron damage affects the upper and lower parts of the face differently

Pyramidal system upper motor neurons originating in the cortex of the frontal lobe supply motor nuclei of the cranial nerves, much as corticospinal fibers supply alpha mo-

tor neurons of the spinal cord. These upper motor neurons are called **corticobulbar neurons** (*bulbar* is a loosely used term referring to just the medulla in some applications and to the medulla, pons, and midbrain in others); their axons accompany the corticospinal tract until they reach the brainstem levels of the nuclei they innervate.

As described in more detail in Chapter 18, corticobulbar fibers originate in the head area of motor cortex and generally project bilaterally to the somatic and branchial motor nuclei of the cranial nerves, or to nearby areas of the reticular formation (see Figure 18-17). This bilateral innervation corresponds to the way in which the muscles of both sides of the head and neck are typically used simultaneously (e.g., pharyngeal muscles during swallowing). The major exception to this pattern involves the muscles of facial expression. The lower motor neurons of each facial motor nucleus project to ipsilateral muscles, so damage to this nucleus or to the facial nerve itself causes weakness of the entire ipsilateral half of the face (Figure 12-9). As in the case of other cranial nerve motor nuclei, the part of the facial nucleus containing motor neurons for the upper part of the face can be activated by motor cortex of either hemisphere (presum-

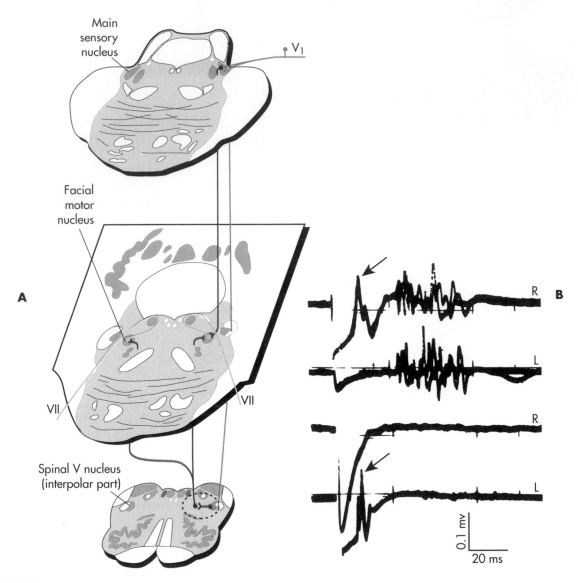

Main sensory nucleus

V_1

Facial motor nucleus

A

VII

VII

Spinal V nucleus (interpolar part)

R B

L

R

L

0.1 mv

20 ms

FIGURE 12-22
A, The connections involved in the blink reflex. **B,** Electrical activity of the orbicularis oculi during a comparable blink reflex elicited by electrical stimulation of the supraorbital nerve in a patient with an infarct in the left lateral medulla (the area outlined by a dotted line in **A**). The upper two traces show the normal responses of the right *(R)* and left *(L)* orbicularis oculi after stimulation of the right supraorbital nerve; there is a brief ipsilateral contraction *(arrow)* mediated by connections involving the trigeminal main sensory nucleus, followed by a more prolonged bilateral contraction mediated by the spinal trigeminal nucleus. Stimulating the left supraorbital nerve (lower two traces) elicits a normal fast ipsilateral response *(arrow)*, but no later response on either side. (**B** From Ongerboer de Visser BW, Kuypers HGJM: Late blink reflex changes in lateral medullary lesions: an electrophysiological and neuro-anatomical study of Wallenberg's syndrome, *Brain* 101:285, 1978.)

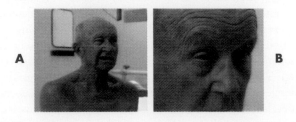

A

B

FIGURE 12-23
Selective weakness of lower facial muscles after corticobulbar damage. This patient had suffered a stroke that resulted in weakness of his left hand (not shown) and the left side of his face. When he tried to bare his teeth **(A)**, weakness of left lower facial muscles was apparent. However, he could raise his eyebrows symmetrically **(B)**.

ably corresponding to the way we typically blink both eyes or wrinkle both sides of the forehead simultaneously). In contrast, just as we can move one side of the mouth independently of the other, the motor neurons for facial muscles below the eye are innervated by many more crossed than uncrossed corticobulbar fibers. The consequence of this pattern is that a lesion of motor cortex or corticobulbar fibers on one side produces weakness of only the lower facial muscles of the opposite side (Figure 12–23). This is a clinical mainstay for distinguishing facial weakness resulting from a supranuclear lesion from that resulting from a nuclear or root lesion.

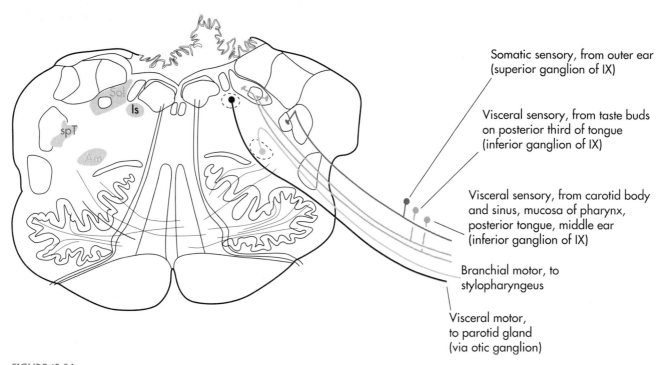

Somatic sensory, from outer ear
(superior ganglion of IX)

Visceral sensory, from taste buds
on posterior third of tongue
(inferior ganglion of IX)

Visceral sensory, from carotid body
and sinus, mucosa of pharynx,
posterior tongue, middle ear
(inferior ganglion of IX)

Branchial motor, to
stylopharyngeus

Visceral motor,
to parotid gland
(via otic ganglion)

FIGURE 12-24

Fiber types in the glossopharyngeal nerve and their peripheral destinations. *Am,* Nucleus ambiguus; *Is,* inferior salivatory nucleus; *Sol,* nucleus of the solitary tract; *spT,* spinal trigeminal nucleus.

The Glossopharyngeal Nerve (IX) Conveys Information From Intraoral Receptors

The glossopharyngeal nerve (Figure 12-24) contains a number of visceral sensory fibers, among them afferents from the carotid body, carotid sinus, medial surface of the eardrum, the walls of the pharynx, and mucous membranes and taste buds of the posterior third of the tongue. The extensive involvement of the glossopharyngeal nerve with intraoral sensation accounts for its name (*glossopharyngeal* is Greek for "tongue and throat"). Most of these visceral sensory fibers enter the solitary tract and synapse in the nucleus of the solitary tract. However, clinical evidence (described shortly) indicates that the fibers conveying information about pain from the pharynx and posterior part of the tongue (or at least collaterals of these fibers) enter the spinal trigeminal tract and terminate in the spinal nucleus. The same may be true of those fibers subserving tactile and temperature sensations; in addition, glossopharyngeal afferents probably also reach the part of the main sensory nucleus concerned with intraoral sensation. This fits with common experience: even though the pharynx is technically a visceral structure, it "feels" like a somatic structure in the way in which we can localize and discriminate stimuli applied there. Thus it is not surprising that the afferents involved should enter the trigeminal system.

Other components of the glossopharyngeal nerve are somatic sensory fibers from the skin of the outer ear; a small group of preganglionic parasympathetic fibers for the parotid gland, arising from scattered cells in the reticular formation of the rostral medulla collectively called the **inferior salivatory nucleus;** and branchial motor fibers for the stylopharyngeus, a small muscle that helps elevate the pharynx during swallowing and speaking. The latter efferents, together with vagal motor neurons for the other laryngeal and pharyngeal muscles, arise from cells in the aptly named **nucleus ambiguus.** This nucleus is located in the ventrolateral medullary tegmentum just dorsal to and roughly coextensive with the inferior olivary nucleus (Figures 12-24 and 12-25), but is sufficiently noncompact that it is difficult to distinguish in myelin-stained sections.

Glossopharyngeal neuralgia is similar in many ways to trigeminal neuralgia; it is rare but particularly distressing. The attacks of pain usually begin in the posterior tongue or the walls of the pharynx and radiate to the vicinity of the ear. One reason this condition is so distressing is that the trigger zone is often on the tongue or pharyngeal wall, and attacks may be set off by simply swallowing or talking. Pharmacological relief is usually available, but in a few rare cases in which it was not, the dorsomedial portion of the spinal trigeminal tract has been transected in the caudal medulla (Figure 12-16). The fact that this surgical procedure is effective provides evidence that the involved pain fibers (technically visceral afferents) travel in the spinal trigeminal tract.

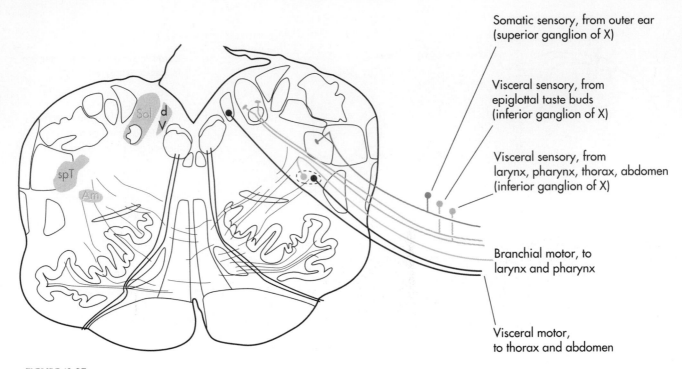

Somatic sensory, from outer ear
(superior ganglion of X)

Visceral sensory, from
epiglottal taste buds
(inferior ganglion of X)

Visceral sensory, from
larynx, pharynx, thorax, abdomen
(inferior ganglion of X)

Branchial motor, to
larynx and pharynx

Visceral motor,
to thorax and abdomen

FIGURE 12-25
Fiber types in the vagus nerve and their peripheral destinations. *Am*, Nucleus ambiguus; *dV*, dorsal motor nucleus of the vagus; *Sol*, nucleus of the solitary tract; *spT*, spinal trigeminal nucleus.

The Vagus Nerve (X) Is the Principal Parasympathetic Nerve

Cranial nerve X, the vagus nerve, is the most widely distributed of the cranial nerves (*vagus* is Latin for "wandering"—fibers of the vagus nerve wander throughout the thoracic and abdominal cavities). The vagus has components and connections similar to, partially overlapping, but more extensive than those of the glossopharyngeal nerve (Figure 12-25). A major collection of preganglionic parasympathetic fibers travels in the vagus nerve to thoracic and abdominal viscera generally. Most of these arise in the **dorsal motor nucleus of the vagus,** which is the principal parasympathetic nucleus of the brain. It is located in the floor of the fourth ventricle just lateral to the hypoglossal nucleus (Figure 12-10), underlying an elevation in the floor of the fourth ventricle called the **vagal trigone.** Additional preganglionic parasympathetic fibers, particularly those to the heart, originate in nucleus ambiguus.

The vagus also contains a large collection of visceral sensory fibers innervating the thoracic and abdominal viscera, including pressure receptors and chemoreceptors of the aortic arch, as well as a few from taste buds of the epiglottis. Vagal afferents innervating the larynx, esophagus, and lower pharynx, like similar fibers from the glossopharyngeal nerve, are thought to enter the spinal trigeminal tract and terminate in the spinal trigeminal nucleus. The remaining vagal visceral sensory fibers enter the solitary tract and terminate in caudal portions of the nucleus of the solitary tract.

Vagal branchial motor fibers arise in nucleus ambiguus and innervate most of the striated muscles of the larynx and pharynx. A clinically useful (though unpleasant for the patient) reflex is the **gag reflex.** Touching the wall of one side of the pharynx in a normal individual elicits the unpleasant bilateral response. The afferent limb is via the glossopharyngeal nerve, whereas the efferent limb is mainly via the vagus. The central connections are not entirely clear and may involve the spinal trigeminal tract and nucleus, the solitary tract and nucleus, or both, in addition to the nucleus ambiguus. Nevertheless the gag reflex, like the blink reflex, can be used to test two cranial nerves (in this case IX and X) and some of their central connections.

The only other component of the vagus nerve is a small collection of somatic sensory fibers from the skin of the outer ear.

The Accessory Nerve (XI) Innervates Neck and Shoulder Muscles

Cranial nerve XI consists of fibers that originate from the very caudal medulla and the anterior horn of the upper five cervical segments, exit just posterior to the dentate ligament, and innervate the sternocleidomastoid and part of the trapezius. These muscles are considered to be at least partially of branchial arch origin (although not all authors agree on this point), which would put accessory nerve fibers in the branchial motor category. In addition

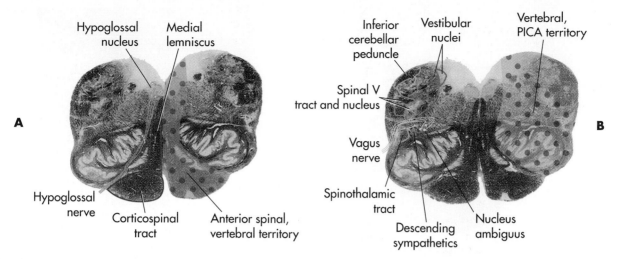

FIGURE 12-26

Medullary syndromes. **A,** Vascular territory typically involved in the medial medullary syndrome (right side of figure), and the structures whose damage would account for the resulting symptoms and signs (left side of figure). **B,** Vascular territory typically involved in the lateral medullary syndrome (right side of figure), and the structures whose damage would account for the resulting symptoms and signs (left side of figure).

to these motor axons, the accessory nerve may include a few muscle afferent fibers.

BRAINSTEM DAMAGE COMMONLY CAUSES DEFICITS ON ONE SIDE OF THE HEAD AND THE OPPOSITE SIDE OF THE BODY

The Brown–Séquard syndrome (see Figure 10-29), which follows hemisection of the spinal cord, demonstrates the possibility of crossed or **alternating** syndromes, in which some symptoms are referred to one side of the body and others to the other side. In the brainstem, most pathways descending to the spinal cord are contralateral to the side on which they terminate, and most pathways ascending from the spinal cord are contralateral to the side on which they arise. However, all the exiting cranial nerves are ipsilateral to the side that they innervate*; in addition, almost all of the cranial nerve nuclei deal with ipsilateral structures. As a result, alternating syndromes, in which long tract symptoms are referred to one side and cranial nerve symptoms to the other side, are the hallmark of brainstem lesions. For example, consider the effects of a lesion involving the medial portion of one side of the rostral medulla (Figure 12-26, *A*), which could be caused by occlusion of a branch of one vertebral or anterior spinal artery. The symptoms involved in the resulting **medial medullary syndrome** include contralateral hemiparesis (damage to the pyramid), contralateral tactile and kines-

thetic deficits (damage to the medial lemniscus), and ipsilateral paralysis with eventual atrophy of the tongue muscles (damage to the hypoglossal nucleus or exiting hypoglossal nerve). This syndrome is also referred to as **alternating hypoglossal hemiplegia.**

More lateral damage at the same brainstem level (which can be caused by occlusion of branches of one vertebral or posterior inferior cerebellar artery) results in the **lateral medullary** (or **Wallenberg's**) **syndrome** (Figure 12-26, *B*). The damaged structures may include the spinothalamic tract, the spinal trigeminal tract, nucleus ambiguus, and descending sympathetic fibers. Symptoms of such damage are loss of pain and temperature sensations over the contralateral body (with relative sparing of tactile sensation), loss of pain and temperature sensations over the ipsilateral face, hoarseness and difficulty in swallowing (as a result of paralysis of ipsilateral laryngeal and pharyngeal muscles), and ipsilateral Horner's syndrome. The inferior cerebellar peduncle and adjacent vestibular nuclei often are included in the lesion, and vertigo, abnormal eye movements, and ipsilateral cerebellar deficits such as ataxia result (see Figure 14-30).

A final example involves a lesion of the cerebral peduncle on one side of the rostral midbrain (Figure 12-27, *A*) as might result from occlusion of branches of one posterior cerebral artery. This damages descending corticospinal fibers, causing contralateral spastic paralysis; it also damages one oculomotor nerve, causing ipsilateral ptosis, pupillary dilation, and lateral strabismus. This symptom complex is called **Weber's syndrome.** Dorsal extension of the damage into the midbrain tegmentum could result in contralateral ataxia (crossed superior cerebellar peduncle) and somatosensory deficits (medial lemniscus, spinothalamic tract).

---

*Even in unusual cases such as efferents to the superior rectus and superior oblique, the crossing occurs within the brainstem, near the cell bodies of origin.

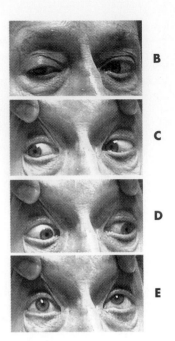

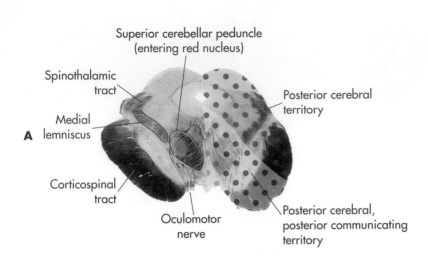

FIGURE 12-27

A, Vascular territory typically involved in the various midbrain syndromes (right side of figure), and the structures whose damage would account for the resulting symptoms and signs (left side of figure). **B-E,** Eye movements of a patient with vascular damage in the right rostral midbrain. At rest **(B)** he had ptosis on the right and his eyes deviated to the right (a way to minimize the diplopia caused by a weak right medial rectus). Gaze to the right **(C)** was preserved, but during attempted gaze to the left **(D)** his right eye failed to adduct fully. Weakness of right eye muscles was also apparent when he attempted to look up **(E).** Downgaze was better preserved and his pupils were equal in size and reactive to light, indicating that not all of the bundles of oculomotor fibers arching through the midbrain tegmentum were affected. The patient also had slight weakness of his left arm and leg, a Babinski sign on the left, and ataxia of his left arm and leg. He recovered completely over a period of about a week.

SUGGESTED READINGS

Beckstead RM, Morse JR, Norgren R: The nucleus of the solitary tract in the monkey: projections to the thalamus and brain stem nuclei, *J Comp Neurol* 190:259, 1980.

Beckstead RM, Norgren R: An autoradiographic examination of the central distribution of the trigeminal, facial, glossopharyngeal and vagal nerves in the monkey, *J Comp Neurol* 184:455, 1979.

Bogousslavsky J, Meienberg O: Eye-movement disorders in brain-stem and cerebellar stroke, *Arch Neurol* 44:141, 1987. *A comprehensive review.*

Brodal A: Central course of afferent fibers for pain in facial, glossopharyngeal and vagus nerves, *Arch Neurol Psychiatry* 57:292, 1947.

Brodal A: *Neurological anatomy in relation to clinical medicine,* ed 3, New York, 1981, Oxford University Press.

Gan R, Noronha A: The medullary vascular syndromes revisited, *J Neurol* 242:195, 1995. *A review of the medial and lateral medullary syndromes and their variants.*

Gauthier JM, Mommay D, Vercher JL: Ocular muscle proprioception and visual localization of targets in man, *Brain* 113:1857, 1990. *The use we make of information from the proprioceptors in extraocular muscles has long been a mystery; it isn't crucial for guiding eye movements. This paper presents one possibility.*

Goodwin GM, Luschei ES: Effects of destroying spindle afferents from jaw muscles on mastication in monkeys, *J Neurophysiol* 37:967, 1974. *In a word, not much. The physiological significance of the mesencephalic nucleus remains obscure.*

Hockman CH, Bieger D, Weerasuriva A: Supranuclear pathways of swallowing, *Prog Neurobiol* 12:15, 1979.

Huang X-F, Törk I, Paxinos G: Dorsal motor nucleus of the vagus nerve: a cyto- and chemoarchitectonic study in the human, *J Comp Neurol* 330:158, 1993.

Jenny AB, Saper CB: Organization of the facial nucleus and corticofacial projection in the monkey: a reconsideration of the upper motor neuron facial palsy, *Neurol* 37: 930, 1987.

Jones EG, Schwark HD, Callahan PA: Extent of the ipsilateral representation in the ventral posterior medial nucleus of the monkey thalamus, *Exp Brain Res* 63:310, 1986.

Kobayashi Y, Matsumura G: Central projections of primary afferent fibers from the rat trigeminal nerve labeled with isolectin B4-HRP, *Neurosci Lett* 217:89, 1996. *Isolectin B4 injected into the trigeminal ganglion selectively labels small-diameter primary afferents, and this study demonstrates nicely the somatotopic arrangement of their terminations in the spinal trigeminal nucleus.*

Kunc Z: Treatment of essential neuralgia of the 9th nerve by selective tractotomy, *J Neurosurg* 23:494, 1965. *Clinical evidence regarding the location of glossopharyngeal pain fibers in the spinal trigeminal tract of humans.*

Leblanc A: *The cranial nerves: anatomy, imaging, vascularisation,* ed 2, Berlin, 1995, Springer-Verlag. *A beautifully illustrated account of the peripheral courses of the cranial nerves and their appearance in clinical images.*

Lowe AA: The neural regulation of tongue movements, *Prog Neurobiol* 15:295, 1980.

Manger PR, Woods TM, Jones EG: Representation of face and intra-oral structures in area 3b of macaque monkey somatosensory cortex, *J Comp Neurol* 371:513, 1996.

Martin MR, Mason CA: The seventh cranial nerve of the rat: visualization of efferent and afferent pathways by cobalt precipitation, *Brain Res* 121:21, 1977.

Matsumoto S et al: A sensory level on the trunk in lower lateral brainstem lesions, *Neurol* 38:1515, 1988. *Clinical evidence about the course of projections from the spinal trigeminal nucleus to the thalamus.*

McCrea RA, Strassman A, Highstein SM: Morphology and physiology of abducens motoneurons and internuclear neurons intracellularly injected with horseradish peroxidase in alert squirrel monkeys, *J Comp Neurol* 243:291, 1986.

McRitchie DA, Törk I: The internal organization of the human solitary nucleus, *Brain Res Bull* 31:171, 1993.

Mizuno N, Nomura S: Primary afferent fibers in the glossopharyngeal nerve terminate in the dorsal division of the principal sensory trigeminal nucleus, *Neurosci Lett* 66:338, 1986.

Ohya A: Responses of trigeminal subnucleus interpolaris neurons to afferent inputs from deep oral structures, *Brain Res Bull* 29:773, 1992.

Olszewski J: On the anatomical and functional organization of the spinal trigeminal nucleus, *J Comp Neurol* 92:401, 1950.

Ongerboer de Visser BW: Afferent limb of the human jaw reflex: electrophysiologic and anatomic study, *Neurol* 32:563, 1982.

Porter JD: Brainstem terminations of extraocular muscle primary afferent neurons in the monkey, *J Comp Neurol* 247:133, 1986.

Porter JD, Guthrie BL, Sparks DL: Innervation of monkey extraocular muscles: localization of sensory and motor neurons by retrograde transport of horseradish peroxidase, *J Comp Neurol* 218:208, 1983.

Rokx JTM, Jüch PJW, van Willigen JD: Arrangements and connections of mesencephalic trigeminal neurons in the rat, *Acta Anat* 127:7, 1986.

Rovit RJ, Murali R, Jannetta PJ, editors: *Trigeminal neuralgia,* Baltimore, 1990, Williams and Wilkins.

Rushton JG, Stevens JC, Miller RH: Glossopharyngeal (vagoglossopharyngeal) neuralgia: a study of 217 cases, *Arch Neurol* 38:201, 1981.

Smith RL: Axonal projections and connections of the principal sensory trigeminal nucleus in the monkey, *J Comp Neurol* 163:347, 1975.

Steindler DA: Trigeminocerebellar, trigeminotectal and trigeminothalamic projections: a double retrograde axonal tracing study in the mouse, *J Comp Neurol* 237:155, 1985.

Stewart WA, King RB: Fiber projections from the nucleus caudalis of the spinal trigeminal nucleus, *J Comp Neurol* 121:271, 1963.

Strassman AM, Potrebic S, Maciewicz RJ: Anatomical properties of brainstem trigeminal neurons that respond to electrical stimulation of dural blood vessels, *J Comp Neurol* 346:349, 1994. *A possible explanation of the pattern of referred pain in response to dural irritation.*

Tamai Y, Iwamoto M, Tsujimoto T: Pathway of the blink reflex in the brainstem of the cat: interneurons between the trigeminal nuclei and the facial nucleus, *Brain Res* 380:19, 1986.

Torvik A: The ascending fibers from the main trigeminal sensory nucleus, *Am J Anat* 100:1, 1957.

Walker AE: The origin, course and terminations of the secondary pathways of the trigeminal nerve in primates, *J Comp Neurol* 71:59, 1939.

Wall M, Wray SH: The one-and-a-half syndrome—a unilateral disorder of the pontine tegmentum: a study of 20 cases and review of the literature, *Neurol* 33:971, 1983.

Warwick R: Representation of the extra-ocular muscles in the oculomotor nuclei of the monkey, *J Comp Neurol* 98:449, 1953.

Way JS: Evidence for the site of the superior salivatory nucleus in the guinea pig: a retrograde HRP study, *Anat Rec* 201:119, 1981.

Young RF: Effect of trigeminal tractotomy on dental sensation in humans, *J Neurosurg* 56:812, 1982. *Tractotomy near the obex causes facial analgesia but no change in dental pain.*

Young RF, Perryman KM: Neuronal responses in rostral trigeminal brain-stem nuclei of macaque monkeys after chronic trigeminal tractotomy, *J Neurosurg* 65:508, 1986. *Evidence that dental pain is processed rostral to the obex, and facial pain caudal to the obex, in the spinal trigeminal nucleus.*

Younge BR: Analysis of trochlear nerve palsies: diagnosis, etiology and treatment, *Mayo Clin Proc* 52:11, 1977.

Zee DS: The organization of the brainstem ocular motor subnuclei, *Ann Neurol* 4:384, 1978. *Speculation on why the motor axons to the superior oblique and superior rectus cross.*

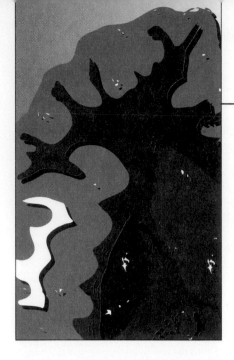

THE CHEMICAL SENSES OF TASTE AND SMELL

Dating back to their origins in some primordial sea, living cells have shared an ability to respond to chemicals, at a minimum detecting and absorbing nutrients. Some cells in or closely associated with the nervous system go beyond this, specializing in detecting certain classes of chemicals adjacent to their membranes and using this information to affect autonomic function, behavior, or perception. These cells fall into four general categories: (1) the myriad visceral chemoreceptors that work in the background, mostly inaccessible to conscious awareness, keeping track of the concentrations of substances such as oxygen, glucose, and neurohormones; (2) **gustatory receptor cells,** or **taste cells,** that mediate the sense of taste; (3) **olfactory receptor neurons** that mediate the sense of smell; and (4) chemosensitive endings, such as some trigeminal endings in mucous membranes, that mediate what has been termed the **common chemical sense**—sensations such as the heat of chili peppers, the sting of ammonia, or the coolness of menthol. The visceral chemoreceptors monitor internal chemical composition, and the other three monitor external chemistry, whether of local air or of substances being considered for ingestion.

Taste, smell, and the common chemical sense, like all the other senses of which we are consciously aware, have both rewarding and warning functions. In this case, the chemical senses are the basis not only of the enjoyment of a meal or a glass of wine, but also of detecting things such as spoiled food or smoke from a fire.

TASTE IS MEDIATED BY RECEPTORS IN TASTE BUDS, INNERVATED BY CRANIAL NERVES VII, IX, AND X

The term "taste" is used in this book as synonymous with the **gustatory** sense, the set of sensations engendered by stimulated taste buds. We commonly assume that this is the same thing as the total sensation we perceive when eating or drinking, but such integrated sensations of **flavor** are actually the result of the combination of three different kinds of input: direct chemical stimulation of taste buds, stimulation of olfactory receptors by vapors from food (Figure 13-7), and stimulation of chemical-sensitive and somatosensory free nerve endings of the trigeminal and other nerves in the mucous membranes of the oral cavity. The latter endings respond to qualities such as the pungency, spiciness, temperature, and texture of food. We have difficulty appreciating the subtleties of food and beverages using just our taste buds, and people with deficits in their sense of olfaction complain that things "taste" bland. Nevertheless, some basic aspects of flavor are encoded by taste receptor cells.

The Tongue Is Covered by a Series of Papillae, Some of Which Contain Taste Buds

The tongue is mostly muscle, but its surface is covered by a series of bumps and folds called **papillae** (Figure

13-1). Most are small conical projections not involved in taste, but **fungiform, foliate,** and **vallate** papillae contain **taste buds** (Figure 13-2). About 200 to 300 fungiform ("mushroom-shaped") papillae are scattered across the surface of the anterior two thirds of the tongue, concentrated on the tip and sides. Typical fungiform papillae contain 3 to 5 taste buds. Foliate ("like a leaf") papillae are the most posterior of a series of about 20 folds on the sides of the posterior tongue; each has 100 to 150 taste buds in its walls. Finally, a series of 8 to 9 vallate or **circumvallate** ("surrounded by a wall") papillae is arranged in a V-shaped line two thirds of the way back along the dorsal surface of the tongue. Each vallate papilla is surrounded by a deep groove in the lingual epithelium (Figure 13-2, *A*), with about 250 taste buds located in the walls of the groove. Hence even though the vallate papillae are few in number, they contain nearly half of the 5000 taste buds found on an average tongue.

Although an "average" tongue contains about 5000 taste buds, the numbers of both papillae and taste buds are surprisingly variable. For example, among normal, healthy individuals, some have as many as 100 times the number of taste buds in their fungiform papillae as others do. This is presumably the basis of the 100-fold variation in threshold concentration for various substances among normal individuals.

Taste buds are usually associated with the tongue, but they are also distributed widely, although in smaller numbers, over the palate and pharynx.★ The pharyngeal and palatal taste buds may be more important for swallowing and for reflex responses to good or bad tastes than for conscious awareness of taste.

Taste receptor cells are modified epithelial cells with neuronlike properties

Each taste bud is an ovoid collection of about 100 modified epithelial cells, most of them taste receptor cells (Figure 13-2, *B-D*). Taste receptor cells are spindle-shaped, with microvillar processes that extend through a small opening, the **taste pore,** where they are exposed to chemical stimuli. At the deep end of the taste bud, the receptor cells make synapses on visceral sensory fibers from the facial, glossopharyngeal, and vagal nerves. Fibers from the facial nerve innervate the taste buds of fungiform and anterior foliate papillae and the palate; fibers from the glossopharyngeal nerve innervate those of val-

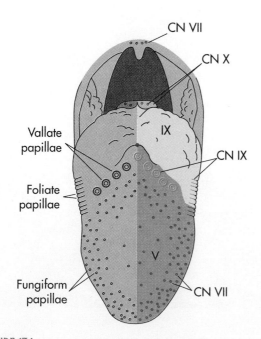

FIGURE 13-1
Distribution and innervation of taste buds, and innervation of the lingual epithelium. The trigeminal nerve *(V)* subserves general sensation from the anterior two thirds of the tongue, and the glossopharyngeal nerve *(IX)* has a similar function for the posterior third of the tongue.

★Different species of animals often adapt to their environments by utilizing elaborate configurations of the same receptor cells used by other species. An example is the star-nosed mole (see Box 9-1). Taste buds provide another example: fish have taste buds on the external surface of their bodies, so they can "taste" the water through which they swim. A single channel catfish may have 100,000 external taste buds—20 times as many as an entire human tongue!

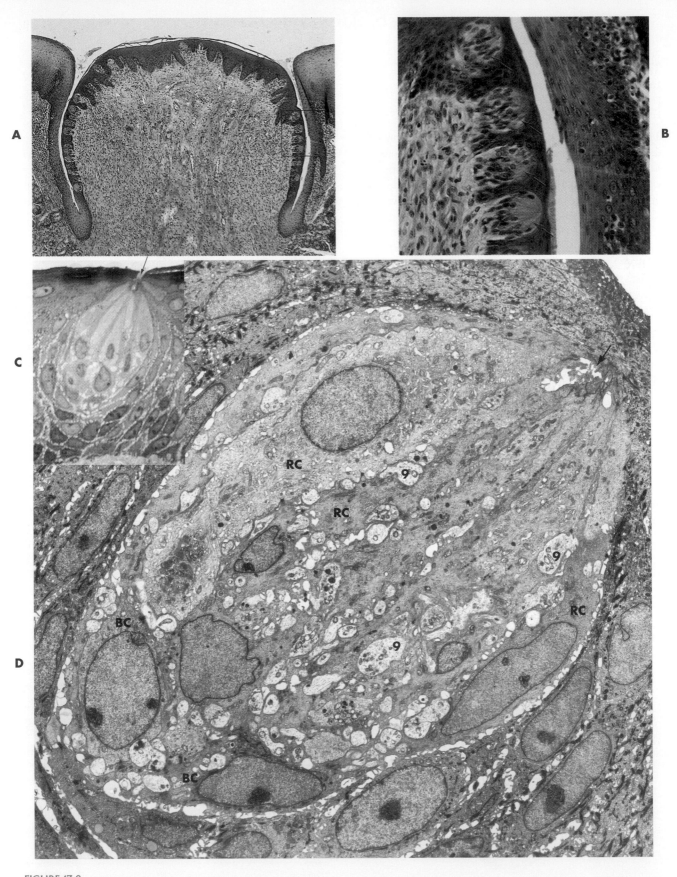

FIGURE 13-2

Morphology of taste buds. **A,** Section of a single vallate papilla from the tongue of a cat. The area outlined in **A** is enlarged in **B,** in which individual taste buds *(arrows)* can be seen just beneath the surface of the papilla. **C,** Light micrograph of a section through the center of a single taste bud from a human fungiform papilla, showing the taste pore *(arrow).* **D,** Electron micrograph of a taste bud from a human circumvallate papilla. The section is not quite through the middle of the taste bud, but the arrow indicates the apex where the taste pore would open in a nearby section. The principal cellular elements are taste receptor cells *(RC)* and basal cells *(BC).* Discrete synapses of the receptor cells onto afferent fibers cannot be seen easily in this micrograph, but numerous glossopharyngeal nerve processes *(9)* are apparent. (**A** and **B** courtesy Dr. Nathaniel T. McMullen, Department of Cell Biology and Anatomy, The University of Arizona College of Medicine. **C** and **D** courtesy Pamela Eller, University of Colorado Health Sciences Center.)

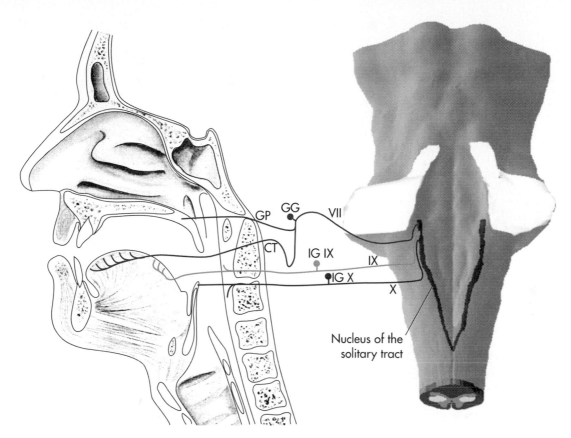

FIGURE 13-3

Innervation of taste buds in different parts of the oral cavity by the facial *(VII)*, glossopharyngeal *(IX)*, and vagus *(X)* nerves. The central processes of all three terminate in rostral parts of the nucleus of the solitary tract. *CT*, Chorda tympani nerve; *GG*, geniculate ganglion; *GP*, greater petrosal nerve; *IG IX*, inferior ganglion of the glossopharyngeal nerve (petrosal ganglion); *IG X*, inferior ganglion of the vagus (nodose ganglion).

late and most foliate papillae and the pharynx; and a few vagal fibers innervate those of the epiglottis and esophagus (Figure 13-3).

Taste receptor cells differentiate from the surrounding lingual epithelium and subsequently depend on chemical interactions with the gustatory nerves for their continued existence; denervation of an area of tongue causes degeneration of its taste buds. Despite this epithelial origin, taste receptor cells have some very neuronlike properties: they contain transduction machinery in their apical membranes, produce receptor potentials in response to appropriate taste stimuli, make typical chemical synapses on the peripheral endings of gustatory nerves, and even produce action potentials when sufficiently depolarized by a receptor potential.★ However, unlike almost all neurons, taste receptor cells have a limited life span. Each lives only a week or two before being replaced by differentiation of **basal cells,** which migrate in from the surrounding epithelium and wait, as their name implies, near the base of the taste bud.

Taste receptor cells utilize a variety of transduction mechanisms to detect sweet, salty, sour, and bitter stimuli

The four basic taste qualities traditionally recognized are sweet, salty, sour, and bitter, but there are probably others.★ Although some areas of the tongue are somewhat more sensitive to one or another—the tip to sweet, the sides to salt and sour, and posterior portions to bitter—in fact all parts of the tongue are sensitive to all four kinds of **tastants.** Corresponding to these multiple taste qualities, taste receptor cells utilize multiple methods to transduce chemical stimuli into electrical signals (Figure 13-4). Some are epithelial mechanisms adapted for use in taste transduction, and others are familiar G protein–coupled mechanisms. Transduction processes include the following:

1. The transduction process for sodium chloride, the prototypical salty stimulus, is ultimately simple. No receptor molecules are involved: Na$^+$ channels in

---

★The role of these action potentials is unclear because taste receptor cells are small enough for receptor potentials to spread electrotonically to their synapses with nerve endings. It has been suggested that the action potentials increase the entry of Ca^{2+} into the cell, enhancing the release of transmitter.

★For example, the flavor-enhancing taste of glutamate (as in monosodium glutamate, or MSG) is probably a separate taste in its own right. This taste is sometimes referred to as *umami*, which is Japanese for "delicious." Cells that respond better to glutamate than to any of the four traditional categories have been found in gustatory relay nuclei and cortex, and glutamate receptors such as the ones in some postsynaptic membranes have been found on some taste cells.

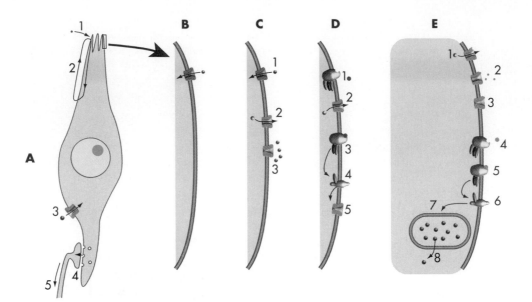

FIGURE 13-4

A sampling of the transduction mechanisms used by taste receptor cells. **A,** Binding of tastant molecules to the apical microvilli of a taste cell *(I)* causes production of a depolarizing receptor potential *(2)*, entry of Ca^{2+} through voltage-gated Ca^{2+} channels *(3)*, release of transmitter onto a peripheral nerve ending *(4)*, and increased firing of the nerve fiber *(5)*. **B,** Na^+ ions flow directly into Na^+ channels. **C,** Protons either flow through Na^+ channels *(I)* or cause normally open K^+ channels *(2)* to close *(3)*. The decreased K^+ conductance causes the membrane potential to move toward the Na^+ equilibrium potential (i.e., depolarize). **D,** Sweet substances bind to G protein–coupled receptors *(I)*. Dissociation of the G protein *(3)* activates an enzyme *(4)* whose product (cyclic AMP) leads to the closing of K^+ channels *(5)* that are normally open *(2)*. **E,** Some bitter substances bind *(2)* to normally open K^+ channels *(I)*, causing them to close *(3)*. Other bitter substances bind to G protein–coupled receptors *(4)*. Dissociation of the G protein *(5)* activates an enzyme *(6)* whose product leads to the release of Ca^{2+} *(8)* from intracellular stores *(7)*.

the apical membranes of taste receptor cells allow inward movement of Na^+ ions, depolarizing the cell (Figure 13-4, *B*).

2. Acids taste sour, and the operative agent is the increased concentration of H^+, which depolarizes receptor cells either by direct movement of protons through Na^+ channels or by blocking the conductance of pH-sensitive apical K^+ channels (Figure 13-4, *C*); again, no receptor molecules are involved.

3. Sweet compounds, in contrast, bind to G protein–coupled receptor molecules that, through a second messenger, cause decreased K^+ conductance in other parts of the cell (Figure 13-4, *D*).

4. Bitter tastes, typical of many toxic substances, serve a protective function and are usually avoided by humans and other animals.★ Bitter-sensitive taste receptor cells use both ligand-gated channels and G-protein-coupled receptors, allowing them to be depolarized by a broad range of chemicals (Figure 13-4, *E*). Some bitter substances, like quinine, bind to ligand-gated K^+ channels and diminish their probability of being open. Other bitter substances bind to G protein–coupled receptor molecules that, through a second messenger, cause release of Ca^{2+} ions from internal stores; the increased Ca^{2+} concentration in turn causes release of transmitter from the taste receptor cell.

Second-Order Gustatory Neurons Are Located in the Nucleus of the Solitary Tract

Chemosensory information not only reaches consciousness as the perception of flavor, but in its role in autonomic responses and the acquisition of food has much closer ties to the hypothalamus and limbic system than do other senses. The second-order neurons that mediate the involvement of taste in all of these connections are located in the nucleus of the solitary tract (see Figure 12-10). The nucleus of the solitary tract, the principal visceral sensory nucleus of the brainstem, receives (via the solitary tract) gustatory afferents as well as the other visceral sensory fibers mentioned in Chapters 12 and 23. However, the gustatory fibers, as well as chemosensitive trigeminal fibers, end separately in lateral and rostral portions of the solitary nucleus (Figures 13-3 and 13-5).

Second-order taste fibers do two things (Figure 13-5). Some participate in reflex activities, such as swallowing★ or coughing, by way of cranial nerve motor nuclei. Others, like fibers in most sensory systems, project to the cerebral cortex by way of the thalamus. In this case, however, the projection is uncrossed. Fibers travel ipsilaterally

---

★Although, of course, many people learn to enjoy the bitterness of things such as the caffeine in coffee and the quinine in tonic water.

★Swallowing is usually not thought of as a reflex activity, but its success depends greatly on sensory input from the oral cavity. For example, try to swallow multiple times in succession, as rapidly as you can, with an empty mouth. Compare this maximum rate to the rate that can be achieved when drinking a beverage.

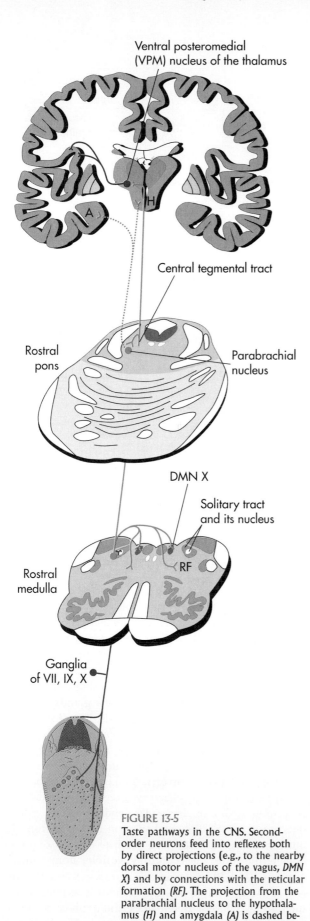

Ventral posteromedial
(VPM) nucleus of the thalamus

Central tegmental tract

Rostral
pons

Parabrachial
nucleus

DMN X

Solitary tract
and its nucleus

Rostral
medulla

RF

Ganglia
of VII, IX, X

FIGURE 13-5
Taste pathways in the CNS. Second-order neurons feed into reflexes both by direct projections (e.g., to the nearby dorsal motor nucleus of the vagus, *DMN X*) and by connections with the reticular formation (*RF*). The projection from the parabrachial nucleus to the hypothalamus (*H*) and amygdala (*A*) is dashed because its existence in primates has not been demonstrated conclusively.

through the central tegmental tract to the most medial part of VPM, where they end adjacent to the uncrossed fibers of the dorsal trigeminal tract (see Figure 12-14). This medial part of VPM then projects to the gustatory cortex, which is located in the insula and the medial surface of the frontal operculum, near the base of the central sulcus. Gustatory cortex projects in turn to orbital cortex of the frontal lobe, where taste information is thought to be integrated with olfactory and other information, and to the amygdala, through which taste information reaches the hypothalamus and limbic system.★

Information About Taste Is Coded by the Pattern of Activity in Populations of Neurons

Sensory systems such as somatic sensation and vision depend on receiving information about specific aspects of a stimulus, highly organized in space and time (e.g., see Figures 3-28, 10-18, and 17-32). Activity in many of the neurons in these systems signals the occurrence of a particular kind of event—particularly its location, as is evident in the detailed topographic maps in places such as somatosensory, visual, and motor cortex (see Figures 3-28 and 17-26). On the other hand, the nervous system also uses combinations of inputs to interpret stimuli, as in the case of Ruffini endings that are involved in the sense of touch but produce no sensation when stimulated in isolation (see Chapter 9). Taste and olfaction emphasize this combinatorial type of processing. Taste stimuli are widely dispersed in the mouth during chewing, and odorants fill the nose during breathing, so spatial localization is less important and we actually use the *touching* of the tongue by a piece of food to localize it (see Box 9-2). Instead the gustatory and olfactory systems together are faced with the task of coding the identities of many thousands of different chemicals, both singly and in mixtures. In principle, this could be accomplished by having many thousands of different receptor types, each particularly sensitive to one chemical. Although the olfactory system does utilize a large number of receptor types (as discussed a little later in this chapter), the chemical senses for the most part use the alternative strategy of coding the identity of a stimulus in terms of the pattern of activity in a large population of neurons with multiple sensitivities. Although this may seem like a cumbersome way to do things, it is actually an efficient system for encoding information about a large variety of potential stimuli using a relatively small number of neurons, similar in principle to using just three kinds of cones as the basis for perceiving hundreds of hues (see Chapter 17).

At every level of the gustatory system, individual cells respond to more than one kind of tastant. Most taste re-

---

★In some animals, taste information reaches the hypothalamus and amygdala more directly, through a projection from the parabrachial nuclei of the brainstem reticular formation. Whether such connections are present in primates like us is still a matter of debate.

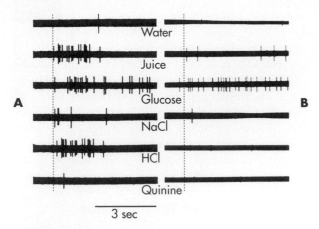

FIGURE 13-6
Responses of single gustatory neurons in the nucleus of the solitary tract (**A**) and the orbital cortex (**B**) of monkeys to tastants applied at the time indicated by the vertical dashed lines. The brainstem neuron responds to multiple tastants, but the cortical neuron is more selective. (**A** from Scott TR et al: Gustatory responses in the nucleus tractus solitarius of the alert cynomolgus monkey, *J Neurophysiol* 55:182, 1986. **B** from Rolls ET, Yaxley S, Sienkiewicz ZJ: Gustatory responses of single neurons in the caudolateral orbitofrontal cortex of the macaque monkey, *J Neurophysiol* 64:1055, 1990.)

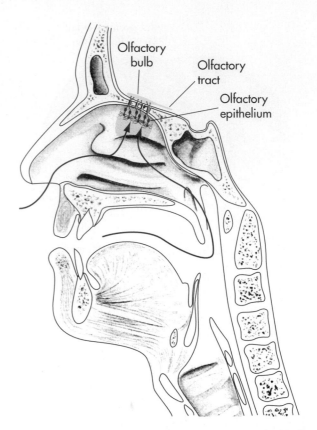

FIGURE 13-7
Location of the olfactory epithelium on the lateral wall of the nasal cavity. The olfactory epithelium continues across the roof of the cavity into a patch of similar size on the nasal septum. Odorants can reach this epithelium either through the nostrils or by way of the oropharynx.

ceptor cells probably contain in their apical membranes more than one of the transduction mechanisms shown in Figure 13-4, although one is likely to predominate in any given cell. Gustatory nerve fibers branch and innervate multiple taste buds that may even be located in multiple papillae, and they too respond to more than one tastant. Here again, one kind of sensitivity usually predominates for any given nerve fiber, in ways that correspond to the relative sensitivities of different areas of the tongue: most facial nerve (chorda tympani) fibers are maximally sensitive to sweet or salty stimuli, and most glossopharyngeal fibers to sour or bitter stimuli. Second-order neurons in the nucleus of the solitary tract are even more broadly tuned (Figure 13-6, *A*). By the time gustatory information reaches higher cortical levels, specific features of a taste stimulus have been extracted and neurons with particular chemical sensitivities are found (Figure 13-6, *B*).

OLFACTION IS MEDIATED BY RECEPTORS THAT PROJECT DIRECTLY TO THE TELENCEPHALON

The other principal player in conscious chemical sensation, the olfactory system, is specialized to detect volatile chemicals or **odorants** drawn into the nasal cavity during breathing or wafting into it from the oropharynx during eating. Although the olfactory sense is relatively less important for visually oriented species like us than for many other animals, it has very impressive capabilities nonetheless. Humans are able to distinguish thousands of different odors—perhaps as many as 10,000, and for trained sniffers even more—some at remarkably low concentrations.

The Axons of Olfactory Receptor Neurons Form Cranial Nerve I

The olfactory system begins peripherally with the **olfactory epithelium,** a pigmented, yellowish patch of cells that occupies about 1 to 2 cm² of the roof and adjacent walls of the nasal cavity on each side (Figure 13-7). Each patch of olfactory epithelium consists of about 5 million receptor cells interspersed with supporting cells and the ducts of small glands (called **Bowman's glands**). Sensory endings of the trigeminal nerve are also found in the olfactory epithelium. The trigeminal endings are responsible for the noxious sensation (not really one of smell) elicited by irritants such as concentrated ammonia. The **olfactory receptor neurons,** unlike taste receptor cells, are true neurons. Each olfactory receptor is a small bipolar neuron, with a single slender dendrite emerging from one end of its cell body and an axon emerging from the other end (Figure 13-8). The dendrite extends to a bulbous termination, the **olfactory vesicle,** from which a series of 10 to 30 immotile cilia spread out over the surface of the epithelium in a layer of mucus secreted by the supporting cells and Bowman's glands. Substances to be smelled diffuse across the mucous layer, either directly or

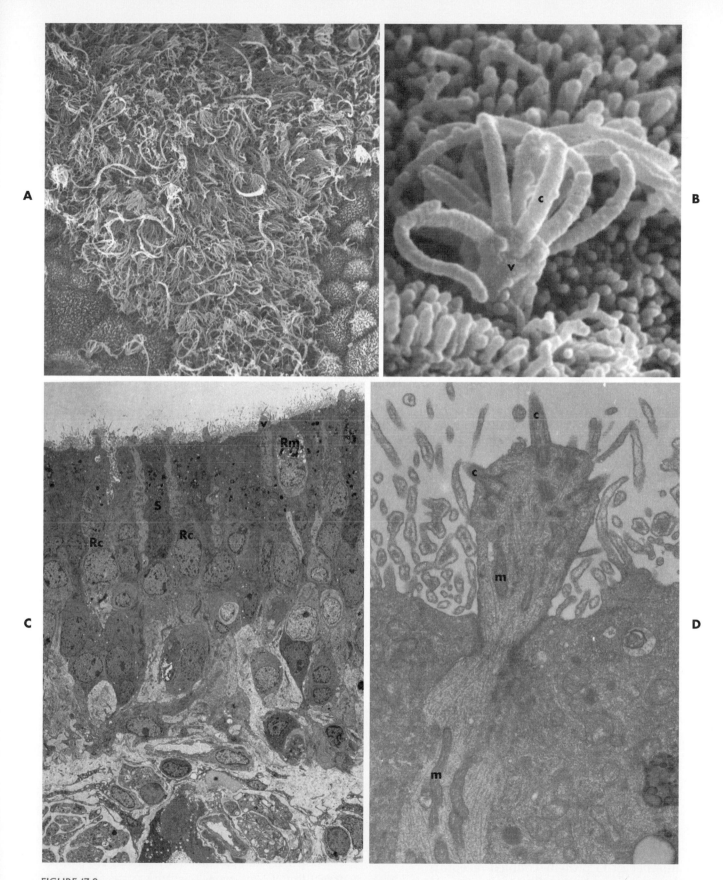

FIGURE 13-8

Human olfactory epithelium. **A**, Low-power scanning electron micrograph, showing the mucosal surface of the epithelium, covered by a felt-work of chemosensory cilia. This area is at the edge of the olfactory epithelium, and nonsensory cells with short microvilli form the adjacent epithelium. **B**, Higher-power view, showing chemosensory cilia *(c)* emerging from a single olfactory vesicle *(v)*. **C**, Transmission electron micrograph, showing ciliated receptor cells *(Rc)*, supporting cells *(S)*, and olfactory vesicles *(v)*. The receptor cell on the right *(Rm)* is of a second type that has microvillar rather than ciliary processes; these are much less numerous than the ciliated receptor cells and are poorly understood. **D**, Higher-magnification micrograph of an olfactory vesicle, showing emerging chemosensory cilia *(c)* and abundant mitochondria *(m)* in and near the vesicle. [**A** and **B** courtesy Dr. Edward E. Morrison, Auburn University College of Veterinary Medicine. **C** and **D** courtesy Pamela Eller, University of Colorado Health Sciences Center.]

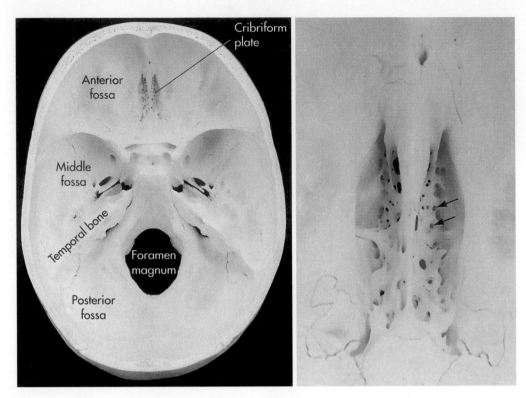

FIGURE 13-9
Cribriform plate of the ethmoid bone, as seen from inside a human skull. Olfactory fila pass through small holes *(arrows)* in the plate to reach the olfactory bulb.

bound to an **odorant-binding protein** in the mucus, and stimulate the chemosensitive cilia of the olfactory receptors.

The unmyelinated axons of the olfactory receptors are among the finest (only 0.2 μm in diameter) and most slowly conducting (0.1 m/sec) axons in the entire nervous system. They collect into a series of about 20 small bundles, the **olfactory fila** (from the Latin *filum* meaning "thread"), which pass through the holes in the cribriform plate of the ethmoid bone (Figure 13-9) and end in the **olfactory bulb.** Collectively the olfactory fila make up the first cranial nerve.

Olfactory receptors are unique among mammalian neurons in that they, like taste receptor cells, are replaced throughout life. Individual receptors have a life span of a month or two, and new receptors arise from undifferentiated basal cells of the olfactory epithelium. No one is quite sure how the axons of such newly formed receptors find their way to the proper synaptic sites in the olfactory bulb.

Olfactory receptor neurons utilize a large number of G protein–coupled receptors to detect a wide range of odors

Distinguishing 10,000 different odors is no mean feat. This is much larger, for example, than the number of tones we can hear or colors we can see, and has long been taken to imply that there are many kinds of olfactory receptor neurons. Recent work has confirmed this, indicating that

there are hundreds, perhaps as many as 1000, closely related olfactory receptor proteins. Each olfactory receptor neuron probably manufactures only one of these proteins, so there may be as many as 1000 different kinds of olfactory receptor neurons. In contrast to the situation in taste receptor cells, however, olfactory receptor neurons apparently all use the same transduction mechanism. All of the olfactory receptor proteins are coupled to G proteins and are structurally similar to other G protein–coupled receptors, such as postsynaptic receptor molecules and rhodopsin in retinal photoreceptors (see Chapter 17). Each olfactory receptor protein binds an array of odorants, an array overlapping but somewhat different from the array bound by other olfactory receptor proteins. This extraordinary diversity of receptor proteins presumably reflects the antiquity and evolutionary importance of olfaction: upwards of 1% of our entire genome is devoted to the specification of olfactory receptor proteins!

The second-messenger cascade set in motion by the binding of an appropriate odorant causes the opening of a cation channel (Figure 13-10). The resulting influx of Na^+ and Ca^{2+} ions produces a depolarizing receptor potential that, if large enough, initiates action potentials in the trigger zone of the receptor neuron (Figure 13-11). The receptor potential soon adapts in most olfactory receptor neurons (Figure 13-12), even if odorant concentration remains constant. This is part of the basis for the common experience of rapidly fading perception of maintained odors.

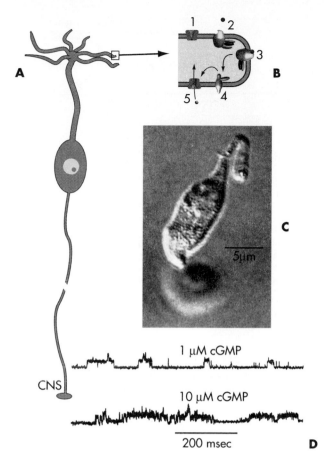

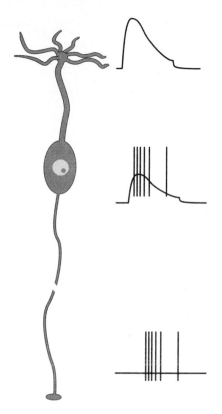

FIGURE 13-10

Chemosensory transduction in olfactory receptor cells. The tip of one chemosensory cilium from the olfactory receptor neuron shown schematically in **A** is enlarged in **B.** Binding of odorant to a G protein–coupled receptor *(2)* sets in motion one or more second-messenger processes *(3, 4)*, resulting in influx of Na⁺ and Ca²⁺ *(5)* through normally closed cation channels *(1)*. Olfactory receptor cation channels are directly gated by the cyclic nucleotides cyclic AMP and cyclic GMP *(cGMP)*. Individual channels can be seen opening and closing **(D)** during application of cyclic GMP, using patch-clamp electrodes applied to single, isolated human olfactory receptor neurons **(C)**. (**C** and **D** from Thüraüf N et al: Cyclic-nucleotide-gated channels in identified human olfactory receptor neurons, *Eur J Neurosci* 8:2080, 1996.)

Olfactory Information Bypasses the Thalamus on Its Way to the Cerebral Cortex

The olfactory bulb develops as an outgrowth from the telencephalon. As a result the olfactory nerve is unique in that it reaches the ipsilateral cerebral hemisphere and does so directly, without a relay in the thalamus. However, the thalamus is part of subsequent stages of olfactory circuitry.

The olfactory nerve terminates in the olfactory bulb

Animals that depend heavily on their sense of smell (called **macrosmatic** animals; from the Greek *osme* meaning "odor") have a well-developed central olfactory apparatus, including a neatly laminated olfactory bulb. In **micros-**

FIGURE 13-11

Transmission of electrical information in olfactory receptor neurons. Receptor potentials produced in chemosensory cilia in response to odorants spread passively through the cell body to the axon initial segment. Action potentials generated there are propagated along the axon and reach synaptic endings in the olfactory bulb.

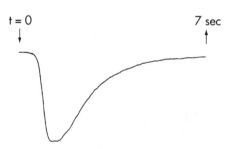

FIGURE 13-12

Adaptation in olfactory receptor neurons, shown by patch-clamp recording of the current flow into a single neuron during continuous application of a mixture of odorants *(arrows)*. Even though the odorant mixture was present continuously for 7 seconds, the current flow was transient. (From Firestein S, Shepherd GM, Werblin FS: Time course of the membrane current underlying sensory transduction in salamander olfactory receptor neurones, *J Physiol* 430:135, 1990.)

matic humans, this lamination is not as apparent, and the olfactory bulb is relatively small and poorly developed. Its most prominent cell type is the **mitral cell,** which has a triangular cell body and was named for its fancied resemblance to a bishop's miter. A mitral cell is configured like a typical cortical pyramidal cell in reverse (compare Figures 1-4, *E* and 13-13); an axon emerges from the pointed side of the pyramid and moves toward the interior of the

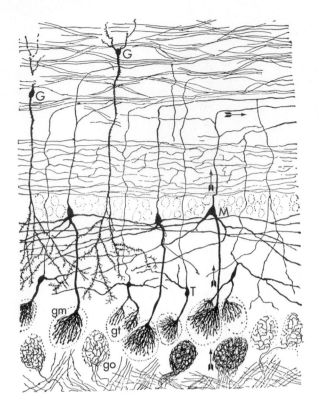

FIGURE 13-13
Glomeruli and neurons of the olfactory bulb. For clarity, most glomeruli in this drawing contain only one type of neural process, either axon terminals of olfactory receptor neurons (*go*), dendrites of mitral cells (*gm*), or dendrites of tufted cells (*gt*). In reality, each glomerulus contains all of these, together with processes of interneurons. *G*, Granule cells; *M*, mitral cells; *T*, tufted cells. (From Ramón y Cajal S: *Histologie du système nerveux de l'homme et des vertébrés,* Paris, 1909, 1911, Maloine.)

bulb to enter the **olfactory tract,** whereas a dendrite emerges from the broad side, ascends to the surface of the bulb, and receives contacts from the incoming axons of olfactory receptors. These dendrites spread out in large spherical arborizations 100 to 200 μm in diameter called **glomeruli.** Olfactory axons terminate in these glomeruli with a great deal of convergence. There are about 1000 glomeruli in each olfactory bulb, and all of the thousands of olfactory receptor neurons that express a given receptor protein project to just one or two of them (Figure 13-14). Hence different odorants activate different collections of glomeruli, which in turn apparently signals the identity of an odorant. The olfactory bulb also contains interneurons (many of them called **granule cells** here as in other regions of the CNS) and a collection of **tufted cells,** which are smaller than mitral cells but also send their dendrites into the glomeruli and their axons into the olfactory tract. The olfactory bulb, like other sensory relays in the CNS, also receives a contingent of efferent fibers that are assumed to regulate or tune its sensitivity in some way. Some are norepinephrine and serotonin inputs from the locus ceruleus and raphe nuclei, similar to those received by other CNS areas. Most, however, arise from

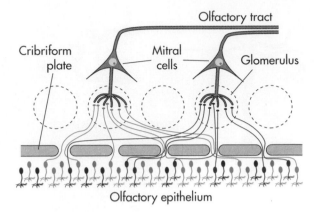

FIGURE 13-14
Sorting of olfactory nerve fibers among glomeruli of the olfactory bulb. Olfactory receptors of different types, each type characterized by one or a few receptor proteins and a restricted range of odor sensitivities (here represented as different colors), are intermingled with each other in a given area of olfactory epithelium. The axon terminals of any given type all converge on one or two glomeruli (which in reality would contain thousands of axon terminals and the dendrites of dozens of mitral and tufted cells).

the **anterior perforated substance** or from the **anterior olfactory nucleus,** a collective name for clusters of cells scattered all along the olfactory tract.

The olfactory bulb projects to olfactory cortex

Axons of mitral and tufted cells proceed caudally in the olfactory tract, giving off collaterals to cells of the anterior olfactory nucleus along the way. Fibers from the anterior olfactory nucleus then project back through the olfactory tracts to both olfactory bulbs (Figure 13-15); crossing fibers do so through the anterior part of the anterior commissure. At the posterior end of the orbital frontal cortex, where the olfactory tract attaches to the base of the brain, some of its fibers end in the anterior perforated substance. (This area forms a distinct elevation called the **olfactory tubercle** in many animals. It is not very obvious in humans but is often referred to as the olfactory tubercle anyway.) Remaining fibers curve laterally as the **lateral olfactory tract** (Figure 13-16, *B*), the principal central projection pathway for the olfactory system.

The lateral olfactory tract travels along the edge of the anterior perforated substance, near the surface of an unusually thin layer of cerebral cortex. When it reaches the lateral border of the anterior perforated substance, it curves up onto the surface of the temporal lobe in the vicinity of the uncus and its remaining fibers disperse and terminate. Along this course from the olfactory bulb, fibers of the olfactory tract end in two general places (Figure 13-15): the primary olfactory cortex and a portion of the amygdala. The primary olfactory cortex consists of the cortex adjacent to the lateral olfactory tract (called **piriform cortex**), an area of cortex covering part of the amygdala (**periamygdaloid cortex**) and a small, anterior region of the parahippocampal gyrus. In addition, the an-

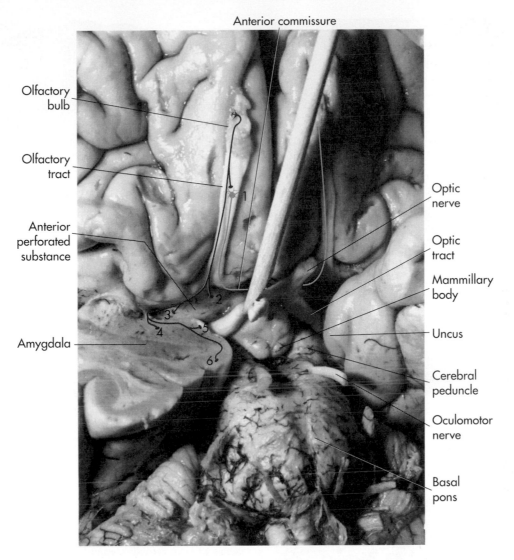

Anterior commissure

Olfactory
bulb

Olfactory
tract

Anterior
perforated
substance

Amygdala

Optic
nerve

Optic
tract

Mammillary
body

Uncus

Cerebral
peduncle

Oculomotor
nerve

Basal
pons

FIGURE 13-15
Central projections of the olfactory bulb. Fibers of the olfactory tract terminate in the anterior olfactory nucleus (*1*), olfactory tubercle (*2*), piriform cortex (*3*), part of the amygdala (*4*), periamygdaloid cortex (*5*), and a small anterior portion of the parahippocampal gyrus (*6*; specifically, a part of the entorhinal cortex, as described further in Chapter 23).

terior olfactory nucleus and olfactory tubercle have a cortexlike structure in many animals and are often included as part of the primary olfactory cortex. These primary receiving sites for olfactory information project in turn to the hypothalamus, to limbic structures such as the hippocampus and the rest of the amygdala, and to the thalamus (Figure 13-17).

Olfactory information reaches other cortical areas via the thalamus

The olfactory system is unique in that no thalamic relay is interposed between receptors and cerebral cortex. However, in this case the initial cortical destination is a distinctive, thin area of cortex (called **paleocortex,** for reasons explained in Chapter 22). The thalamus does become involved in the pathway from olfactory bulb to olfactory association cortex. One such area is located posteriorly on

the orbital surface of the frontal lobe, extending onto the anterior insula (adjacent to gustatory cortex). The primary olfactory cortex sends information to this cortical area through a relay in the thalamus (the **dorsomedial nucleus;** see Chapter 16), as well as through direct projections. The net result of this sequence of connections is that olfactory receptor neurons, like taste buds, wind up represented in the ipsilateral cerebral hemisphere. Hence the chemical senses are at the opposite end of a spectrum from somatic sensory and motor systems, in which a given part of the body is represented primarily in the contralateral cerebral hemisphere. Other sensory systems are somewhere in between, as in the partly crossed–partly uncrossed representation of each ear (see Chapter 14) and eye (see Chapter 17).

Neurons of the olfactory bulb and primary olfactory cortex, like neurons in early stages of the gustatory system, respond to multiple odorants. Neurons of olfactory asso-

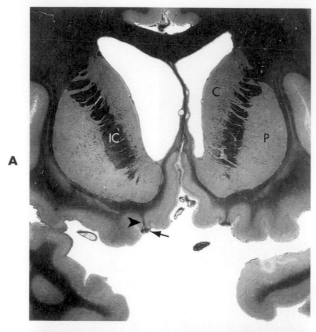

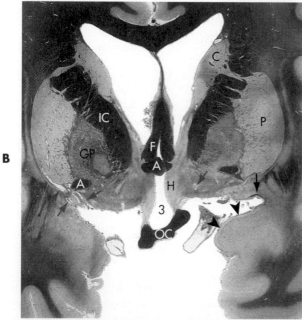

FIGURE 13-16
Course of the lateral olfactory tract. **A,** Near the site where the olfactory tract *(arrow)* attaches to the base of the brain, fibers *(arrowhead)* that arose in the anterior olfactory nucleus leave and move toward the anterior commissure (or arrive from the contralateral anterior olfactory nucleus). **B,** Just posterior to the level of **A,** the lateral olfactory tract *(arrow)* curves ventrally onto the surface of the temporal lobe, headed for the periamygdaloid cortex *(arrowheads)* and other targets indicated in Figure 13-15. This section passes through the anterior perforated substance, named for the many small perforating or ganglionic arteries that penetrate the brain in this area *(colored arrows)*. *3,* Third ventricle; *A,* anterior commissure; *C,* caudate nucleus; *F,* fornix; *GP,* globus pallidus; *H,* hypothalamus; *IC,* internal capsule; *P,* putamen.

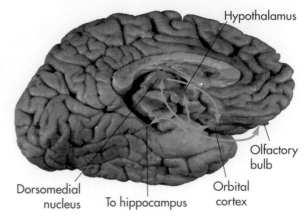

FIGURE 13-17
Projections of the primary olfactory cortex.

ciation cortex, like those of gustatory association cortex, are more likely to respond only to selected stimuli. Areas of orbital cortex have even been found in which neurons respond to the smell or the taste or the sight of a particular kind of food.

Conductive and Sensorineural Problems Can Affect Olfactory Function

Although our sense of smell is exquisitely sensitive and allows some remarkable discriminations, it is less well developed in humans (and less important in everyday life) than in many other species. Someone deprived of the sense of smell (i.e., rendered **anosmic**) by disease or injury is likely to complain less of loss of olfaction than of a taste disorder. (As noted earlier, much of what we attribute to our sense of taste actually depends on the aromas of what we eat and drink.) However, testing olfaction can sometimes provide useful diagnostic clues. For example, tumors growing at the base of the skull beneath the orbital surface of the frontal lobe can become quite large before they cause any symptoms other than unilateral anosmia.

Two general kinds of processes can disrupt the sense of smell: processes that prevent odorants from reaching the olfactory epithelium (**conductive** olfactory deficit) and processes that damage olfactory receptor neurons or parts of the olfactory CNS (**sensorineural** olfactory deficit). Conductive olfactory deficits can be caused by things like nasal polyps, septal deviations, and inflammations. Sensorineural olfactory deficits are most commonly a consequence of head injuries or neurodegenerative conditions such as Parkinson's or Alzheimer's diseases. The olfactory fila may be torn loose from the olfactory bulb as a consequence of head trauma and be unable to regrow through a scarred cribriform plate, or olfactory areas at the base of the brain may be damaged by slight movement of the brain across the base of the skull. In addition, for unknown reasons some patients suffer permanent damage to olfactory receptor neurons after a severe upper respiratory infection.

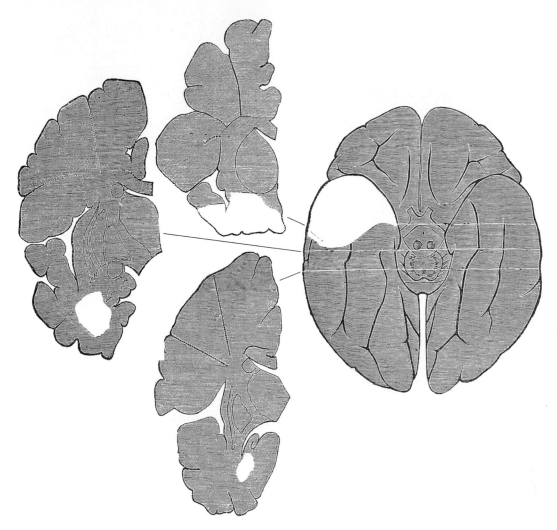

FIGURE 13-18

A classic case of uncinate seizures. A 53-year-old woman began to have spells during which she would have hallucinations of a small woman "who was rather agreeable and was always flitting about the kitchen; she always saw the same woman in every paroxysm. She never thought it was anything but a vision, but was very worried about it." At the same time she would have illusions of very unpleasant odors, variously described as "burning dirty stuff" or a "nasty dreadful smell," and a feeling of suffocation. Between the seizures her sense of smell was intact bilaterally. Subsequently she developed weakness and somatosensory changes on the left, and died. At autopsy "a tumour the size of a tangerine orange" was found that occupied the indicated parts of her brain. (From Jackson JH, Beevor CE: Case of tumour of the right temporo-sphenoidal lobe bearing on the localisation of the sense of smell and on the interpretation of a particular variety of epilepsy, *Brain* 12:346, 1889.)

Patients with anosmia of sensorineural origin are likely to have an intact common chemical sense and be able to perceive a range of volatile substances such as ammonia or menthol, most but not all of which are irritating.*

Conversely, *excess* activity in olfactory structures can also cause disturbances. Piriform cortex has been directly identified as functionally important olfactory cortex in humans because electrical stimulation there causes olfactory sensations. Clues pointing in the same direction were provided in the nineteenth century by the British neurologist Hughlings Jackson, who noted that seizures originating in the vicinity of the uncus may begin with an illusion of smell or taste, most often an unpleasant one (Figure 13-18). The seizure may go on to include motor phenomena such as chewing movements or smacking of the lips and alterations of consciousness such as a "dreamy state" or a feeling of déjà vu. Seizures of this type are still known as **uncinate seizures.**

SUGGESTED READINGS

Axel R: The molecular logic of smell, *Sci Am* 273(4):154, 1995.

Barlow LA, Chien C-B, Northcutt RG: Embryonic taste buds develop in the absence of innervation, *Devel* 122:1103, 1996.

Beckstead RM, Morse JR, Norgren R: The nucleus of the solitary tract in the monkey: projections to the thalamus and brain stem nuclei, *J Comp Neurol* 190:259, 1980.

Beckstead RM, Norgren R: An autoradiographic examination of the central distribution of the trigeminal, facial, glossopharyngeal and vagal nerves in the monkey, *J Comp Neurol* 184:455, 1979.

Beidler LM, Smallman RL: Renewal of cells within taste buds, *J Cell Biol* 27:263, 1965.

---

*Hence substances like these are *not* useful for testing olfaction, and common odorants such as coffee are used instead.

Buck L, Axel R: A novel multigene family may encode odorant receptors: a molecular basis for odor recognition, *Cell* 65:175, 1991. *The initial description of the very large family of genes now thought to code olfactory receptor proteins.*

Chaudhari N et al: The taste of monosodium glutamate: membrane receptors in taste buds, *J Neurosci* 16:3817, 1996. *Evidence that some taste cells have G protein–coupled glutamate receptors in their membranes, and that these receptors are involved in tasting MSG.*

Collings VB: Human taste response as a function of locus of stimulation on the tongue and soft palate, *Percep Psychophys* 16:169, 1974.

Deems DA et al: Smell and taste disorders: a study of 750 patients from the University of Pennsylvania Smell and Taste Center, *Arch Otolaryngol Head Neck Surg* 117:519, 1991. *Although 66% of the patients complained of a taste deficit, fewer than 4% actually had one.*

Doty RL, editor: *Handbook of olfaction and gustation*, New York, 1995, Marcel Dekker, Inc. *A recent, extensive review of both basic and clinical aspects of the chemical senses.*

Doty RL et al: Olfactory dysfunction in patients with head trauma, *Arch Neurol* 54:1131, 1997.

Eichenbaum H et al: Selective olfactory deficits in case H.M., *Brain* 106:459, 1983. *H.M. is a famous patient who had the anterior parts of both temporal lobes removed. A severe memory impairment resulted, as discussed in Chapter 23. In addition, he lost his ability to identify odors, even though his ability to detect odors was unimpaired.*

Finger TE, Silver WL: *Neurobiology of taste and smell*, New York, 1987, John Wiley & Sons. *A review of the comparative anatomy and physiology of the chemical senses.*

Gonzalez C et al: Carotid body chemoreceptors: from natural stimuli to sensory discharges, *Physiol Rev* 74:829, 1994. *One example of the array of chemoreceptors of which we are not consciously aware.*

Graziadei PPC, Monti Graziadei GA: Neurogenesis and neuron regeneration in the olfactory system of mammals. I. Morphological aspects of differentiation and structural organization of the olfactory sensory neurons, *J Neurocytol* 8:1, 1979.

Henkin RI, Christiansen RL: Taste localization on the tongue, palate and pharynx of normal man, *J Appl Physiol* 22:316, 1967.

Höfer D, Püschel B, Drenkhahn D: Taste receptor-like cells in the rat gut identified by expression of α-gustducin, *Proc Natl Acad Sci* 93:6631, 1996. *The same transduction mechanisms used by taste receptor cells may be used for local signaling by cells in the intestinal wall.*

Hughlings Jackson J, Beevor CE: Case of tumour of the right temporo-sphenoidal lobe bearing on the localisation of the sense of smell and on the interpretation of a particular variety of epilepsy, *Brain* 12:346, 1889.

Imfeld TM, Schroeder HE: Palatal taste buds in man: topographical arrangement in islands of keratinized epithelium, *Anat Embryol* 185:259, 1992.

Jean A: Brainstem organization of the swallowing network, *Brain Behav Evol* 25:109, 1984.

Kinnamon SC, Cummings TA: Chemosensory transduction mechanisms in taste, *Ann Rev Physiol* 54:715, 1992.

Lalonde ER, Eglitis JA: Number and distribution of taste buds on the epiglottis, pharynx, larynx, soft palate and uvula in a human newborn, *Anat Rec* 140:91, 1961.

Lawrence C: Dysgeusia ("cognate, dis-gusting"), *Lancet* 348:1102, 1996. *A first-person account of the distorted and disagreeable sensations that can accompany diminution of taste.*

McRitchie DA, Törk I: The internal organization of the human solitary nucleus, *Brain Res Bull* 31:171, 1993.

Menini A, Picco C, Firestein S: Quantal-like current fluctuations induced by odorants in olfactory receptor cells, *Nature* 373:435, 1995. *Preliminary physiological evidence that olfactory receptor cells can respond to the binding of a single odorant molecule.*

Miller IJ Jr: Variation in human fungiform taste bud densities among regions and subjects, *Anat Rec* 216:474, 1986.

Miller IJ Jr, Reedy FE Jr: Variations in human taste bud density and taste intensity perception, *Physiol Behav* 47:1213, 1990.

Mombaerts P et al: Visualizing an olfactory sensory map, *Cell* 87:675, 1996. *Technically elegant experiments providing a visual demonstration of the convergence of a multitude of olfactory neurons with the same putative receptor protein onto just two glomeruli.*

Moran DT et al: The fine structure of the olfactory mucosa in man, *J Neurocytol* 11:721, 1982.

Mori K, Yoshihara Y: Molecular recognition and olfactory processing in the mammalian olfactory system, *Prog Neurobiol* 45:585, 1995.

Morrison EE, Costanzo RM: Morphology of the human olfactory epithelium, *J Comp Neurol* 297:1, 1990.

Nakamura T, Gold GH: A cyclic nucleotide-gated conductance in olfactory receptor cilia, *Nature* 325:442, 1987. *"These data suggest a remarkable similarity between the mechanisms of olfactory and visual transduction and indicate considerable conservation of sensory transduction mechanisms."*

Norgren R: Gustatory system. In Paxinos G, editor: *The human nervous system*, San Diego, 1990, Academic Press.

Price JL: Olfactory system. In Paxinos G, editor: *The human nervous system*, San Diego, 1990, Academic Press.

Price JL, Slotnick BM: Dual olfactory representation in the rat thalamus: an anatomical and electrophysiological study, *J Comp Neurol* 215:63, 1983.

Rolls ET, Baylis LL: Gustatory, olfactory, and visual convergence within the primate orbitofrontal cortex, *J Neurosci* 14:5437, 1994.

Schiffman SS: Taste and smell losses in normal aging and disease, *JAMA* 278:1357, 1997.

Schul R, Slotnick BM, Dudai Y: Flavor and the frontal cortex, *Behav Neurosci* 110:760, 1996.

Scott TR et al: Gustatory responses in the nucleus tractus solitarius of the alert cynomolgus monkey, *J Neurophysiol* 55:182, 1986.

Seiden AM, editor: *Taste and smell disorders*, New York, 1997, Thieme Medical Publishers.

Shepherd GM, Greer CA: Olfactory bulb. In Shepherd GM, editor: *The synaptic organization of the brain*, ed 4, New York, 1998, Oxford University Press.

Shikama Y et al: Localization of the gustatory pathway in the human midbrain, *Neurosci Lett* 218:198, 1996.

Slotnick BM, Kaneko N: Role of mediodorsal thalamic nucleus in olfactory discrimination learning in rats, *Science* 214:91, 1981.

Stone LM et al: Taste receptor cells arise from local epithelium, not neurogenic ectoderm, *Proc Natl Acad Sci* 92:1916, 1995.

Torre V et al: Transduction and adaptation in sensory receptor cells, *J Neurosci* 15:7757, 1995. *A nice discussion of unifying themes in the transduction mechanisms used by different kinds of receptors.*

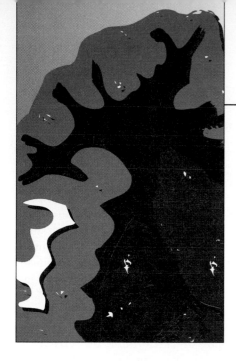

HEARING AND BALANCE: THE EIGHTH CRANIAL NERVE

Hearing and balance functionally are very different senses, but they begin peripherally in very similar ways. The eighth cranial nerve carries two special sensory components, one in a **cochlear division** and one in a **vestibular division.** Both divisions innervate elaborate end organs containing specialized mechanoreceptors (called **hair cells** because of their appearance), but the end organs are such that the two divisions respond to different types of mechanical stimuli. The cochlear division carries information about sound, whereas the vestibular division signals position and movement of the head.

AUDITORY AND VESTIBULAR RECEPTOR CELLS ARE LOCATED IN THE WALLS OF THE MEMBRANOUS LABYRINTH

The structures innervated by the eighth nerve are embedded in the temporal bone (Figure 14-1), where the receptor cells form parts of the walls of a convoluted, membranous tube that is suspended within a bony tube (Figure 14-2).

The Membranous Labyrinth Is Suspended Within the Bony Labyrinth, a Cavity in the Temporal Bone

The walls of the bony tube are formed by the hardest bone in the body—the petrous ("rocklike") portion of the temporal bone. Because the tube consists of so many twists and turns, it is called the **bony labyrinth.** The coiled **cochlea** (Latin for "snail shell") extends anteriorly from an enlargement called the **vestibule,** to which three **semicircular canals** are attached. The **membranous labyrinth,** the membranous tube suspended within the bony labyrinth, mostly follows the same contours (Figure 14-2). Hence there is a **cochlear duct** within the bony cochlea and a **semicircular duct** within each semicircular canal. However, the vestibule contains two enlargements of the membranous labyrinth, the **utricle** (to which the semicircular ducts attach) and the **saccule** (which is connected to the cochlear duct).

The bony labyrinth is filled with **perilymph,** which is similar in composition to CSF (and therefore to extracellular fluid generally; that is, low K^+ concentration and high

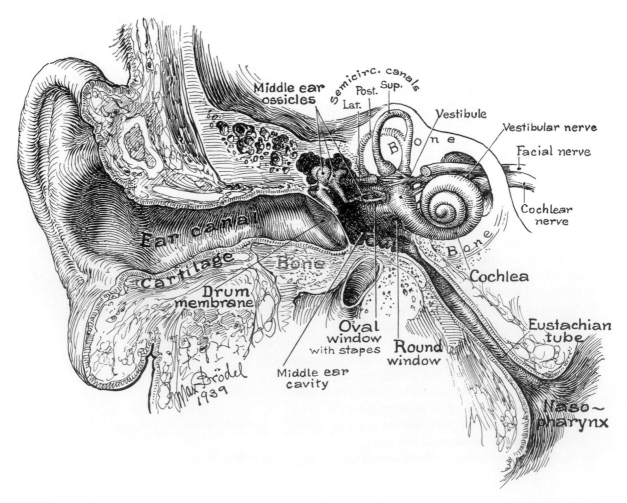

FIGURE 14-1
The outer, middle, and inner ears, showing the bony labyrinth embedded in the temporal bone. The semicircular canals labeled "lateral" and "superior" in this drawing are called *horizontal* and *anterior*, respectively, in this chapter. (From Brödel M: *Three unpublished drawings of the anatomy of the human ear,* Philadelphia, 1946, WB Saunders.)

Na$^+$ concentration); the subarachnoid space around the brain is actually continuous with the perilymphatic space of the bony labyrinth through a tiny canal in the temporal bone. The membranous labyrinth, in contrast, is filled with **endolymph,** a peculiar fluid that is similar in ionic composition to intracellular fluids (that is, high K$^+$ concentration and low Na$^+$ concentration). As might be expected from this difference in fluid composition, the membranous labyrinth is a continuous, closed system in which every part communicates with every other part (like CSF in the ventricles). A system of tight junctions joins the cells in the walls of the membranous labyrinth, forming a diffusion barrier between endolymph and perilymph. The receptor cells of the labyrinth (hair cells) form part of this diffusion barrier and, as discussed a little later in this chapter, the resulting voltage and concentration gradients across parts of their membranes are important in the transduction process.

Endolymph is actively secreted, circulates through the membranous labyrinth, and is reabsorbed

Endolymph is produced continuously by specialized cells in several locations in the membranous labyrinth, using an active pumping mechanism that results in a positive electrical potential inside the membranous labyrinth. Much like CSF, endolymph has a path of circulation and reabsorption. It flows from the semicircular ducts into the utricle and from the cochlear duct into the saccule. The ducts interconnecting the utricle and saccule meet in a Y-shaped junction, through which endolymph flows into the **endolymphatic duct,** leaves the labyrinth, and reaches the **endolymphatic sac** in the dura covering the temporal bone, where it is reabsorbed. Just as obstruction of CSF flow causes expansion of the ventricles and neurological symptoms, obstruction of endolymph flow causes ballooning of the membranous labyrinth and otological symptoms. **Ménière's disease** is characterized by transient attacks of vertigo, nausea, and hearing loss accompanied by ringing in the ears **(tinnitus),** and its defining anatomical feature is swelling of the membranous labyrinth (referred to as **endolymphatic hydrops**). Although there are probably multiple etiologies of Ménière's disease, many cases are thought to be caused by defective circulation or absorption of endolymph.

Auditory and Vestibular Receptors Are Hair Cells

Hair cells of the labyrinth were named for the array of a hundred or so specialized microvilli that project as a bundle from one end of the cell into the endolymphatic interior of the membranous labyrinth (Figure 14-3); the other end of the hair cell synapses on peripheral processes of eighth nerve fibers, which in turn convey auditory and

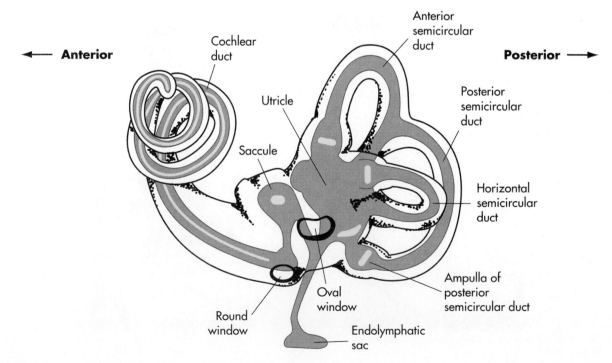

FIGURE 14-2

Membranous labyrinth of the left ear as seen through an outline of the bony labyrinth. Pale green areas indicate the locations of patches or strips of hair cells in the wall of the membranous labyrinth. The endolymphatic sac is located beneath the dura on the surface of the temporal bone. It contains no receptor cells but rather is the principal site of absorption of endolymph. [Modified from Warwick R, Williams PLW, editors: *Gray's anatomy*, Br ed 35, Philadelphia, 1973, WB Saunders.]

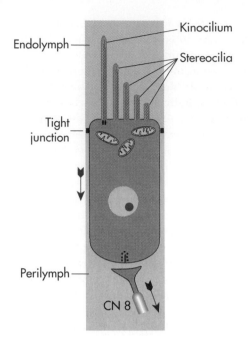

FIGURE 14-3
Schematic view of a typical hair cell. Tight junctions near the microvillar end of the cell join the hair cell to neighboring supporting cells and form part of the diffusion barrier between endolymph and perilymph (Figures 14-4 and 14-12). Hence each hair cell is bathed partly in endolymph and partly in perilymph. Transduction channels are located near the tips of the stereocilia, and *arrows* indicate the direction of information flow.

vestibular information to the CNS. Hair cell microvilli, somewhat illogically referred to as **stereocilia,** are arranged asymmetrically: they are lined up in graduated rows, so that the tallest are toward one side of the hair cell. Adjacent to the tallest stereocilia of each hair cell in the semicircular ducts, utricle, and saccule is a single true cilium, the **kinocilium.** Cochlear hair cells have kinocilia that degenerate during fetal development, indicating that these processes play no essential role in the transduction process; kinocilia may instead be important for establish-

Table 14-1	Locations and Functions of Hair Cells			
Location of hair cells	Part of labyrinth	Gelatinous material	Stimulus transduced
Organ of Corti	Cochlea	Tectorial membrane	Sound
Cristae	Semicircular ducts	Cupula	Angular acceleration
Maculae	Utricle, saccule	Otolithic membrane	Linear acceleration

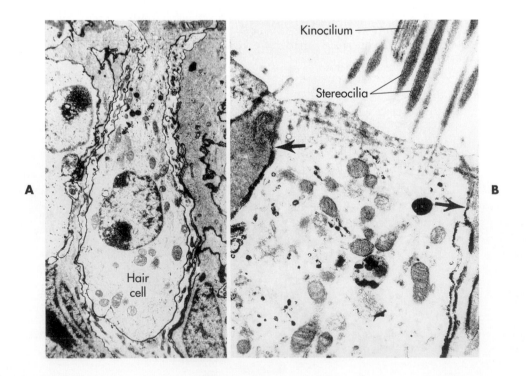

FIGURE 14-4
Part of the membranous labyrinth of a guinea pig after a tracer substance (horseradish peroxidase) had been injected into the cisterna magna. **A,** Electron micrograph of the saccular macula; dark reaction product outlines all the cellular elements of the macula. **B,** Higher-magnification micrograph of the apical end of the hair cell shown in **A;** reaction product fills extracellular space up to, but not beyond, junctional complexes *(arrows)* that separate the perilymphatic and endolymphatic spaces. (Courtesy Dr. David L. Asher.)

ing the anatomical asymmetry of hair cells, or for some mechanical connections of the hair cells in which they persist.

Hair cells are grouped into six discrete clusters in different parts of the labyrinth (Figure 14-2, Table 14-1), and fundamental aspects of the arrangement of each cluster are the same. The stereocilia of the hair cells (and the kinocilium, when present) protrude into the endolymphatic space inside the membranous labyrinth and are associated with a specialized mass of gelatinous material, one for each cluster of hair cells. Typically the association is a physical connection. Movement of the gelatinous mass relative to the hair cells causes deflection of stereocilia that in turn causes a receptor potential, through a transduction mechanism described a little later.

In sections through the labyrinth (e.g., Figure 14-9) it often looks as though the hair cells and associated structures are bathed in the endolymph that fills the membranous labyrinth. However, it has long been reasoned that this is unlikely because it would mean (among other things) that eighth nerve fibers reaching the bases of hair cells would also be passing through endolymph. Endolymph has such a high K^+ concentration that standard nerve fibers could not work in its presence. In fact, the real barrier between endolymph and perilymph is a series of tight junctions near the tops of the hair cells, between them and neighboring supporting cells. Because perilymph is continuous with the CSF of subarachnoid space, marker substances introduced into the cisterna magna infiltrate the sensory epithelia of the labyrinth and surround the hair cells, stopping only at the array of tight junctions (Figure 14-4). Hence the stereocilia and the apical surfaces of hair cells are exposed to endolymph, whereas other surfaces of the hair cells, as well as the nerve fibers they contact, are bathed in perilymph (Figure 14-9, *E*).

Hair cells have mechanosensitive transduction channels

Stereocilia are packed full of cross-linked actin filaments (Figure 14-5, *C*), which makes them rigid. In response to mechanical deformation they do not bend, but rather pivot at their bases where they are attached to the hair cell. Various linking molecules interconnect neighboring stereocilia, so the whole hair bundle moves as a unit in response to mechanical stimuli. Some of these links are symmetrical, connecting a given stereocilium to all of its neighbors. However, fine filamentous connections called **tip links** extend from the tip of each stereocilium only to its next tallest neighbor (Figure 14-5). Tip links are thought to have a special role in the transduction process, which (at least in a conceptual sense) is remarkably straightforward (Figure 14-6). A mechanically gated cation channel is located at one or both ends of each tip link and is normally open part of the time. Deflecting the hair bundle toward the tallest stereocilia stretches the tip

links, increasing the probability of channel opening. The channels are permeable to most small cations, and because K^+ ions are the most abundant cations in the endolymph they flow down the electrical gradient from the positive endolymph into the negative interior of the hair cells. The resulting inward K^+ current depolarizes the hair cells,[*] causes the opening of voltage-gated Ca^{2+} channels and increased release of transmitter onto eighth nerve endings. The excitatory transmitter (probably glutamate) then causes an increased firing frequency in the eighth nerve fibers. Deflecting the hair bundle in the opposite direction decreases the tension on the tip links; the transduction channels close, baseline K^+ current stops, the hair cells hyperpolarize, and transmitter release and firing rate diminish. Deflecting the hair bundle in a perpendicular direction (i.e., parallel to the rows of stereocilia) has no effect on the tip links and so does not cause a receptor potential.

Subtle differences in the physical arrangements of hair cells determine the stimuli to which they are most sensitive

Hair cells in all parts of the labyrinth use the same basic transduction mechanism, initiated by movement of a gelatinous mass and deflection of stereocilia. The critical variable in different parts of the labyrinth is the physical coupling between the gelatinous masses and the stereocilia. It is remarkable that variations in the way these gelatinous masses are made up and arranged, and the way in which different parts of the membranous labyrinth are suspended mechanically, allow some hair cells to respond to sound, others to head movement, and still others to head position.

THE COCHLEAR DIVISION OF THE EIGHTH NERVE CONVEYS INFORMATION ABOUT SOUND

The auditory system faces a basic mechanical problem because the sound vibrations that it must detect are propagated in air, whereas the auditory receptor cells (like other elements of the nervous system) live in a fluid-filled environment. Water is harder to move than air, and nearly all of the sound energy incident on a simple air-water interface is reflected. Fluids in small channels like the labyrinth are even harder to move, with the result that if the auditory receptor organ (the **organ of Corti**) and its fluid surroundings were mechanically coupled to the outside world by a simple

---

[*]Increased K^+ conductance in typical neurons causes K^+ efflux and hyperpolarization, reflecting the fact that the K^+ equilibrium potential is typically around -90 mv. However, because of the high K^+ concentration in endolymph, the K^+ equilibrium potential across the membranes of stereocilia is about 0 mv.

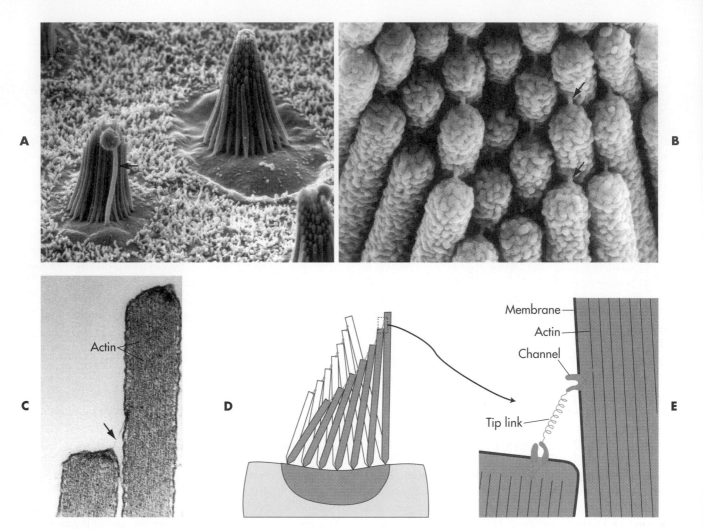

FIGURE 14-5

Stereocilia and tip links. **A,** Scanning electron micrograph of the tops of hair cells in the saccule of a bullfrog, showing the graduated arrays of stereocilia extending from each. Ajdacent to the tallest stereocilia is the single kinocilium *(arrow)*, which has a characteristic bulbous tip in this species. **B,** Higher-magnification micrograph of a group of stereocilia. Each stereocilium is connected to its next taller neighbor by a filamentous tip link *(arrows)*. **C,** Longitudinal transmission electron micrograph through parts of two stereocilia, showing the actin filaments filling them and the tip link interconnecting them. **D,** Apparent mechanism of action of stereocilia and tip links. Deflecting the hair bundle toward the tallest stereocilia stretches the tip links. As indicated in **E,** this stretch increases the probability of cation channels at one or both ends of the tip links being open. (Courtesy Drs. David Corey and G.M.G. Shepherd, Howard Hughes Medical Institute, Harvard Medical School.)

membrane, it would receive no more than 0.1% of the sound energy that fell on the membrane. One major task of the air-filled **outer** and **middle ears** (Figure 14-1) therefore is to transfer sound as efficiently as possible to the fluid-filled **inner ear.**

The Outer and Middle Ear Convey Air-Borne Vibrations to the Fluid-Filled Inner Ear

The outer ear is basically a complicated funnel consisting of the **auricle** (or **pinna**) and the **external auditory meatus** or **canal;** it conducts sound to the **tympanic membrane.** Sound-induced vibrations are transferred along a chain of three small bones, or **ossicles,** that traverse the middle ear cavity (an air-filled

cavity in the temporal bone). The handle of the **malleus** is attached to the medial surface of the tympanic membrane, so movements of this membrane are transferred directly to the malleus. The malleus in turn is attached to the **incus,** which is attached to the **stapes,** so sound-induced vibrations eventually reach the oval-shaped footplate of the stapes. The footplate of the stapes occupies a hole in the temporal bone called the **oval window;** on the other side of the oval window is the perilymph-filled vestibule of the bony labyrinth. The vestibule leads directly to the cochlea, which contains the organ of Corti. Thus vibration of the tympanic membrane ultimately results in movement of the fluids of the inner ear.

The chain of middle ear ossicles acts as a lever system with a small mechanical advantage, so a given force at the

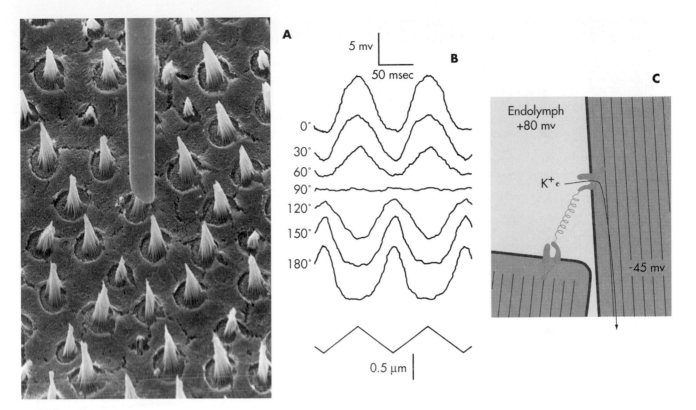

FIGURE 14-6

Transduction in hair cells. The otolithic membrane (Figure 14-25) was removed from the macula of a bullfrog's saccule; a glass micropipette was then slipped over a bundle of stereocilia (**A**) and used to wiggle it in various directions. **B**, Receptor potentials were simultaneously recorded using a second micropipette (not shown). The bottom trace indicates the time course of 0.5-μm movements, and the traces above show the dependence of the resulting receptor potentials on the direction of deflection. Movement toward the kinocilium (0°) produces a depolarizing receptor potential, movement away (180°) a hyperpolarizing receptor potential. Movement perpendicular to the plane of the tip links (90°) has no effect on the hair cell. **C**, Stretching a tip link opens cation channels in the stereocilia. Even though the K⁺ concentration in endolymph is about the same as that inside the stereocilia, the positive endolymphatic potential and the negative membrane potential of the hair cell combine to form a large electrical driving force that moves K⁺ ions through these open cation channels. (**A** and **B** from Shotwell SL, Jacobs R, Hudspeth AJ: Directional sensitivity of individual vertebrate hair cells to controlled deflection of their hair bundles, *Ann NY Acad Sci* 374:1, 1981. **C** modified from a drawing provided by Drs. David Corey and G.M.G. Shepherd, Howard Hughes Medical Institute, Harvard Medical School.)

tympanic membrane results in a slightly greater force at the footplate of the stapes. More importantly, the active, or moving, area of the tympanic membrane is about 15 times that of the footplate of the stapes. The net result of the mechanical advantage and the size difference is that stapedial vibrations have a much greater force *per unit area* of the footplate; this force is sufficient to move the perilymph, and more than 60% of the sound energy incident on the tympanic membrane is successfully transferred to the inner ear. Hence the middle ear apparatus acts as a transformer, much as an electrical transformer alters the voltage and current of a source to better match the requirements of a particular circuit. The effectiveness of this system is quite extraordinary. At threshold at 3000 Hz (the frequency to which we are most sensitive) the tympanic membrane moves a distance somewhat less than the diameter of a single hydrogen atom.★ By the time such a threshold vibra-

tion of the tympanic membrane reaches the cochlear hair cells it deflects their stereocilia through an angle of only about 0.003°. Bending the Empire State Building through an angle of 0.003° would deflect its top by less than an inch!★ From this threshold we can hear over a 10 million-fold range of sound pressure levels before sounds become painfully loud. (It is cumbersome to keep track of all the zeros in numbers like this so, as described in Box 14-1, a logarithmic **decibel** scale is used to express sound pressure levels.) In addition, although we are most sensitive at about 3000 Hz, the frequency range of human hearing in healthy young adults extends from about 20 Hz to 20,000 Hz (Box 14-1). All of this is accomplished with a surprisingly small number of nerve fibers: in contrast to the million or so axons in an optic nerve, there are only about 30,000 fibers in a human cochlear nerve. Somehow, analysis by the CNS of the information carried by these 30,000 fibers enables us to detect and interpret the myriad sounds of nature, music, and human language.

★This is as sensitive as an ear can usefully be made. Under ideal conditions in a very quiet setting, blood can actually be heard flowing through the vessels near the ear. If ears were much more sensitive, we would be distracted by hearing noise generated by air molecules colliding with the tympanic membrane!

★An Americanization of an Eiffel Tower analogy presented by A.J. Hudspeth in *Nature* 341:397, 1989.

Box 14-1   The Frequency and Intensity Range of Human Hearing

Because the range of sound levels over which we have useful hearing is so vast, a logarithmic scale has been devised to indicate the volume of one sound relative to some standard. The unit in this scale as originally defined is the **bel,** named for Alexander Graham Bell, the inventor of the telephone:

(14-1)

$$\text{intensity (in bels)} = \log \frac{I}{I_0}$$

where I is the intensity of the sound in question and I_0 is a reference intensity (usually the threshold for normal hearing).

Bels are large units, representing large changes in sound intensities, so tenths of bels, or **decibels (dB),** are used instead:

(14-2)

$$\text{intensity (in dB)} = 10\log \frac{I}{I_0}$$

In practice, it is much easier to measure the pressure level of a sound than its intensity. Because intensity is proportional to the square of the pressure, decibels are 20 times the log of the pressure ratio (seemingly contrary to the implication of the term *deci*bel):

(14-3)

$$dB = 10\log \frac{I}{I_0} = 10\log \frac{P^2}{P_0^2} = 20\log \frac{P}{P_0}$$

where P is the pressure of the sound in question and P_0 is a reference pressure (usually the threshold for normal hearing).

So a sound pressure level ten million times greater than threshold is 140 dB above threshold (Figure 14-7):

(14-3)

$$20\log \frac{10^7}{1} = 20 \times 7 = 140 \text{ dB}$$

Multiple mechanical properties of the outer, middle, and inner ear collaborate to determine the sensitivity of ears to sounds of various frequencies. The combined result of all these factors is that we are most sensitive in the 1000- to 3000-Hz range important for spoken language, somewhat less sensitive at higher frequencies, and much less sensitive at lower frequencies (Figure 14-8).

Decibel scale

0	Threshold of hearing
10	Rustle of leaves
20	Sound-treated studio
30	Very quiet room at home, whispered speech
40	Library
50	Very quiet office
60	Normal speech
70	Typical traffic noise
80	Typical factory noise
90	Subway train
100	Chain saw, loud orchestra
110	Personal stereo headphones
120	Threshold of discomfort, rock concert
130	Jet takeoff
140	Threshold of pain

FIGURE 14-7

The decibel levels (relative to the normal threshold of hearing) of a variety of sounds. (Courtesy Dr. Theodore J. Glattke, Department of Speech and Hearing Sciences, The University of Arizona.)

Two tiny muscles attached to the middle ear bones modulate the transmission of vibrations to the inner ear. One, the **tensor tympani,** is attached to the handle of the malleus; when it contracts, it increases the tension on the tympanic membrane and decreases the transmission of vibrations through the ossicular chain. The other muscle, the **stapedius,** is attached to the neck of the stapes; it too decreases the transmission of vibrations when it contracts. The tensor tympani receives motor innervation from the trigeminal nerve and the stapedius from the facial nerve; both muscles are involved in certain auditory reflexes to be described shortly.

The Cochlea Is the Auditory Part of the Labyrinth

The auditory part of the inner ear, like the vestibular part, consists of a portion of the endolymph-filled membranous labyrinth suspended within a portion of the perilymph-filled bony labyrinth.

The bony part is the cochlea, which coils through 2¾ turns from its relatively broad base to its apex. The cochlea lies on its side in the temporal bone, with its base facing medially and posteriorly (Figure 14-24), but for the sake of simplicity it is usually discussed as though it sits upright on its base. The cochlea has a core of spongy bone

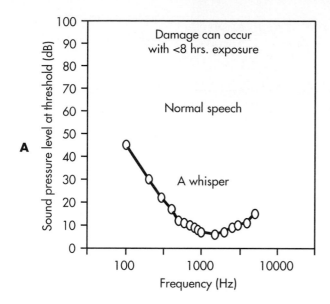

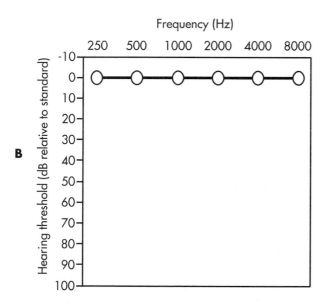

FIGURE 14-8
A, Variation of the threshold of hearing with sound frequency, expressed as decibels relative to the threshold sound pressure level at the most effective frequency. **B,** A normal audiogram obtained with an audiometer, which compensates for the frequency dependence in **A.** Readings displaced downward from this level (Figure 14-20) would indicate hearing loss (i.e., that a greater than normal sound pressure level was required for hearing at that frequency). (Courtesy Dr. Theodore J. Glattke, Department of Speech and Hearing Sciences, The University of Arizona.)

called the **modiolus,** from which the **osseous spiral lamina** projects like the threads of a screw (Figure 14-9). A winding cavity within the modiolus parallels the spiral lamina and houses the **spiral ganglion,** which contains the cell bodies of the primary auditory afferent fibers. The central processes of these cells collect at the base of the cochlea to form the cochlear division of the eighth nerve; the peripheral processes pass in bundles through a series of canals in the osseous spiral lamina to innervate the auditory receptors.

The cochlear duct (the auditory portion of the membranous labyrinth) is firmly anchored to the bony labyrinth in such a way that the duct is triangular in cross section (Figure 14-9, *C*). One corner of the triangle is attached to the osseous spiral lamina, and the other two corners are attached to the outer wall of the bony cochlea. The result is that the cochlear duct and osseous spiral lamina act as a partition between two perilymphatic spaces (except at the apex of the cochlea, where perilymph can pass from one space to the other through a small opening called the **helicotrema**). The perilymphatic space above the cochlear duct is called the **scala vestibuli** because it is directly continuous with the perilymph of the vestibule. The space below the cochlear duct is called the **scala tympani** because it ends blindly at the **secondary tympanic membrane** (or **round window membrane**). The space enclosed by the cochlear duct is filled with endolymph and is called the **scala media.** Each of the three walls of the cochlear duct has a different structure (Figure 14-9, *D*). The thin **vestibular** (or **Reissner's**) **membrane** borders the scala vestibuli and probably serves mainly as a barrier between the endolymph and perilymph, playing no great role in the mechanical properties of the cochlea. The **spiral ligament,** thickened periosteal tissue adhering to the outer wall of the bony cochlea, forms the second wall. It includes on its endolymph-facing surface the **stria vascularis,** a specialized area rich in capillaries that produces most of the endolymph in the membranous labyrinth. Finally, the **basilar membrane** spans the gap between the edge of the osseous spiral lamina and the spiral ligament, completing the "floor" of the cochlear duct and separating the scala media from the scala tympani.

Vibrations reaching the stapes footplate are transferred to the perilymph adjacent to the scala vestibuli. Although perilymph is incompressible, the round window membrane is elastic, allowing these vibrations to enter the labyrinth. When the stapes footplate moves inward, the round window membrane bulges out; when the footplate moves outward, the membrane is drawn inward. In the process, small quantities of perilymph are displaced within the cochlea. Most of this energy passes directly from the scala vestibuli to the scala tympani, deforming the cochlear duct (Figure 14-10). The cochlear duct contains the auditory receptors, and this deformation stimulates some of them. Static pressure changes and vibrations of very low frequency simply move a little perilymph through the helicotrema and do not deform the cochlear duct.

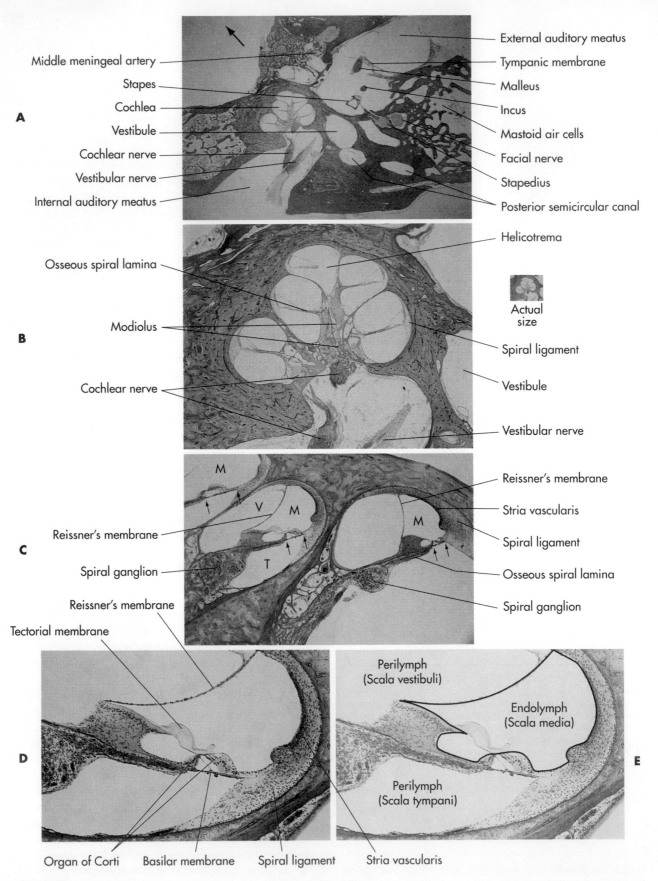

Middle meningeal artery
Stapes
Cochlea
Vestibule
Cochlear nerve
Vestibular nerve
Internal auditory meatus

External auditory meatus
Tympanic membrane
Malleus
Incus
Mastoid air cells
Facial nerve
Stapedius
Posterior semicircular canal

A

Osseous spiral lamina

Modiolus

Cochlear nerve

B

Helicotrema

Actual size

Spiral ligament

Vestibule

Vestibular nerve

C

M
V
M
M
T

Reissner's membrane
Spiral ganglion

Reissner's membrane
Stria vascularis
Spiral ligament
Osseous spiral lamina
Spiral ganglion

Reissner's membrane
Tectorial membrane

D

E

Perilymph (Scala vestibuli)
Endolymph (Scala media)
Perilymph (Scala tympani)

Organ of Corti   Basilar membrane   Spiral ligament   Stria vascularis

FIGURE 14-9

The temporal bone and cochlea. **A,** Horizontal section of the right temporal bone of a 39-year-old woman, shown at about 2.5 times actual size. The section was rotated slightly counterclockwise so that the orientation of the cochlea would correspond to that in other parts of the figure; anterior is indicated by the *arrow.* **B,** An enlarged view of the cochlea in **A. C,** One side of another human cochlea, cutting through the scala media (*M*) three times; the basal turn is toward the right, the apical turn toward the left. The width of the basilar membrane (*arrows*) increases progressively going from the base to the apex. *T,* Scala tympani; *V,* scala vestibuli. **D** and **E,** Enlargement of the scala media from the middle turn of the section in **C.** The dark line in **E** indicates the location of the band of junctional complexes that restrict diffusion between endolymph and perilymph. [**A** and **B** courtesy Dr. David L. Asher. **C-E** courtesy Dr. Allen L. Bell, Anatomy Department, University of New England College of Osteopathic Medicine.]

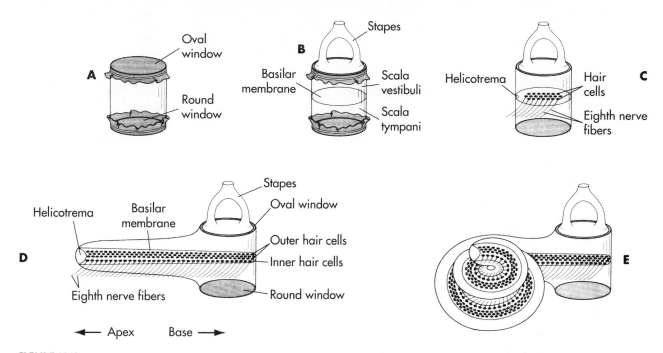

FIGURE 14-10

Building a cochlea, step by step. **A,** The bony cochlea represented as a rigid cylinder, its contents of perilymph, cochlear duct, and endolymph by fluid, and the oval and round windows by two elastic membranes; pushing on one of the membranes would displace some fluid and cause the other membrane to bulge out. **B,** Addition of a pistonlike stapes to push or pull on the oval window and of an interposed, elastic basilar membrane (representing the scala media). Now pushing on the stapes would displace not only the round window membrane, but also the basilar membrane. **C,** Addition of hair cells to the basilar membrane and of a helicotrema connecting the scala vestibuli and scala tympani. Pushing on the stapes quickly would still displace both the basilar and round window membranes, but a steady push or pull would cause perilymph to move slowly through the helicotrema and allow the basilar membrane to resume its initial position. **D,** Stretching out the basilar membrane and making it narrower near the oval and round windows provides an array of hair cells coupled to sections of the basilar membrane with differing resonant frequencies. **E,** Coiling up the elongated cochlea completes the model. (Redrawn from Kiang NYS: Stimulus representation in the discharge patterns of auditory neurons. In Tower DB, editor: *The nervous system,* vol 3, New York, 1975, Raven Press.)

Traveling waves in the basilar membrane stimulate hair cells in the organ of Corti, in locations that depend on sound frequency

Three basic parameters that must be encoded by the auditory system during its initial analysis of a sound are the intensity, frequency, and location of the stimulus. The intensity of a sound, like intensity in other sensory systems, is coded by the rate of action potential firing in populations of nerve fibers and by the numbers of nerve fibers responding. Frequency is indicated largely by the particular part of the organ of Corti that is most active, through a mechanism described in this section. Analysis of the location of a sound, as discussed a little later in this chapter, depends heavily on a comparison of sounds reaching the two ears and so is accomplished in the CNS.

The organ of Corti (Figures 14-11 and 14-12) is a strip of hair cells and supporting cells about 35 mm long that rests on the basilar membrane. The hair cells are arranged in two groups, a single row of about 3500 **inner hair cells** near the edge of the osseous spiral lamina and a band of about 15,000 **outer hair cells** three to five cells wide, directly above the flexible basilar membrane. The two groups are separated by a space called the **tunnel of**

Corti, through which the peripheral processes of eighth nerve fibers must pass on their way to the outer hair cells. The stereocilia of the outer hair cells are inserted into the gelatinous **tectorial membrane** so that vibration of the basilar membrane causes oscillations of the hairs and therefore oscillation of the membrane potential of the hair cells. Anatomical evidence indicates that the stereocilia of the inner hair cells are not attached to the tectorial membrane and that these hair cells may be stimulated directly by movement of endolymph within the cochlear duct.

A pressure pulse delivered to the scala vestibuli by movement of the stapes causes a **traveling wave** of deformation to move along the basilar membrane (Figure 14-13, *A* and *B*), much as waves spread from the site of a pebble dropping into a body of water. However, because the mechanical properties of the basilar membrane vary progressively along the length of the basilar membrane, the traveling wave reaches peak amplitude at a location that depends on the frequency of the stimulus. The basilar membrane is about 100 μm wide and relatively stiff at the base of the cochlea, and about 500 μm wide and relatively floppy at the apex (Figure 14-9, *C*). The entire basilar membrane responds to intense, low-frequency

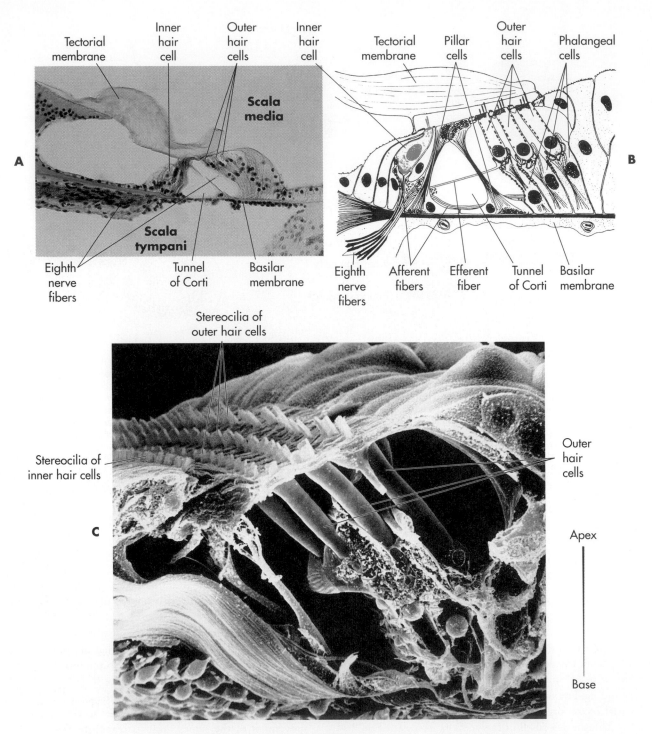

FIGURE 14-11

Structure of the organ of Corti. **A,** Light micrograph of a human organ of Corti (enlarged from Figure 14-9, *D*). **B,** Drawing of a cross section of the organ of Corti. Of the several types of supporting cells in the organ of Corti, two in particular make major contributions to its mechanical stability. The pillar cells produce microtubule-filled processes (Figure 14-12, *A*) that frame the tunnel of Corti. The phalangeal cells form cup-shaped, microtubule-filled structures that support the outer hair cells (Figure 14-12, *B*); thin processes of these cells also extend to the tops of the outer hair cells, where their platelike expansions fill the spaces between outer hair cells, forming the reticular lamina. **C,** Scanning electron micrograph of the organ of Corti of a guinea pig. The tectorial membrane has been removed, and the stereocilia of the three rows of outer hair cells can be seen protruding into scala media; normally these stereocilia would be embedded in the tectorial membrane. No inner hair cells are present in this view, but their stereocilia can also be seen protruding into scala media. The inset to the right of **C** shows the actual size of an unrolled basilar membrane. (**A** courtesy Dr. Allen L. Bell, Anatomy Department, University of New England College of Osteopathic Medicine. **B** from Northern JL: *Hearing disorders,* ed 2, Boston, 1984, Little, Brown & Co. **C** from Bredberg G. In Evans EF, Wilson JP, editors: *Psychophysics and physiology of hearing,* New York, 1977. © Academic Press, Inc. [London] Ltd.)

A   **B**

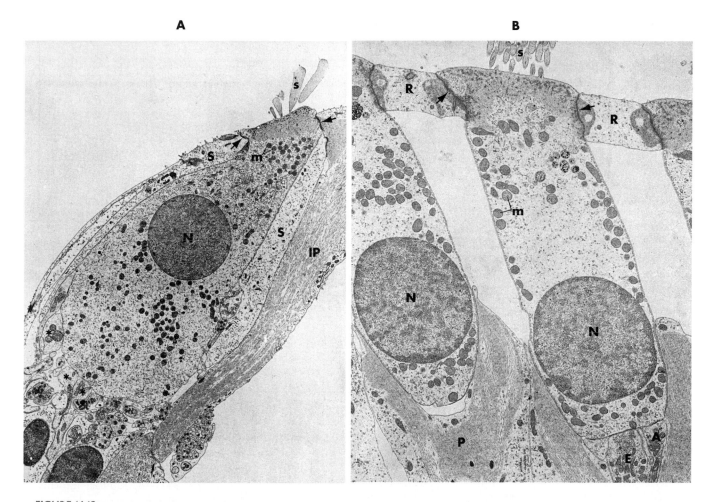

FIGURE 14-12

Electron micrographs of monkey hair cells. **A,** Inner hair cells have a flask-shaped cell body, round nucleus *(N)*, abundant mitochondria *(m)*, and the expected tuft of stereocilia *(s)* protruding into the scala media. The cell body is flanked by supporting cells *(S)* and at its base the cell makes synaptic contacts with endings of eighth nerve fibers (*). Nearby a microtubule-filled process of a special kind of supporting cell, an inner pillar cell *(IP)*, forms one side of the tunnel of Corti. Junctional complexes *(arrows)* near the apex of the inner hair cell separate the endolymph of the scala media from the extracellular fluids in the organ of Corti. **B,** Outer hair cells also have abundant mitochondria *(m)* and round nuclei *(N)*, but their cell bodies are cylindrical and exposed directly to fluid-filled extracellular spaces. The bases of the cells form synaptic contacts with both afferent *(A)* and efferent *(E)* nerve endings and are supported by cup-shaped, microtubule-rich processes of outer phalangeal cells *(P)*. Thin processes of the outer phalangeal cells (not seen in this section) end as platelike expansions attached by junctional complexes *(arrows)* to the tops of the outer hair cells, forming the reticular lamina *(R)* that mechanically supports the top of this part of the organ of Corti. (From Kimura RS: Sensory and accessory epithelia of the cochlea. In Friedmann I, Ballantyne J, editors: *Ultrastructural atlas of the inner ear,* London, 1984, Butterworths.)

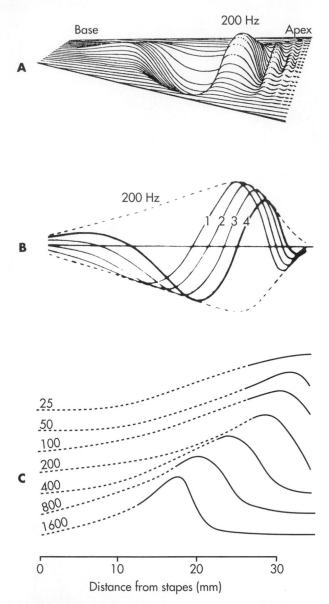

FIGURE 14-13

Traveling waves in the basilar membrane. **A,** Three-dimensional representation of the displacement of a model basilar membrane at one instant in time during the traveling wave in response to 200-Hz vibration. (The amplitude of the displacement is greatly exaggerated for clarity.) **B,** The displacements seen along the longitudinal midline of a human basilar membrane at a series of successive instants (*1–4*) in response to a 200-Hz tone. The dashed lines show the envelope of the displacements over time. Individual traveling waves move from the base to the apex of the cochlea, but their envelope has a maximum at one point along the length of the basilar membrane. **C,** The envelopes of the traveling waves produced by tones of successively higher frequency peak progressively closer to the base of the cochlea. (**A** from Tonndorf J: Shearing motion in scala media of cochlear models, *J Acoust Soc Am* 32:238, 1960. **B** and **C** redrawn from von Békésy G: *Experiments in hearing,* New York, 1960, McGraw-Hill.)

sounds, but closer to threshold it is driven most effectively by sounds of progressively higher frequencies as one moves from the apex to the base of the cochlea (Figure 14-13, *C*). Because the organ of Corti (which contains the auditory receptor cells) rests on the basilar membrane, different receptor cells respond best to sounds of different frequencies.★ Individual eighth nerve fibers respond to a broad range of frequencies when the sound is intense, but are sharply tuned to a narrow range of frequencies at threshold (Figure 14-14). This mechanical tuning of the basilar membrane is the beginning of a **tonotopic organization** within the auditory system, quite analogous to the somatotopic organization of the somatosensory system; in this case particular frequencies are mapped in an orderly fashion onto particular areas of relay nuclei and auditory cortex (Figure 14-18).

Vibrations of the basilar membrane are amplified by outer hair cells

The sensitivity of individual cochlear nerve fibers at their preferred frequencies is much greater—by more than a thousandfold for some fibers—than can be accounted for by the mechanical tuning of different parts of the basilar membrane (Figure 14-14, *A*), and it has been known for some time that some active process must add energy to the vibration of the basilar membrane in the area of maximum amplitude of the traveling wave (Figure 14-14, *B*). The source of this added energy appears to be the outer hair cells.

Despite the fact that there are many more outer than inner hair cells, most spiral ganglion cells receive their input only from inner hair cells. About 90% of all cochlear nerve fibers receive their entire input from single inner hair cells; 20 different auditory afferents may receive synaptic input from one inner hair cell. In contrast, the remaining 10% of the auditory afferents branch repeatedly and each innervates multiple outer hair cells. This pattern of innervation implies that most of the auditory information conveyed to the CNS originates from inner hair cells. Nevertheless, the outer hair cells contribute substantially to the sensitivity of the inner hair cells. For example, certain ototoxic drugs that selectively destroy the outer hair cells cause the auditory threshold to rise by a factor of 10^3 to 10^4. The probable mechanism for the added sensitivity is suggested by the observation that outer hair cells are contractile (Figure 14-15), so that oscillations of their membrane potential resulting from vibration of the basilar membrane cause the cells themselves to change their lengths. Although the details are not yet clear, this vibration in turn is thought to increase the mechanical stimulation of the inner hair cells, thus increasing the magnitude of the receptor potentials produced by them.

★Low frequencies vibrate large extents of the basilar membrane, and additional information about low frequencies is provided by multiple eighth nerve fibers all firing in phase with the sound wave.

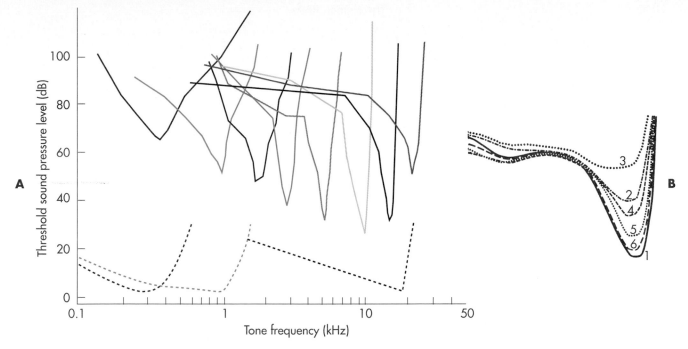

FIGURE 14-14
Tuning of the frequency response of individual cochlear nerve fibers by a combination of the mechanical properties of the basilar membrane and an active amplification mechanism. **A,** Threshold vs. frequency plots for eight different guinea pig cochlear nerve fibers. Each responds over a range that extends far into the low-frequency range if sound is loud, but has a much narrower range of maximum sensitivity. The dotted curves at the bottom show the expected mechanical tuning of the basilar membrane (on an arbitrary scale); all three lack the sharply tuned portion of the curves demonstrated for cochlear nerve fibers. **B,** The tuning curve of a single eighth nerve fiber of a cat before *(1)* and during *(2, 3)* instillation of a metabolic inhibitor (potassium cyanide) into the inner ear. The sharply tuned portion of the tuning curve is lost, indicating that it depends on some active metabolic process. After washing out the cyanide, the sharp tuning is regained *(4–6)*. [**A** redrawn from Evans EF: The frequency response and other properties of single fibres in the guinea-pig cochlear nerve, *J Physiol* 226:263, 1972. **B** from Evans EF, Klinke R: Reversible effects of cyanide and furosemide on the tuning of single cochlear nerve fibres, *J Physiol* 242:129P, 1974.]

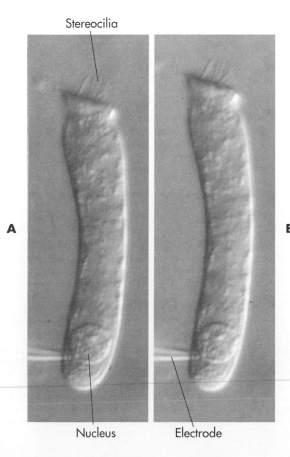

FIGURE 14-15
Electrically induced length changes in an isolated outer hair cell from a guinea pig. A microelectrode was used to depolarize **(A)** and hyperpolarize **(B)** the cell, causing it to shorten and lengthen. (Courtesy Dr. M. Holley, University of Bristol.)

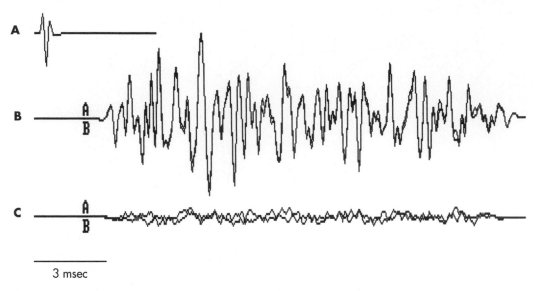

FIGURE 14-16

Otoacoustic emissions. In response to 82-dB clicks (**A**) delivered to the right ear, that ear emits sound of about 19-dB sound pressure level for about 15 msec (**B**). In contrast, a similar click delivered to the same patient's left ear elicits no otoacoustic emissions (**C**), indicating damage to the middle ear apparatus or outer hair cells. Both **B** and **C** show superimposed average responses to two series of 1000 clicks (*A* and *B*), demonstrating how reproducible the response is. (Courtesy Dr. Theodore J. Glattke, Department of Speech and Hearing Sciences, The University of Arizona.)

If motion of the outer hair cells can enhance the vibration of the basilar membrane, then it might be expected that these vibrations could travel backward through the perilymph and middle ear ossicles to vibrate the tympanic membrane slightly. A vibrating tympanic membrane would behave like a tiny loudspeaker, producing sound. This can in fact be recorded as **otoacoustic emissions** (Figure 14-16). For several milliseconds after a brief sound stimulus, a sensitive microphone in the external auditory meatus can detect faint sounds emitted by the ear itself. Because the production of otoacoustic emissions requires a normal middle ear, as well as inner ear function up to and including the hair cells, it is now the basis of important audiological tests. Measuring otoacoustic emissions is particularly useful for testing the hearing of infants, who are obviously unable to respond verbally to sounds the way adults can.

Auditory Information Is Distributed Bilaterally in the CNS

Auditory primary afferents, whose cell bodies are located in the spiral ganglion of the modiolus, enter the brainstem at the pontomedullary junction. There each fiber bifur-cates and sends one branch to the **dorsal cochlear nucleus** and one branch to the **ventral cochlear nucleus.** These cochlear nuclei form a continuous band of cells that covers the dorsal and lateral aspects of the inferior cerebellar peduncle (Figure 14-17, *C*).

Sensory systems characteristically analyze multiple aspects of a stimulus, such as the color and brightness of a visual stimulus or the shape and texture of a somatosensory stimulus. Similarly, the auditory system analyzes things such as the frequency (perceived as pitch), intensity, and location of a sound. Some aspects of this auditory analysis are initiated in the cochlea and involve a fairly straightforward CNS pathway (described shortly), but determining the location of a sound source involves additional processing at the level of the brainstem.

Some fibers from the cochlear nuclei (mainly from the dorsal cochlear nucleus) loop over the top of the inferior cerebellar peduncle, cross the midline with a rostral inclination, and join the **lateral lemniscus,** the major ascending auditory pathway of the brainstem. The lateral lemniscus is somewhat diffuse as it forms in the caudal pons, but in the rostral pons it forms a flattened band (the Greek word *lemniskos* means "ribbon") on the lateral sur-

FIGURE 14-17

The ascending auditory pathway. **A,** Major components of the lateral lemniscus, in which some fibers represent the contralateral ear (*red*), some the ipsilateral ear (*green*), and some both ears (*blue*). *C–H* indicate the planes of the sections shown in **C-H. B,** Overview of the entire auditory pathway, ending in the transverse temporal gyri on the superior surface of the temporal lobe. **C-H,** Brainstem cross sections at the levels indicated in **A,** showing components of the ascending auditory pathway. **I,** The lateral sulcus spread open to reveal the transverse temporal gyri. *4,* Fourth ventricle; *A,* cerebral aqueduct; *CP,* cerebral peduncle; *ICP,* inferior cerebellar peduncle; *ML,* medial lemniscus; *PAG,* periaqueductal gray; *RN,* red nucleus; *S,* spinothalamic tract; *SB,* brachium of the superior colliculus; *SC,* superior colliculus; *SCP,* superior cerebellar peduncle; *SN,* substantia nigra; *VI,* abducens nucleus. (**B** modified from a drawing by Max Brödel in Rothman L, Crowe SJ, editors: *The 1940 year book of eye, ear, nose, and throat,* Chicago, 1940, Year Book Medical Publishers, Inc.)

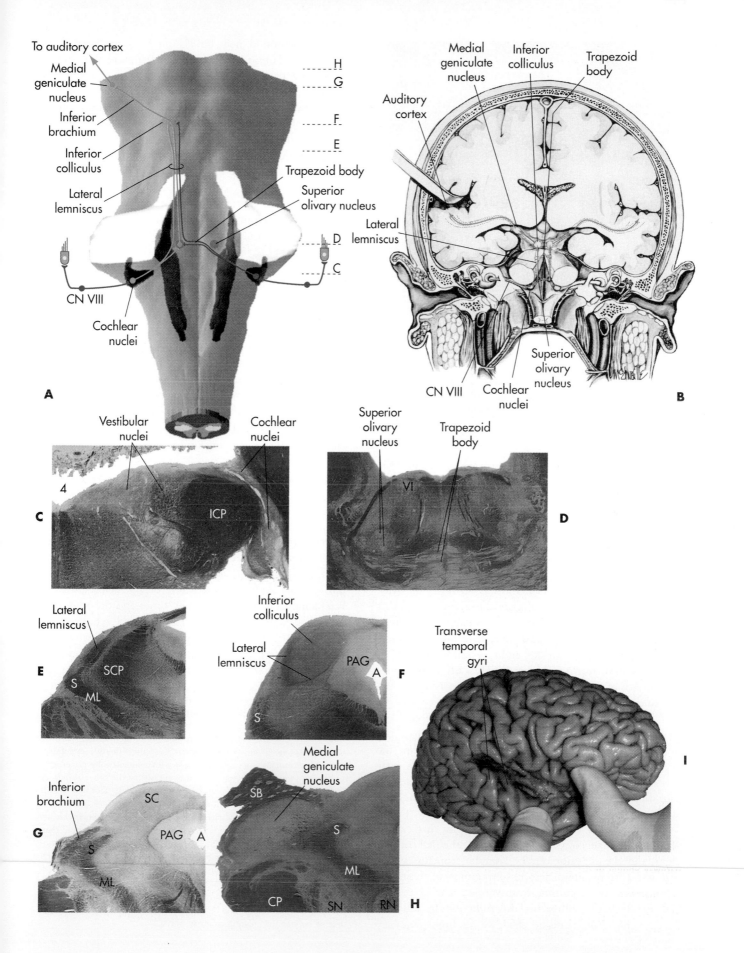

A

To auditory cortex
Medial geniculate nucleus
Inferior brachium
Inferior colliculus
Lateral lemniscus
CN VIII
Cochlear nuclei
H
G
F
E
D
C
Trapezoid body
Superior olivary nucleus

B

Medial geniculate nucleus
Inferior colliculus
Trapezoid body
Auditory cortex
Lateral lemniscus
CN VIII
Cochlear nuclei
Superior olivary nucleus

C

Vestibular nuclei
Cochlear nuclei
4
ICP

D

Superior olivary nucleus
Trapezoid body
VI

E

Lateral lemniscus
SCP
S
ML

F

Inferior colliculus
Lateral lemniscus
PAG
A
S

G

Inferior brachium
SC
PAG
A
S
ML

H

Medial geniculate nucleus
SB
S
ML
CP
SN
RN

I

Transverse temporal gyri

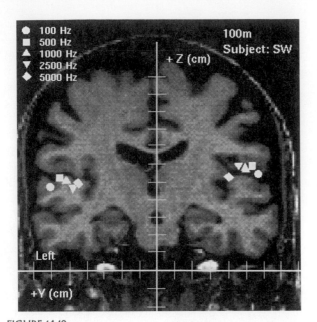

FIGURE 14-18
Tonotopic mapping in human primary auditory cortex, demonstrated by applying 500-msec tone bursts at 5 different sound frequencies to one ear while mapping the magnetic field changes produced by neuronal current flow in primary auditory cortex. (From Cansino S, Williamson SJ, Karron D: Tonotopic organization of human auditory association cortex, *Brain Res* 663:38, 1994.)

face of the tegmentum (Figure 14-17, *E*). A smaller number of efferents from the cochlear nuclei do not cross the midline, but instead join the ipsilateral lateral lemniscus; hence each lateral lemniscus carries some information from both ears. Virtually all fibers of the lateral lemniscus terminate in the inferior colliculus. The inferior colliculus then gives rise to the **brachium** (Latin for "arm") **of the inferior colliculus** (or **inferior brachium**), which assumes a superficial position and terminates in the **medial geniculate nucleus,** a portion of the thalamus that protrudes in a posterior direction, overlapping the midbrain. Fibers from the medial geniculate nucleus project tonotopically to the primary auditory cortex, located in the **transverse temporal gyri** (of **Heschl**) on the superior surface of the temporal lobe, mostly buried in the lateral sulcus (Figures 14-17, *I* and 14-18).

A much larger number of efferents from the cochlear nuclei, all from the ventral cochlear nucleus, pass beneath the inferior cerebellar peduncle. Some join the lateral lemniscus of each side and proceed to the inferior colliculus. Many, however, are involved in sound localization and end in the **superior olivary nucleus,** at the rostral end of the facial motor nucleus (Figure 14-17, *D*). There are two general strategies that can be used to localize sounds coming from the left or the right, and the superior olivary complex contains a medial and a lateral subnucleus corresponding to these two strategies. A sound coming from the left reaches the left ear slightly before it reaches the right ear. In addition, because the head creates a "shadow" for high-frequency

sounds, the sound may be a little bit more intense at the left ear. Sound localization can therefore be accomplished by comparing the time of arrival and the intensity of a sound at the two ears.* The time-of-arrival comparison, which is begun in the medial superior olive, is more effective for low frequencies and for terrestrial animals with relatively large heads (like us). We have a correspondingly large medial superior olive and small lateral superior olive. Fibers from the ventral cochlear nuclei of both sides converge on the medial superior olive of each side, providing the anatomical substrate for binaural comparison. Crossing from one cochlear nucleus to the contralateral superior olivary nucleus occurs in the **trapezoid body** (Figure 14-17, *D*), a large collection of second-order fibers that pass through and ventral to the medial lemnisci.† Each superior olivary nucleus then projects through the lateral lemniscus to the ipsilateral inferior colliculus.

Each lateral lemniscus thus conveys information from both ears, both because the cochlear nuclei project bilaterally and because the superior olive receives bilateral input. One consequence is that damage to the auditory pathway at any level rostral to the cochlear nuclei does not cause deafness in either ear. Rather, it causes problems with localizing sounds and may cause difficulties in separating sounds from background noise.

Activity in the ascending auditory pathway generates electrical signals that can be measured from the scalp

A brief sound causes a series of electrical waves, in the nanovolt range, that can be recorded from the surface of the head. The signals are so small that they are normally buried in background electrical noise, but when the same brief stimulus is presented many times and the responses are averaged, the waves can be measured reproducibly. Early peaks of the waveform represent electrical activity in the eighth nerve arriving at the cochlear nuclei, and later peaks represent combined activity at successive sites in the

---

*This method works well for determining the horizontal position of a sound, but is of little help in telling up from down or in front from behind. Some animals (e.g., owls) have one ear located higher than the other, so that even sounds in the sagittal plane affect the two ears differently. Most animals (e.g., cats and dogs) with symmetrically placed ears can create interaural differences by moving one or the other auricle or by cocking their heads. Humans take advantage of the fact that sounds coming from different directions in the sagittal plane are distorted in characteristic ways by the auricle. For example, high frequencies are attenuated more by the auricle when coming from behind the head than when coming from in front. The CNS apparently compares what something sounds like to what it *ought* to sound like, and uses this comparison to help determine elevation.
†Historically the term *trapezoid body* was used to refer to the trapezoid-shaped area of the brainstem containing both the medial lemnisci and the crossing auditory fibers. The term is now used in a functional sense, referring only to the crossing auditory fibers.

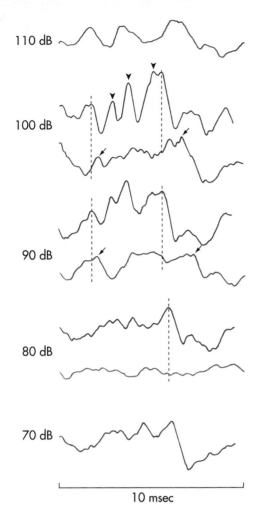

110 dB

100 dB

90 dB

80 dB

70 dB

10 msec

FIGURE 14-19
Brainstem auditory evoked responses in response to sounds presented to the right *(red traces)* or left *(blue traces)* ear of a 42-year-old man who complained of hearing loss in his left ear. Sounds in the right ear elicited a response with a series of well-defined peaks *(arrowheads, dashed lines)* at normal latencies. Using two of these peaks as reference points *(dashed lines)*, it can be seen that the corresponding peaks elicited by sounds in the left ear *(arrows)* were smaller and delayed. This patient had an acoustic neuroma (Figure 14-20, *D*). (Courtesy Dr. Theodore J. Glattke, Department of Speech and Hearing Sciences, The University of Arizona.)

auditory pathway. Because this pathway extends from the pontomedullary junction to the temporal lobes, abnormalities in the **brainstem auditory evoked response** can be helpful in localizing lesions (Figure 14-19).

Middle Ear Muscles Contract in Response to Loud Sounds

As noted earlier, contraction of the stapedius stiffens the ossicular chain and alters the transmission of vibrations. When a loud sound enters one ear, both stapedius muscles contract in a reflex fashion; an individual with a damaged facial nerve may complain that sounds are too loud in the ipsilateral ear (a condition known as **hyperacusis**). The pathway involved is from one ventral cochlear nucleus to

both superior olivary nuclei and from there to both facial motor nuclei. It is possible to test this reflex arc in a useful clinical procedure. When the stapedius contracts, less low-frequency sound energy incident on the eardrum is transferred along the ossicular chain, and more is reflected back from the eardrum. By measuring changes in the amount of a test sound reflected back from one eardrum when a loud sound is introduced into the contralateral ear, the stapedius reflex can be analyzed quantitatively.

The physiological function of the stapedius reflex is a matter of some dispute. The most common view is that it protects the inner ear from damage caused by excessively loud sounds. Clearly this could work only for chronic noise because a brief loud sound would be over before the stapedius could contract. However, no chronic noise of sufficient intensity to activate the reflex exists in nature, except near large waterfalls. A second view of the reflex is that it helps the inner ear extract meaningful sounds from noisy backgrounds. Stapedial contraction selectively impedes the transmission of low frequencies and so could selectively reduce the effects of low-frequency noise.

The function of the tensor tympani in auditory processes is less clear. This muscle too is activated bilaterally in some individuals in response to a loud sound in one ear, but only if the sound is extremely loud. Thus for most individuals in most physiological situations, only the stapedius is active. The tensor tympani contracts bilaterally in response to something touching the face, in response to startling stimuli (auditory or not), and before speech production, but the function of the contraction in these situations is obscure.

Conductive and Sensorineural Problems Can Affect Hearing

Basic aspects of hearing can be tested simply by measuring an individual's thresholds for hearing a series of pure tones of different frequencies, presented either through earphones (**air conduction**) or by way of a vibrator applied to the mastoid process or forehead (**bone conduction**). Plotting threshold sound levels for each frequency, relative to the average thresholds for a normal population of young subjects, yields an **audiogram** (Figure 14-20, *A*).

Just as in the case of olfaction, two general kinds of processes can cause loss of hearing: processes that prevent sound from reaching the labyrinth (**conductive** hearing loss) and processes that damage hair cells, cochlear nerve fibers, or the cochlear nuclei (**sensorineural** hearing loss★). Comparing audiograms obtained by air conduction and bone conduction can often help distinguish between the two. Hearing normally by air conduction requires

---

★Because damage to the auditory pathway at levels rostral to the cochlear nuclei does not cause substantial hearing loss in either ear, sensorineural hearing loss in one ear implies damage to the cochlea, eighth nerve, or cochlear nuclei. More sophisticated tests are required to assess changes in hearing resulting from damage at more rostral sites.

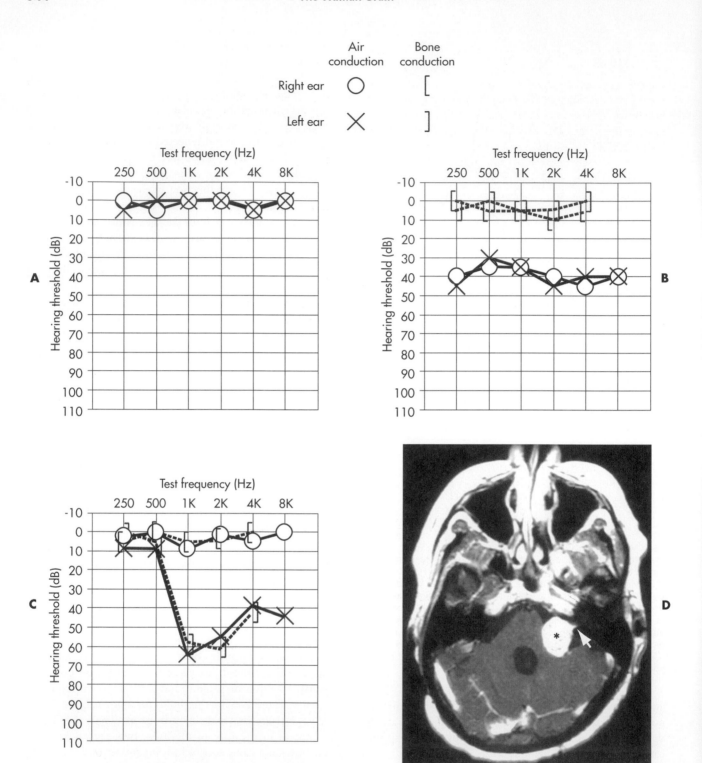

FIGURE 14-20

Normal and abnormal audiograms. **A**, A normal audiogram, showing only the results obtained by air conduction. Although hearing by air conduction is normally more sensitive than hearing by bone conduction, the audiometric procedure compensates for the difference. Hence curves for hearing by bone conduction would normally be more or less superimposed on those for hearing by air conduction. **B**, Audiometric results for a patient with bilateral conductive hearing loss caused by chronic otitis media (middle ear infections). Hearing by bone conduction is normal, but hearing by air conduction is impaired. **C**, Audiometric results for the same patient whose brainstem auditory evoked responses are shown in Figure 14-19. Hearing in the right ear is normal, but thresholds for the left ear are elevated whether air conduction or bone conduction is used. **D**, An MRI of a 67-year-old woman with an acoustic neuroma. The tumor (*) presses against the left side of the brainstem and extends laterally *(arrow)* into the internal auditory meatus. Although commonly called *acoustic neuromas,* these tumors are more properly referred to as *vestibular schwannomas,* because they usually arise from Schwann cells in the vestibular division of the eighth nerve. (**A-C** courtesy Dr. Theodore J. Glattke, Department of Speech and Hearing Sciences, The University of Arizona. **D** courtesy Dr. Raymond F. Carmody, Department of Radiology, The University of Arizona College of Medicine.)

normal function of the outer, middle, and inner ears. Hence hearing loss measured by air conduction could be the result of damage at any of these sites. Hearing by bone conduction, in contrast, involves direct transmission of vibrations from the skull to the fluids of the inner ear, bypassing the outer and middle ears. Hence hearing loss measured by bone conduction indicates a sensorineural problem. Someone who hears normally by bone conduction but not by air conduction (Figure 14-20, B) is therefore likely to have a conductive hearing loss. Typical causes are accumulation of fluid in the middle ear as a result of infection, or bony growths that impede vibration of the middle ear ossicles (otosclerosis). In contrast, someone with hair cell damage (e.g., from ototoxic drugs) or cochlear nerve damage (e.g., from an acoustic neuroma) would have comparable hearing losses measured by either air or bone conduction (Figure 14-20, C).

THE VESTIBULAR DIVISION OF THE EIGHTH NERVE CONVEYS INFORMATION ABOUT LINEAR AND ANGULAR ACCELERATION OF THE HEAD

One universal task for living creatures is keeping track of their orientation relative to the outside world. Mobile creatures have the added task of adjusting their orientation in response to self-generated or externally imposed movements. Vertebrates seem to have come up with an adaptation to meet these needs long ago. All jawed vertebrates have basically similar vestibular labyrinths, featuring three semicircular canals on each side of the head together with two or more **otolithic organs.** In every case the three semicircular canals are approximately orthogonal to each other, with one in a roughly horizontal plane and the other two in more or less vertical planes (Figure 14-21). The vestibular portion of the human bony labyrinth consists of a central area called the **vestibule** and three semicircular canals—**horizontal, anterior**, and **posterior**—that are attached to the vestibule (Figure 14-1). Within each semicircular canal is a semicircular duct,* which is the corresponding part of the membranous labyrinth. Within the vestibule are the two otolithic organs, the utricle and the saccule, each a dilation of the membranous labyrinth. The semicircular ducts and otolithic organs are suspended within the bony labyrinth rather than being stretched across it like the cochlear duct. Pressure changes caused by movement of the stapes are therefore equally distributed throughout the perilymph surrounding the vestibular parts of the membranous labyrinth and do not deform them, except in certain unusual pathological conditions.

---

*Although the term *semicircular canal* technically is supposed to designate a part of the bony labyrinth, it is often used interchangeably to refer to either a bony semicircular canal or a membranous semicircular duct.

The Semicircular Ducts Detect Angular Acceleration

Each semicircular duct communicates at both ends with the utricle. At one end of each duct is a dilation called an **ampulla.** Each ampulla contains a **crista,** a transversely oriented ridge of tissue covered by supporting cells and sensory hair cells (Figure 14-22). As in other parts of the labyrinth, each hair cell bears a graduated array of stereocilia (here accompanied by a kinocilium) embedded in a gelatinous mass. In this case the gelatinous mass, called a **cupula,** covers the crista and extends across the ampulla as a partition. All the hair cells of a given crista are aligned with their kinocilia facing in the same direction, so deflection of the cupula in one direction causes the afferents that innervate that crista to increase their firing rate, and deflection in the opposite direction causes them to decrease their firing rate. The hair cells of the horizontal canal have their kinocilia facing the utricle, so deflecting the cupula of this canal toward the utricle causes an increased firing rate. In contrast, the hair cells of the anterior and posterior canals have their kinocilia facing away from the utricle.

The most straightforward way to deflect a cupula is to rotate its semicircular duct about an axis perpendicular to it (like a wheel on an axle). As such a rotation begins, the endolymph lags behind because of inertia; this motion of duct and endolymph relative to one another deflects the cupula and stimulates the hair cells (Figure 14-23, A). However, as the rotation continues, the endolymph "catches up" because of factors such as friction and the elasticity of the cupula, and the stimulation ceases (Figure 14-23, B). At the end of the rotation, the endolymph continues to move for a short time (again because of inertia), and the cupula bulges in the opposite direction (Figure 14-23, C). Thus each semicircular canal responds best to *changes* in the speed of rotation in a particular plane (i.e., angular acceleration). Because the three semicircular canals are arranged in roughly orthogonal planes (Figure 14-24), and because most head movements have a rotational component, movements in any direction can be detected. The fact that the semicircular canals cannot detect maintained rotation is not a great disadvantage because (except at amusement parks) we usually do not experience maintained rotations.

The relative orientations of the three semicircular canals should be noted in Figure 14-24. The horizontal canal, as its name implies, is roughly horizontal (actually, it is tilted backward about 30°), whereas the anterior and posterior canals are roughly vertical. However, the anterior and posterior canals are also arranged at an angle of about 45° to the sagittal plane. The anterior canal of one side is therefore parallel to the posterior canal of the other side, so movements that affect one will affect the other. Thus the horizontal canals of the two sides form a functional pair, whereas the anterior canal of one side forms a functional pair with the posterior canal of the other side.

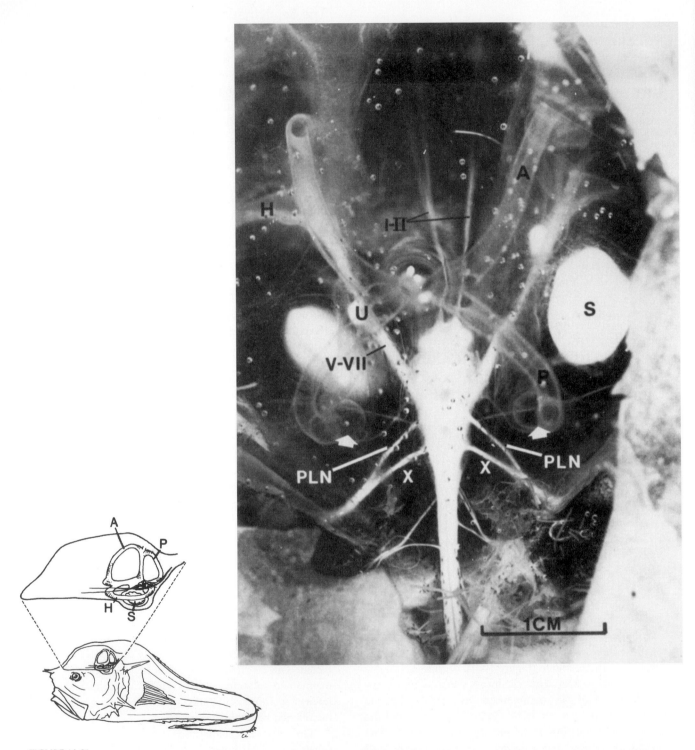

FIGURE 14-21

A striking illustration of the arrangement of vertebrate semicircular canals. *Acanthonus armatus* (drawn at the bottom left) is a species of small, deep-water fish that has particularly large semicircular canals and a particularly tiny brain. The photograph is a view into the cranial cavity from above; the orthogonally arranged anterior, posterior, and horizontal semicircular canals (*A, P,* and *H*) can be seen clearly. The large otoliths of the utricle (*U*) and especially the saccule (*S*) are also evident. Each saccular otolith weighed about four times as much as the fish's entire brain! *I, II, V, VII,* and *X* are cranial nerves; *PLN,* posterior lateral line nerve, which innervates sensory receptors along the fish's side. (From Fine ML, Horn MH, Cox B: *Acanthonus armatus,* a deep-sea teleost with a minute brain and large ears, *Proc Roy Soc Lond* B230:257, 1987.)

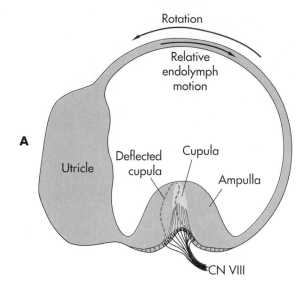

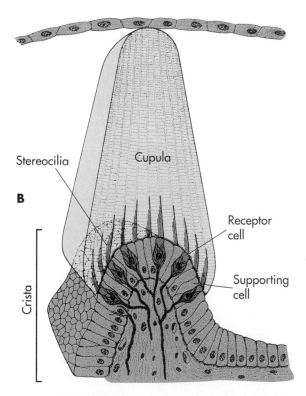

FIGURE 14-22
Two views of the interior of an ampulla. **A,** The arrangement of the cupula as a diaphragm across the endolymph-filled ampulla. Rotation in an appropriate plane causes endolymph to push against the cupula and deform it, which in turn causes deflection of hair cell stereocilia. **B,** An enlargement of a crista and cupula, showing the relationship of hair cells, their bundles of stereocilia, and the cupular diaphragm. (**A** modified from Melvill Jones G, Milsum JH: Spatial and dynamic aspects of visual fixation, *IEEE Trans Biomed Eng* 12:54, 1965. **B** modified from Wersäll J: Studies on the structure and innervation of the sensory epithelium of the cristae ampullares in the guinea pig, *Acta Otolaryngol* [Suppl] 126:1, 1956.

The Utricle and Saccule Detect Linear Acceleration

There are no cristae in the utricle and saccule, but each has in its wall a patch of supporting cells and hair cells called a **macula.** The utricular macula, lying at the bottom of the utricle, is roughly horizontal when one (or one's head) is in an upright posture. The saccular macula is on the medial wall of the saccule and is roughly vertical. The sensory hairs of the macular receptors are also embedded in a gelatinous membrane similar in composition to the cupula. However, in the case of each macula the gelatinous substance also contains minute crystals of calcium carbonate called **otoconia** or **otoliths*** and so is called an **otolithic membrane** (Figure 14-25), from which the otolithic organs get their name. The otoconia make the otolithic membrane denser than endolymph, so the membrane flops around and stays flopped when the position of the head changes. This stimulates the hair cells, which then signal the new position of the head. In this case the macula is responding to the force of gravity, but it responds equally well to other linear accelerating forces, such as those experienced in elevators and automobiles.

As might be expected from the orientation of its macula, the utricle is most sensitive to tilts beginning from a head-upright position. The saccule, in contrast, is more sensitive to tilts beginning from a head-sideways position. The hair cells of a given macula are arranged with their kinocilia facing in several different directions, so any tilt stimulates some cells more than others. The result is that every different head position causes a unique pattern of activity in the branches of the eighth nerve that innervate the utricle and saccule.

Vestibular Primary Afferents Project to the Vestibular Nuclei and the Cerebellum

Vestibular primary afferents have their cell bodies in the **vestibular** (or **Scarpa's**) **ganglion** in the internal auditory meatus. Their peripheral processes end about the hair cells just described. Their central processes enter the brainstem at the pontomedullary junction. Some proceed directly to the cerebellum, passing through the **juxtarestiform body,** which is located on the medial aspect of the inferior cerebellar peduncle. They end in the **flocculus, nodulus,** and nearby areas, as discussed in more detail in Chapter 20. Most primary vestibular afferents, however, end in the vestibular nuclei of the rostral medulla and caudal pons (Figure 14-26).

Four vestibular nuclei have been distinguished on the basis of their histology and connections: the **inferior,**

---

*Technically speaking, the very small crystals in the human otolithic membrane are otoconia (Greek for "ear dust"), whereas the somewhat larger concretions of some other vertebrates are otoliths (Greek for "ear stones"). However, the two terms are often used interchangeably.

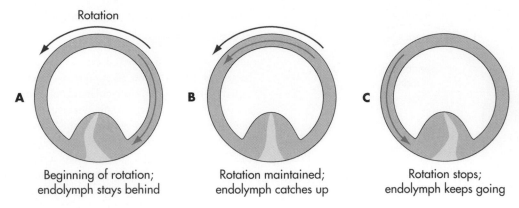

FIGURE 14-23
Relative movement of semicircular ducts, endolymph, and cupula at the beginning of rotation (**A**), during maintained rotation (**B**), and at the end of rotation (**C**).

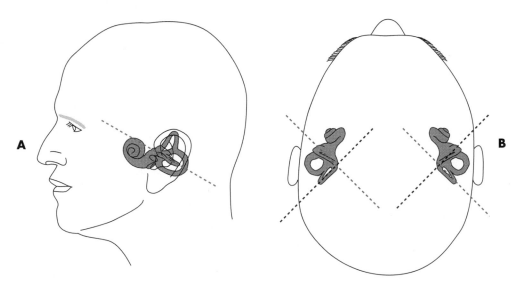

FIGURE 14-24
Orientation of different parts of the labyrinth (not drawn to scale), as seen from the left (**A**) and from above (**B**).

medial, lateral (or **Deiters'**), and **superior vestibular nuclei** (Figure 14-26). Each particular semicircular canal and otolithic organ has its own pattern of termination in the vestibular nuclei, and each vestibular nucleus has its own pattern of secondary connections. For the sake of simplicity, these patterns, for the most part, are ignored in this account and the vestibular nuclear complex treated as a uniform entity.

Inputs to the vestibular nuclei (in addition to primary vestibular afferents) include projections from the cerebellum (by way of the juxtarestiform body), the spinal cord, and the contralateral vestibular nuclei (Figure 14-26). The cerebellar projections arise directly from the flocculonodular lobe and indirectly from other cerebellar areas as well, as discussed further in Chapter 20. Input from the spinal cord makes reasonable sense because it would be difficult to adjust posture properly in response to a movement or a tilt without knowledge of the current orienta-

tion of the body. A small amount of this information travels with the posterior spinocerebellar tract as direct spinovestibular fibers, but most of it reaches the vestibular nuclei indirectly via relays in the cerebellum or reticular formation. Finally, the left and right vestibular apparatus normally function together as a coordinated pair, and the vestibular nuclear complexes of the two sides are extensively interconnected.

The Vestibular Nuclei Project Primarily to the Spinal Cord, Cerebellum, and Nuclei of Cranial Nerves III, IV, and VI

The connections of the vestibular nuclei are varied and widespread but not surprising in view of their function. We use the vestibular system principally to regulate posture and to coordinate eye and head movements; the anatomical substrates of these functions are connections

Surface of
hair cell

Tip of
kinocilium

Bundle of
stereocilia

Otoconia

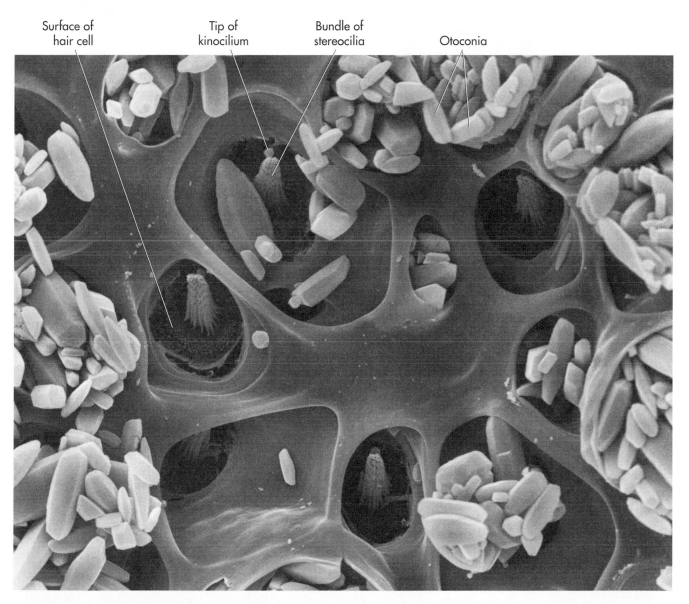

FIGURE 14-25
Scanning electron micrograph of the otolithic membrane of the saccule of a bullfrog. Bundles of sensory hairs, each bundle consisting of a single kinocilium and numerous stereocilia, can be seen projecting from individual hair cells into holes in the otolithic membrane. These holes are enlarged as a result of preparation for electron microscopy; in life the hair bundles are embedded directly in the otolithic membrane. (From Corey DP, Hudspeth AJ: Response latency of vertebrate hair cells, *Biophys J* 26:499, 1979.)

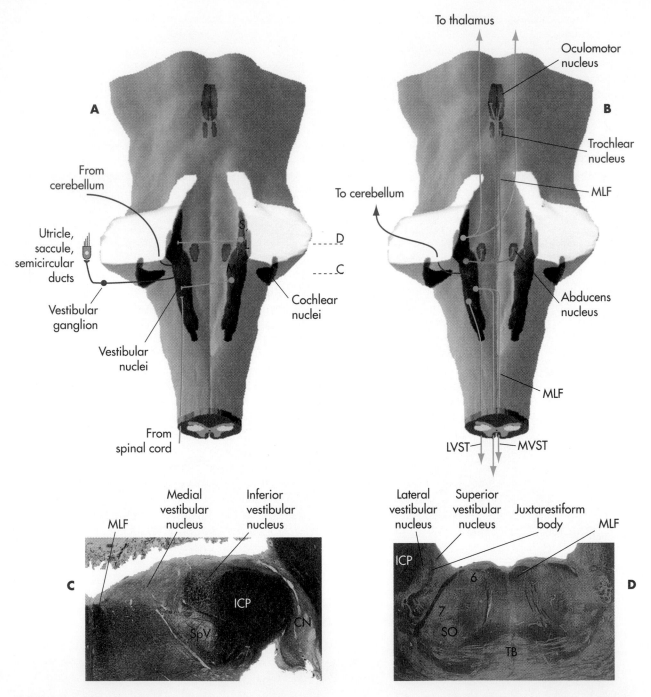

FIGURE 14-26

Inputs to (**A**) and outputs from (**B**) the vestibular nuclei. *C* and *D* refer to the planes of the brainstem cross sections indicated in **A** and shown in **C** and **D**, showing the vestibular nuclei. *6*, Abducens nucleus; *7*, facial motor nucleus; *CN*, cochlear nuclei; *I*, inferior vestibular nucleus; *ICP*, inferior cerebellar peduncle; *L*, lateral vestibular nucleus; *LVST*, lateral vestibulospinal tract; *M*, medial vestibular nucleus; *MLF*, medial longitudinal fasciculus; *MVST*, medial vestibulospinal tract; *S*, superior vestibular nucleus; *SpV*, spinal trigeminal nucleus; *SO*, superior olivary nucleus; *TB*, trapezoid body.

with the spinal cord and with the motor nuclei of the extraocular muscles. The cerebellum is also involved in both these functions, and correspondingly there are substantial interconnections between it and the vestibular nuclei. We also have a conscious awareness of movement through space; there is a corresponding vestibular projection through the thalamus to cerebral cortex. Finally, there are connections between the vestibular nuclei and the reticular formation (including visceral centers of the reticular formation, as anyone who has been seasick can attest).

Secondary fibers arising in the vestibular complex project (Figure 14-26) to (1) parts of the cerebellum, including the same areas as do primary vestibular afferents (again, via the juxtarestiform body); (2) the thalamus; (3) the spinal cord, in the lateral and medial vestibulospinal tracts; (4) the motor nuclei of the extraocular muscles; and (5) the vestibular apparatus. (This is in addition to the previously mentioned projections to the reticular formation and the contralateral vestibular nuclei.)

Vestibular projections to the thalamus, and from there to the cerebral cortex, have been a matter of some controversy. The thalamic relay seems to be in a small nucleus in the inferior part of the thalamus near VPL and VPM. Secondary vestibular fibers reach the thalamus bilaterally, some by traveling with the auditory fibers of the lateral lemniscus and others by traversing the reticular formation near the MLF. Several cortical areas receive vestibular information from the thalamus; their relative roles are not completely understood. One is located in the parietal lobe at the junction between the intraparietal and postcentral sulci, and another in the depths of the central sulcus; both are near the portion of the postcentral gyrus where the head is represented. This makes sense, as the somatosensory cortex of the postcentral gyrus is concerned with conscious appreciation of body position. Another, which may be most directly concerned with vestibular information, is in a posterior part of the insula near auditory cortex.

Vestibulospinal fibers influence antigravity muscles and neck muscles

The **lateral vestibulospinal tract** arises in the lateral vestibular nucleus and sends excitatory projections to the motor neurons for antigravity muscles at all levels of the ipsilateral spinal cord, where it is located in the ventral part of the lateral funiculus. This is the principal route by which the vestibular system brings about postural changes to compensate for tilts and movements of the body. If as a child (or an adult) you ever spun yourself around until you felt dizzy and then proceeded to stagger, you have experienced the effects of exaggerated activity in your lateral vestibulospinal tract.

The **medial vestibulospinal tract** arises mainly in the medial vestibular nucleus and reaches both sides of the cervical spinal cord by projecting caudally through the MLF. It is responsible for stabilizing head position as we do

things like walk around, and for coordinating head movements with eye movements.

The vestibular nuclei participate in the vestibuloocular reflex

The most critically important function of the vestibular system is not to mediate awareness of movement or to adjust posture, but rather to help generate eye movements that compensate for head movements. Retinal photoreceptors, as discussed in Chapter 17, use a second-messenger transduction process that is relatively slow, and clear vision of images that move across the retina is impossible. The nervous system, as described further in Chapter 21, exerts considerable effort to keep images from moving around on the retina.

Many secondary vestibular fibers project directly through the MLF and through the adjacent reticular formation to the motor neurons of the oculomotor, trochlear, and abducens nuclei. This forms the basis of the **vestibuloocular reflex** (VOR), by means of which a person's gaze can stay fixed on an object even though the head is moving or being moved. One might think that this is a form of visual tracking, but the reflex is faster than visual tracking,★ works even in the dark in normal individuals, and works relatively poorly in individuals with bilateral vestibular damage (Figure 14-27); thus it seems clear that the vestibular division of cranial nerve VIII forms the afferent limb. Each semicircular canal has connections via the vestibular nuclei that are appropriate to cause eye deviation in its own plane. This is most easily understood in the case of the horizontal canal. Imagine rotating to the left about a vertical axis. This would cause the cupula of the left horizontal canal to bulge toward the utricle (Figure 14-28), hence depolarizing the hair cells of this canal and increasing the firing rate of the eighth nerve fibers that innervate them. Excitatory connections with the left vestibular nuclei and from there to the right abducens nucleus result in deviation of both eyes to the right (Figure 14-28), compensating for the rotation. Other combinations of semicircular canals and extraocular muscles are similarly straightforward, although more difficult to visualize. For example, rotating forward and to the right in the plane of the right anterior canal causes contraction of the right superior rectus and left inferior oblique, which in turn causes compensatory elevation and rotation of both eyes. As in the case of spinal reflexes, VOR circuitry includes

---

★You can demonstrate this to yourself easily by comparing the speeds of visual tracking and the vestibuloocular reflex. Hold your index finger up at arm's length in front of you. Keeping your head still, track the finger visually as you move it back and forth more and more rapidly, and note the speed at which it becomes blurred. Now hold the finger still and watch it, using the vestibuloocular reflex, while wagging your head back and forth. It should be apparent that the VOR is capable of much higher velocities.

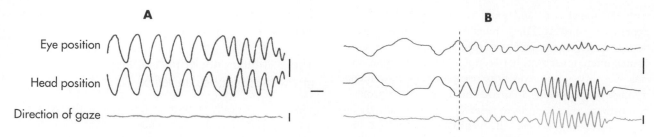

FIGURE 14-27

Normal and abnormal vestibuloocular reflexes. The surface of the cornea is electrically positive relative to the back of the eye, so deviation of an eye toward a nearby electrode will cause the electrode to become more positive relative to a distant electrode. This is used clinically to record eye movements. These traces show the position of the eyes in the horizontal plane *(blue)*, the position of the same individual's head *(blue)*, and *(green)* the sum of these two positions, which corresponds to the net direction in which the individual is looking. By convention, an upward deflection indicates movement to the right. **A,** A normal individual moved her head back and forth while trying to maintain her gaze fixed on a stationary target. Notice that as her head moves in one direction, her eyes move through an equal but opposite angle, so the direction of gaze does not change. This is the normal vestibuloocular reflex. **B,** A patient with bilateral loss of vestibular hair cells (caused by ototoxicity of the streptomycin used to treat her for pneumonia) attempts to do the same thing. At the slow head velocities at the beginning of the recording, she was able to use visual feedback to generate compensatory eye movements. However, once head velocity reached about $50°$/sec *(dashed line)*, the lack of a vestibuloocular reflex made it impossible to generate large enough compensatory eye movements. As a result the direction of gaze began to oscillate in phase with head movement, and the patient had a disturbing visual illusion of the world moving. All vertical scale marks correspond to $40°$, and the horizontal scale mark to 1 sec. (Redrawn from Atkin A, Bender MB: Ocular stabilization during oscillatory head movements, *Arch Neurol* 19:559, 1968.)

inhibitory connections to the motor neurons for antagonist muscles (Figure 14-28).

A vestibuloocular reflex is not always a good thing to have, and the VOR, like stretch and other reflexes, is modifiable. For example, we do a lot of our looking by using head movements in combination with eye movements. Unless the VOR were suppressed during the part of a gaze shift mediated by head turning, a counterrotation of the eyes would be generated and the direction of gaze would not change. Another example is compensating for the effects of eyeglasses, which change the relationship between head movement and the movement of images across the retina. All of this is addressed by the flocculus, which adjusts the gain of the VOR as necessary. In fact the degree of plasticity of this reflex, as discussed further in Chapter 20, is quite remarkable: in some experimental situations it can actually reverse direction.

Nystagmus can be physiological or pathological

During head rotations that are too large to be compensated for by the vestibuloocular reflex, the VOR is periodically interrupted by very rapid eye movements in the opposite direction (Figure 14-29). The resulting back-and-forth eye movements, with a slow phase in one direction and a fast phase in the other, are a form of **nystagmus** (from a Greek word meaning "to nod off," referring to the way a sleepy person's head sags slowly and then snaps back upright while trying to stay awake). The eye movements of nystagmus may be horizontal, vertical, or torsional; they may have a faster component in one direction, or the movements in both directions may have the same speed. Nystagmus of certain types is a normal physiological response to stimulation of the vestibular or visual system, but spontaneous or exaggerated nystagmus can be characteristic of some kinds of neuropathology (Figure 14-30).

An example of normal physiological nystagmus is the one just described—horizontal nystagmus, with a fast component in one direction, induced by rotation. In this case the nystagmus is named for the direction of rapid movement (e.g., if the eyes move slowly to the right and then rapidly back to the left, it would be called **nystagmus to the left,** or **left-beating nystagmus**). Left-beating **rotatory nystagmus** would be seen at the beginning of rotation to the left (Figures 14-28 and 14-29, *B*), ensuring a stable image on the retina except during the brief "reset" movements of the fast phase. When the rotation stopped, the cupula would be deflected in the opposite direction (Figure 14-23, *C*), fooling the brainstem into thinking the direction of rotation had reversed, and a brief period of right-beating **postrotatory nystagmus** would ensue. The response during sustained rotation, when there is no cupular deflection (Figure 14-23, *B*), depends on the conditions of illumination. In the dark or with the subject's eyes closed, nystagmus would cease; with visual input, for reasons explained below, left-beating nystagmus might continue throughout the rotation.

The same movement of endolymph that underlies rotatory nystagmus can be produced by instilling cool or warm water into a subject's ear, causing endolymphatic convection currents that, in turn, induce nystagmus. Consider an individual whose head is tilted back about 60°, bringing the horizontal semicircular canals into a vertical plane. Cool water instilled into the right ear causes the endolymph in the right horizontal canal to cool and sink, causing a convection current of endolymph in a clockwise direction (viewed from the top of the head). This movement of endolymph relative to the canal is the same movement that is produced at the onset of rotation of the individual to the left (Figure 14-29, *C*), and the response of this single semicircular canal is sufficient to cause nystagmus to the left. This is called **caloric nys-**

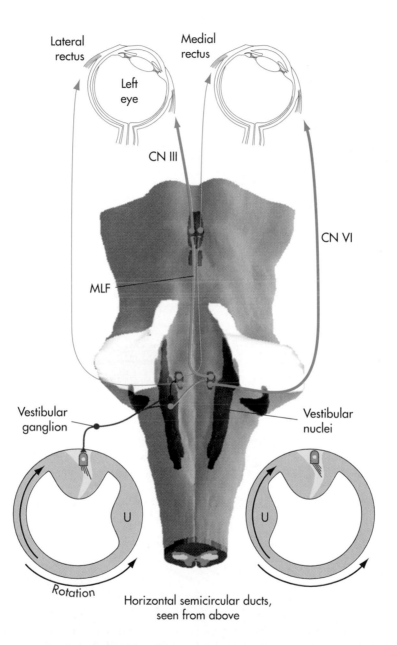

FIGURE 14-28
The pathway of the vestibuloocular reflex underlying the response to rotation to the left. Excitation of the left horizontal semicircular duct causes increased contraction of the right lateral rectus and left medial rectus, by way of excitatory interneurons *(green)* in the left vestibular nuclei; simultaneously, motor neurons for the left lateral rectus and right medial rectus (the antagonist muscles) are inhibited, by way of inhibitory interneurons *(red)*. Notice that this rotation also causes bulging of the cupula of the right horizontal semicircular canal *away from* the utricle, thus hyperpolarizing the hair cells of this canal. Although its connections are not shown in the figure, this would have a complementary effect (e.g., less excitation of motor neurons for the left lateral rectus and right medial rectus).

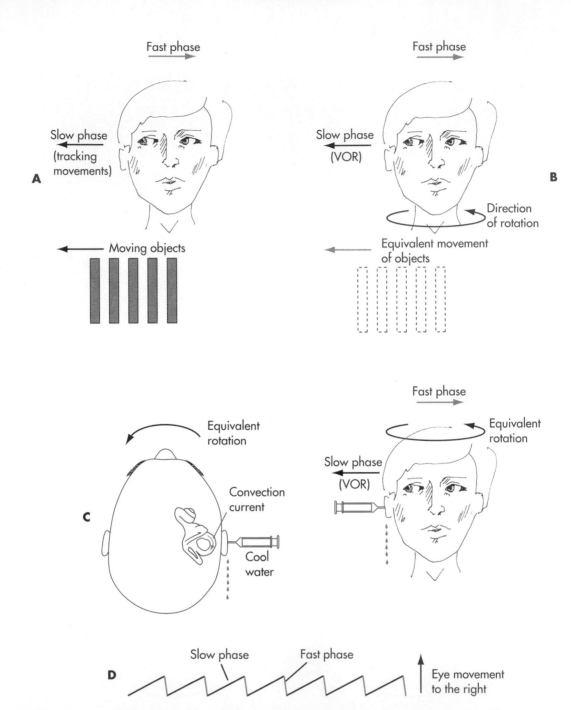

FIGURE 14-29

Three different ways to cause nystagmus with its fast phase to the left. **A,** Movement of a series of objects to an individual's right causes slow tracking eye movements to the right followed by rapid "reset" movements to the left. **B,** Rotation to the left is equivalent, as far as retinal image movement is concerned, to movement of objects to the right. The result is nystagmus to the left, as in **A.** If the individual's eyes are open, visual movement continues throughout the rotation, and the nystagmus may persist. If the eyes are closed, the nystagmus is mediated only by the vestibular system and is transient. The direction of nystagmus reverses at the end of rotation in either condition. **C,** Cool water instilled into the right ear causes the same movement of endolymph in the right horizontal semicircular duct as does the rotation in **B.** The result again is nystagmus to the left. **D,** Idealized electrical recording of horizontal nystagmus with its fast phase to the left.

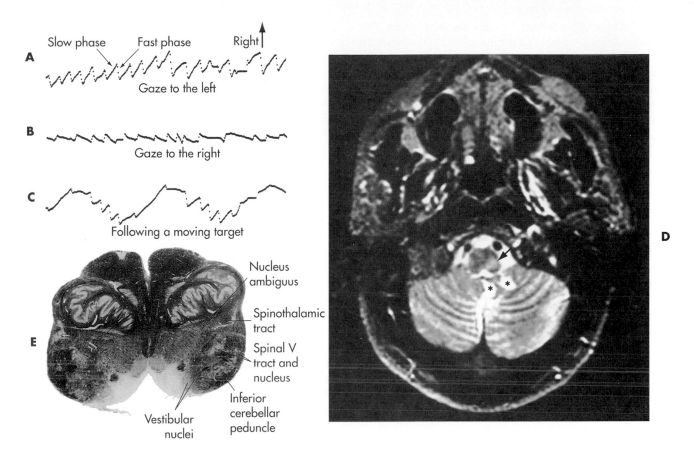

FIGURE 14-30

Pathological nystagmus caused by brainstem damage. A 62-year-old man developed the abrupt onset of vertigo and nausea. He was found to have spontaneous nystagmus to the left that increased when he looked to the left **(A)** and changed to right-beating nystagmus when he looked to the right **(B)**. Smooth tracking of moving targets was severely impaired when the target moved to the left **(C)** because his nystagmus was accentuated by gaze in this direction. He also had signs of left-sided cerebellar damage (see Chapter 20): intention tremor on the left, incoordination of the left arm on finger to nose testing, and slight left dysdiadochokinesia. He was markedly off balance and could hardly even sit up because of nausea that worsened with movement of his head. **D**, A T2-weighted axial MRI showed increased signal intensity in the left lateral medulla *(arrow)* and left paramedian cerebellum *(asterisks)*, both areas supplied by the posterior inferior cerebellar artery (PICA; see Figure 11-26). **E**, A section of the rostral medulla in a plane similar to **D**. In this case of lateral medullary (or Wallenberg's) syndrome, damage to the vestibular nuclei, inferior cerebellar peduncle, and cerebellum produced the findings described. Other structures likely to be damaged in such a case, and the resulting deficits, include the spinal trigeminal tract and nucleus (ipsilateral facial analgesia), spinothalamic tract (analgesia of the contralateral side of the body), and nucleus ambiguus (hoarseness, ipsilateral palatal and pharyngeal weakness). In addition, damage to fibers descending from the hypothalamus to the intermediolateral cell column of the spinal cord could cause ipsilateral Horner's syndrome. (Courtesy Dr. Terry Fife, St. Joseph's Hospital and Regional Medical Center and The University of Arizona College of Medicine.)

tagmus, and its mechanism is the same as that of rotationally induced vestibular nystagmus.*

Finally, because the whole purpose of vestibular nystagmus is to keep images from moving on the retina, it is not surprising that a similar pattern of eye movements can be elicited by moving visual stimuli. Consider the reflex eye movements that occur when a person sits in a rapidly moving train, vaguely watching regularly spaced telephone poles fly by. The person's eyes tend to slowly fol-

low a particular pole toward the rear of the train and then flick back toward the front of the train to find a new pole to fixate on. In the case of an individual seated on the right side of the train, this would constitute nystagmus to the left (Figure 14-29, *A*). Because it is induced by moving visual stimuli, it is called **optokinetic nystagmus** (OKN). Fortunately it is not necessary to use trains and telephone poles to demonstrate optokinetic nystagmus clinically; a rotating striped drum or a moving piece of striped cloth usually suffices. Optokinetic nystagmus accounts for the continued nystagmus during sustained rotation if the lights are on.

The pathway involved in vestibular nystagmus primarily involves the MLF for connections rostral to the abducens nucleus. The slow phase is simply a reflection of direct VOR connections from the vestibular nuclei to the abducens, trochlear, and oculomotor nuclei. The fast

---

*This gravitational model seems so logical that it has been accepted without much question since caloric nystagmus was first described in 1908. However, the era of space flight has allowed demonstrations that caloric nystagmus can be elicited in orbiting astronauts, who are experiencing nearly zero gravity. However, its properties under these conditions are somewhat different from normal, and the current consensus is that caloric nystagmus is mostly the result of convection currents and partly the result of a direct thermal effect of some sort.

phase, like fast eye movements in general (see Chapter 21), requires timing signals that originate from the reticular formation. One consequence is that a comatose patient with depressed function of the reticular formation, but with an otherwise intact brainstem, may show only the slow phase of caloric nystagmus—that is, caloric stimulation produces only a tonic deviation of the eyes in the direction of the slow phase of the expected nystagmus. Abnormalities of this conjugate deviation can therefore be of some value in determining the location of structural damage in the brainstem of a comatose patient. Turning the head of a comatose individual from side to side can elicit similar conjugate lateral eye movements. The movements in this case are those appropriate to keep both eyes pointed in the same forward direction relative to the trunk (e.g., head movement to the right causes contraversive eye movements to the left). These are called **doll's head eye movements** (or the **oculocephalic reflex**) and mostly represent no more than a vestibuloocular reflex that is normally suppressed when a conscious individual moves head and eyes to one side simultaneously to look at something. The afferent limb of the oculocephalic reflex probably also includes proprioceptors of the neck because some reflex movement can still be elicited from patients with nonfunctional labyrinths.

At the termination of rotation to the left, nystagmus with its fast phase to the right is seen in a normal individual, as discussed above. In addition, trying to point at something with closed eyes results in deviation of the arm to the left; this is called **past pointing.** There is also a tendency to fall to the left when walking. The lateral vestibulospinal tract ordinarily is quite important in directing the changes in muscle tone that correspond to the postural changes involved in balance; postrotatory past pointing and a tendency to fall demonstrate exaggerated activity in this tract.

Conditions that make the cupula sensitive to gravity cause nystagmus and illusions of movement

A normal cupula has the same density as its endolymphatic surroundings, so gravity causes no movement of the cupula relative to its crista, and the semicircular ducts are insensitive to head position. Conditions that change the relative densities of cupula and endolymph would be expected to make the semicircular ducts gravity-sensitive, resulting in illusions of movement in response to certain orientations of the head. This is the commonly accepted explanation for the positionally dependent **vertigo** (illusions of movement) and nystagmus seen during and after excessive alcohol consumption (Figure 14-31). As blood alcohol levels rise, alcohol initially leaves the capillaries and infiltrates the cupulae, making them less dense than surrounding endolymph. During this period, holding the head in a position that allows cupular deflection by attempted flotation causes nystagmus. This lasts for several

hours, until the alcohol concentrations of cupulae and endolymph equilibrate and the nystagmus stops. Subsequently, after blood alcohol levels drop, alcohol leaves the cupulae first. This makes them *more* dense than endolymph and causes several hours of positionally dependent nystagmus in the opposite direction.

Age or trauma can cause detachment of otoconia in the utricle, making them free to move into a semicircular duct and either stick to or collide with a cupula. The posterior duct is most often affected, with the result that orienting the head with the cupula of this canal in a horizontal plane (typically by rolling over in bed) causes a brief episode of vertigo and nystagmus. This syndrome is called **benign positional vertigo**—benign because in most patients the otoconia work their way out of the semicircular duct and the symptoms vanish. For patients with persistent symptoms, a series of positioning maneuvers can usually speed the return of the otoconia to the utricle.

Efferents control the sensitivity of hair cells

Some fibers arising in or near the vestibular nuclei project back through the eighth nerve and end on the hair cells of the vestibular apparatus. These efferents are another example of the widespread phenomenon of feedback from a higher level to a lower level of a sensory system. The role of such efferents, in general, is poorly understood, and the vestibular system is no exception. One common suggestion is that the efferents could compensate for self-generated activity in the sensory system. For example, the horizontal semicircular canals receive the same stimulation if you rotate your head as they do if someone begins to rotate the chair in which you are sitting. However, the reflex postural adjustments to the two rotations are quite different. If the efferent system compensated for the hair cell response to self-generated rotation, the reflex postural adjustments would be eliminated. There is some experimental evidence that this may be the case, but there is also evidence that this is not the principal role of the efferents.

Similarly, neurons near the superior olivary nucleus project through the eighth nerve to cochlear hair cells. The efferent neurons ending on outer hair cells (Figure 14-12, *B*) influence their contractility and so alter the sensitivity of the regions of the cochlea that they innervate.

The Vestibular, Proprioceptive, and Visual Systems Collectively Mediate Position Sense

The vestibular system is not the only source of information about the position and motion of the head in space. The visual system also plays a major role, and in most situations is actually dominant. Most of us have experienced an illusion of movement when we were stationary and a nearby large object (such as a train on the next track) moved. It should also be noted that the vestibular apparatus can give no information about the position of the *body*, so additional information is required for tasks such as

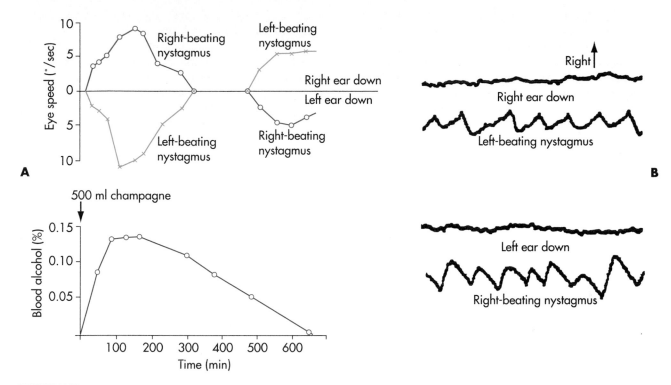

FIGURE 14-31

Induction of nystagmus by alteration of the relative density of the cupula and endolymph. **A,** During the period of peak blood alcohol levels after ingestion of half a liter of champagne, placing the head in a right-ear-down position (parts of the curve above the horizontal axis) causes nystagmus with its fast phase to the right; a left-ear-down position causes nystagmus with its fast phase to the left. As blood alcohol levels drop, alcohol levels in the cupulae and endolymph equilibrate; the nystagmus ceases and is then followed by a period in which the nystagmus reverses direction. **B,** Ingestion of heavy water (deuterium oxide), which is *more* dense than normal cupulae and endolymph, has just the opposite effect. Before drinking heavy water, the subject has no nystagmus in either head position (upper trace of each pair). Thirty minutes after drinking 200 ml of heavy water, the subject has left-beating nystagmus when the right ear faces down and right-beating nystagmus when the left ear faces down (lower trace of each pair). (**A** redrawn from Aschan G, Bergstedt M: Positional alcohol nystagmus (PAN) in man following repeated alcohol doses, *Acta Otolaryngol Suppl* 330:15, 1975. **B** from Money KE, Myles WS: Heavy water nystagmus and effects of alcohol, *Nature* 247:404, 1974.)

reaching with a hand for a seen object. Much of the additional information is provided by mechanoreceptors in the neck that detect the orientation of the head relative to the body. If the first three cervical dorsal roots of a monkey are anesthetized bilaterally, severe disorientation results, involving not only eye-hand coordination but also such basic activities as walking and climbing.

Vestibular, visual, and somatosensory inputs are normally combined seamlessly to produce our sense of orientation and movement. If one of the three is defective, the remaining two are adequate for most functions. For example, humans can compensate reasonably well for total loss of vestibular function, as long as visual cues are available. However, loss of two of the three systems is disabling. This is the basis of **Romberg's sign**, the greatly increased swaying and loss of balance caused by closing the eyes in a patient with defective vestibular or somatosensory function.

SUGGESTED READINGS

Baloh RW, Halmagyi GM, editors: *Disorders of the vestibular system,* New York, 1996, Oxford University Press.

Baloh RW, Honrubia V: *Clinical neurophysiology of the vestibular system,* ed 2, Philadelphia, 1990, F.A. Davis Company.

Bender MB, Feldman M: Visual illusions during head movement in lesions of the brain stem, *Arch Neurol* 17:354, 1967.
An interesting discussion of what happens if a patient's vestibular apparatus is damaged so that it is impossible to tell if movement of a visual image is caused by head movement or motion in the outside world.

Borg E, Counter SA: The middle-ear muscles, *Sci Am* 261(2):74, 1989.

Bottini G et al: Identification of the central vestibular projections in man: a positron emission tomography activation study, *Exp Brain Res* 99:164, 1994.

Boyle R: Activity of medial vestibulospinal tract cells during rotation and ocular movement in the alert squirrel monkey, *J Neurophysiol* 70:2176, 1993.

Bracchi F et al: Multiday recordings from the primary neurons of the statoreceptors of the labyrinth of the bullfrog, *Acta Otolaryngol Suppl* 334, 1975. *Technically astonishing experiments in which continuous recordings were made from single utricular primary afferents of a bullfrog aboard a rocket that blasted off and put the frog in orbit for a few days.*

Brandt T, Daroff RB: The multisensory physiological and pathological vertigo syndromes, *Ann Neurol* 7:195, 1980. *Stimulation or dysfunction of the vestibular, visual, or somatosensory systems can cause illusions of movement.*

Brandt TH, Dieterich M, Danek A: Vestibular cortex lesions affect the perception of verticality, *Ann Neurol* 35:403, 1994.

Clinical evidence that an important area of vestibular cortex in humans is located in the posterior insula.

Bredberg G, Ades HW, Engström H: Scanning electron microscopy of the normal and pathologically altered organ of Corti, *Acta Otolaryngol Suppl* 301:3, 1972. *Pretty pictures from a variety of mammals.*

Brindley GS: How does an animal that is dropped in a nonupright posture know the angle through which it must turn in the air so that its feet point to the ground? *J Physiol* 180:20P, 1965. *Briefly, it remembers which way was up when you let go of it. The paper isn't much longer than its title.*

Clark DL, Kreutzberg JR, Chee FKW: Vestibular stimulation influence on motor development in infants, *Science* 196:1228, 1977.

Cohen LA: Role of eye and neck proprioceptive mechanisms in body orientation and motor coordination, *J Neurophysiol* 24:1, 1961.

Dallos P, Popper AN, Fay RR, editors: *The cochlea,* New York, 1996, Springer-Verlag.

Dieterich M, Brandt TH, Fries W: Otolith function in man: results from a case of otolith Tullio phenomenon, *Brain* 112:1377, 1989. *A remarkable case of a patient whose stapes footplate popped through the oval window, where it could push against the utricle. Loud sounds subsequently caused nystagmus and loss of balance.*

Fekix H et al: Morphological features of human Reissner's membrane, *Acta Otolaryngol* 113:321, 1993.

Fernández C, Goldberg JM, Abend WK: Response to static tilts of peripheral neurons innervating otolith organs of the squirrel monkey, *J Neurophysiol* 35:978, 1972.

Fine ML, Horn MH, Cox B: *Acanthonus armatus,* a deep-sea teleost fish with a minute brain and large ears, *Proc R Soc Lond* B230:257, 1987. *"Acanthonus armatus, a deep-water benthopelagic fish, has, per unit body weight, the smallest brain and largest semicircular canals of any known teleost and possibly any vertebrate."*

Friedmann I, Ballantyne J, editors: *Ultrastructural atlas of the inner ear,* London, 1984, Butterworth & Co.

Goldberg JM, Fernández C: Efferent vestibular system in the squirrel monkey: anatomical location and influence on afferent activity, *J Neurophysiol* 43:986, 1980.

Hudspeth AJ: How the ear's works work, *Nature* 341:397, 1989. *A review of the biophysics of hair cells by one of the major investigators in this area.*

Jenkins WM, Masterton RB: Sound localization: effects of unilateral lesions in the central auditory system, *J Neurophysiol* 47:987, 1982.

de Jong PTVM et al: Ataxia and nystagmus induced by injection of local anesthetics in the neck, *Ann Neurol* 1:240, 1977.

Kemp DT: Stimulated acoustic emissions from within the human auditory system, *J Acoust Soc Am* 64:1386, 1978. *The original description of evoked otoacoustic emissions, which for a while were known as "Kemp echoes."*

Klinke R, Schmidt CL: Efferent influence on the vestibular organ during active movements of the body, *Pflügers Arch* 318:325, 1970. *Clever experiments giving a hint about a goldfish's use for the efferent fibers in its vestibular nerve.*

Lang W, Büttner-Ennever JA, and Büttner U: Vestibular projections to the monkey thalamus: an autoradiographic study, *Brain Res* 177:3, 1979.

Lee D, Lishman R: Vision in movement and balance, *New Scientist* 65:59, 1975. *A popularized but fascinating account of how easy it is to confuse one's position sense by presenting conflicting visual and vestibular inputs.*

Lidén G, Peterson JL, Harford ER: Simultaneous recording of changes in relative impedance and air pressure during acoustic and non-acoustic elicitation of the middle-ear reflexes, *Acta Otolaryngol Suppl* 263:208, 1970.

Living without a balancing mechanism, *N Engl J Med* 246:458, 1952. *A first-hand account by an anonymous physician of the remarkable compensation we can achieve after bilateral damage to the vestibular apparatus.*

Mahoney T, Vernon J, Meikle M: Function of the acoustic reflex in discrimination of intense speech, *Arch Otolaryngol* 105:119, 1979.

Middlebrooks JC, Green DM: Sound localization by human listeners, *Ann Rev Psychol* 42:135, 1991.

Moore JK: The human auditory brain stem: a comparative view, *Hearing Res* 29:1, 1987.

Moore JK, Osen KK: The cochlear nuclei in man, *Am J Anat* 154:393, 1979.

Naitoh Y et al: Projections of the individual vestibular end-organs in the brain stem of the squirrel monkey, *Hearing Res* 87:141, 1995.

Osterhammel P, Terkildsen K, Zilstorff K: Vestibular habituation in ballet dancers, *Adv Otorhinolaryngol* 17:158, 1970. *How do people who rotate for a living do it?*

Pickles JO: *An introduction to the physiology of hearing,* ed 2, London, 1988, Academic Press.

Robinette MS, Glattke TJ: *Clinical applications of otoacoustic emissions,* New York, 1997, Thieme Medical Publishers, Inc.

Rudge P, Bronstein AM: Investigations of disorders of balance, *J Neurol Neurosurg Psych* 59:568, 1995.

Ryan A, Dallos P: Effect of absence of cochlear outer hair cells on behavioral auditory threshold, *Nature* 253:44, 1975.

Scharf B et al: On the role of the olivocochlear bundle in hearing: a case study, *Hearing Res* 75:11, 1994.

Sharp JA, Barber HO, editors: *The vestibulo-ocular reflex and vertigo,* New York, 1993, Raven Press.

Shaw MD, Baker R: The locations of stapedius and tensor tympani motoneurons in the cat, *J Comp Neurol* 216:10, 1983.

Simpson JI, Graf W: Eye-muscle geometry and compensatory eye movements in lateral-eyed and frontal-eyed animals, *Ann NY Acad Sci* 374:20, 1981. *Pitching to one side or the other requires vertical compensatory eye movements in rabbits but torsional eye movements in us, even though both species have semicircular canals arranged similarly. This fascinating paper provides an explanation.*

Spoendlin H: The innervation of the organ of Corti, *J Laryngol Otol* 81:717, 1967.

Spoendlin H, Schrott A: Analysis of the human auditory nerve, *Hearing Res* 43:25, 1989.

von Baumgarten R et al: Effects of rectilinear acceleration and optokinetic and caloric stimulations in space, *Science* 225:208, 1984.

Von Békésy G: *Experiments in hearing,* New York, 1960, McGraw-Hill. *A large collection of clever and skillful experiments by the grand master of auditory physiology.*

Wilson VJ, Jones GM: *Mammalian vestibular physiology,* New York, 1979, Plenum Press.

Yates BJ: Vestibular influences on the autonomic nervous system, *Ann NY Acad Sci* 781:458, 1996. *We don't often think of it, but vestibular-autonomic interactions are involved not just in conditions such as motion sickness but also in functions such as regulation of blood pressure as we go from sitting to standing.*

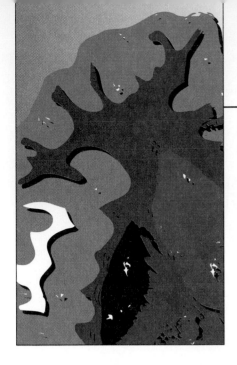

ATLAS OF THE HUMAN BRAINSTEM*

This series of five chapters on the functional anatomy of the brainstem concludes here, with a summary of the principal contents of the brainstem at each level (Figures 15-1 to 15-3), a series of transverse sections of the brainstem (Figures 15-4 to 15-9), and brief descriptions of structures indicated in these sections.

*Parts of this chapter were modified from Nolte J, Angevine JB Jr: *The human brain in photographs and diagrams*, St. Louis, 1995, Mosby.

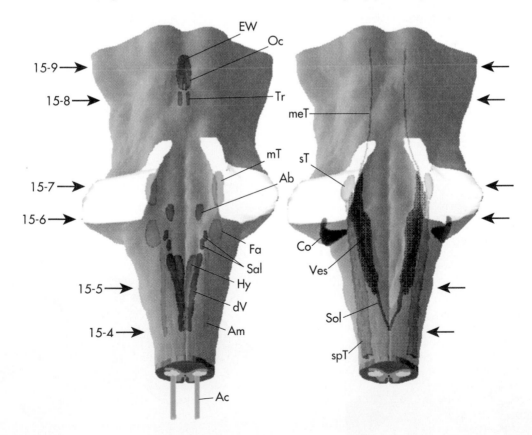

FIGURE 15-1
Three-dimensional reconstructions of the brainstem, with motor *(left)* and sensory *(right)* cranial nerve nuclei indicated. *Arrows* indicate the planes of the sections shown in Figures 15-4 to 15-9. *Ab,* Abducens nucleus; *Ac,* accessory nucleus; *Am,* nucleus ambiguus; *Co,* cochlear nuclei; *dV,* dorsal motor nucleus of the vagus; *EW,* Edinger-Westphal nucleus; *Fa,* facial motor nucleus; *Hy,* hypoglossal nucleus; *meT,* mesencephalic nucleus of the trigeminal; *mT,* trigeminal motor nucleus; *Oc,* oculomotor nucleus; *Sal,* salivatory nuclei; *Sol,* nucleus of the solitary tract; *spT,* spinal trigeminal nucleus; *sT,* trigeminal main sensory nucleus; *Tr,* trochlear nucleus; *Ves,* vestibular nuclei.

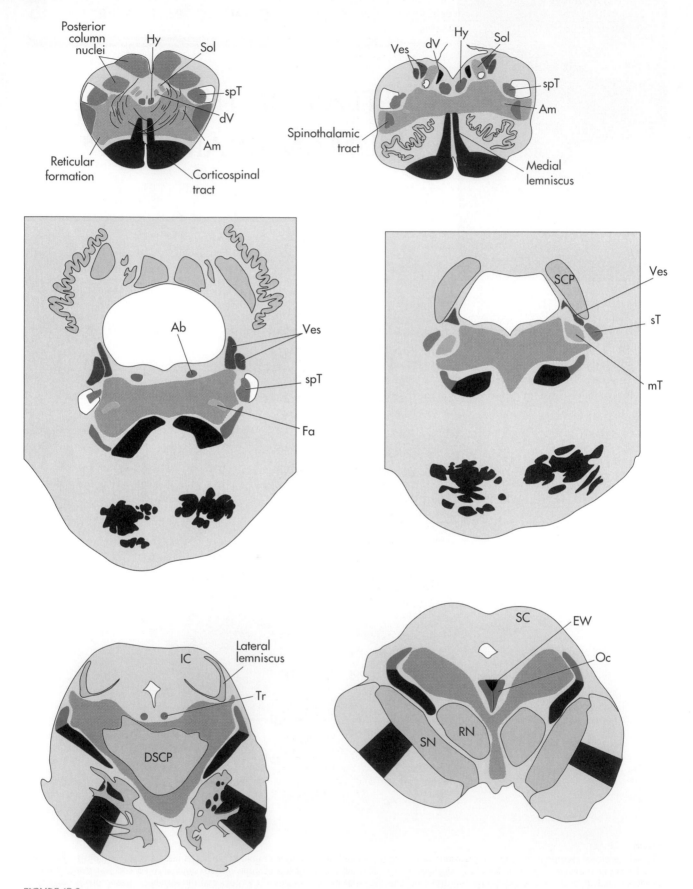

FIGURE 15-2
Schematic views of the transverse sections of the brainstem shown photographically in Figures 15-4 to 15-9, each enlarged to about three times its actual size. Major tracts and cranial nerve nuclei are indicated. *DSCP*, Decussation of the superior cerebellar peduncles; *IC*, inferior colliculus; *RN*, red nucleus; *SC*, superior colliculus; *SCP*, superior cerebellar peduncle; *SN*, substantia nigra; other abbreviations as in Figure 15-1. (Modified from Nolte J, Angevine JB Jr: *The human brain in photographs and diagrams*, St. Louis, 1995, Mosby.)

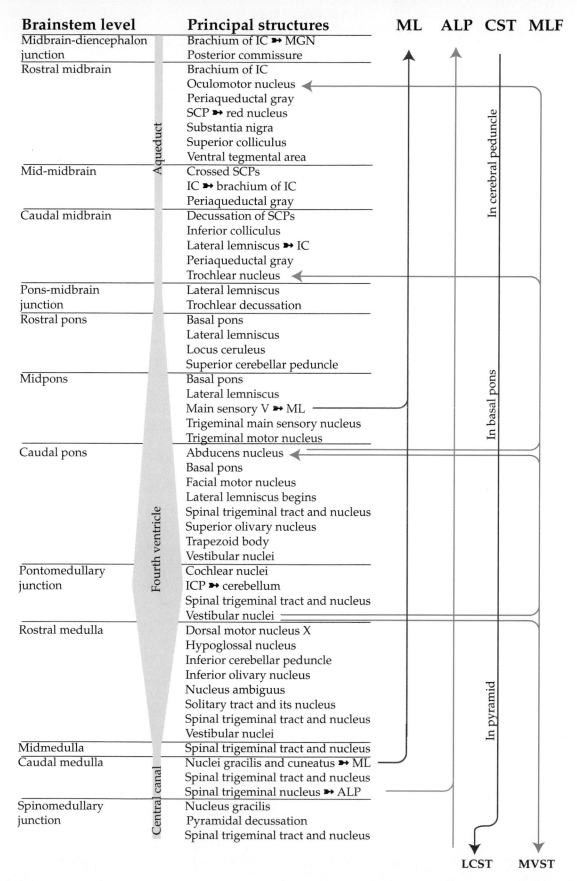

Brainstem level	Principal structures	ML	ALP	CST	MLF
Midbrain-diencephalon junction	Brachium of IC ➤ MGN				
	Posterior commissure				
Rostral midbrain	Brachium of IC				
	Oculomotor nucleus				
	Periaqueductal gray				
	SCP ➤ red nucleus				
	Substantia nigra				
	Superior colliculus				
	Ventral tegmental area				
Mid-midbrain	Crossed SCPs				
	IC ➤ brachium of IC				
	Periaqueductal gray				
Caudal midbrain	Decussation of SCPs				
	Inferior colliculus				
	Lateral lemniscus ➤ IC				
	Periaqueductal gray				
	Trochlear nucleus				
Pons-midbrain junction	Lateral lemniscus				
	Trochlear decussation				
Rostral pons	Basal pons				
	Lateral lemniscus				
	Locus ceruleus				
	Superior cerebellar peduncle				
Midpons	Basal pons				
	Lateral lemniscus				
	Main sensory V ➤ ML				
	Trigeminal main sensory nucleus				
	Trigeminal motor nucleus				
Caudal pons	Abducens nucleus				
	Basal pons				
	Facial motor nucleus				
	Lateral lemniscus begins				
	Spinal trigeminal tract and nucleus				
	Superior olivary nucleus				
	Trapezoid body				
	Vestibular nuclei				
Pontomedullary junction	Cochlear nuclei				
	ICP ➤ cerebellum				
	Spinal trigeminal tract and nucleus				
	Vestibular nuclei				
Rostral medulla	Dorsal motor nucleus X				
	Hypoglossal nucleus				
	Inferior cerebellar peduncle				
	Inferior olivary nucleus				
	Nucleus ambiguus				
	Solitary tract and its nucleus				
	Spinal trigeminal tract and nucleus				
	Vestibular nuclei				
Midmedulla	Spinal trigeminal tract and nucleus				
Caudal medulla	Nuclei gracilis and cuneatus ➤ ML				
	Spinal trigeminal tract and nucleus				
	Spinal trigeminal nucleus ➤ ALP				
Spinomedullary junction	Nucleus gracilis				
	Pyramidal decussation				
	Spinal trigeminal tract and nucleus				

LCST   MVST

FIGURE 15-3

Principal structures at different brainstem levels. Only the levels containing the major parts of structures are indicated. Many structures extend a short distance into adjacent levels (e.g., the nucleus of the solitary tract extends a bit into the caudal medulla and caudal pons). Raphe nuclei and other elements of the reticular formation are not indicated in the table, but are present at all brainstem levels. *ALP*, Anterolateral pathway; *CST*, corticospinal tract; *IC*, inferior colliculus; *ICP*, inferior cerebellar peduncle; *LCST*, lateral corticospinal tract; *ML*, medial lemniscus; *MLF*, medial longitudinal fasciculus; *MGN*, medial geniculate nucleus; *MVST*, medial vestibulospinal tract; *SCP*, superior cerebellar peduncle.

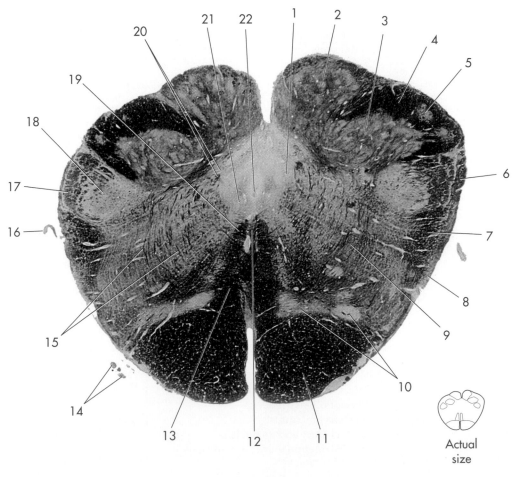

20 19 18 17 16 15 14 21 22 1 2 3 4 5 6 7 8 9 10 13 12 11

Actual
size

FIGURE 15-4

FIGURE 15-4

Caudal medulla (close to the level of the obex).

1. Dorsal motor nucleus of the vagus. The caudal end of the nucleus of origin of most preganglionic parasympathetic neurons for thoracic and abdominal viscera.
2. Nucleus gracilis. Site of termination of fasciculus gracilis and the origin of the leg portion of the medial lemniscus.
3. Nucleus cuneatus. Site of termination of fasciculus cuneatus and the origin of the arm portion of the medial lemniscus.
4. Fasciculus cuneatus. Uncrossed primary afferents, carrying tactile and proprioceptive information from the arm.
5. Lateral cuneate nucleus. Arm equivalent of Clarke's nucleus. Proprioceptive primary afferents travel through fasciculus cuneatus to reach the lateral cuneate nucleus, which then gives rise to uncrossed cuneocerebellar fibers that enter the cerebellum through the inferior cerebellar peduncle.
6. Posterior spinocerebellar tract. Uncrossed fibers from Clarke's nucleus, carrying proprioceptive information from the leg that will reach the ipsilateral half of the cerebellar vermis through the inferior cerebellar peduncle.
7. Anterolateral pathway. Mostly-crossed fibers from the spinal posterior horns and intermediate gray conveying pain and temperature information to the thalamus (spinothalamic tract), reticular formation, and midbrain.
8. Anterior spinocerebellar tract. Crossed fibers from lumbosacral spinal gray matter, carrying proprioceptive and other information from the leg. This tract stays in approximately the same position until the rostral pons, where it moves over the surface of the superior cerebellar peduncle (Figure 15-7) and turns posteriorly into the cerebellum.
9. Location of nucleus ambiguus. Lower motor neurons for laryngeal and pharyngeal muscles and preganglionic parasympathetic neurons for the heart.
10. Inferior olivary nucleus (medial accessory nucleus). The inferior olivary complex gives rise to climbing fibers that end in the contralateral half of the cerebellum (see Chapter 20). Those from the accessory nuclei project mainly to the vermis and flocculus, those from the principal inferior olivary nucleus to the cerebellar hemisphere.

11. Pyramid. Corticospinal fibers from the ipsilateral precentral gyrus and adjacent areas of cerebral cortex.
12. Raphe nuclei. Widely projecting serotonergic neurons that collectively blanket the CNS. Those in caudal brainstem levels such as this project mainly to the spinal cord.
13. Medial lemniscus, the principal ascending pathway for tactile and proprioceptive information. Originates in the contralateral posterior column nuclei and terminates in the thalamus (VPL).
14. Hypoglossal nerve fibers, on their way to the muscles of the ipsilateral half of the tongue.
15. Crossing fibers from the nuclei gracilis and cuneatus forming the medial lemniscus, the principal ascending pathway for tactile and proprioceptive information.
16. Fibers of the vagus nerve, on their way to muscles of the ipsilateral half of the larynx and pharynx. These caudal filaments of the vagus are sometimes considered separately as the cranial part of the accessory nerve.
17. Spinal trigeminal tract. Primary afferents from the ipsilateral side of the face, at this level conveying information about pain and temperature.
18. Spinal trigeminal nucleus (caudal nucleus). Site of termination of part of the spinal trigeminal tract, and the origin of part of the anterolateral pathway. At this level, the nucleus has the appearance of the spinal posterior horn, has a component similar to the substantia gelatinosa, and processes pain and temperature information.
19. Medial longitudinal fasciculus (MLF). At this level, the fibers of the medial vestibulospinal tract.
20. Solitary tract and its nucleus. Primary afferents conveying visceral information from cranial nerves VII, IX, and X (as well as some chemosensory information from the trigeminal nerve) travel through the solitary tract to reach the surrounding nucleus of the solitary tract. Only information from viscera reaches this caudal level.
21. Hypoglossal nucleus. Lower motor neurons for the ipsilateral half of the tongue.
22. Central canal. Merges rostrally with the fourth ventricle and caudally with the central canal of the spinal cord.

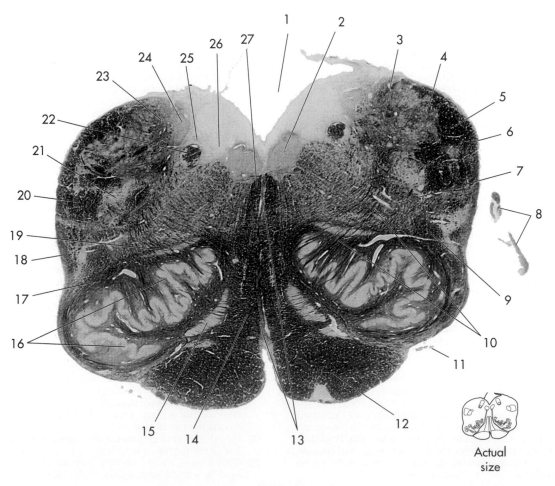

Actual
size

FIGURE 15-5

FIGURE 15-5

Rostral medulla.

 1. Fourth ventricle.
 2. Hypoglossal nucleus. Lower motor neurons for the ipsilateral half of the tongue.
 3. Nucleus cuneatus. Site of termination of fasciculus cuneatus and the origin of the arm portion of the medial lemniscus.
 4. Lateral cuneate nucleus. Arm equivalent of Clarke's nucleus. Proprioceptive primary afferents travel through fasciculus cuneatus to reach the lateral cuneate nucleus, which then gives rise to uncrossed cuneocerebellar fibers that enter the cerebellum through the inferior cerebellar peduncle.
 5. Inferior cerebellar peduncle. By the time it enters the cerebellum, it contains crossed olivocerebellar fibers, the uncrossed posterior spinocerebellar tract, vestibulocerebellar fibers, and other cerebellar afferents.
 6. Posterior spinocerebellar tract entering the inferior cerebellar peduncle. Uncrossed fibers from Clarke's nucleus, carrying proprioceptive information from the leg to the ipsilateral half of the cerebellar vermis.
 7. Location of nucleus ambiguus. Lower motor neurons for laryngeal and pharyngeal muscles and preganglionic parasympathetic neurons for the heart.
 8. Vagus nerve (CN X).
 9. Anterolateral pathway. Mostly-crossed fibers from the spinal posterior horns and intermediate gray conveying pain and temperature information to the thalamus (spinothalamic tract), reticular formation, and midbrain.
10. Olivocerebellar fibers. Cross the midline as internal arcuate fibers, join the inferior cerebellar peduncle, and end in the cerebellar cortex as climbing fibers.
11. Hypoglossal nerve fibers, on their way to the muscles of the ipsilateral half of the tongue.
12. Pyramid. Corticospinal fibers from the ipsilateral precentral gyrus and adjacent areas of cerebral cortex.
13. Raphe nuclei. Serotonergic neurons that at this level are one source of descending pain-control fibers to the spinal cord.
14. Medial lemniscus, the principal ascending pathway for tactile and proprioceptive information. Originates in the contralateral posterior column nuclei and terminates in the thalamus (VPL).
15. Inferior olivary nucleus (medial accessory nucleus). The inferior olivary complex gives rise to climbing fibers that end in the contralateral half of the cerebellum (see Chapter 20). Those from the accessory nuclei project mainly to the vermis and flocculus, those from the principal inferior olivary nucleus to the cerebellar hemisphere.
16. Inferior olivary nucleus (principal nucleus). The inferior olivary complex gives rise to climbing fibers that end in the contralateral half of the cerebellum (see Chapter 20). Those from the accessory nuclei project mainly to the vermis and flocculus, those from the principal inferior olivary nucleus project to the cerebellar hemisphere.
17. Fibers of the central tegmental tract reaching the inferior olivary nucleus.
18. Anterior spinocerebellar tract. Crossed fibers from lumbosacral spinal gray matter, carrying proprioceptive and other information from the leg. This tract stays in approximately the same position until the rostral pons, where it moves over the surface of the superior cerebellar peduncle (Figure 15-7) and turns posteriorly into the cerebellum.
19. Inferior olivary nucleus (dorsal accessory nucleus). The inferior olivary complex gives rise to climbing fibers that end in the contralateral half of the cerebellum (see Chapter 20). Those from the accessory nuclei project mainly to the vermis and flocculus, those from the principal inferior olivary nucleus project to the cerebellar hemisphere.
20. Spinal trigeminal tract. Primary afferents from the ipsilateral side of the face, including those on their way to the caudal nucleus conveying information about pain and temperature.
21. Spinal trigeminal nucleus (interpolar nucleus). Some primary afferents of the spinal trigeminal tract, including those carrying information about dental pain, end here.
22. Solitary tract. Primary afferents conveying visceral information from cranial nerves VII, IX, and X (as well as some chemosensory information from the trigeminal nerve) to the surrounding nucleus of the solitary tract.
23. Inferior vestibular nucleus with bundles of vestibular primary afferents running through it.
24. Medial vestibular nucleus. Site of origin of the medial vestibulospinal tract (among other connections).
25. Nucleus of the solitary tract. Site of termination of the visceral primary afferents in the solitary tract.
26. Dorsal motor nucleus of the vagus. Most of the preganglionic parasympathetic neurons for thoracic and abdominal viscera.
27. Medial longitudinal fasciculus (MLF). At this level, the fibers of the medial vestibulospinal tract.

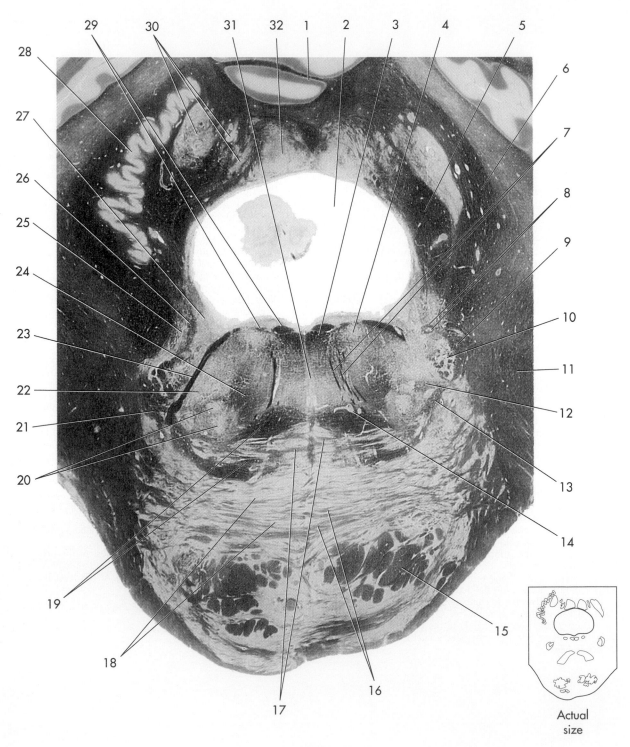

Actual
size

FIGURE 15-6

FIGURE 15-6
Caudal pons.
1. Vermis of the cerebellum. The zone of cerebellar cortex straddling the midline.
2. Fourth ventricle.
3. Medial longitudinal fasciculus (MLF). At this level, fibers from vestibular nuclei and abducens interneurons, active in coordinating eye movements.
4. Abducens nucleus. Contains the lower motor neurons for the ipsilateral lateral rectus, as well as the interneurons that project through the contralateral MLF to medial rectus motor neurons.
5. Superior cerebellar peduncle. Fibers from the deep cerebellar nuclei to the contralateral red nucleus and thalamus (ventral lateral nucleus [VL]).
6. Inferior cerebellar peduncle entering the cerebellum. Contains crossed olivocerebellar fibers, the uncrossed posterior spinocerebellar tract, vestibulocerebellar fibers, and other cerebellar afferents.
7. Abducens nerve fibers, on their way to the ipsilateral lateral rectus.
8. Solitary tract and its nucleus. Primary afferents conveying visceral information from cranial nerves VII, IX, and X (as well as some chemosensory information from the trigeminal nerve) travel through the solitary tract to reach the surrounding nucleus of the solitary tract. Only gustatory information reaches this rostral level.
9. Spinal trigeminal tract. Primary afferents from the ipsilateral side of the face, including those on their way to the caudal nucleus conveying information about pain and temperature.
10. Spinal trigeminal nucleus (oral nucleus). Some primary afferents of the spinal trigeminal tract, particularly those carrying tactile information, end here.
11. Middle cerebellar peduncle. Fibers from contralateral pontine nuclei that end as mossy fibers in all areas of cerebellar cortex.
12. Lateral lemniscus. Ascending auditory fibers from the cochlear and superior olivary nuclei, representing both ears.
13. Anterolateral pathway. Mostly-crossed fibers from the spinal posterior horns and intermediate gray conveying pain and temperature information to the thalamus (spinothalamic tract), reticular formation, and midbrain.
14. Errant avian.
15. Corticospinal, corticobulbar, and corticopontine fibers, from ipsilateral cerebral cortex.
16. Pontocerebellar fibers, from pontine nuclei of one side to the opposite middle cerebellar peduncle.

17. Trapezoid body. Crossing auditory fibers, primarily from the ventral cochlear nucleus.
18. Pontine nuclei. Source of pontocerebellar fibers that cross the midline and form the middle cerebellar peduncle.
19. Medial lemniscus. The principal ascending pathway for tactile and proprioceptive information. Originates in the contralateral posterior column nuclei, terminates in the thalamus (VPL).
20. Superior olivary nucleus. First site of convergence of fibers representing the two ears and the source of many of the fibers of the lateral lemniscus.
21. Anterior spinocerebellar tract. Crossed fibers from lumbosacral spinal gray matter, carrying proprioceptive and other information from the leg. This tract stays in approximately the same position until the rostral pons, where it moves over the surface of the superior cerebellar peduncle (Figure 15-7) and turns posteriorly into the cerebellum.
22. Facial motor nucleus. Lower motor neurons for ipsilateral muscles of facial expression.
23. Facial nerve fibers. Most of them are on their way to ipsilateral muscles of facial expression.
24. Central tegmental tract. Descending fibers from the red nucleus to the inferior olivary nucleus, together with fibers to and from different levels of the reticular formation.
25. Lateral vestibular nucleus, source of the lateral vestibulospinal tract.
26. Juxtarestiform body. Fibers of the inferior cerebellar peduncle interconnecting the vestibular nuclei and cerebellum.
27. Superior vestibular nucleus.
28. Dentate nucleus. The deep nucleus connected to the cerebellar hemisphere and the source of most of the fibers in the superior cerebellar peduncle.
29. Internal genu of the facial nerve. Facial nerve fibers, most of them on their way to ipsilateral muscles of facial expression.
30. Interposed nucleus. The deep cerebellar nucleus connected to the paravermal or intermediate zone of cerebellar cortex.
31. Raphe nuclei. Widely projecting serotonergic neurons that collectively blanket the CNS. Those in intermediate brainstem levels such as this are one source of descending pain-control fibers to the spinal cord, and also project to other brainstem levels and the cerebellum.
32. Fastigial nucleus. The deep cerebellar nucleus connected to the vermis.

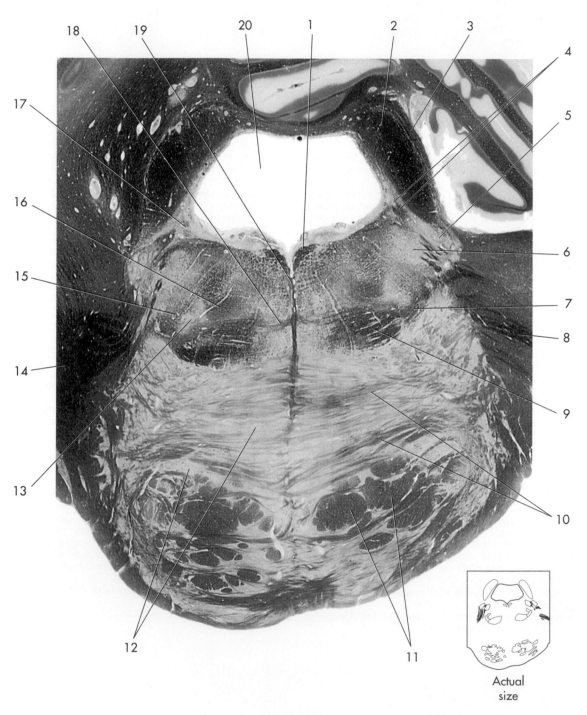

FIGURE 15-7

FIGURE 15-7

Midpons.
1. Medial longitudinal fasciculus (MLF). At this level, the fibers are from vestibular nuclei and abducens interneurons and are active in coordinating eye movements.
2. Superior cerebellar peduncle. Fibers from the deep cerebellar nuclei to the contralateral red nucleus and thalamus (VL).
3. Anterior spinocerebellar tract. Crossed fibers from lumbosacral spinal gray matter, carrying proprioceptive and other information from the leg.
4. Mesencephalic trigeminal tract and nucleus. Processes of primary afferent cell bodies in the mesencephalic trigeminal nucleus travel through the tract, leave the brainstem, and innervate mechanoreceptors in and around the mouth.
5. Trigeminal main sensory nucleus. Site of termination of large-diameter trigeminal afferents; site of origin of the uncrossed dorsal trigeminal tract and of part of the medial lemniscus.
6. Trigeminal motor nucleus. Lower motor neurons for ipsilateral muscles of mastication.
7. Anterolateral pathway. Mostly-crossed fibers from the spinal posterior horns and intermediate gray conveying pain and temperature information to the thalamus (spinothalamic tract), reticular formation, and midbrain.
8. Trigeminal nerve. Somatosensory (and some chemosensory) fibers from the ipsilateral half of the head; efferents to ipsilateral muscles of mastication.
9. Medial lemniscus. The principal ascending pathway for tactile and proprioceptive information. Originates in the contralateral posterior column nuclei and terminates in the thalamus (VPL).
10. Pontocerebellar fibers, from pontine nuclei of one side to the opposite middle cerebellar peduncle.
11. Corticospinal, corticobulbar, and corticopontine fibers from ipsilateral cerebral cortex.
12. Pontine nuclei. Source of pontocerebellar fibers that cross the midline and form the middle cerebellar peduncle.
13. Superior olivary nucleus. First site of convergence of fibers representing the two ears and the source of many of the fibers of the lateral lemniscus.
14. Middle cerebellar peduncle. Fibers from contralateral pontine nuclei that end as mossy fibers in all areas of cerebellar cortex.
15. Lateral lemniscus. Ascending auditory fibers from the cochlear and superior olivary nuclei.
16. Central tegmental tract. Descending fibers from the red nucleus to the inferior olivary nucleus, together with fibers to and from different levels of the reticular formation.
17. Superior vestibular nucleus.
18. Trapezoid body. Crossing auditory fibers, primarily from the ventral cochlear nucleus.
19. Raphe nuclei. Widely projecting serotonergic neurons that collectively blanket the CNS. Those in rostral brainstem levels such as this project mainly to the cerebrum and cerebellum.
20. Fourth ventricle.

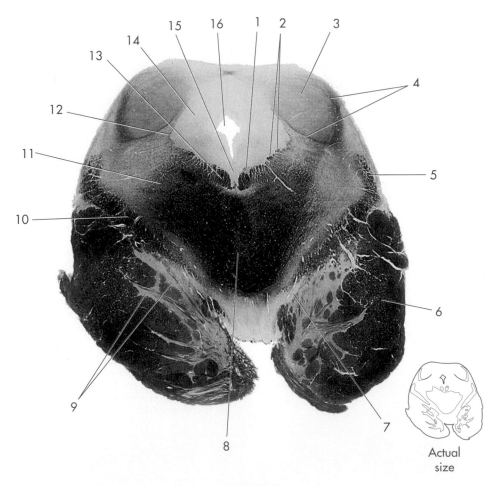

FIGURE 15-8

Actual
size

FIGURE 15-8

Caudal midbrain.

1. Trochlear nucleus. Lower motor neurons for the contralateral superior oblique muscle.
2. Trochlear nerve fibers, on their way to the contralateral superior oblique (after crossing in the trochlear decussation at the pons-midbrain junction).
3. Inferior colliculus. Site of termination of the lateral lemniscus and site of origin of the brachium of the inferior colliculus, which carries auditory information to the medial geniculate nucleus.
4. Lateral lemniscus ending in the inferior colliculus, the next stop in the central auditory pathway.
5. Anterolateral pathway. Mostly-crossed fibers from the spinal posterior horns and intermediate gray conveying pain and temperature information to the thalamus (spinothalamic tract), reticular formation, and midbrain.
6. Basis pedunculi (of the cerebral peduncle), right at the junction between the cerebral peduncle and the basal pons. Descending corticospinal, corticobulbar, and corticopontine fibers from ipsilateral cerebral cortex.
7. Substantia nigra. The very caudal end of the compact part, containing dopaminergic neurons whose axons terminate in the caudate nucleus and putamen.

8. Decussation of the superior cerebellar peduncles. Fibers from the deep cerebellar nuclei to the contralateral red nucleus and thalamus (VL).
9. Pontine nuclei. Source of pontocerebellar fibers that cross the midline and form the middle cerebellar peduncle.
10. Medial lemniscus. The principal ascending pathway for tactile and proprioceptive information. Originates in the contralateral posterior column nuclei and terminates in the thalamus (VPL).
11. Central tegmental tract. Descending fibers from the red nucleus to the inferior olivary nucleus, together with fibers to and from different levels of the reticular formation.
12. Mesencephalic trigeminal tract. Processes of cell bodies in the adjacent mesencephalic trigeminal nucleus that innervate mechanoreceptors in and around the mouth.
13. Medial longitudinal fasciculus (MLF). At this level, the fibers are from vestibular nuclei and abducens interneurons and are active in coordinating eye movements.
14. Periaqueductal gray. Site of origin of the descending pain control pathway that relays in nucleus raphe magnus (among other connections).
15. Raphe nuclei. Widely projecting serotonergic neurons that collectively blanket the CNS. Those in rostral brainstem levels such as this project mainly to the cerebrum.
16. Cerebral aqueduct.

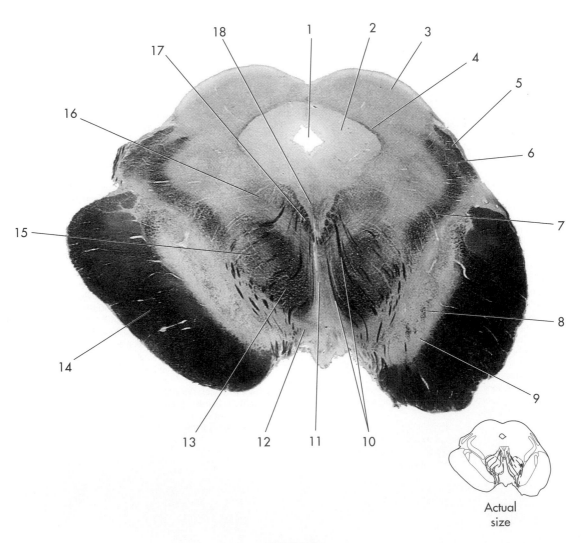

Actual
size

FIGURE 15-9

FIGURE 15-9
Rostral midbrain.
1. Cerebral aqueduct.
2. Periaqueductal gray. Site of origin of the descending pain control pathway that relays in nucleus raphe magnus (among other connections).
3. Superior colliculus. Involved in visual attention and eye movements and site of termination of most fibers of the superior brachium.
4. Mesencephalic trigeminal tract. Processes of cell bodies in the adjacent mesencephalic trigeminal nucleus that innervate mechanoreceptors in and around the mouth.
5. Brachium of the inferior colliculus. Ascending auditory fibers on their way from the inferior colliculus to the medial geniculate nucleus.
6. Anterolateral pathway. Mostly-crossed fibers from the spinal posterior horns and intermediate gray conveying pain and temperature information to the thalamus (spinothalamic tract), reticular formation, and midbrain.
7. Medial lemniscus. The principal ascending pathway for tactile and proprioceptive information. Originates in the contralateral posterior column nuclei and terminates in the thalamus (VPL).
8. Substantia nigra (compact part). Dopaminergic neurons whose axons terminate in the caudate nucleus and putamen.
9. Substantia nigra (reticular part). Site of termination of fibers from the caudate nucleus and putamen and site of origin of fibers to the thalamus, superior colliculus, and reticular formation.
10. Oculomotor nerve fibers. Axons of lower motor neurons and preganglionic parasympathetic neurons for the ipsilateral medial, superior and inferior recti, inferior oblique, levator palpebrae, pupillary sphincter, and ciliary muscle.

11. Raphe nuclei. Widely projecting serotonergic neurons that collectively blanket the CNS. Those in rostral brainstem levels such as this project mainly to the cerebrum.
12. Ventral tegmental area. Dopaminergic neurons whose axons terminate in limbic and frontal cortical sites.
13. Crossed superior cerebellar peduncle entering the red nucleus. Fibers from the contralateral deep cerebellar nuclei, on their way to the red nucleus and thalamus (VL).
14. Basis pedunculi (of cerebral peduncle). Descending corticospinal, corticobulbar, and corticopontine fibers from ipsilateral cerebral cortex.
15. Red nucleus. Receives inputs from the contralateral deep cerebellar nuclei via the superior cerebellar peduncle, and projects primarily to the inferior olivary nucleus, via the central tegmental tract.
16. Central tegmental tract. Descending fibers from the red nucleus to the inferior olivary nucleus, together with fibers to and from different levels of the reticular formation.
17. Medial longitudinal fasciculus (MLF). At this level, the fibers are from vestibular nuclei and abducens interneurons and are active in coordinating eye movements.
18. Oculomotor nucleus. Lower motor neurons for the ipsilateral medial and inferior recti and inferior oblique muscles, the contralateral superior rectus muscle, and the levator palpebrae of both sides; preganglionic parasympathetic neurons for the pupillary sphincter and the ciliary muscle.

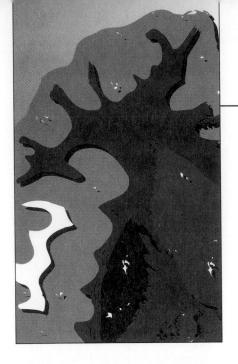

THE THALAMUS AND INTERNAL CAPSULE: GETTING TO AND FROM THE CEREBRAL CORTEX

The diencephalon, mostly hidden from view between the cerebral hemispheres (Figure 16-1, *A*), constitutes only about 2% of the CNS by weight. Nevertheless, it has extremely widespread and important connections, and the great majority of sensory, motor, and limbic pathways involve one or more relays in the diencephalon. Most motor and limbic pathways also involve telencephalic structures that are discussed in later chapters, so this chapter provides only a general overview of the connections of diencephalic nuclei. A more detailed consideration of these connections in terms of functional systems is provided in subsequent chapters. In addition, a series of sections demonstrating major structures of both the diencephalon and the telencephalon is provided in Chapter 24. Nearly all the connections between the cerebral cortex and subcortical structures, prominently including the diencephalon, travel through the internal capsule, so an overview of this structure is provided here as well.

THE DIENCEPHALON INCLUDES THE EPITHALAMUS, SUBTHALAMUS, HYPOTHALAMUS, AND THALAMUS

The diencephalon (Figure 16-1, *B*) is conventionally divided into four parts, each of which includes the term *thalamus* (from the Greek word meaning "inner chamber")

as part of its name.* These parts are (1) the **epithalamus,** which includes the **pineal gland** and a few nearby neural structures; (2) the **dorsal thalamus,** which is usually referred to simply as the **thalamus;** (3) the **subthalamus;** and (4) the **hypothalamus.**

The only part of the diencephalon that can be seen on an intact brain is the inferior surface of the hypothalamus (see Figures 3-14 and 3-15), which includes the **mammillary bodies** and the **infundibular stalk.** However, the entire medial surface of the diencephalon, much of which forms each wall of the third ventricle, can be seen on a hemisected brain (Figure 16-2). Superiorly the diencephalon borders the subarachnoid space of the transverse cerebral fissure; inferiorly, as previously noted, it is also exposed to subarachnoid space. Laterally it is bounded by the internal capsule (see Figures 3-17 to 3-19). The caudal boundary of the diencephalon is a plane through the posterior commissure and the caudal edge of the mammillary bodies; the rostral boundary is a plane through the anterior commissure and the optic chiasm. These rostral and caudal boundaries are approximate and semiarbitrary and are used only for purposes of discussion. Functionally con-

*A few other structures, most notably the globus pallidus, are derived embryologically from the diencephalon but usually are not considered part of it in discussions of the adult brain.

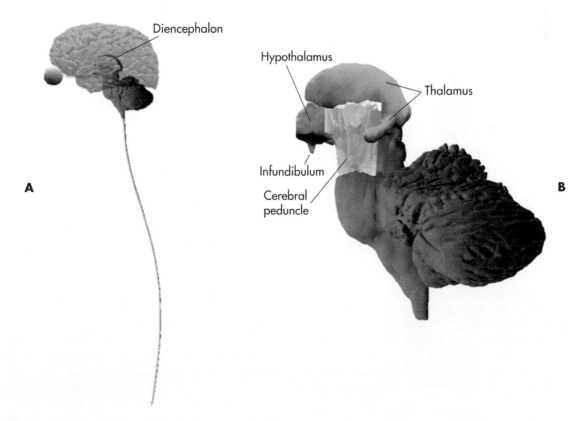

A **B**

FIGURE 16-1
Three-dimensional reconstructions of the diencephalon. **A,** The entire CNS, showing the diencephalon *(green)* almost completely surrounded by the cerebral hemispheres. **B,** The diencephalon, brainstem, and cerebellum, with the cerebral hemispheres removed.

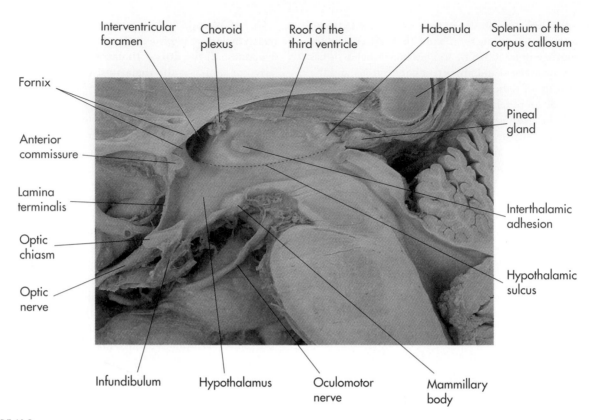

Fornix
Anterior commissure
Lamina terminalis
Optic chiasm
Optic nerve
Interventricular foramen
Choroid plexus
Roof of the third ventricle
Habenula
Splenium of the corpus callosum
Pineal gland
Interthalamic adhesion
Hypothalamic sulcus
Infundibulum
Hypothalamus
Oculomotor nerve
Mammillary body

FIGURE 16-2
Close-up photograph of the medial surface of a hemisected brain, illustrating parts of the diencephalon and some surrounding structures. [Modified from Nolte J, Angevine JB Jr: *The human brain in photographs and diagrams,* St. Louis, 1995, Mosby.]

tinuous neural tissue extends through both boundaries; in addition (as noted in earlier chapters), certain thalamic nuclei protrude through the posterior boundary to a position alongside the midbrain.

As a consequence of the cephalic flexure, the axis of the diencephalon is inclined about 80° with respect to the axis of the brainstem (see Figure 3-1). This means that sections cut in a plane similar to that used in the last few chapters (i.e., perpendicular to the long axis of the brainstem) are at a peculiar angle to the diencephalon. Therefore in this and subsequent chapters, sections cut in horizontal and coronal planes are shown (Figure 16-3).★

The Epithalamus Includes the Pineal Gland and the Habenular Nuclei

The **pineal gland** is a midline, unpaired structure situated just rostral to the superior colliculi. It somewhat resembles a pine cone in shape—hence its name. Because each of us has only one pineal gland, which is located

deep within the brain, it was thought for a time that this organ might be the seat of the soul. This now seems unlikely because pineal tumors do not cause the changes one would expect to find associated with distortion of the soul; rather, these tumors compress the midbrain and cause the changes one would expect to find associated with distortion of this part of the brainstem. Early findings may include hydrocephalus (because of the squeezing shut of the aqueduct) and various defects of eye movements and pupillary reactions (because of damage to the oculomotor and trochlear nuclei and pathways ending in them). In addition, pineal tumors may cause changes in sexual development, giving a clue to at least one of its possible functions. The pineal arises as an evagination from the roof of the diencephalon; in fish, amphibians, and many reptiles, it contains photoreceptor cells similar to those of the eye. In these species it is suspected of monitoring day length and season and participating in the regulation of circadian and circannual rhythms (although there are probably other functions as well). The pineal gland of birds and mammals contains no photoreceptors and consists of a collection of secretory cells **(pinealocytes),** some glial cells, and a rich vascular network. Nevertheless, it still receives a light-regulated input by way of a circuitous pathway that begins in the retina and, after one or more relays in the hypothalamus, reaches the intermediolateral cell column of the spinal cord. Preganglionic sympathetic fibers from

---

★The horizontal sections are oriented with the anterior portion at the top of the picture because this is the way CT and MRI scans are conventionally oriented. One result, which can sometimes cause confusion, is that anterior parts of the brainstem also are situated toward the top of the picture; this is upside down relative to the way the brainstem was pictured in Chapters 11-15.

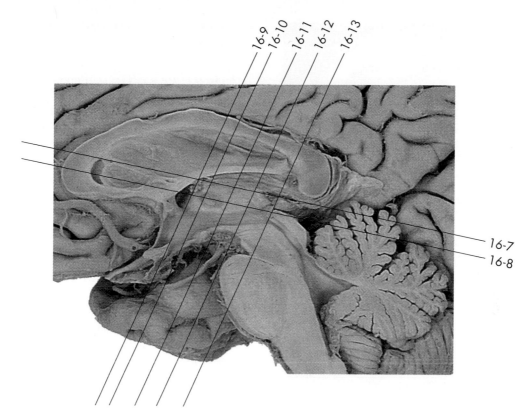

FIGURE 16-3

Approximate planes of section of various photographs in this chapter. (This is not the brain used for any of the sections shown in this chapter, so some details may not quite correspond.) [Modified from Nolte J, Angevine JB Jr: *The human brain in photographs and diagrams*, St. Louis, 1995, Mosby.]

the spinal cord then synapse on postganglionic neurons of the superior cervical ganglion, which in turn send their axons to the pineal.

The mammalian pineal is an endocrine gland involved in reproductive cycles and other functions and has no known neural output. It secretes a hormone derived from serotonin, called **melatonin,** at relatively high rates during darkness. A role for melatonin has been suggested in circadian rhythms and sleep induction, and in many species it has an antigonadotropic effect. Light, by way of the neural pathway just described, causes a decrease in melatonin production. Thus increasing day lengths cause a decrease in melatonin production, which in turn causes an increase in gonadal function. This system is of considerable importance in mammals with prominent seasonal sexual cycles, but its effects in humans are not clear. It has been reported, however, that nonparenchymal pineal tumors, which presumably destroy pinealocytes, tend to be associated with precocious puberty, as though the production of some antigonadotropic substance had been halted. The converse has been reported as well—that parenchymal pineal tumors tend to be associated with hypogonadism. These tumors are quite rare, however, and the routine clinical importance of the pineal arises from the fact that after the age of 17 calcareous concretions accrue

in it. This makes it opaque to x-rays and hence a useful radiological landmark (Figure 16-4) because it normally lies in the midline, and slight shifts in its position can be indicative of expanding masses of various types.

The pineal gland is attached to the dorsal surface of the diencephalon by a stalk. Caudally at the base of the stalk is the posterior commissure; rostrally is a small swelling on each side called a **habenula** (Figures 16-2 and 16-12). Underlying each habenula are the **habenular nuclei.** The two habenulae are interconnected by the small **habenular commissure.** Each habenula receives one major input bundle, the **stria medullaris thalami,** and gives rise to one major output bundle with the awesome name of **habenulointerpeduncular tract** (or **fasciculus retroflexus**). The stria medullaris thalami (Figures 16-7 and 16-11) underlies a horizontal ridge on the dorsomedial surface of the thalamus to which the roof of the third ventricle is attached. The habenulointerpeduncular tract, as its name implies, extends from the habenula to the **interpeduncular nucleus,** located between the cerebral peduncles, and to other parts of the midbrain reticular formation. The fibers of the stria medullaris thalami originate in various limbic structures, so the pathway through the habenula is one route through which the limbic system can influence the brainstem reticular formation.

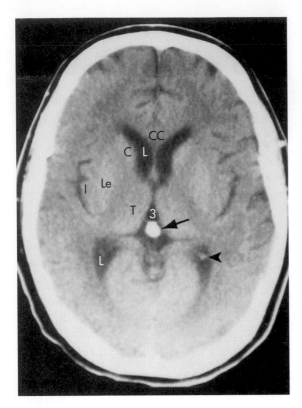

FIGURE 16-4
Uncontrasted CT of a normal 58-year-old-man. Calcium deposits in the pineal gland (*arrow*) and in the glomus (enlarged region of choroid plexus in the atrium of the lateral ventricle; *arrowhead*) make them x-ray dense and hence apparent in CTs, even without contrast. *3,* Third ventricle; *C,* caudate nucleus; *CC,* corpus callosum; *I,* insula; *L,* lateral ventricle; *Le,* lenticular nucleus; *T,* thalamus. (Courtesy Dr. Raymond F. Carmody, Department of Radiology, The University of Arizona College of Medicine.)

The Subthalamus Includes the Subthalamic Nucleus and the Zona Incerta

Parts of the midbrain tegmentum continue into the diencephalon as the subthalamus. This area is completely surrounded by neural tissue and is located inferior to the thalamus, lateral to the hypothalamus, and medial to the basis pedunculi and internal capsule (Figures 16–11 and 16–12). The subthalamus contains rostral portions of the red nucleus and substantia nigra and is traversed by somatosensory pathways on their way to the thalamus as well as by several pathways involving the cerebellum and basal ganglia (the latter pathways are discussed in Chapters 19 and 20). In addition, the subthalamus contains the **subthalamic nucleus** and **zona incerta** (Figure 16–11). The subthalamic nucleus is a lens-shaped, biconvex structure located just medial and superior to portions of the basis pedunculi and internal capsule. This nucleus is interconnected with the basal ganglia, as discussed in Chapter 19. The zona incerta is a small mass of gray matter intervening between the subthalamic nucleus and the thalamus. It appears to be a rostral continuation of the midbrain reticular formation and has rather widespread

connections (including direct projections to the cerebral cortex), although its function is largely unknown.

THE THALAMUS IS THE GATEWAY TO THE CEREBRAL CORTEX

The thalamus is a large, egg-shaped, nuclear mass with a posterior appendage (Figures 16-1, *B* and 16-5), making up about 80% of the diencephalon. It extends anteriorly to the interventricular foramen, superiorly to the transverse cerebral fissure, and inferiorly to the hypothalamic sulcus; posteriorly it overlaps the midbrain (Figure 16-13). The thalamus is part of a remarkably large number of pathways; all sensory pathways relay in the thalamus, and many of the anatomical circuits used by the cerebellum, basal ganglia, and limbic structures also involve thalamic relays. These various systems utilize more or less separate portions of the thalamus, which has therefore been subdivided into a series of nuclei.

Thalamic nuclei can be distinguished from each other both by their topographical locations within the thalamus and by the patterns of their inputs and outputs.

The Thalamus Has Anterior, Medial, and Lateral Divisions Defined by the Internal Medullary Lamina

The topographical organization of the thalamus is shown in Figure 16-6 and Table 16-1. A thin, curved sheet of myelinated fibers, the **internal medullary lamina,** divides most of the thalamus into medial and lateral groups of nuclei (Figures 16-7 and 16-8). Anteriorly the internal medullary lamina bifurcates and encloses an anterior group of nuclei, usually referred to collectively as the **anterior nucleus,** which borders on the interventricular foramen. The medial group similarly contains a single large nucleus, the **dorsomedial (DM) nucleus.***

The lateral group of nuclei composes the bulk of the thalamus and is further subdivided into a dorsal tier and a ventral tier. The dorsal tier consists of the **lateral dorsal (LD)** nucleus (Figure 16-11), the **lateral posterior (LP)** nucleus (Figure 16-12), and the large **pulvinar** (Figure 16-13). The lateral posterior nucleus is continuous with the pulvinar; both nuclei have somewhat similar connections, so the two together are sometimes referred to as the **pulvinar-LP complex.** The bulk of the ventral tier consists of three nuclei arranged along an anterior-posterior line: the **ventral anterior (VA) nucleus** (Figure 16-9), the **ventral lateral (VL) nucleus** (Figures 16-10 and 16-11), and the **ventral posterior (VP) nucleus** (Figures 16-11 and 16-12). The ventral posterior nucleus is customarily subdivided into the **ventral posterolateral (VPL) nucleus** and **ventral posteromedial (VPM) nucleus.** VPL is the somatosensory relay nucleus for the

---

*Also referred to by many as the **mediodorsal (MD) nucleus.**

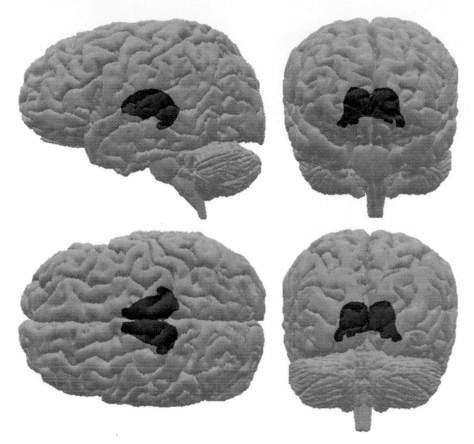

FIGURE 16-5
The location and orientation of the thalamus in the center of the cerebrum.

body and VPM for the head. VA and VL are involved in motor control circuits that include the cerebellum and basal ganglia. The **lateral geniculate nucleus** (visual system) and **medial geniculate nucleus** (auditory system) are located posterior to these ventral tier nuclei and inferior to the pulvinar and protrude posteriorly alongside the midbrain (Figure 16-13). These two nuclei are most conveniently considered as a posterior extension of the ventral tier, although they are sometimes referred to as a separate thalamic subdivision.

Intralaminar nuclei are embedded in the internal medullary lamina

At certain locations within the thalamus the internal medullary lamina splits and encloses groups of cells. These nuclei are collectively called the **intralaminar nuclei,** the two largest of which are the **centromedian (CM)** and **parafascicular (PF) nuclei** (Figure 16-12). The centromedian nucleus is a large, round nucleus located medial to VPL/VPM; VPM conforms to the rounded shape of the centromedian nucleus, and for this reason the VPM was once called the *semilunar* or *arcuate nucleus.* The parafascicular nucleus is located medial to the centromedian nucleus and received its name from the fact that the habenulointerpeduncular tract (fasciculus retroflexus) passes through it.

Table 16-1	Topographical Subdivisions of the Thalamus and Their Principal Nuclei	
Subdivision	Principal nucleus or nuclei	Common abbreviation
Anterior division	Anterior	
Medial division	Dorsomedial	DM
Lateral division	Dorsal tier	
	Lateral dorsal	LD
	Lateral posterior	LP
	Pulvinar	
	Ventral tier	
	Ventral anterior	VA
	Ventral lateral	VL
	Ventral posterior	
	Ventral posterolateral	VPL
	Ventral posteromedial	VPM
	Medial geniculate	MGN
	Lateral geniculate	LGN
Intralaminar nuclei	Centromedian	CM
	Parafascicular	PF
	Others	
	Reticular nucleus	
Reticular nucleus		

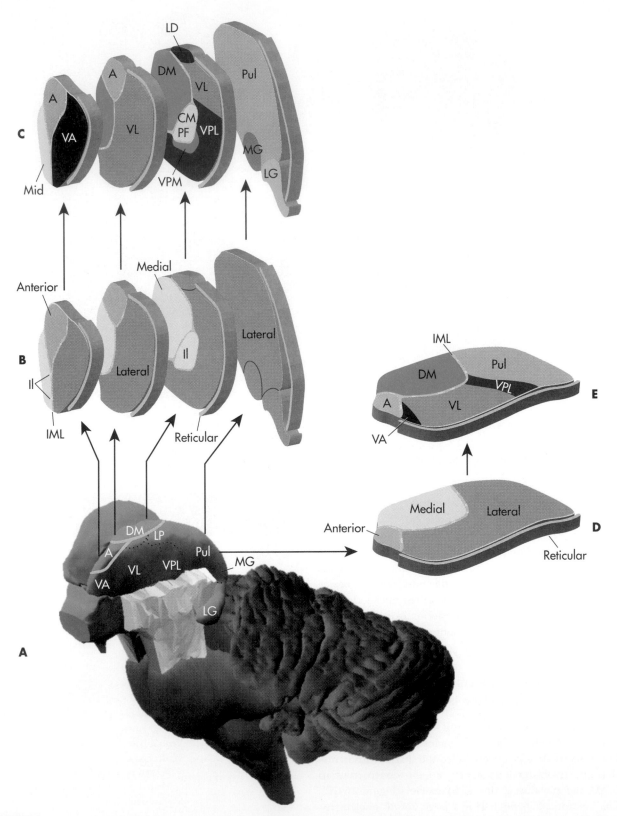

FIGURE 16-6

Topographical subdivisions of the thalamus. **A,** Lateral view of the left thalamus as seen from slightly above and in front. The reticular nucleus has been removed; ordinarily it would cover the entire lateral surface. **B** and **C,** Same as **A** but exploded into four pieces to show the internal arrangement of topographical subdivisions (**B**) and the major nuclei of each subdivision (**C**). The most anterior sliced surface corresponds approximately to Figure 16-9; the most posterior sliced surface corresponds approximately to Figure 16-13. **D** and **E,** A horizontal slab corresponding approximately to Figure 16-7 showing the internal arrangement of topographical subdivisions (**D**) and the major nuclei of each subdivision (**E**). *A,* Anterior nucleus; *CM,* centromedian nucleus (the largest intralaminar nucleus); *DM,* dorsomedial nucleus; *Il,* intralaminar nuclei; *IML,* internal medullary lamina; *LD,* lateral dorsal nucleus; *LG,* lateral geniculate nucleus; *LP,* lateral posterior nucleus; *MG,* medial geniculate nucleus; *Mid,* midline nuclei; *PF* parafascicular nucleus; *Pul,* pulvinar; *VA,* ventral anterior nucleus; *VL,* ventral lateral nucleus; *VPL,* ventral posterolateral nucleus; *VPM,* ventral posteromedial nucleus.

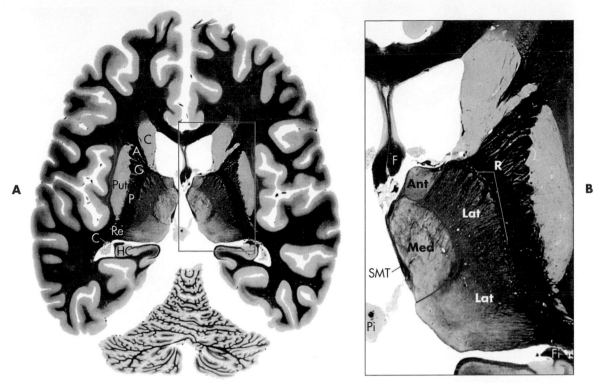

FIGURE 16-7

Topographical subdivisions of the thalamus, as seen in a horizontal section at the level of the stria medullaris thalami *(SMT)*. **A,** The entire section shown at about two thirds actual size. **B,** Enlargement of the area indicated in **A,** showing the demarcation of anterior *(Ant)*, medial *(Med)*, and lateral *(Lat)* divisions by the internal medullary lamina (drawn in red). The lateral surface of the thalamus is covered by the reticular nucleus *(R)*. *A,* Anterior limb of the internal capsule; *C,* caudate nucleus (the head of the caudate anteriorly and the tail of the caudate posteriorly); *F,* fornix; *Fi,* fimbria (fibers associated with the hippocampus that will join the fornix); *G,* genu of the internal capsule; *HC,* hippocampus; *P,* posterior limb of the internal capsule; *Pi,* pineal gland; *Put,* putamen; *Re,* retrolenticular part of the internal capsule. [Modified from Nolte J, Angevine JB Jr: *The human brain in photographs and diagrams,* St. Louis, 1995, Mosby.]

The thalamic reticular nucleus partially surrounds the thalamus

The lateral surface of the thalamus is covered by a second curved sheet of myelinated fibers called the **external medullary lamina.** The thin shell of cells that intervenes between the external medullary lamina and the internal capsule is the **thalamic reticular nucleus*** (Figures 16-7 to 16-13). The reticular nucleus looks continuous inferiorly with the zona incerta (Figure 16-11), but this continuity is of no apparent functional significance.

Midline nuclei cover the ventricular surface of the thalamus

A thin layer of cells, essentially a rostral continuation of parts of the periaqueductal gray, covers portions of the medial surface of the thalamus. These cells constitute the **midline nuclei** of the thalamus (not to be confused with the dorsomedial nucleus). The midline nuclei of the two sides fuse in the interthalamic adhesion, when it is present.

*Both the thalamic reticular nucleus and the brainstem reticular formation were named for their reticulated appearance, but they are distinct from each other in anatomical location and in patterns of connections.

Patterns of Input and Output Connections Define Functional Categories of Thalamic Nuclei

Thalamic nuclei are often thought of as simply pipelines through which information flows to the cerebral cortex, and for much of the time this is a reasonable approximation of what they do. The thalamus also has a second role, however, that is presumably the reason for its continued existence. Successive stages in most neural pathways participate in transforming information or extracting features. For example, neurons at different levels of the retina and of visual cortical areas have different receptive fields, some emphasizing color, others contrast or movement (see Chapter 17). Thalamic neurons, in contrast, are not sites at which substantial changes in receptive fields develop. Rather, the thalamus is the site where decisions are implemented about which information should reach the cerebral cortex for further processing. This general role is reflected in the physiological properties of thalamic neurons, and the particular type of information affected by a thalamic nucleus is a function of its input and output connections.

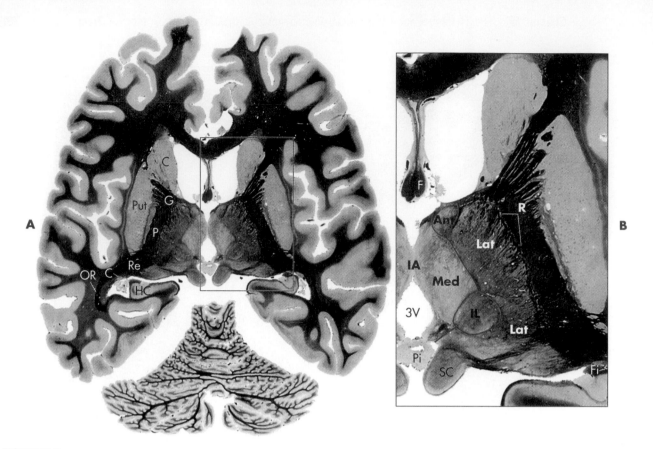

FIGURE 16-8

Topographical subdivisions of the thalamus, as seen in a horizontal section at a midthalamic level. **A,** The entire section shown at about two thirds actual size. **B,** Enlargement of the area indicated in **A,** showing the demarcation of anterior *(Ant),* medial *(Med),* lateral *(Lat),* and intralaminar *(IL)* divisions by the internal medullary lamina (drawn in red). The lateral surface of the thalamus is covered by the reticular nucleus *(R). 3V,* Third ventricle; *C,* caudate nucleus (the head of the caudate anteriorly and the tail of the caudate posteriorly); *F,* fornix; *Fi,* fimbria (fibers associated with the hippocampus that will join the fornix); *G,* genu of the internal capsule; *HC,* hippocampus; *IA,* interthalamic adhesion (location of midline nuclei); *OR,* optic radiation (fibers on their way from the thalamus to visual cortex); *P,* posterior limb of the internal capsule; *Pi,* pineal gland; *Put,* putamen; *Re,* retrolenticular part of the internal capsule. [Modified from Nolte J, Angevine JB Jr: *The human brain in photographs and diagrams,* St. Louis, 1995, Mosby.]

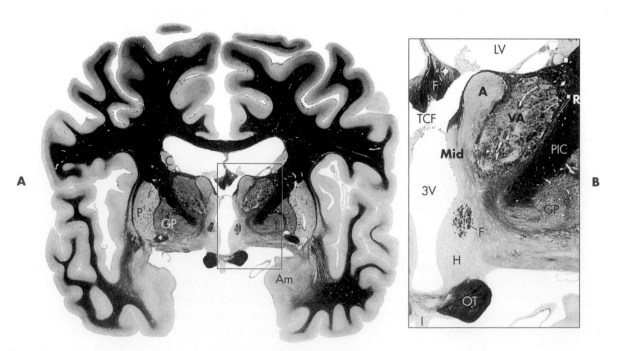

FIGURE 16-9

Coronal section through the anterior thalamus, near the interventricular foramen. **A,** The entire section shown at about 80% actual size. **B,** Enlargement of the area indicated in **A,** showing the anterior *(A),* midline *(Mid),* reticular *(R),* and ventral anterior *(VA)* nuclei. *3V,* Third ventricle; *,* anterior commissure (just before its fibers turn medially and cross the midline); *Am,* amygdala; *C,* caudate nucleus; *F,* fornix; *GP,* globus pallidus; *H,* hypothalamus; *I,* infundibulum; *LV,* lateral ventricle; *OT,* optic tract; *P,* putamen; *PIC,* posterior limb of the internal capsule; *TCF,* transverse cerebral fissure.

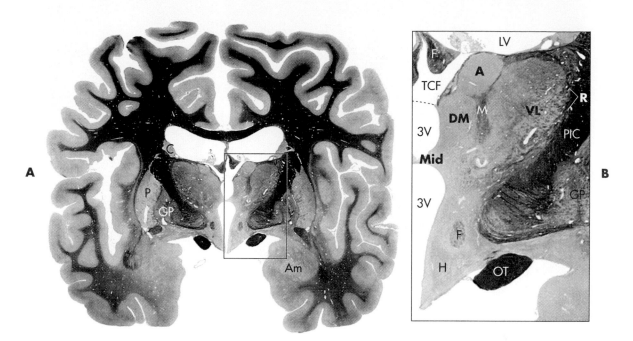

FIGURE 16-10

Coronal section through the anterior thalamus. **A,** The entire section shown at about 80% actual size. **B,** Enlargement of the area indicated in **A,** showing the anterior *(A),* dorsomedial *(DM),* midline *(Mid),* reticular *(R),* and ventral lateral *(VL)* nuclei. *3V,* Third ventricle; *Am,* amygdala; *C,* caudate nucleus; *F,* fornix; *GP,* globus pallidus; *H,* hypothalamus; *LV,* lateral ventricle; *M,* mammillothalamic tract (entering the anterior nucleus); *OT,* optic tract; *P,* putamen; *PIC,* posterior limb of the internal capsule; *TCF,* transverse cerebral fissure. [Modified from Nolte J, Angevine JB Jr: *The human brain in photographs and diagrams,* St. Louis, 1995, Mosby.]

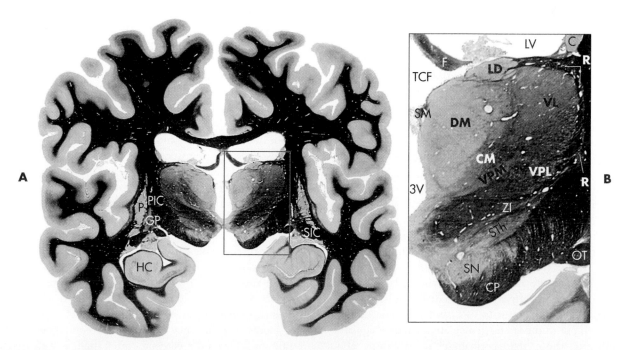

FIGURE 16-11

Coronal section through the midthalamus. **A,** The entire section shown at about 80% actual size. **B,** Enlargement of the area indicated in **A,** showing the centromedian *(CM),* dorsomedial *(DM),* lateral dorsal *(LD),* reticular *(R),* ventral lateral *(VL),* ventral posterolateral *(VPL),* and ventral posteromedial *(VPM)* nuclei. *3V,* Third ventricle; *C,* caudate nucleus; *CP,* cerebral peduncle; *F,* fornix; *GP,* globus pallidus; *HC,* hippocampus; *LV,* lateral ventricle; *OT,* optic tract; *P,* putamen; *PIC,* posterior limb of the internal capsule; *SIC,* sublenticular part of the internal capsule; *SM,* stria medullaris thalami; *SN,* substantia nigra; *STh,* subthalamic nucleus; *TCF,* transverse cerebral fissure; *ZI,* zona incerta. [Modified from Nolte J, Angevine JB Jr: *The human brain in photographs and diagrams,* St. Louis, 1995, Mosby.]

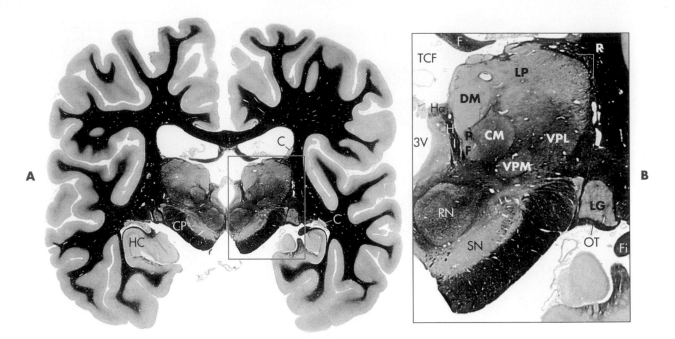

FIGURE 16-12
Coronal section through the posterior thalamus. **A,** The entire section shown at about 80% actual size. **B,** Enlargement of the area indicated in **A,** showing the centromedian *(CM)*, dorsomedial *(DM)*, lateral geniculate *(LGN)*, lateral posterior *(LP)*, reticular *(R)*, ventral posterolateral *(VPL)*, and ventral posteromedial *(VPM)* nuclei. *3V,* Third ventricle; *C,* caudate nucleus; *CP,* cerebral peduncle; *F,* fornix; *Fi,* fimbria (fibers associated with the hippocampus that will join the fornix); *Ha,* habenula; *HC,* hippocampus; *HI,* habenulointerpeduncular tract; *OT,* optic tract (entering the lateral geniculate nucleus); *RN,* red nucleus; *SN,* substantia nigra; *TCF,* transverse cerebral fissure. (Modified from Nolte J, Angevine JB Jr: *The human brain in photographs and diagrams,* St. Louis, 1995, Mosby.)

All thalamic nuclei (except the reticular nucleus) are variations on a common theme

The thalamic reticular nucleus is developmentally not really part of the thalamus and has distinctive anatomical and physiological properties. It is nevertheless considered part of the thalamus because of its location and its extensive involvement in thalamic function, as described a little later in this chapter. All other thalamic nuclei are a mixture of projection neurons, whose axons provide the output from the thalamus, and small inhibitory interneurons that use GABA as a neurotransmitter (Figure 16-14, *A*). Projection neurons account for about 75% of all thalamic neurons, although the relative proportions of projection neurons and interneurons vary in different nuclei.

Inputs to the thalamus can be divided into two broad categories, referred to here as **specific inputs** and **regulatory inputs** (Figure 16-14, *A*). Specific inputs are those conveying the information that a given thalamic nucleus may pass on to its outputs. The medial lemniscus, for example, is a specific input to VPL, and the optic tract is a specific input to the lateral geniculate nucleus. Regulatory inputs are those that contribute to decisions about whether and in what form information leaves a thalamic nucleus. The source of regulatory inputs is broadly similar from one thalamic nucleus to another: most come from the cortical area to which a given thalamic nucleus projects, some come from the thalamic reticular nucleus, and

the remainder include diffuse cholinergic, noradrenergic, and serotonergic endings from the brainstem reticular formation. Although thalamic nuclei are usually thought of primarily in terms of their specific inputs, these are in fact greatly outnumbered by the regulatory inputs—a reflection of the distinctive role of the thalamus. This is nicely illustrated by the lateral geniculate nucleus, in which fewer than 20% of the synapses on its projection neurons come from optic tract fibers and half or more come from visual cortex.

Distinctive patterns of outputs and specific inputs allow thalamic nuclei (other than the reticular nucleus) to be grouped into three categories. **Relay nuclei** receive well-defined bundles of specific input fibers and project to particular functional areas of the cerebral cortex (Figure 16-14, *B*); their role is to deliver information from particular functional systems to appropriate cortical areas. **Association nuclei** were originally so named because they project to cortical areas traditionally referred to as *association areas* (see Chapter 22), but they have characteristic patterns of inputs as well. They receive major contingents of specific inputs from the cerebral cortex itself, as well as some from a variety of subcortical structures (Figure 16-14, *C*). Although the precise role of thalamic association nuclei is not understood, they are likely to be important in the distribution and gating of information *between* cortical areas. Finally, although here too the details are not under-

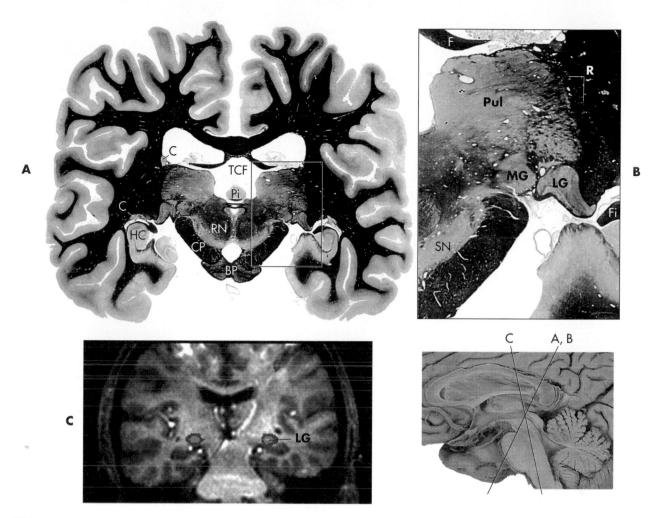

FIGURE 16-13
Coronal section through the posterior thalamus. **A,** The entire section shown at about 80% actual size. **B,** Enlargement of the area indicated in **A,** showing the lateral *(LGN)* and medial geniculate *(MGN)* and reticular *(R)* nuclei and the pulvinar *(Pul).* **C,** fMRI data from a subject watching a red and black checkerboard in which the squares reversed color 8 to 10 times per second, superimposed on a T1-weighted coronal slice at a level similar to that shown in **A.** The stimulus activates not only occipital cortex above and below the calcarine sulcus (see Figure 6-19, *C*), but also the lateral geniculate nucleus *(LG).* The inset at the bottom right shows the relative planes of section in **A, B,** and **C.** *BP,* Basal pons; *C,* caudate nucleus; *CP,* cerebral peduncle; *F,* fornix; *Fi,* fimbria (fibers associated with the hippocampus that will join the fornix); *HC,* hippocampus; *Pi,* pineal gland; *RN,* red nucleus; *SN,* substantia nigra; *TCF,* transverse cerebral fissure. [Modified from Nolte J, Angevine JB Jr: *The human brain in photographs and diagrams,* St. Louis, 1995, Mosby. **C** from Chen W et al: Mapping of lateral geniculate nucleus activation during visual stimulation in human brain using fMRI, *Magn Reson Med* 39:89, 1998.

stood, the intralaminar and midline nuclei seem to have a special role in the function of the basal ganglia and limbic system. Their specific inputs come from a wide array of sites, prominently including parts of the basal ganglia and limbic system, and they project not only to areas of cerebral cortex, but even more prominently to parts of the basal ganglia and limbic system (Figure 16-14, *D*).

Thalamic projection neurons have two physiological states

The function of the thalamus as a gateway to the cerebral cortex depends on a combination of ion channels in its projection neurons that allows these neurons to function in two distinctly different physiological states. Projection

neurons that are slightly depolarized are in a **tonic mode** and behave like typical neurons described elsewhere in this book. Slight additional depolarization causes a train of action potentials, and slight hyperpolarization causes their cessation (Figure 16-15, *A* and *B*). Neurons in the tonic mode can faithfully transmit to the cortex information reaching them via specific inputs, using trains of action potentials whose frequency is a function of input magnitude. Projection neurons hyperpolarized beyond the tonic range enter a **burst mode,** characterized by the availability of special voltage-gated Ca^{2+} channels. Slight depolarization of a neuron in the burst mode causes transient opening of the voltage-gated Ca^{2+} channels, followed by their inactivation (similar to the opening and closing of voltage-gated Na^+ channels that underlies action poten-

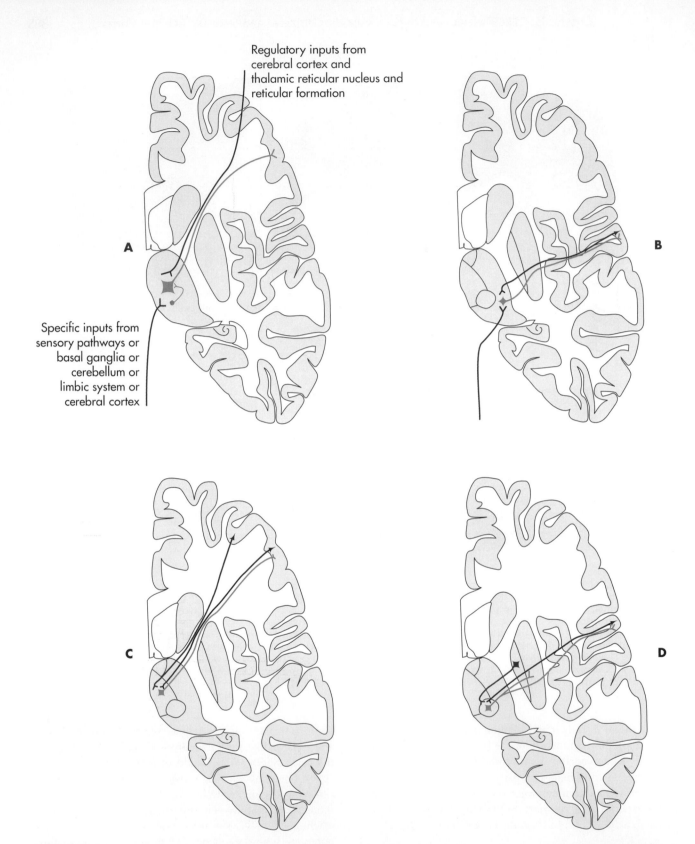

Regulatory inputs from
cerebral cortex and
thalamic reticular nucleus and
reticular formation

A

Specific inputs from
sensory pathways or
basal ganglia or
cerebellum or
limbic system or
cerebral cortex

B

C

D

FIGURE 16-14

Organization of the thalamus. **A,** Overview of the contents and connections of thalamic nuclei (except the reticular nucleus), shown in a schematic horizontal section through one cerebral hemisphere. Thalamic nuclei contain projection neurons *(green)* and inhibitory interneurons *(orange)* in varying proportions. Axons of projection neurons reach the cerebral cortex (and, depending on the nucleus, other sites as well). Each nucleus receives a characteristic set of specific inputs *(blue)*, usually from one principal source. Each nucleus also receives an array of regulatory inputs *(red)*, most prominently from the cortical area to which it projects. **B,** Relay nuclei receive specific inputs from subcortical pathways (e.g., the medial lemniscus) and project to a well-defined functional area of cortex. **C,** Association nuclei receive major specific inputs from association cortex (e.g., prefrontal cortex) and project to related association areas. **D,** Intralaminar and midline nuclei receive distinctive sets of specific inputs (typically from basal ganglia or limbic structures) and project not only to the cerebral cortex, but also to basal ganglia or limbic structures.

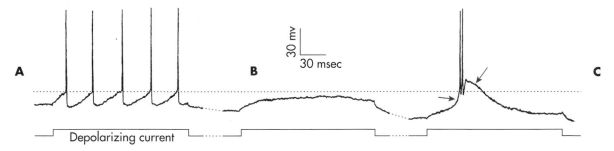

FIGURE 16-15
Effects of membrane potential on the physiological state of a projection neuron from the lateral geniculate nucleus of a cat. Three depolarizing current pulses of the same magnitude were injected into the neuron, starting from three different membrane potential levels; threshold for initiation of action potentials is indicated by the dotted red line. **A,** Starting from -55 mv, the voltage-gated Ca²⁺ channels are inactive, and depolarization initiates a train of action potentials. **B,** Starting from -60 mv, the voltage-gated Ca²⁺ channels are still inactive, but the depolarization is insufficient to bring the membrane to threshold. **C,** Starting from -70 mv, the voltage-gated Ca²⁺ channels are active, and the depolarization causes them to open and then inactivate and close; the Ca²⁺ influx causes an additional slow, depolarizing wave *(arrows)* sufficient to initiate a brief burst of action potentials. (Modified from Sherman SM, Guillery RW: Functional organization of thalamocortical relays, *J Neurophysiol* 76:1367, 1996.)

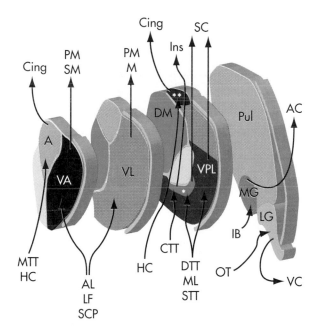

FIGURE 16-16
Major specific inputs to and outputs from relay nuclei. Thalamic nuclei: *, Ventral posteromedial nucleus; **, lateral dorsal nucleus; *A*, anterior nucleus; *DM*, dorsomedial nucleus; *LG*, lateral geniculate nucleus; *MG*, medial geniculate nucleus; *Pul*, pulvinar; *VA*, ventral anterior nucleus; *VL*, ventral lateral nucleus; *VPL*, ventral posterolateral nucleus. Input pathways and structures: *AL*, Ansa lenticularis (Chapter 19); *CTT*, central tegmental tract; *IB*, brachium of the inferior colliculus; *DTT*, dorsal trigeminal tract; *HC*, hippocampus; *LF*, lenticular fasciculus (Chapter 19); *ML*, medial lemniscus; *MTT*, mammillothalamic tract; *OT*, optic tract; *SCP*, superior cerebellar peduncle (Chapter 20); *STT*, spinothalamic tract. Cortical destinations: *AC*, Auditory cortex; *Cing*, cingulate gyrus; *Ins*, insula; *M*, primary motor cortex (precentral gyrus); *PM*, premotor cortex (Chapter 18); *SC*, somatosensory cortex; *SM*, supplementary motor area (Chapter 18); *VC*, visual cortex.

tials). The transient influx of Ca²⁺ ions while the channels are open causes a depolarizing wave that may be sufficient to trigger a burst of action potentials (Figure 16-15, *C*). The duration of the inactivation of the voltage-gated Ca²⁺ channels is 100 msec or longer, so bursts of action potentials can only occur a few times per second. Hence neurons in this mode are unable to transmit information about specific inputs accurately.

The functional mode of a thalamic projection neuron at any given moment is determined largely by its regulatory inputs. Focusing attention, whether on a stimulus or a task or a thought, presumably involves placing the appropriate thalamic projection neurons in the tonic mode. The burst mode, in contrast, may have more than one function. During most phases of sleep, projection neurons are in the burst mode, dominated by rhythmic waves of depolarization (see Figure 22-25) and effectively unable to transmit information about their specific inputs. During wakefulness, however, many projection neurons are also in the burst mode. In this case, the amplification provided by the voltage-gated Ca²⁺ channels may make these neurons particularly sensitive to the occurrence of an event, even though they would be unable to participate in the analysis of its details.

There are relay nuclei for sensory, motor, and limbic systems

Relay nuclei and their connections are indicated in Figures 16-16 and 16-17 and Table 16-2. They include the sensory relay nuclei (VPL/VPM and the geniculate nuclei) and several others as well, because parts of the motor and limbic systems also have thalamic relays. VL and VA are the motor relay nuclei, receiving the superior cerebellar peduncle and various outputs from the basal ganglia and projecting to motor and premotor cortex. The anterior nucleus is the principal relay nucleus for the limbic system, receiving the **mammillothalamic tract** (Figure 16-10) and projecting to the cingulate gyrus. The mammillothalamic tract, as its name implies, arises in the mammillary body. The cingulate gyrus is a prominent component of the limbic lobe (see Figure 3-11). The way in which this pathway fits into the limbic system as a whole

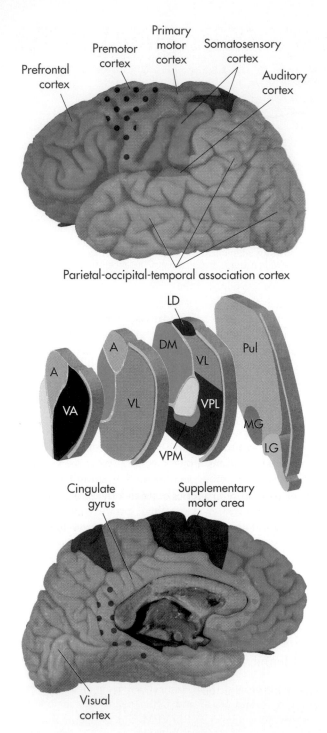

FIGURE 16-17

Principal cortical projection areas of relay and association nuclei. The major thalamic nucleus associated with each cortical area is indicated by the color coding, but projection areas are not nearly as exclusive as this figure implies. The pulvinar, for example, also projects to visual cortex and to parts of prefrontal cortex; these inputs are simply overshadowed by those from the lateral geniculate and dorsomedial nuclei, respectively.

is detailed in Chapter 23. The lateral dorsal (LD) nucleus also projects to the cingulate gyrus, and in this and other ways closely resembles the anterior nucleus. Therefore, in spite of the fact that a discrete input tract does not end in it, some authors have begun to refer to LD as a relay nucleus functionally related to the anterior nucleus.

As a general rule, the cerebral cortex is more important for the proper functioning of sensory systems in humans than it is in other mammals. For example, cats deprived of somatosensory cortex or visual cortex retain a significant portion of their previous somatosensory or visual capabilities, and rats treated similarly retain even more. Nevertheless, it is sometimes claimed that sensory stimuli, particularly somatosensory stimuli, "enter consciousness" in humans at the level of the thalamus. When the somatosensory cortex in humans is destroyed, the remaining awareness of stimuli is very crude, consisting mainly of an ability by the individual to recognize the fact of being touched or receiving a painful stimulus. The ability to localize the stimulus or to discriminate its intensity is severely impaired. These conclusions are based mainly on studies of humans who have sustained damage to one parietal lobe, but it seems doubtful that the remaining sensory capabilities are in fact a result of consciousness at the level of the thalamus ipsilateral to the lesion. In most cases it appears that the remaining capabilities could be a result of slight bilaterality in the function of the contralateral thalamus and parietal lobe.

The dorsomedial nucleus and pulvinar are the principal association nuclei

There are two great areas of association cortex in the human brain (Figure 16-17). One is the **prefrontal cortex,** anterior to the motor areas of the frontal lobe. The second is the **parietal-occipital-temporal association cortex** occupying the area surrounded by the primary somatosensory, visual, and auditory cortices. Corresponding to these two areas are two large association nuclei or nuclear complexes (Figure 16-17). The dorsomedial nucleus is interconnected with the prefrontal cortex and is involved in prefrontal functions such as affect and foresight, as described further in Chapters 22 and 23. Bilateral damage to the dorsomedial nucleus or to its connections with the frontal lobe has effects similar in some ways to those of prefrontal lobectomy. Major inputs to the dorsomedial nucleus, in addition to those from prefrontal cortex, come from various elements of the limbic system, such as the amygdala.

The pulvinar/LP complex is interconnected with the parietal-occipital-temporal association cortex. The major inputs to this complex, aside from those arising in association cortex, come from parts of the visual system. The pulvinar is the largest nucleus in the human thalamus and is better developed in humans than in any other mammal. One would expect that a nucleus this large and this highly

Table 16-2   Specific Inputs To and Cortical Outputs From Thalamic Relay and Association Nuclei

Type	Nucleus	Specific inputs	Cortical output
Relay	Anterior	Mammillothalamic tract, hippocampus	Cingulate gyrus
	Lateral dorsal (LD)	Hippocampus	Cingulate gyrus
	Ventral anterior and ventral lateral (VA/VL)★	Basal ganglia, cerebellum	Motor areas
	Ventral posterolateral (VPL)	Medial lemniscus (body), Spinothalamic tract (body)	Somatosensory cortex
	Ventral posteromedial (VPM)	Medial lemniscus (face), Spinothalamic tract (face), Central tegmental tract (taste)	Somatosensory cortex, Insula
	Medial geniculate (MGN)	Brachium of the inferior colliculus	Auditory cortex
	Lateral geniculate (LGN)	Optic tract	Visual cortex
Association	Dorsomedial† (DM)	Prefrontal cortex, olfactory and limbic structures	Prefrontal cortex
	Lateral posterior (LP)	Parietal lobe	Parietal lobe
	Pulvinar	Parietal, occipital, and temporal lobes	Parietal, occipital, and temporal lobes

★Basal ganglia outputs go mostly to VA and cerebellar outputs mostly to VL, but the two are considered together as a combined motor relay nucleus in this account.
†Also commonly referred to as the *mediodorsal nucleus (MD)*.

developed in humans would have an important, well-defined function. Unfortunately, the role of the pulvinar (and of LP) is largely unknown at this time. There are hints that it may be involved in some aspects of visual perception or attention, and there are occasional reports of language deficits after damage to it, but in general no particular syndrome and no obvious sensory deficits follow damage to the pulvinar/LP complex.

Intralaminar nuclei project to both the cerebral cortex and the basal ganglia

The midline and intralaminar nuclei have long been considered to form a nonspecific system that projects to widespread areas of the cerebral cortex and produces general changes in cortical function. However, more recent work with improved anatomical techniques indicates that, although the connections of these nuclei do not have the point-to-point precision seen with relay nuclei, there is nevertheless a considerable degree of specificity. The inputs to these nuclei as a group are from diverse sources, including multiple cortical areas, the basal ganglia, cerebellum, brainstem reticular formation, and spinothalamic and spinoreticulothalamic fibers carrying information about dull, aching pain. However, each nucleus has a specific pattern of inputs. Similarly, as a group the midline and intralaminar nuclei have widespread projections to multiple cortical areas, the basal ganglia, and limbic structures, but each individual nucleus has its own specific pattern of projections. For example, the centromedian nucleus pro-

jects to the putamen and to motor cortex, whereas the parafascicular nucleus projects to the caudate nucleus and to prefrontal cortex. As described in Chapter 19, the basal ganglia participate in a series of parallel anatomical circuits through the thalamus and cerebral cortex, each loop involving a different motor, cognitive, or affective function. Although the details and the functional implications are far from understood, it seems likely that individual midline and intralaminar nuclei affect particular circuits of the basal ganglia or limbic system. Because the basal ganglia and limbic system collectively affect most cortical functions, collective changes in the activity of the midline and intralaminar nuclei would be expected to have the widespread effects traditionally ascribed to these nuclei.

The thalamic reticular nucleus projects to other thalamic nuclei and not to the cerebral cortex

The thalamic reticular nucleus, unlike all other thalamic nuclei, has no projections to the cerebral cortex. Rather, the reticular nucleus is a sheet of neurons that receive inputs from the cortex and from thalamic projection neurons and send inhibitory (GABA) projections back to the thalamus (Figure 16-18). Inspection of Figure 16-9 reveals that axons traveling from thalamus to cortex or from cortex to thalamus must traverse the reticular nucleus. As they do so, these fibers give off collaterals to the reticular nucleus. For example, the portion of the reticular nucleus adjacent to VPL/VPM receives convergent inputs from somatosensory

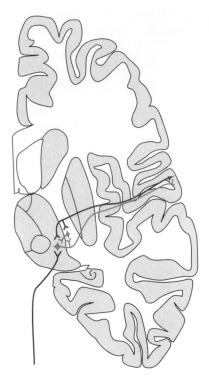

FIGURE 16-18
Connection pattern of the thalamic reticular nucleus. Most or all axons entering or leaving the thalamus, except for specific inputs, give off collaterals to neurons of the reticular nucleus. Each small area of the reticular nucleus in turn sends inhibitory projections to a restricted area of the thalamus.

fibers on their way to the postcentral gyrus, and from regulatory fibers on their way from the postcentral gyrus to VPL/VPM. The output of each portion of the reticular nucleus goes to that thalamic nucleus from which it receives its input. This makes the reticular nucleus an important source of regulatory inputs to the thalamus.

Small Branches of the Posterior Cerebral Artery Provide Most of the Blood Supply to the Thalamus

Inspection of a hemisected brain (see Figure 6-14) reveals that the anterior and middle cerebral arteries and their branches near the circle of Willis are anterior to most of the thalamus. The blood supply of the thalamus is therefore mostly from branches of the posterior cerebral artery (see Figure 6-20). Specifically, branches of the posterior choroidal artery supply some dorsomedial regions, and most of the rest of the thalamus is supplied by small ganglionic or perforating arteries arising from the posterior cerebral and posterior communicating arteries. These ganglionic arteries are sometimes divided into two groups: a **posteromedial** group arising from the posterior cerebral and posterior communicating arteries within the circle of Willis and a **posterolateral** group arising from the posterior cerebral artery distal to the circle. The pos-

teromedial (sometimes also called **thalamoperforant** arteries) group supplies medial and anterior portions of the thalamus as well as the subthalamus. The posterolateral group (sometimes also called **thalamogeniculate** arteries) supplies most of the posterior and lateral thalamus. Finally, the anterior choroidal artery often sends a few small branches to the subthalamus and to ventral regions of the thalamus, particularly the lateral geniculate nucleus.

Damage to the thalamus most often occurs as a result of vascular accidents, particularly involving the thalamogeniculate arteries. The damage frequently involves other structures in addition to the thalamus (e.g., the adjacent internal capsule), and a large collection of deficits with far-reaching consequences may result from relatively small lesions in this area. Characteristically, a type of dysesthesia results from damage more or less restricted to the posterior thalamus. The condition is somewhat similar to trigeminal neuralgia in that paroxysms of intense pain may be triggered by somatosensory stimuli. This pain may spread to involve one entire half of the body. It is usually resistant to pain-killing drugs and is called **thalamic pain.** In addition, those stimuli that do not cause a pain attack may be perceived abnormally; their intensity (and even their modality) may be distorted, and they may seem unusually uncomfortable or pleasant. The cause may be selective damage to the fast-pain spinothalamic fibers that end in VPL/VPM, with sparing of the slow-pain spinothalamic and spinoreticulothalamic fibers that end in other nuclei. Extensive damage to the posterior thalamus also causes total (or nearly total) loss of somatic sensation in the contralateral head and body. After a period of time, some appreciation of painful, thermal, and gross tactile stimuli usually returns. Functions customarily associated with the medial lemniscus tend to be more severely and permanently impaired. Discriminative tactile sensibility may be abolished, position sense may be greatly impaired, and a sensory type of ataxia (resulting from the loss of proprioception) may persist. The combination of thalamic pain, hemianesthesia, and sensory ataxia, all contralateral to a posterior thalamic lesion, is called the **thalamic syndrome.** It is often accompanied by mild and transient paralysis (a result of damage to corticospinal fibers in the adjacent internal capsule) and by various types of residual involuntary movements (a result of damage to nearby basal ganglia).

INTERCONNECTIONS BETWEEN THE CEREBRAL CORTEX AND SUBCORTICAL STRUCTURES TRAVEL THROUGH THE INTERNAL CAPSULE

The large collection of thalamocortical and corticothalamic fibers just described need a route by which to travel from their origins to their destinations. This route is provided by the **internal capsule,** a compact bundle of fibers in the cleft (Figure 16-19) between the thalamus

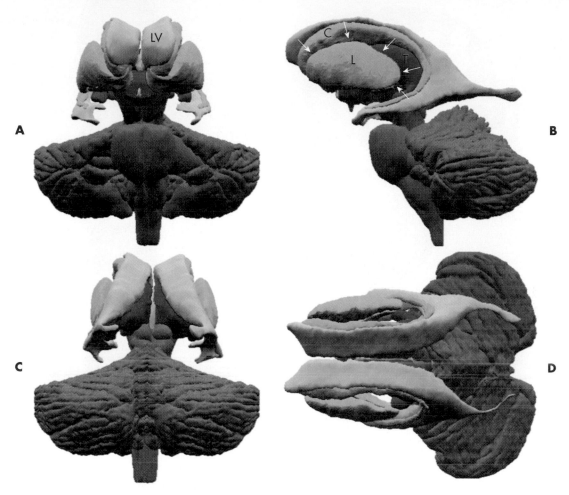

FIGURE 16-19
Three-dimensional reconstruction of the diencephalon, basal ganglia, lateral ventricles *(LV)*, brainstem, and cerebellum, seen from in front **(A)**, the left side **(B)**, the rear **(C)**, and above **(D)**. The cleft through which the internal capsule passes, bounded by the thalamus *(T)* medially and the caudate *(C)* and lenticular *(L)* nuclei laterally, is indicated by arrows in **B** but is apparent in all four views.

(medially) and the putamen, globus pallidus, and head of the caudate nucleus (laterally). Almost all the neural traffic to and from the cerebral cortex passes through the internal capsule. As Figures 16-7 and 16-8 indicate, the internal capsule is in a convenient location for fibers entering or leaving the thalamus. In addition to these, other fibers descend from the cortex through the internal capsule and then through the cerebral peduncle to reach pontine nuclei **(corticopontine fibers),** motor nuclei of cranial nerves and other brainstem sites **(corticobulbar fibers),** and spinal cord motor neurons and interneurons **(corticospinal fibers).** Still other fibers project from the cerebral cortex through the internal capsule to additional subcortical targets, such as various parts of the basal ganglia, for example, the putamen and the caudate nucleus. All of these fibers fan out as the **corona radiata** just above the internal capsule and mingle with other fiber bundles interconnecting different cortical areas in the **centrum semiovale** of each hemisphere (Figure 16-20).

The three-dimensional shape of the internal capsule is a bit difficult to visualize, but the beautiful dissections shown in Figures 16-21 and 16-22 should help. The internal capsule is a continuous sheet of fibers that forms the medial boundary of the lenticular nucleus and then continues around posteriorly and inferiorly to partially envelop this nucleus. Inferiorly many of the fibers in the internal capsule funnel down into the cerebral peduncle. Superiorly they all fan out into the corona radiata, in which they travel through the centrum semiovale to reach their cortical origins or destinations. Thus the entire fiber system is shaped like a trumpet with a large notch cut out of its bell (Figure 16-22); the flared-out bell corresponds to the region where the fibers of the internal capsule spread out to form the corona radiata, and the notch corresponds to the location where this continuous sheet of fibers is interrupted in an intact brain by the lateral sulcus. The narrowest part of the trumpet corresponds to the cerebral peduncle, and in an intact brain the lenticular nucleus sits where a mute would sit in a trumpet.

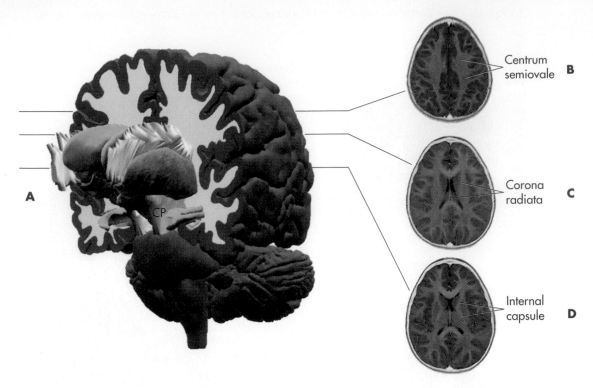

FIGURE 16-20
Three-dimensional reconstruction **(A)** of the internal capsule emerging above its cleft as the corona radiata, and of part of it emerging below the cleft as the cerebral peduncle *(CP)*. **B-D** show horizontal MR images at three different levels of this fiber system. **(B-D,** Modified from Nolte J, Angevine JB Jr: *The human brain in photographs and diagrams*, St. Louis, 1995, Mosby.)

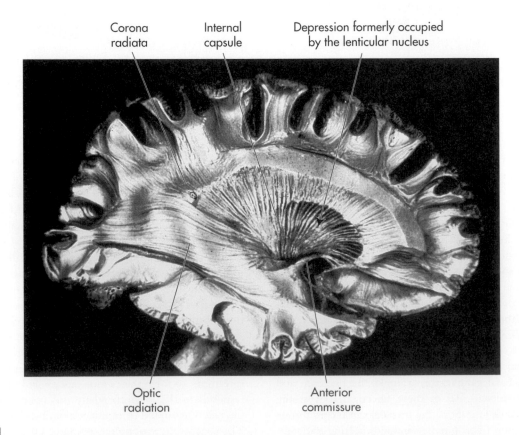

FIGURE 16-21
Dissection of the right cerebral hemisphere from its lateral aspect. Most of the cerebral cortex, including that of the insula, was removed. The lenticular nucleus (putamen and globus pallidus) was then removed, revealing the internal capsule. The internal capsule outlines the former location of the lenticular nucleus, and its fibers then continue into the corona radiata. The fibers of the anterior commissure can also be seen collecting from the temporal lobe and projecting toward the midline. [From Ludwig E, Klingler J: *Atlas cerebri humani*, Boston, 1956, Little, Brown & Co.]

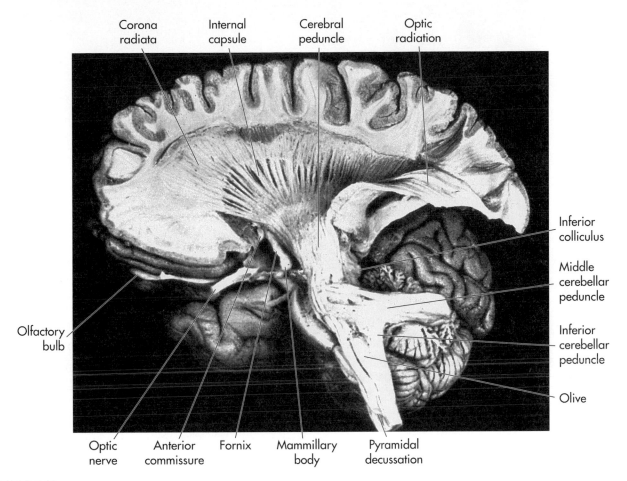

FIGURE 16-22
Dissection of the left cerebral hemisphere from its lateral aspect. This dissection is similar to that of Figure 16-23 except that the temporal lobe has also been removed so that the continuity of the internal capsule and the cerebral peduncle can be seen. The flared-out, trumpet-shaped progression from the cerebral peduncle, through the internal capsule, and into the corona radiata is shown here about as well as it can be. The entire course of the pyramidal tract from the corona radiata through the medullary pyramid can also be seen, as can the origin of the middle cerebellar peduncle in the basal part of the pons. [From Ludwig E, Klingler J: *Atlas cerebri humani*, Boston, 1956, Little, Brown & Co.)

The Internal Capsule Has Five Parts

The internal capsule is divided into five regions on the basis of the relationship of each part to the lenticular nucleus (Figures 16-7 and 16-8). The **anterior limb** is the portion between the lenticular nucleus and the head of the caudate nucleus. The **posterior limb** is the portion between the lenticular nucleus and the thalamus. The **genu** is the portion at the junction of the anterior and posterior limbs. Because this junction occurs at the anterior end of the thalamus, the genu is adjacent to the interventricular foramen (at the anterior end of the thalamus) and to the venous angle (see Figure 6-29). The **retrolenticular part** is the portion posterior to the lenticular nucleus. The **sublenticular part** is the portion inferior to the lenticular nucleus. The demarcation of the anterior and posterior limbs is distinct at the genu, but the transition from the posterior limb to the retrolenticular part to the sublenticular part is gradual, and dividing lines between these portions are somewhat arbitrary. Because the internal capsule is a continuous, curved sheet of fibers, it is not possible to see all of its parts in any one section, no mat-

ter what the plane of the section is. It is possible to see the first four parts mentioned above in a single horizontal section (Figures 16-7 and 16-8), but to get a clear idea of the sublenticular part, it is usually necessary to use coronal sections (Figure 16-11).

By and large, the contents of each portion of the internal capsule can be inferred from its anatomical location (Figure 16-23). Major components are as follows:

1. The anterior limb contains the fibers interconnecting the anterior nucleus and the cingulate gyrus and those interconnecting the dorsomedial nucleus and prefrontal cortex. Also included are some of the fibers projecting from the frontal lobe to the ipsilateral pontine nuclei **(frontopontine fibers).**
2. The posterior limb contains fibers interconnecting VA and VL with the motor and premotor cortex. It also contains the corticospinal and corticobulbar fibers and the somatosensory fibers projecting from VPL/VPM to the postcentral gyrus. It was thought for many years that the corticospinal tract is located in the anterior portion of the posterior limb near

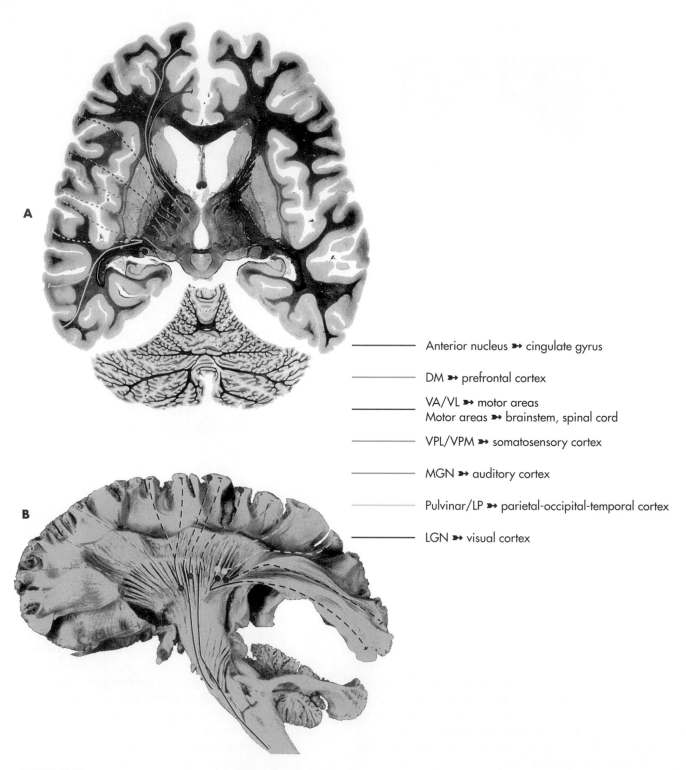

Anterior nucleus ➤➤ cingulate gyrus

DM ➤➤ prefrontal cortex

VA/VL ➤➤ motor areas
Motor areas ➤➤ brainstem, spinal cord

VPL/VPM ➤➤ somatosensory cortex

MGN ➤➤ auditory cortex

Pulvinar/LP ➤➤ parietal-occipital-temporal cortex

LGN ➤➤ visual cortex

FIGURE 16-23

Principal components of the various parts of the internal capsule, as seen in a horizontal section (**A**) and in the dissection from Figure 16-22. The thalamic cell bodies indicated schematically in **B** would actually be on the other side of the internal capsule. Not all elements can be seen in both parts of the figure. For example, the anterior nucleus and the pulvinar are not present in the plane of section shown in **A**, so no cell bodies are indicated; neither cingulate nor auditory cortex is present in the dissection shown in **B**, so no projections to them are indicated. (**A** modified from Nolte J, Angevine JB Jr: *The human brain in photographs and diagrams*, St. Louis, 1995, Mosby; **B** modified from Ludwig E, Klingler J: *Atlas cerebri humani*, Boston, 1956, Little, Brown & Co.)

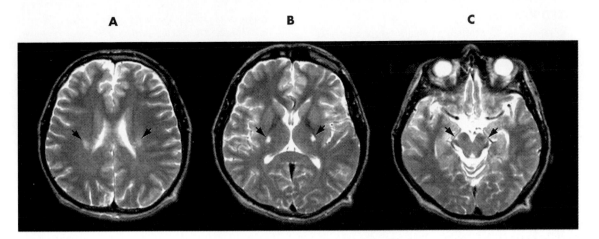

FIGURE 16-24
A dramatic demonstration of the location of the corticospinal tract in the corona radiata (**A**), internal capsule (**B**), and cerebral peduncle (**C**). These T2-weighted MR images are from a 34-year-old patient with motor neuron disease (also called *amyotrophic lateral sclerosis,* or *Lou Gehrig's disease*), in which both upper and lower motor neurons degenerate. Increased signal intensity corresponding to the corticospinal tracts is apparent at all three levels *(arrows).* (From Thorpe JW et al: Brain and spinal cord MRI in motor neuron disease, *J Neurol Neurosurg Psychiatry* 61:314, 1996.)

the genu. For most of their course, however, these fibers are actually located in the posterior third of the posterior limb adjacent to the somatosensory projections (Figure 16-24).

3. The genu is a transition zone between the anterior and posterior limbs and contains some frontopontine fibers as well as many of the fibers interconnecting VA and VL with the motor and premotor cortex. Corticobulbar fibers to motor nuclei of cranial nerves are also located near the genu.

4. The retrolenticular part of the internal capsule contains most of the fibers interconnecting the thalamus with posterior portions of the cerebral hemisphere. These include the fibers passing in both directions between the parietal-occipital-temporal association cortex and the pulvinar/LP complex. They also include part of the **optic radiation.** The optic radiation is the large collection of visual system fibers projecting from the lateral geniculate nucleus to the banks of the calcarine sulcus. The portion in the retrolenticular part of the internal capsule ends in the superior bank of the calcarine sulcus. As explained in the next chapter, these are the fibers conveying information from inferior portions of the visual fields. Finally, the retrolenticular part also contains additional corticopontine fibers, principally from the parietal lobe.

5. The sublenticular part of the internal capsule is continuous with the retrolenticular part and contains the remainder of the optic radiation (i.e., those fibers ending in the inferior bank of the calcarine sulcus and carrying information about superior visual fields). The sublenticular part also contains the **auditory radiation,** whose fibers pass laterally from the medial geniculate nucleus under the

lenticular nucleus and lateral sulcus and then turn superiorly to end in the superior temporal gyrus (see Figure 14-17, *B*).

Small Branches of the Middle Cerebral Artery Provide Most of the Blood Supply to the Internal Capsule

The blood supply of the internal capsule is from two principal sources, the **lateral striate arteries** and the **anterior choroidal artery** (see Figure 6-20). The lateral striate (or **lenticulostriate**) arteries are the collection of fine ganglionic branches of the proximal portion of the middle cerebral artery and supply most of the anterior limb, genu, and posterior limb (see Figure 6-7). The anterior limb and genu also receive part of their supply from ganglionic branches of the anterior cerebral and anterior communicating arteries, particularly from a relatively large one called the **recurrent artery** (of **Heubner**), or **medial striate artery.** The anterior choroidal artery supplies inferior and posterior regions of the internal capsule. It overlaps the lateral striate arteries in supplying the posterior limb and provides most of the supply of the retrolenticular and sublenticular parts. Ganglionic branches of the posterior cerebral artery also help supply the retrolenticular and sublenticular parts.

Small strokes in the internal capsule could obviously have major consequences. Hemorrhage of a lateral striate artery in the vicinity of the posterior limb can result in contralateral spastic paralysis and hemianesthesia. If the retrolenticular and sublenticular parts are also involved, visual deficits would be added to the symptoms. The auditory radiations would be damaged as well, but this would produce relatively minor deficits because of the bilateral nature of the central auditory pathways.

The fox jumped.

SUGGESTED READINGS

Aggleton JP, Desimone R, Mishkin M: The origin, course, and termination of the hippocampothalamic projections in the macaque, *J Comp Neurol* 243:409, 1986.

Brzezinski A: Melatonin in humans, *New Engl J Med* 336:186, 1997.

Chung C-S et al: Thalamic haemorrhage, *Brain* 119:1873, 1996.

Craig AD et al: A thalamic nucleus specific for pain and temperature sensation, *Nature* 372:770, 1994.

Erisir A, Van Horn SC, Sherman SM: Relative numbers of cortical and brainstem inputs to the lateral geniculate nucleus, *Proc Nat Acad Sci* 94:1517, 1997.

Erlich SS, Apuzzo MLJ: The pineal gland: anatomy, physiology and clinical significance, *J Neurosurg* 63:321, 1985.

Giguere M, Goldman-Rakic PS: Mediodorsal nucleus: areal, laminar, and tangential distribution of afferents and efferents in the frontal lobe of rhesus monkeys, *J Comp Neurol* 277:195, 1988.

Gillilan LA: The arterial and venous blood supplies to the forebrain (including the internal capsule) of primates, *Neurol* 18:653, 1968.

Groenewegen HJ, Berendse HW: The specificity of the 'non-specific' midline and intralaminar thalamic nuclei, *Trends Neurosci* 17:52, 1994.

Groothius DR, Duncan GW, Fisher CM: The human thalamo-cortical sensory path in the internal capsule: evidence from a small capsular hemorrhage causing a pure sensory stroke, *Ann Neurol* 2:328, 1977.

Guido W, Weyand T: Burst responses in the thalamic relay cells of the awake behaving cat, *J Neurophysiol* 74:1782, 1995. *Elegant though technically demanding experiments demonstrating some of the factors that influence the response mode of lateral geniculate projection neurons during normal behavior.*

Guillery RW: Anatomical evidence concerning the role of the thalamus in corticocortical communication: a brief review, *J Anat* 187:583, 1995. *A well-written account of current views of the connections of thalamic association nuclei.*

Guillery RW, Feig SL, Lozsádi DA: Paying attention to the thalamic reticular nucleus, *Trends Neurosci* 21:28, 1998.

Ilinsky IA, Kultas-Ilinsky K: Sagittal cytoarchitectonic maps of the Macaca mulatta thalamus with a revised nomenclature of the motor-related nuclei validated by observations on their connectivity, *J Comp Neurol* 262:331, 1987.

Jones EG: *The thalamus,* New York, 1985, Plenum Press. *A well-written, profusely illustrated review of the comparative anatomy and physiology of the thalamus.*

Jones EG, Leavitt RY: Retrograde axonal transport and the demonstration of non-specific projections to the cerebral cortex and striatum from thalamic intralaminar nuclei in the rat, cat, and monkey, *J Comp Neurol* 154:349, 1974.

Kolmac CI, Mitrofanis J: Organisation of the reticular thalamic projection to the intralaminar and midline nuclei, *J Comp Neurol* 377:165, 1997.

Langworthy OR, Fox HM: Thalamic syndrome: syndrome of the posterior cerebral artery: a review, *Arch Intern Med* 60:203, 1937.

Lin C-S et al: A major direct GABAergic pathway from zona incerta to neocortex, *Science* 248:1553, 1990.

Ludwig E, Klingler J: *Atlas cerebri humani,* Boston, 1956, Little, Brown & Co., Inc. *A collection of remarkable dissections of human brains. Formalin-fixed brains were frozen and thawed once or twice, which for some reason makes dissection much easier. (This ac-counts for the spongy appearance of the cortex in Figures 16-21 and 16-22.) The actual dissections were done with jeweler's forceps and wooden probes.*

Mikol J et al: Connections of laterodorsal nucleus of the thalamus. II. Experimental study in Papio papio, *Brain Res* 138:1, 1977.

Montero UM: A quantitative study of synaptic contacts on interneurons and relay cells of the cat lateral geniculate nucleus, *Exp Brain Res* 86:257, 1991.

Mountcastle VB, Henneman E: The representation of tactile sensibility in the thalamus of the monkey, *J Comp Neurol* 97:409, 1952. *An early physiological demonstration of the mapping of the body surface onto VPL/VPM.*

Plets C et al: The vascularization of the human thalamus, *Acta Neurol Belg* 70:687, 1970. *Long and detailed.*

Pritchard TC et al: Projections of thalamic gustatory and lingual areas in the monkey, *Macaca fascicularis*, *J Comp Neurol* 244:213, 1986.

Reiter RJ, editor: *The pineal and reproduction: progress in reproductive biology,* vol 4, Basel, 1978, S. Karger.

Robertson RT, Thompson SM, Kaitz SS: Projections from the pretectal complex to the thalamic lateral dorsal nucleus of the cat, *Exp Brain Res* 51:157, 1983.

Romanski LM et al: Topographic organization of medial pulvinar connections with the prefrontal cortex in the rhesus monkey, *J Comp Neurol* 379:313, 1997.

Ross ED: Localization of the pyramidal tract in the internal capsule by whole brain dissection, *Neurol* 30:59, 1980.

Rousseaux M et al: Disorders of smell, taste, and food intake in a patient with a dorsomedial thalamic infarct, *Stroke* 27:2328, 1996.

Russchen FT, Amaral DG, Price JL: The afferent input to the magnocellular division of the mediodorsal thalamic nucleus in the monkey, Macaca fascicularis, *J Comp Neurol* 256:175, 1987.

Sadikot AF, Parent A, François C: The centre médian and parafascicular thalamic nuclei project respectively to the sensorimotor and associative-limbic territories in the squirrel monkey, *Brain Res* 510:161, 1990.

Sandson TA et al: Frontal lobe dysfunction following infarction of the left-sided medial thalamus, *Arch Neurol* 48:1300, 1991.

Sherman SM, Guillery RW: Functional organization of thalamocortical relays, *J Neurophysiol* 76:1367, 1996. *An outstanding review of the circuitry, physiology and probable modes of operation of thalamic relay and association nuclei.*

Sugitani M: Electrophysiological and sensory properties of the thalamic reticular neurones related to somatic sensation in rats, *J Physiol* 290:79, 1979.

Ulrich DJ, Tamamaki N, Sherman SM: Brainstem control of response modes in neurons of the cat's lateral geniculate nucleus, *Proc Nat Acad Sci* 87:2560, 1990.

Walker AE: *The primate thalamus,* 1938, University of Chicago Press. *An early (and historically important) exposition of the thalamic terminology commonly used today.*

Whitsel BL et al: Thalamic projections to S-I in macaque monkey, *J Comp Neurol* 178:385, 1978. *The microarchitecture of the projection from VPL/VPM to the cortex, giving some idea of how remarkably detailed this projection is.*

Wilkins RH, Brody IA: The thalamic syndrome, *Arch Neurol* 20:560, 1969. *A brief introduction to (and excerpted translation of) the original work (Dejerine J, Roussy G: Le syndrome thalamique, Rev Neurol 14:521, 1906).*

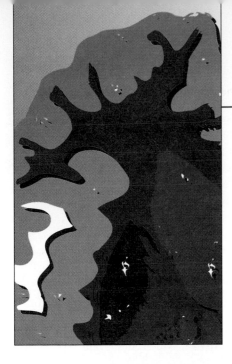

C H A P T E R   17

THE VISUAL SYSTEM

It is clear from everyday experience that we are a visually oriented species. Although it is arguable which of our senses is the most important, loss of the visual sense is certainly a greater handicap for humans than loss of, for example, the olfactory or gustatory sense. Partly because of its importance (and partly for anatomical and technical reasons to be discussed later), a great deal of research has been done on the visual system. Currently, we probably know more about the visual system than about any other sensory system, and there is considerable promise that with further study we will be able to understand in some detail how this portion of the CNS actually works.

Some lizards, fish, and amphibians have a photosensitive pineal organ that constantly stares up at the sky as a sort of "third eye." In mammals, however, all photic information originates in the **rods** and **cones** of the **retina** and then is conveyed to the brain by way of the axons of the output cells (called **ganglion cells**) of the retina. These axons, together with the axons of higher-order cells on which they synapse, form a visual pathway that begins in the eyes anteriorly and ends in the occipital lobes posteriorly. Throughout most of this course a precise **retinotopic** arrangement of fibers is maintained so that particular small regions of the retina are represented in particular small regions of more central parts of the pathway. Damage at many different locations within this system can result in visual deficits, and a knowledge of the anatomy involved makes it possible to understand these deficits. Conversely, the same knowledge is frequently helpful in deducing the site of a lesion.

THE EYE HAS THREE CONCENTRIC TISSUE LAYERS AND A LENS

Eyes and cameras both need to deal with similar sets of issues—regulating the amount of light reaching the photosensitive surface, focusing on near and far objects, maintaining a stable relationship between the focusing apparatus and the photosensitive surface, and recording the pattern of incoming light—so, not surprisingly, they have many analogous components. On the other hand, the retina is part of an outgrowth of the diencephalon (Figure 17-1), and one result of this origin is numerous parallels between the eye and the brain and meninges. The eye can be thought of as formed from three roughly spherical, concentric tissue layers with a lens suspended inside them (Figure 17-2). Each layer contributes to different structures in different parts of the eye (Table 17-1).

The outermost tissue layer is continuous with the dura mater. Like the dura, it is a feltwork of collagenous connective tissue. Most of this layer forms the **sclera,** the "white of the eye," which continues posteriorly as the sheath of the optic nerve. Beginning at a circular transition zone called the **limbus,** the anterior one sixth of this layer is the transparent **cornea,** which admits light to the eye.

The heavily vascularized middle layer, the **uvea★** or **uveal tract,** is similar in some ways to the arachnoid and pia. This is the principal route through which blood vessels and nerves (other than the optic nerve) travel within the wall of the eye. Over most of its extent the uvea is sandwiched between the sclera and the retina as the densely pigmented **choroid.** Choroidal capillaries supply retinal photoreceptors, and choroidal pigment absorbs stray light (much like the flat black paint job inside a camera does). The uvea continues anteriorly to form the bulk of the **ciliary body** (containing the **ciliary muscle**) and the **stroma** of the **iris.**

The innermost layer is an outgrowth of the CNS and is itself a two-part structure, reflecting its origin from the two layers of infolded optic cup (Figure 17-1). Over most of its extent, this layer comprises the **retina,** which lines the choroid. The outer portion of the retina, adjacent to the choroid, is the **retinal pigment epithelium,** whereas the inner portion, adjacent to the interior of the

---

★*Uvea* is Latin for "grape." This part of the eye apparently received its name for the aperture in its anterior portion that lets the rays in.

Table 17-1 Derivatives of the Three Tissue Layers of the Eye

Layer	Posterior to ora serrata	Between ora serrata and limbus	Anterior to limbus
Fibrous outer layer	Sclera	Sclera	Cornea
Vascular middle layer (uveal tract)	Choroid	Ciliary body (vascular core) Ciliary muscle	Iris (stroma)
Inner layer (neuroepithelial double layer)	Neural retina Retinal pigment epithelium	Ciliary body (double-layered ciliary epithelium)	Iris (posterior epithelial layers) Pupillary dilator Pupillary sphincter

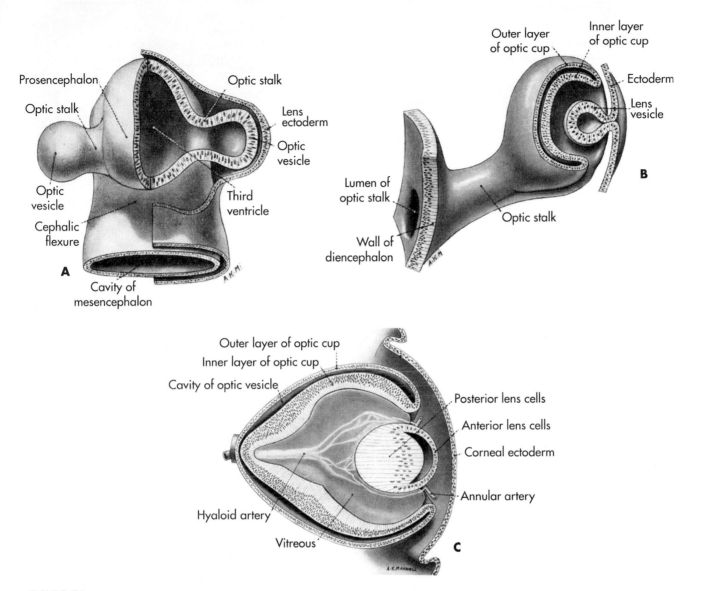

FIGURE 17-1

Embryological development of the eye. **A,** At about 4 weeks, the optic vesicle of each side has evaginated from the prosencephalon in this head-on view. **B,** At about 5 weeks, the initially spherical optic vesicle has folded in on itself to form the two-layered optic cup; the optic cup partially envelops the lens vesicle, which is derived from surface ectoderm. **C,** At about 6 weeks, the lens vesicle has pinched off, and additional surface ectoderm has begun to form the surface of the cornea. The outer layer of the two-layered optic cup will go on to form the retinal pigment epithelium; the inner layer will form the neural retina. Anteriorly both layers will grow around farther in front of the lens and participate in the formation of the iris and ciliary body. The hyaloid and annular arteries are transient embryological structures helping to supply the eye as it develops. The annular artery later merges with the network of choroidal capillaries. The distal parts of the hyaloid artery degenerate and the proximal parts persist as the central retinal artery. (From Hamilton WJ: *Textbook of human anatomy,* ed 2, St. Louis, 1976, Mosby.)

eye, is the **neural retina.** Under normal conditions no space exists between the pigment epithelium and the neural retina in the adult. However, the mechanical connections between the two are not very strong, and under certain circumstances this potential space opens, constituting **retinal detachment.** Retinal receptors are metabolically dependent on pigment epithelial cells and on the adjacent choroidal vasculature, so detached areas stop working. The photosensitive retina ends anteriorly at a serrated border (the **ora serrata**), but the same two layers continue as the double-layered **ciliary epithelium** covering the ciliary body and the double layer of pigmented epithelium covering the posterior surface of the iris.

Intraocular Pressure Maintains the Shape of the Eye

Cameras have rigid bodies, designed to keep film in some stable position relative to the lens. In contrast, the shape of the eye (and position of the retina) is maintained in much the same way as inflating a soccer ball maintains its shape. The collagenous sclera and cornea correspond to the wall of the soccer ball, and intraocular fluid pressure replaces air pressure. The pressure is generated by a now-familiar process of fluid production, circulation, and reabsorption (Figure 17-3). The ciliary body functions as a small outpost of choroid plexus, secreting **aqueous humor** across the

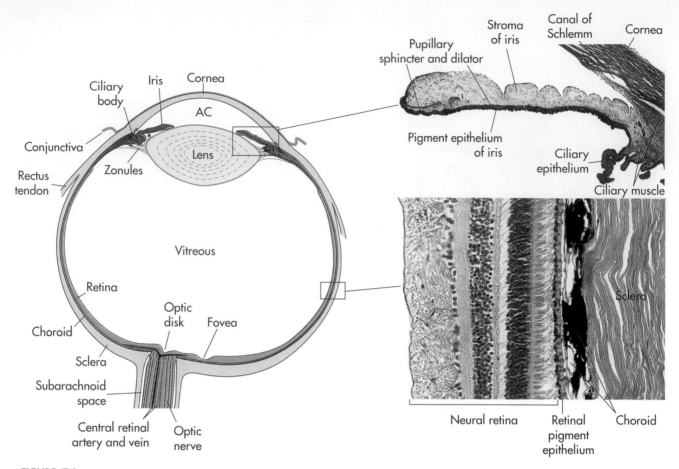

FIGURE 17-2
General structure of the eye as seen in a horizontal section, with histological sections of the iris and ciliary body (upper inset) and the wall of the eye (lower inset). *AC*, Anterior chamber; *, posterior chamber. (Lower inset courtesy Dr. Allen L. Bell, Anatomy Department, University of New England College of Osteopathic Medicine.)

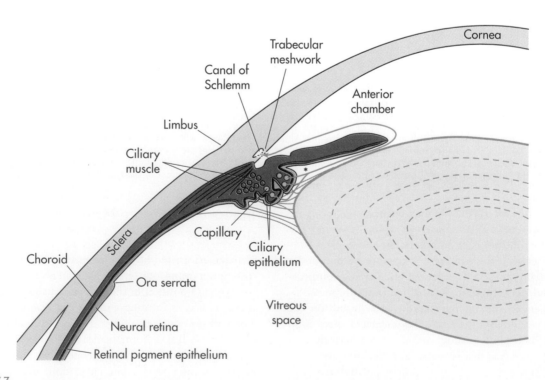

FIGURE 17-3
Production and circulation of aqueous humor. Components filtered through fenestrated ciliary capillaries are transported across the ciliary epithelium, enter the posterior chamber (*), move through the pupil into the anterior chamber, pass through the trabecular meshwork, and enter the canal of Schlemm.

ciliary epithelium and into the **posterior chamber,** the space between the iris and the lens. Pushed along by hydrostatic pressure, the aqueous humor passes through the pupil and into the **anterior chamber,** filters through the collagenous **trabecular meshwork** (analogous to arachnoid granulations) at the iridocorneal angle and enters the **canal of Schlemm,** which communicates directly with the venous drainage of the eye. The production rate (about $2\mu l/min$) is sufficient to completely replace the aqueous humor about 15 times a day. The space behind the lens, constituting most of the intraocular volume, is filled with gelatinous **vitreous** (Latin for "glassy") **humor,** so the resistance to aqueous outflow afforded by the trabecular meshwork causes a pressure of about 15 mm Hg that is transmitted throughout the eye, maintaining its shape.

In much the same way that blocking CSF circulation or reabsorption causes increased intracranial pressure, headache, and neural damage, processes that interfere with circulation or reabsorption of aqueous humor cause the painful condition of **glaucoma,** and ultimately retinal damage.

The Cornea and Lens Focus Images on the Retina

Focusing an image requires refraction of light across one or more interfaces where there is a change in refractive index. The aqueous and vitreous humors have a refractive index only slightly lower than that of the lens, so the lens accounts for only a relatively small proportion of the refractive power of the eye; its major role is adjusting the focus of the eye for near and far objects, as described below. Hence for nonaquatic vertebrates like us, most of the refraction occurs at the front surface of the cornea.★ This accounts for our ability to see 90° or more to the side (Figure 17-29).

One can imagine a variety of strategies for changing the focus of an optical device to **accommodate** to near objects—moving the photosensitive surface, moving the refractive elements, or changing the shape of the refractive elements. Different animals have adapted each of these strategies. Conventional cameras are adjusted for near or far objects by moving their lenses closer to or farther from the film; similarly, fish have intraocular muscles that move the lens back and forth. Arthropods cannot move or deform lenses that are part of the exoskeleton, but some have muscles that move the retina closer to or farther from the lens. Some animals have muscles attached to the cornea that can change its curvature. Terrestrial vertebrates use intraocular muscles to change the shape of the lens. Our lens is suspended by strands of connective tissue called **zonules,** attached at one end to the lens and at the other end to the ciliary body. At rest, the tension of this zonular

suspension keeps the lens slightly flattened and the eye focused on distant objects. The ciliary muscle (Figure 17-3) has some fibers oriented circumferentially that act as a kind of sphincter; contraction of these fibers pulls the ciliary attachment points of the zonules toward the center of the pupil and relaxes some of the tension in the zonular suspension. Other ciliary muscle fibers are oriented parallel to the surface of the eye; contraction of these pulls the ciliary attachment points partly anteriorly and partly toward the center of the pupil, again relaxing some of the tension in the zonular suspension. Hence, somewhat counterintuitively, contraction of the ciliary muscle allows the lens to fatten as the eye accommodates to near objects: the posterior surface of the lens is embedded in the vitreous humor and does not move, but the anterior surface bulges out slightly.

The Iris Affects the Brightness and Quality of the Image Focused on the Retina

The range of light intensities over which we have useful vision, from starlight to bright sunlight, is an astonishing 10^{12} or so—a million million-fold.★ This is a much greater range of intensities than receptor potentials and frequencies of action potentials can encode directly, so there are mechanisms for adapting visual sensitivity to the ambient illumination. Most of these mechanisms depend on the physiology and wiring of retinal neurons, but in addition the iris plays a role in regulating the amount of light reaching the retina. The two posterior epithelial layers are densely pigmented, and in brown-eyed individuals the stroma contains substantial additional pigment, so essentially all light reaching the retina must first pass through the **pupil,** the aperture in the middle of the iris.

The size of the pupil is controlled by two smooth muscles in the iris (Figure 17-2), both highly unusual in being derived from the same layers of neural ectoderm that give rise to the retina. The circumferentially arranged **pupillary sphincter†** encircles the pupil, at what was embryologically the edge of the optic cup. The **pupillary dilator,** whose fibers are arranged like spokes radiating from the sphincter, is located at the interface between the pigment epithelial layers and the stroma. The sphincter is the stronger of the two, and reflex connections (Figure 17-36) mediated by the optic and oculomotor nerves constrict the pupil in response to increased levels of illumination. The pupillary sphincter can contract by about 80%, much more than other muscles and enough to vary the diameter of the pupil from about 8 mm to 1.5 mm. However, this corresponds to only about a thirtyfold change in area,

---

★Fish and other aquatic animals obviously cannot use this mechanism. Instead, they have much larger, more spherical lenses, and adaptations to increase the difference in refractive index between the lens and the intraocular fluids.

★Continuing the camera analogy, this corresponds to about 40 f-stops. Pupillary constriction can only account for about 4 f-stops.

†Signs of this optic cup origin are found in the many species, including many fish and amphibians and even some mammals, whose pupillary sphincters contain visual pigment and contract autonomously in response to light.

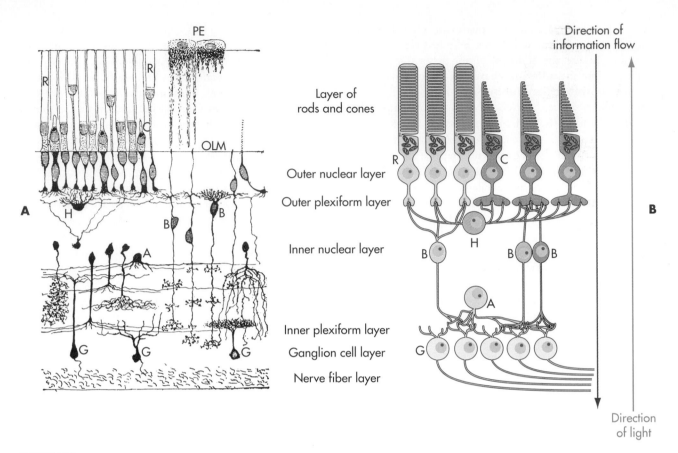

FIGURE 17-4

Cell types and their arrangement in the retina. **A,** Drawing of Golgi-stained cells of the frog retina. **B,** Schematic illustration of a generalized vertebrate retina showing retinal layers. *A,* Amacrine cell; *B,* bipolar cell; *C,* cone; *G,* ganglion cell; *H,* horizontal cell; *OLM,* outer limiting membrane; *PE,* pigment epithelium; *R,* rod. (**A** from Ramón y Cajal S: *Histologie due système nerveux de l'homme et des vertébrés,* vol 2, Paris, 1911, Maloine.)

consistent with the idea that retinal mechanisms play the major role in adjusting visual sensitivity.

In addition to decreasing the amount of light reaching the retina, a smaller pupil improves the optical performance of the eye (just as, within limits, a smaller aperture improves the optical performance of a camera lens). This is particularly important when focusing on near objects (Figures 17-37 and 17-38).

THE RETINA CONTAINS FIVE MAJOR NEURONAL CELL TYPES

One reason so much research has been done on the visual system is the overall anatomical simplicity of the neural retina relative to other parts of the nervous system. Although it contains hundreds of millions of neurons, there are only five basic types involved in the processing of visual information, and their patterns of interconnections are fundamentally the same throughout the retina.

The five cell types have their somata neatly arranged in three layers and make most of their synapses in two additional layers. In each synaptic zone, one cell type brings visual information in, another type carries information out, and a third type serves as a laterally interconnecting element.

A simplified, schematic illustration of these basic connection patterns is shown in Figure 17-4. Starting peripherally, the photoreceptor cells, stimulated by light, project to the first layer of synapses where they terminate on the aptly named **bipolar** and **horizontal cells.** The bipolar cells then project to the next layer of synapses, whereas the horizontal cells spread laterally and interconnect receptors, bipolar cells, and other horizontal cells. In the second layer of synapses, bipolar cells terminate on ganglion cells and **amacrine cells.**★ Axons of the ganglion cells leave the eye as the **optic nerve,** whereas processes of the amacrine cells spread laterally and interconnect bipolar cells, ganglion cells, and other amacrine cells.

Retinal Neurons and Synapses Are Arranged in Layers

The entire retina is conventionally described as a 10-layered structure, beginning with the pigment epithelium (Figure 17-5); five of these layers are the layers of cell bodies and synapses mentioned above. In naming these layers, the term **nuclear** refers to cell bodies and the term **plex-**

★*Amacrine* is Greek for "without a long process," referring to the fact that most amacrine cells do not have a conventional axon.

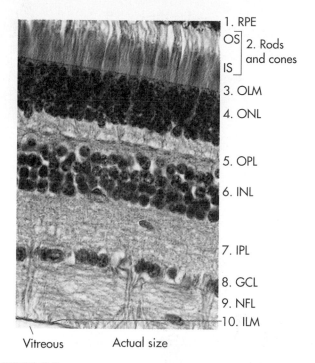

1. RPE
OS
IS
2. Rods and cones
3. OLM
4. ONL
5. OPL
6. INL
7. IPL
8. GCL
9. NFL
10. ILM

Vitreous   Actual size

FIGURE 17-5
Light micrograph of human retina. The entire retina is only 200 to 300 µm thick. *GCL,* Ganglion cell layer; *ILM,* inner limiting membrane; *INL,* inner nuclear layer; *IPL,* inner plexiform layer; *IS,* inner segments; *NFL,* nerve fiber layer; *OLM,* outer limiting membrane; *ONL,* outer nuclear layer; *OPL,* outer plexiform layer; *OS,* outer segments; *RPE,* retinal pigment epithelium. (Courtesy Dr. Allen L. Bell, Anatomy Department, University of New England College of Osteopathic Medicine.)

iform to synaptic zones. **Inner** and **outer** refer to the number of synapses by which a structure is separated from the brain, so that, for example, photoreceptors are "outer" with respect to bipolar cells. The 10 layers of the retina are as follows:

1. The **retinal pigment epithelium** is a single layer of polygonal, pigmented cells. One side of each cell adjoins the choroid, whose capillaries supply the avascular first two layers of the retina. The other side of each cell forms numerous fine processes that partially surround the outer portions of the receptor cells and obliterate the space that existed embryonically within the wall of the optic cup. Pigment epithelial cells are intimately involved metabolically with the receptors. They also play a role in absorbing light that has passed through the retina.

2. **Rods** and **cones** are the two different types of vertebrate photoreceptor. Each consists of several regions (Figure 17-6): an **outer segment,** an **inner segment,** a cell body, and a synaptic terminal. Strictly speaking, "rod" or "cone" refers to only the outer segment plus the inner segment of a photoreceptor cell, but in common usage these terms are often used to refer to entire receptors.

The outer segment of a rod is relatively long and cylindrical, whereas that of a cone (except in the fovea) is shorter and tapered (Figures 17-6 and 17-7). Each type of outer segment is filled with hundreds of flattened membranous sacs, or **disks.** In cones, the interior of many of these disks is continuous with extracellular space, but in rods, almost all of the disks have pinched off from the external membrane and are wholly intracellular. The major protein constituent of the outer segment membranes of both rods and cones is the visual pigment, which is called **rhodopsin** in rods. (There is no universally accepted name for the visual pigments of cones, and they are often called *rhodopsins* as well, or simply **cone pigments**). Hence photons traversing the outer segment of a rod or cone must pass through hundreds or thousands of sheets of membrane, each full of visual pigment molecules. As one might expect from this localization of visual pigment, the outer segment is the site of visual transduction; photons absorbed here cause a receptor potential that then spreads to the rest of the cell. Note that the photosensitive portion of the receptor cells is located in the part of the neural retina that is farthest removed from incoming light (i.e., the retina is inverted with respect to the path of light through it). This curious situation is universally true among vertebrates. However, this does not detract from visual sensitivity or acuity because the retina is thin (Figure 17-5) and transparent (Figure 17-8) and because other anatomical modifications, discussed shortly, are found in the retinal area of greatest acuity.

Each outer segment is connected to its inner segment by a narrow ciliary stalk. The inner segments contain, among other organelles, a very prominent collection of mitochondria. These mitochondria are thought to supply the energy necessary for processes associated with transduction and for the synthesis of visual pigments. These pigments are continually renewed, being synthesized in the inner segment, transported through the ciliary stalk, and incorporated into disk membranes. "Old" disks at the apical ends of the outer segments of rods and cones are then phagocytosed by the pigment epithelium. (Certain types of retinal degeneration are probably caused by a defect in this renewal-phagocytosis process.)

As discussed later in this chapter, rods mediate low-acuity, monochromatic vision in dim light, whereas cones mediate high-acuity color vision, but require more light to do so.

3. The **outer limiting membrane** was so named because it has the appearance of a distinct line when viewed with a light microscope. However, electron microscopy has revealed it to be a row of intercellular junctions (Figure 17-6, *B*). Elongated specialized glial cells called **Müller cells** span almost the entire retina, ending distally at the bases of the inner segments of the rods and cones. Here adjacent Müller processes and inner segments are joined by junctional complexes, which collectively form the outer limiting membrane.

4. The **outer nuclear layer** consists of the cell bodies of the rods and cones.

5. The **outer plexiform layer** is the relatively thin synaptic zone in which receptors terminate on horizontal

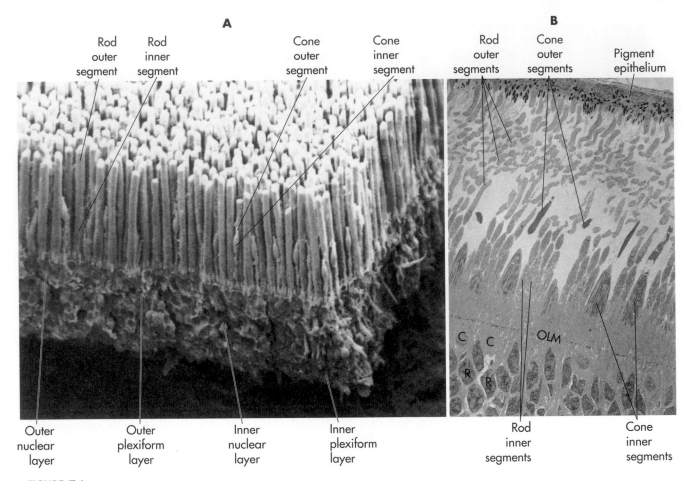

A

Rod outer segment | Rod inner segment | Cone outer segment | Cone inner segment

B

Rod outer segments | Cone outer segments | Pigment epithelium

Outer nuclear layer | Outer plexiform layer | Inner nuclear layer | Inner plexiform layer

Rod inner segments | Cone inner segments

FIGURE 17-6
Electron micrographs of rods and cones. **A,** Scanning electron micrograph of the retina of a bullfrog. **B,** Electron micrograph of the photoreceptor layer of a rhesus monkey's retina. This section was taken from a region near the fovea but not in it, so both rods and cones are plentiful. The outer limiting membrane is actually a row of intercellular junctions. The insertion of the tips of rod outer segments into the pigment epithelial layer is apparent. (**A** from Steinberg RH: Scanning electron microscopy of the bullfrog's retina and pigment epithelium, *Z Zellforsch* 143:451, 1973. **B** courtesy Dr. David Moran and Pamela Eller, University of Colorado Health Sciences Center.)

and bipolar cells and in which processes of horizontal cells spread laterally. The rods and cones synapse on separate subpopulations of bipolar cells and on different regions of some horizontal cells (Figures 17-20 and 17-21).

6. The **inner nuclear layer** contains the cell bodies of all the retinal interneurons as well as those of the Müller cells. The nuclei of horizontal cells are found near its distal edge, those of bipolar cells in the middle, and those of amacrine cells near its proximal edge. Bipolar cells conduct visual information through this layer, projecting to the second synaptic zone.

7. The **inner plexiform layer** is the relatively thick synaptic zone in which bipolar cells terminate on amacrine and ganglion cells, and processes of amacrine cells spread laterally. The actual pattern of interconnections is somewhat more complex than that shown in Figure 17-4. The amacrine cells provide one example of this added complexity: based on neurochemical and anatomical characteristics, more than 30 different types, each presumed to have a somewhat distinctive function, have been described.

8. The **ganglion cell layer** contains the cell bodies of the ganglion cells, whose dendrites ramify in the inner plexiform layer and whose axons leave the eye as the optic nerve. This cell layer is considerably thinner than either the outer or the inner nuclear layer in most retinal locations, reflecting the fact that there are about 5 million cones and about 100 million rods in a human retina but only about 1 million ganglion cells. Clearly a good deal of convergence is involved in retinal processing, but the convergence is not uniform across the retina. As discussed shortly, some regions are specialized for high acuity and have little convergence, whereas other regions are specialized for high sensitivity and have a great deal of convergence.

Visual information travels in several parallel streams, just as somatosensory information travels rostrally through the spinal cord and brainstem in multiple parallel pathways. In the case of the visual system, the axons of several anatomically and functionally distinct classes of ganglion cells share the same optic nerve in their course toward the brain. In the primate visual system, approximately 80% of

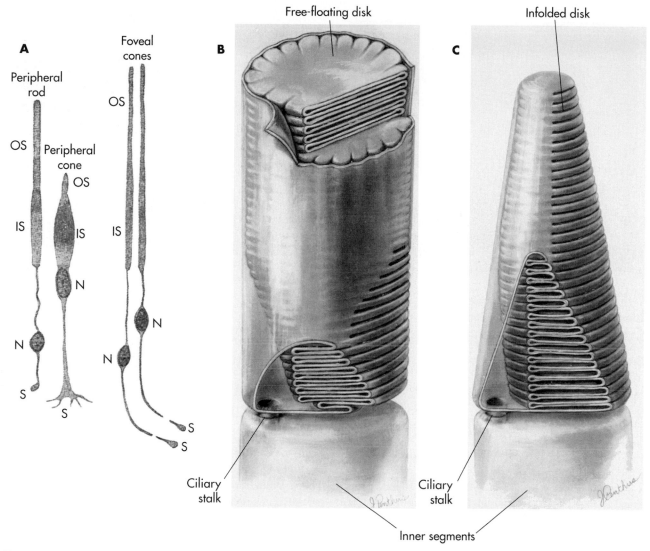

FIGURE 17-7

Ultrastructural differences between the outer segments of rods and cones. **A** shows the general shape of peripheral rods and cones and foveal cones dissociated from a human retina. *IS,* Inner segment; *N,* nucleus in cell body; *OS,* outer segment; *S,* synaptic ending. **B,** Rod outer segment (cut off toward the top to be the same length as the cone outer segment in **C**); note that some disks toward the base of the outer segment are open to the outside world but that most disks are pinched off and completely surrounded by cytoplasm. **C,** Cone outer segment; note that this outer segment tapers toward its apex (hence its name) and that all of its disks are infoldings of the plasma membrane with their interiors still continuous with extracellular space. (**A** from Ramón y Cajal S: *Histologie due système nerveux de l'homme et des vertébrés,* vol 2, Paris, 1911, Maloine. **B** and **C** courtesy Dr. Richard W. Young, University of California at Los Angeles.)

all ganglion cells form a single class of small cells that are particularly responsive to the colors of visual objects and to details of their shapes. Some general aspects of the distinctive connections of this and other ganglion cell classes are mentioned later in this chapter.

9. The **nerve fiber layer** is the collection of axons of ganglion cells, which converge like spokes toward the **optic disk** or **optic papilla** (located posteriorly and slightly medial to the midline of the eye [Figure 17-2]), where they form the optic nerve. The central retinal artery, a branch of the ophthalmic artery, traverses the optic nerve and enters the eye at the optic disk. Hence the retina has a dual blood supply, with outer layers supplied by the choroidal circulation (also fed by the ophthalmic artery) and inner layers by the central retinal artery.

10. The **inner limiting membrane** is a thin basal lamina that intervenes between the vitreous and the proximal ends of the Müller cells.

The Retina Is Regionally Specialized

Cross sections through the retina do not have the same appearance at all locations. For example, no photoreceptors, interneurons, or ganglion cells are present at the optic disk, where the axons of ganglion cells leave the

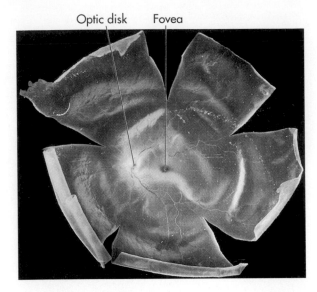

FIGURE 17-8
An isolated human neural retina. (Courtesy Dr. Dennis M. Dacey, University of Washington School of Medicine.)

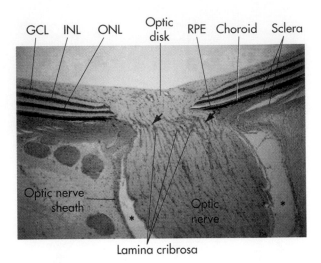

FIGURE 17-9
Light micrograph of a human optic disk, showing the absence of neuronal layers at this location. *Arrows* indicate bundles of optic nerve fibers passing through the lamina cribrosa, the perforated scleral zone adjacent to the optic disk. *, Subarachnoid space surrounding optic nerve; *GCL*, ganglion cell layer; *INL*, inner nuclear layer; *ONL*, outer nuclear layer; *RPE*, retinal pigment epithelium. (Courtesy Dr. Allen L. Bell, Anatomy Department, University of New England College of Osteopathic Medicine.)

eye to form the optic nerve (Figure 17-9). These axons originate near the vitreous, so they must turn posteriorly and traverse the retina before passing through the sclera. Because there are no photoreceptors at the optic disk, we are blind to any object whose image falls on this part of the retina. Although the **blind spot** can easily be demonstrated (Figure 17-10), we have no awareness as we walk around of a blank spot in visual space. One might think this is because the left eye can see the part of the visual field that falls on the right eye's blind spot, and vice versa (Figure 17-29). This cannot be the explanation, though, because we are unaware of the blind spot even with one eye closed. The real reason is that our nervous system simply "fills it in." We are actually quite skillful at this, and patients with damage to their visual systems can become blind in surprisingly large areas of their visual fields without being aware of it.

Beginning near the lateral edge of the optic disk is a circular portion of the retina, about 5 mm in diameter, in which many of the cells contain a yellow pigment (Figure 17-8). This gives the area a yellowish color when examined with appropriate illumination and has led to its being called the **macula lutea** (Latin for "yellow spot"), often shortened to **macula.** In the center of the macula is a depression about 1.5 mm in diameter, called the **fovea,** which is particularly rich in cones. In the central part of the fovea is a pit, only about 350 μm across, which contains only elongated cones (no rods) and is directly in line with the visual axis (Figure 17-11). The central fovea is specialized for vision of the highest acuity; all the neurons and capillaries that are present elsewhere (and that light would otherwise traverse before

reaching the receptors) are collected around the edges of the fovea. Specialized interneurons called **midget bipolar cells** receive their inputs from individual foveal cones. These bipolars in turn contact individual **midget ganglion cells,** so that an anatomical basis for highly detailed foveal vision is maintained.★

The fovea is one extreme in a changing rod/cone distribution across the retina (Figure 17-12). The packing density of cones decreases sharply outside the fovea, whereas that of the rods increases, reaching a maximum just outside the macula. From here to the edge of the retina, the cone density remains at a low level, and the rod density slowly declines as well (Figure 17-13). Given the properties of rods and cones, it follows from these distributions that the fovea is used for high-acuity color vision in reasonably bright light, whereas extrafoveal regions function at lower light levels.

★One might think it advantageous to continue the anatomical specializations of the fovea, such as small, tightly packed photoreceptors and no convergence, throughout the retina; this would give us highly detailed vision over our entire field of view. However, as Wässle and Boycott point out (*Physiol Rev* 71:447, 1991), foveal vision requires so much cerebral cortex (e.g., Figures 17-26 and 17-27) that using foveal specializations throughout the retina would necessitate 100 times as much cerebral cortex as we presently have available in our entire cerebrum! Hence we use a very small fovea, together with precisely controlled eye movements that allow us to aim it at objects of interest (see Chapter 21).

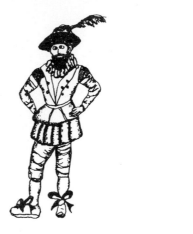

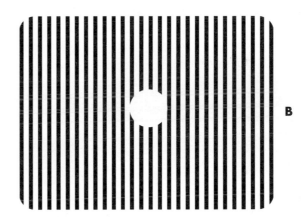

FIGURE 17-10

How to demonstrate your right eye's blind spot to yourself. **A,** Close your left eye, hold the book at arm's length, stare fixedly at the spot on the left side of the figure, and slowly move the book toward you. At some point about a foot from your face, the bearded gentleman will lose his head. **B,** Demonstration of how the CNS "fills in" the blind spot. As in part **A** above, close your left eye, stare at the black spot with your right eye, and move the book slowly toward you. When the image of the hole in the striped pattern falls on your blind spot, your brain will try to convince you that there are stripes where none exist. (**A** based on a technique of King Charles II, as recounted by Rushton WAH: King Charles II and the blind spot, *Vision Res* 19:255, 1979.)

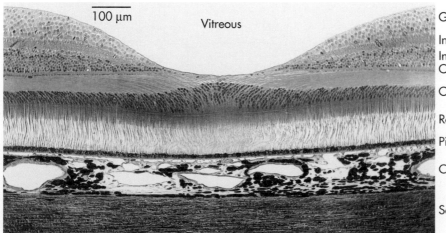

FIGURE 17-11

Fovea of a rhesus monkey. Note that all retinal elements (except the photoreceptors, which are all cones in the center of the fovea) are displaced to either side so that light only needs to pass through the outer nuclear layer before reaching the cones. The nerve fiber layer is scanty in this region because the axons of more laterally placed ganglion cells arc around the fovea on their way to the optic disk. (From Fine BS, Yanoff M: *Ocular histology,* ed 2, New York, 1979, Harper & Row.)

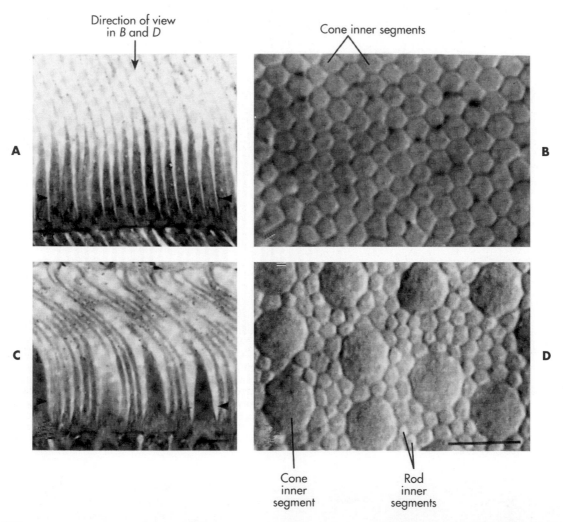

FIGURE 17-12

Differential distribution of rods and cones in the human retina. **A** and **C** show standard histological sections parallel to the long axes of photoreceptor inner and outer segments in the fovea (**A**) and the midperipheral retina (**C**). **B** and **D** show the array of photoreceptors in comparable areas of another retina viewed end-on, using a special video microscopy technique (Nomarski differential interference contrast) that allows focusing on a particular cross-sectional plane of the sample. In this case, the plane of focus is one that cuts through the photoreceptor inner segments at the level indicated by the arrowheads in **A** and **C**. In the fovea (**B**) all the inner segments are of closely packed, slender cones, whereas in the midperipheral retina (**D**) the inner segments of fatter cones are interspersed among the rod inner segments. Scale mark in **D** = 10 μm. (From Curcio CA et al: Human photoreceptor topography, *J Comp Neurol* 292:497, 1990.)

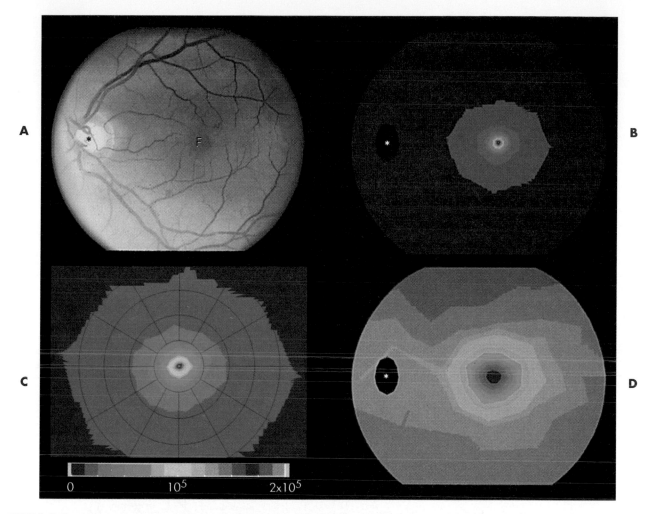

FIGURE 17-13
Differential distribution of rods and cones in the human retina. **A,** Funduscopic view of the left retina. Arteries and veins emerge from the optic disk (*) and arc around the fovea *(F)*. **B** and **D** show the distributions of cones and rods, respectively, in an area of retina comparable to that shown in **A.** Note the absence of photoreceptors in the optic disk (*), the foveal concentration of cones (shown enlarged in **C**), and the perifoveal concentration of rods. The scale at the lower left shows the number of cells per mm². (**A** courtesy Dr. Christine A. Curcio, Department of Ophthalmology, University of Alabama at Birmingham. **B-D** modified from Curcio CA et al: Human photoreceptor topography, *J Comp Neurol* 292:497, 1990.)

RETINAL NEURONS TRANSLATE PATTERNS OF LIGHT INTO PATTERNS OF CONTRAST

Analogies between eyes and cameras mostly cease at the level of the retina. Cameras and film are generally designed to produce accurate maps of patterns of illumination. The impression that our visual system does the same is largely illusory. On the contrary, visual systems are specialized to recognize significant objects and features in visual scenes in spite of changes in angle of view, distance, and illumination. Receptor potentials in the array of retinal photoreceptors are the beginning of a neural process in which patterns of light are dissected into their components—areas of motion, boundaries between light and dark areas, boundaries between areas of different color, and other features—and the abstracted properties somehow reassembled into a unified perception. The brain in

effect makes its "best guess" in interpreting patterns of light, and the results are sometimes inaccurate or go considerably beyond the information received by the eye (Figure 17-14). The blind spot of which we are unaware is one example; another is the feeling that we have sharp, clear, color vision throughout our visual fields, whereas this is only true for a small central region (Figure 17-17).

Photoreceptors Utilize G-protein–Coupled Ion Channels to Produce Hyperpolarizing Receptor Potentials

Rhodopsin and cone pigments are members of the same family of G-protein–coupled receptors that mediate many postsynaptic effects and some other sensory transduction processes, such as olfaction. In the case of rods and cones, the ligand of the receptor protein **opsin,** rather than being a neurotransmitter or an odorant, is a vitamin A de-

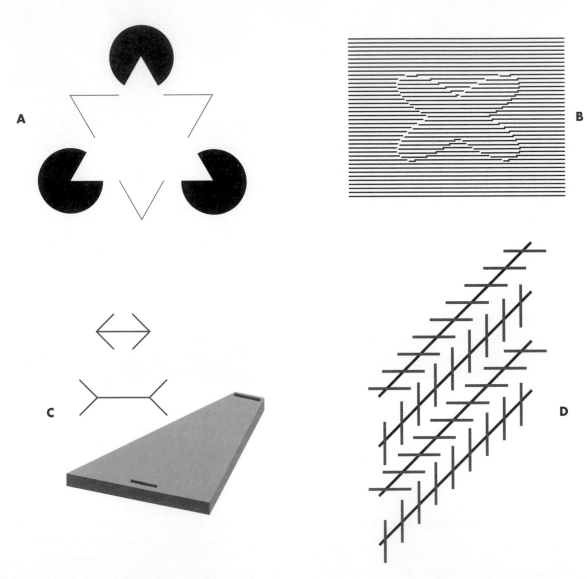

FIGURE 17-14
Some simple visual illusions. **A,** A Kanizsa figure, in which an illusory figure (here a white triangle) seems to be located in front of other objects, partially occluding them. In fact, nothing is there except black lines and notched disks. **B,** Slight displacement of some line segments causes the illusory appearance of a raised surface. **C,** Misperception of line length. In the Müller-Lyer illusion, the upper of the two horizontal lines appears shorter, even though both are the same length. The oppositely directed angles at the ends of these lines may give false perspective cues; the two lines on the apparent three-dimensional surface are also equal in length. **D,** The Zöllner illusion. All four black lines are actually parallel to each other.

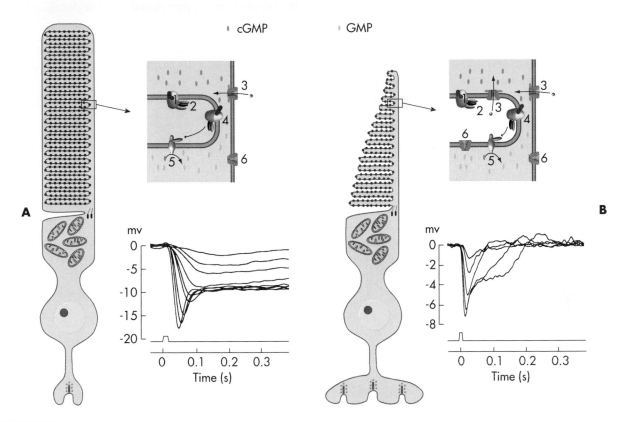

FIGURE 17-15

Phototransduction in rods **(A)** and cones **(B).** In the dark, rhodopsin and cone pigments *(I)* bind II-*cis* retinal, transducin is inactive *(2),* and cGMP-gated cation channels are open *(3).* Light isomerizes II-*cis* retinal to all-*trans* retinal *(4),* activating transducin, which in turn activates an enzyme (phosphodiesterase) that hydrolyzes cGMP *(5).* Decreased availability of cGMP causes the cGMP-gated cation channels to close *(6)* and the photoreceptors to hyperpolarize. The voltage records show the responses of a monkey rod *(left)* and red cone *(right)* to IO-msec flashes of increasing intensity. The light intensity for the cone records was several thousand times greater than for the rod records, resulting in the absorption of about 40 times as many photons per flash by the cone. It can be seen that cone responses are faster, briefer, and less sensitive than rod responses. (Voltage records from Schneeweis DM, Schnapf JL: Photovoltage of rods and cones in the macaque retina, *Science* 268:1053, 1995.)

rivative **(11-*cis* retinal)** that enables the photopigments to absorb visible light. Slight differences among the opsins of rods and each of the three types of cones results in differences in the wavelengths absorbed preferentially by each photopigment (Figure 17-18, *A*). The only effect of light in the phototransduction process is to isomerize 11-*cis* retinal to all-*trans* retinal, which shortly thereafter dissociates from opsin. Isomerization of retinal causes a conformational change in the opsin to which it is bound, and opsin in its altered conformation activates nearby molecules of **transducin,** a G protein (Figure 17-15). Each activated transducin in turn activates phosphodiesterase, an enzyme that hydrolyzes **cyclic guanosine monophosphate (cGMP).** This seemingly cumbersome process results in great amplification. Absorption of a single photon by one of the hundred million rhodopsins in a rod can activate hundreds of transducins; each transducin-activated phosphodiesterase can hydrolyze about a thousand cGMP molecules per second.

The surface membranes of rod and cone outer segments contain cGMP-gated cation channels. In the dark, the cGMP concentration is relatively high, the cation channels are open most of the time, and a current carried

mainly by Na$^+$ flows into the outer segment (Figure 17-16). As a result rods and cones have a relatively depolarized resting potential of about –40 mv in the dark, and release neurotransmitter (glutamate) at a steady rate onto processes of bipolar and horizontal cells. Light-induced hydrolysis of cGMP causes cation channels to close, the membrane hyperpolarizes toward the potassium equilibrium potential, and transmitter release declines.★

Rods function in dim light

Rods carry this amplification mechanism to an extreme, producing small but detectable electrical responses to single photons. Absorption of one photon by a dark-adapted rod causes transient closure of several hundred cation channels in the surface membrane, about a million ions are prevented from entering (Figure 17-16), and there is a

---

★In a sense, therefore, our photoreceptors are really "darkness receptors," depolarizing and releasing more transmitter as the level of illumination decreases. Presumably because we spend less than half our time in darkness this arrangement is not as metabolically inefficient as it sounds at first.

small, brief decrease in the rate of transmitter release. This sensitivity comes at a price, however. Rods can respond only up to about moonlight levels of light intensity; they are saturated in room light and daylight. In addition, rod responses are slow (Figure 17-15, *A*). Finally, the responses of multiple rods must be pooled to produce meaningful changes in the firing rate of ganglion cells in response to dim light. Particularly in the peripheral retina, the output of thousands of rods converges on hundreds of bipolar cells before ultimately reaching single ganglion cells; hence spatial resolution in dim light is relatively poor.

All of our retinal rods contain the same rhodopsin, making them incapable of discriminating color. Even though rhodopsin absorbs 500 nm light more effectively than light of other wavelengths, every photon absorbed sets in motion the same G-protein–coupled cascade. Hence a dim 500-nm stimulus causes the same receptor potential as a brighter 600-nm stimulus.

Populations of cones signal spatial detail and color

Cones have smaller outer segments, less visual pigment, and smaller, briefer single-photon responses than rods. All of this makes cones less sensitive (but faster) than rods (Figure 17-15, *B*), and they require moonlight or greater levels of illumination to function effectively. Hence we use rods to see by starlight (**scotopic** vision), both rods and cones in moonlight (**mesopic** vision), and only cones for anything brighter than moonlight (**photopic** vision).

There is considerably less convergence in cone pathways than in rod pathways. This contributes further to the lower sensitivity of the cone system because individual ganglion cells collect information from only a small number of cones. However, it also makes possible the resolution of fine spatial detail. Acuity is highest in the fovea (Figure 17-17), where midget ganglion cells have receptive fields with centers the size of a single cone.

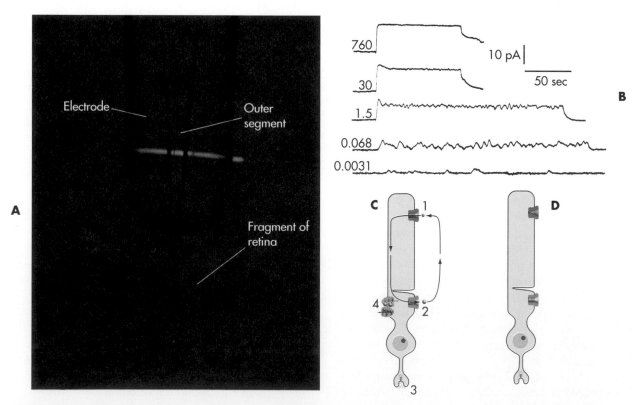

FIGURE 17-16
Current flows into retinal rods in the dark, and changes in this current flow in response to light. **A,** Drawing a single rod outer segment into a tightly fitting suction electrode allows all the current flowing into the outer segment to be recorded, both in the dark and in response to small slits of light. **B,** Reduction in current flow (upward deflections) in response to light of increasing intensity (given in photons/μm²/sec). The dimmest light causes transient reductions reflecting channel closings in response to absorption of single photons; the brightest light completely terminates the current that flows in the dark. **C,** In the dark, current flows into the outer segment *(1)* through normally open Na⁺ channels and flows out of the inner segment *(2)* through normally open K⁺ channels. The resulting depolarization causes tonic release of glutamate from the receptor's synaptic terminal *(3)*. Ionic concentration gradients are maintained by Na⁺/K⁺ pumps in the inner segment *(4)*. In response to light **(D),** the Na⁺ channels close, the receptor hyperpolarizes, and glutamate release slows or ceases. (**A** courtesy Dr Denis A. Baylor, Department of Neurobiology, Stanford University School of Medicine. **B** from Baylor DA, Lamb TD, Yau K-Y: Responses of retinal rods to single photons, *J Physiol* 288:613, 1979.)

In contrast to the single class of retinal rods, cones come in three varieties defined by the wavelength of light each absorbs most efficiently (Figure 17-18, *A*). Hence there are **long-wavelength, middle-wavelength,** and **short-wavelength** cones, also commonly referred to as **red,**★ **green,** and **blue** cones. The absorption peak is determined by the kind of opsin a particular cone makes; each of the cone opsins binds the same 11-*cis* retinal as rhodopsin does. Multiple populations of cones are the starting point for color vision. Even though individual cones, like individual rods, can only report the numbers of photons absorbed and not their wavelength, the relative levels of activity of multiple populations of cones provide information about wavelength (Figure 17-18, *B*). The **trichromatic** nature of our color vision is indicated by the fact that any color in the spectrum can be matched by some combination of three primary colors (e.g., red, green, and blue) that stimulates the three populations of cones the same relative amounts as the test stimulus. The genes for the red and green cone pigments are located next to each other on the X chromosome, and unequal crossing over during meiosis can cause one X chromosome to wind up with a missing or defective red or green gene. As a result, about 2% of the male population is red-green **color blind** because of lack of the red or green pigment (conditions

called **protanopia** and **deuteranopia,** respectively). The incidence in females is much lower because they are likely to have at least one X chromosome with normal red and green genes. Lack of the blue cone pigment **(tritanopia)** is rare, and because the blue gene is located on chromosome 7, is equally uncommon in males and females.

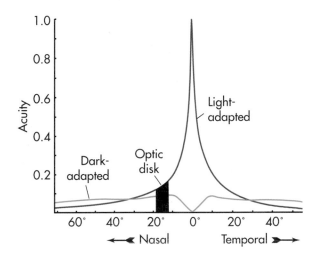

FIGURE 17-17
Spatial acuity of different retinal regions under different conditions of illumination. When using cones in bright light, acuity is highest in the fovea but falls off rapidly. When using rods in dim light acuity is always less than with foveal cone vision, and is zero in the fovea because no rods are present there. (Redrawn from Ruch T, Patten HD, editors: *Physiology and biophysics,* ed 20, Philadelphia, 1979, WB Saunders Company.)

★Red cones are still referred to as "red" because they are the most important for distinguishing colors at the red end of the spectrum, even though they absorb maximally in the yellow range.

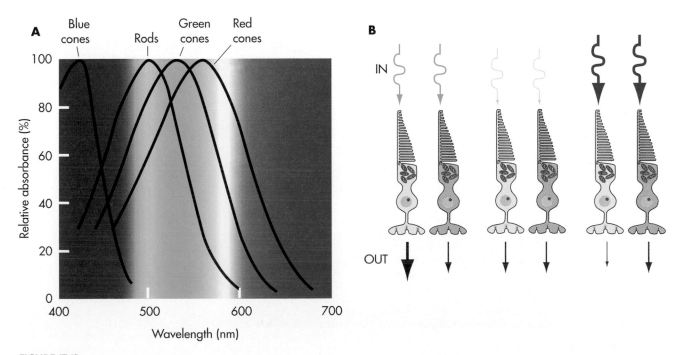

FIGURE 17-18
A, Absorption spectra of rod and cone visual pigments. **B,** Schematic indication of the necessity for multiple cone types to discriminate wavelengths. "Red" cones produce receptor potentials of the same size in response to moderate green light, dim yellow light, or bright red light. Green cones, however, produce receptor potentials of progressively decreasing size. Hence wavelength can be discriminated by comparing the outputs of different classes of cones.

Ganglion Cells Have Center-Surround Receptive Fields

The visual system can be viewed as a series of synapses beginning in the outer plexiform layer and extending to and beyond the visual association areas of the occipital, temporal, and parietal lobes. At each level a certain amount of information processing takes place, so cortical neurons respond best to stimuli that are quite different from those best able to stimulate individual rods and cones. A cell at any given level in the visual system, like a cell in the somatosensory system, can be characterized by its **receptive field,** which in this case refers to the retinal area in which changing conditions of illumination produce an alteration of the cell's activity. By extension, receptive fields of visual neurons can also be defined in terms of the particular part of the outside world whose image falls on this region of the retina. One initially surprising observation about the receptive fields of the bipolar cells and more proximal neurons is that the intensity of illumination is relatively unimportant in determining a cell's level of activity. Rather, the important parameter is the contrast between different areas of the receptive field. That is, the visual system is especially attuned to the detection of borders be-

tween light and dark areas, or between areas of different color. This is in large part responsible for the fairly constant appearance of objects despite varying illumination. For example, the words on this page do not change their appearance when looked at in room light or sunlight, despite the fact that more light is reflected from the print in sunlight than from the white background in room light.

Recordings from individual ganglion cells show that their receptive fields are composed of two concentric, roughly circular zones. Illumination of the central area (the **center**) causes either an increase or a decrease in the background firing rate (Figure 17-19), whereas illumination of the peripheral area (the **surround**) has the opposite effect; hence there are **ON-center** and **OFF-center** receptive fields. Simultaneous illumination of both center and surround causes relatively little change in firing rate because the antagonistic effects of the two areas tend to cancel each other. Cells of different functional classes vary in the sizes of their receptive fields, their color sensitivity, and some temporal aspects of their responses, but not in their basic center-surround organization. Thus even at the level of the ganglion cell, the contrast between two different areas of the receptive fields is of paramount importance.

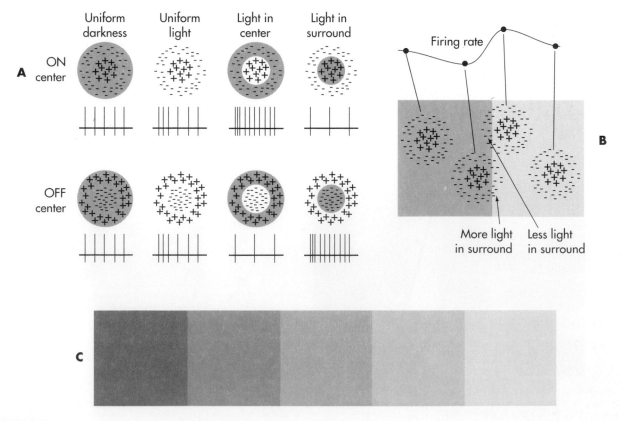

FIGURE 17-19

Center-surround characteristics of retinal ganglion cells. **A,** ON-center and OFF-center ganglion cells are named for their response to light in the center of the receptive field. **B,** The antagonistic surround (in this case using an ON-center cell as an example) results in an accentuation of the change in firing rate when an area of contrast moves across the receptive field. **C,** One result of this enhanced contrast sensitivity is the family of illusions called *Mach bands.* Each square is a uniform shade of gray (you can verify this by covering up all but one square), but the darkness and lightness on either side of a transition appear exaggerated.

Center-surround receptive fields are formed in the outer plexiform layer

The properties of the center of center-surround receptive fields reflect the "straight-through" receptor-bipolar-ganglion cell path. The properties of the surround result at least partially from the influence of receptors in the surround on receptors in the center by way of horizontal cells (Figure 17-20). Thus the basic spatial organization of ganglion cell receptive fields occurs in the outer plexiform layer. Further lateral interactions in the inner plexiform layer, mediated by amacrine cells, are thought to enhance the center-surround effect and to modify such things as the temporal characteristics of the ganglion cell response. For example, some ganglion cells respond only transiently to a change in illumination, whereas others show a maintained change in discharge rate. Many lower vertebrates have much more complex ganglion cell receptive fields, and there is a corresponding increase in the thickness of the inner plexiform layer and a proliferation of amacrine cell synapses.

Every point in the visual field is represented by both ON-center and OFF-center ganglion cells. This means that in the fovea, for example, each cone synapses on two midget bipolar cells (Figure 17-20), one of which depolarizes and one of which hyperpolarizes in response to increases in light intensity (and vice versa). The two midget bipolar cells synapse on two midget ganglion cells, with the result that one of the ganglion cells fires faster whether light intensity increases or decreases. This presumably enhances the speed of visual processing: it takes much less time to determine that a cell's firing rate has increased than to determine that it has decreased.

Rod and cone signals reach the same ganglion cells

The entire range of light intensities, from scotopic threshold to bright sunlight, is signaled by the same population of ganglion cells. Cone signals reach ganglion cells by the

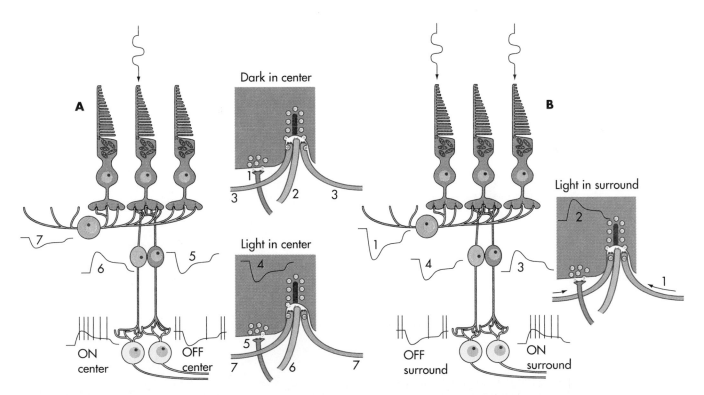

FIGURE 17-20
Formation of center-surround receptive fields at the level of bipolar cells, using foveal cones and midget bipolar cells as examples. A, Formation of receptive field centers. In the dark, photoreceptors are depolarized and release glutamate onto the superficial synapses made by OFF-center bipolar cells (1), and onto the invaginating processes of ON-center bipolar cells (2) and horizontal cells (3). Because of the nature of the postsynaptic receptor molecules, glutamate hyperpolarizes the processes of ON-center bipolar cells and depolarizes the other two kinds of processes. Hence in the dark, ON-center bipolar cells are relatively hyperpolarized, and horizontal cells and OFF-center bipolar cells are relatively depolarized. Light in the receptive field center hyperpolarizes the cone (4), decreases glutamate release, and reverses all of these polarizations: OFF-center bipolar cells (as their name implies) hyperpolarize (5), and the ganglion cells to which they project fire more slowly; ON-center bipolar cells depolarize (6); horizontal cells also hyperpolarize (7) but only moderately because glutamate is still being released onto their other processes. B, Role of horizontal cells in formation of the antagonistic surround. Light delivered to cones surrounding the central cone of A causes a large hyperpolarization of horizontal cells (1) because of diminished glutamate release on many of their processes. This in turn causes diminished release of GABA from horizontal cell processes, depolarizing the synaptic terminals of the central cone (2). This causes increased glutamate release (as though it just got darker in the center of the receptive field), depolarization of the OFF-center bipolar cell (3), and hyperpolarization of the ON-center bipolar cell.

circuitry just described. Rods use a more circuitous route that enables them to cleverly "hitch a ride" on parts of the cone circuitry (Figure 17-21). At mesopic levels, gap junctions between rods and cones open and rod receptor potentials flow directly into the synaptic terminals of cones. At scotopic levels, rod signals reach special bipolar cells dedicated to rod function, which then transmit this information through amacrine cells to cone bipolar cells.

HALF OF THE VISUAL FIELD OF EACH EYE IS MAPPED SYSTEMATICALLY IN THE CONTRALATERAL CEREBRAL HEMISPHERE

Ganglion cell axons travel in the optic nerve to the **optic chiasm,** where they undergo a partial decussation and enter one or the other **optic tract.** Most of the fibers in each optic tract then terminate in the **lateral geniculate nucleus,** which is the thalamic relay nucleus for vision. Geniculate fibers travel through the internal capsule and corona radiata to the primary visual cortex in the banks of the calcarine sulcus. In addition, a considerable number of optic tract fibers project to the midbrain and a few to the hypothalamus. Throughout this pathway, the numbers of fibers and areas of representation for the macula are disproportionately large for the macula's actual size. This reflects the relatively small amount of convergence in the macula, which in turn reflects its specialization for high acuity.

Fibers From the Nasal Half of Each Retina Cross in the Optic Chiasm

The unmyelinated axons of ganglion cells collect at the optic disk, pierce the sclera in a region called the **lamina cribrosa** (Figure 17-9), and acquire myelin sheaths, forming the optic nerve. The optic nerve is, by embryology and adult anatomy, actually a tract of the CNS and as such has meningeal coverings much like other areas. The sclera continues as its dural sheath, lined in turn by arachnoid and pia. The subarachnoid space around the optic nerve communicates with subarachnoid space generally; increases in intracranial pressure are transmitted to the optic

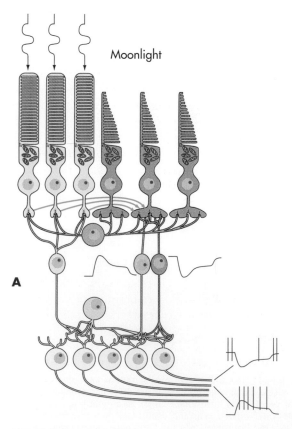

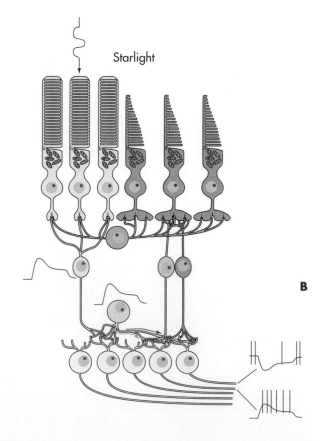

Moonlight

Starlight

A

B

FIGURE 17-21

Rod signals reach ganglion cells through a remarkable system of modifiable gap junctions and special amacrine cells. At mesopic levels **(A),** gap junctions between rod and cone terminals open *(green arrows)* and rod receptor potentials gain access to the cone circuitry described in Figure 17-20. At scotopic levels **(B),** rod signals reach rod bipolar cells, which hyperpolarize in response to glutamate and depolarize in response to light. Rod bipolar cells terminate on processes of special amacrine cells, in turn depolarizing them. Gap junctions open between amacrine cell processes and the synaptic terminals of cone ON-center bipolar cells *(green arrow),* allowing rod signals access to this branch of the cone circuitry. Other processes of the same amacrine cells make inhibitory chemical synapses on the synaptic terminals of cone OFF-center bipolar cells *(red arrow)* and also on dendrites of OFF-center ganglion cells.

nerve. Such an increase in pressure can cause detectable swelling of the optic disk. This swelling, called **pa-pilledema,** can be a valuable diagnostic sign.

Just anterior to the infundibular stalk, the two optic nerves partially decussate in the optic chiasm. All fibers from the nasal half of each retina cross to the contralateral optic tract; all fibers from the temporal half of each retina pass through the lateral portions of the chiasm without crossing and enter the ipsilateral optic tract. The result is that each optic tract contains the fibers arising in the temporal retina of the ipsilateral eye and the nasal retina of the contralateral eye. As indicated in Figure 17-22, this apparently curious partial decussation is exactly appropriate for delivering all the information from the contralateral visual field to each optic tract. Also, because much of the basis for depth perception involves a comparison of the slightly different views seen by our two eyes, it is necessary to bring together information from comparable areas of the two retinas, which the optic chiasm accomplishes.

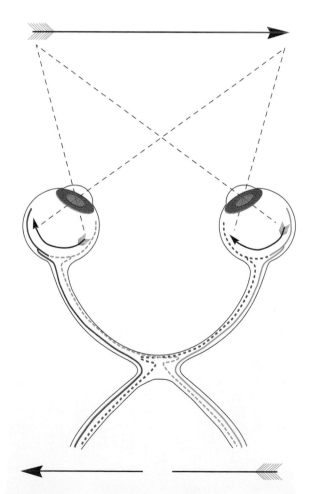

FIGURE 17-22
Schematic diagram illustrating the formation of the optic chiasm and tracts. All information from the temporal side of a vertical line passing through a given fovea enters the ipsilateral optic tract; all information from the nasal side crosses in the chiasm and enters the contralateral optic tract. The result, as indicated, is that each optic tract "looks" at the contralateral visual field.

From the optic tract to the visual cortex, cells and fibers representing corresponding areas of the two retinas (i.e., fibers carrying information about the same area in the visual field) are located near each other, with the result that damage to the optic tract or more central parts of the pathway tends to cause comparable visual deficits in both eyes.★

Most Fibers of the Optic Tract Terminate in the Lateral Geniculate Nucleus

The optic tract curves posteriorly around the cerebral peduncle, and most of its fibers terminate in the lateral geniculate nucleus (Figures 16-13 and 17-23). This is a six-layered, dome-shaped nucleus in which the optic fibers terminate in a precise **retinotopic** pattern. The pattern is about the same in each layer so that a given point in the visual field is represented in a column of cells extending through all six layers. However, each layer receives input from only one eye: layers 1 (most inferior), 4, and 6 (most superior) from the contralateral eye and layers 2, 3, and 5 from the ipsilateral eye (Figure 17-23, *C*). Consistent with this anatomical arrangement, electrical recordings from the lateral geniculate nucleus reveal few cells that can be activated by both eyes.

Layers 3 to 6 contain small neurons that receive their inputs from the numerically dominant class of small ganglion cells sensitive to color and form. In view of its small neurons these layers are referred to as the **parvocellular layers** and this entire subdivision of the visual system as the **parvocellular system.** Layers 1 and 2 contain larger neurons that receive their inputs from a separate class of larger ganglion cells that are more sensitive to movement and contrast. This subdivision, including the **magnocellular layers** (1 and 2) of the lateral geniculate nucleus, is referred to as the **magnocellular system.**

The Lateral Geniculate Nucleus Projects to Primary Visual Cortex

Fibers arising in the lateral geniculate nucleus project through the retrolenticular and sublenticular parts of the internal capsule, curve around the lateral wall of the lateral ventricle (Figures 17-24 and Figure 17-30), and terminate in the cortex adjacent to the calcarine sulcus. The optic radiation is sometimes called the **geniculocalcarine tract,** reflecting its origin and termination. Not all of these fibers pass directly backward to the occipital lobe. Rather, they form a broad sheet covering much of the

---

★The retinotopic arrangement in the optic tract is only approximate because fibers sort themselves not only by retinal origin but also by functional type. This is presumably the basis of clinical reports that partial optic tract damage, though uncommon, causes deficits mainly involving only selected aspects of visual function, such as color vision, or more extensive deficits in one eye than the other.

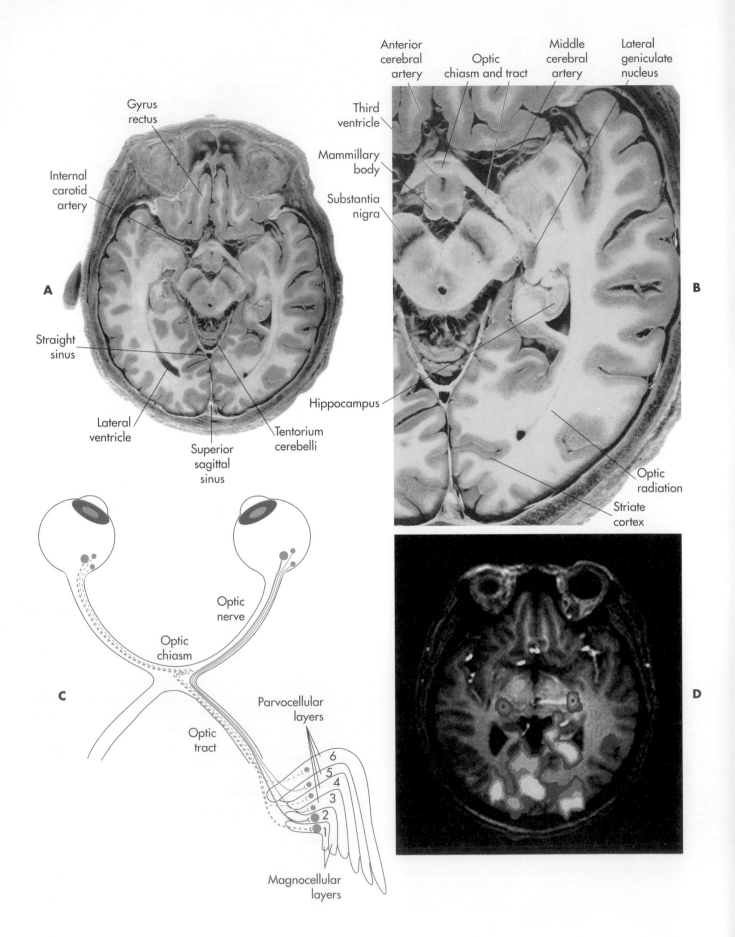

A

Gyrus rectus

Internal carotid artery

Straight sinus

Lateral ventricle

Superior sagittal sinus

Tentorium cerebelli

B

Anterior cerebral artery

Optic chiasm and tract

Middle cerebral artery

Lateral geniculate nucleus

Third ventricle

Mammillary body

Substantia nigra

Hippocampus

Optic radiation

Striate cortex

C

Optic nerve

Optic chiasm

Optic tract

Parvocellular layers

6
5
4
3
2
1

Magnocellular layers

D

FIGURE 17-23
Delivery of visual information to the lateral geniculate nucleus. **A,** A horizontal section (enlarged in **B**) just above the confluence of the sinuses, showing most of the visual pathway. **C,** The projection from the retina to the lateral geniculate nucleus, indicating how information traveling in the magnocellular and parvocellular pathways, as well as information from the two eyes, remains segregated at the level of the lateral geniculate. Notice, however, that all information from a given point in the visual field ends up in a column that extends through all six geniculate layers. **D,** fMRI data from a subject watching a red and black checkerboard in which the squares reversed color 8 to 10 times per second, superimposed on a T1-weighted horizontal slice at a level similar to that shown in **A.** The stimulus activates not only occipital cortex posteriorly, but also the lateral geniculate nuclei (*). [**A** and **B** courtesy Dr. John T. Willson, University of Colorado Health Sciences Center. **D** from Chen W et al: Mapping of lateral geniculate nucleus activation during visual stimulation in human brain using fMRI, *Magn Reson Med,* 39:89, 1998.)

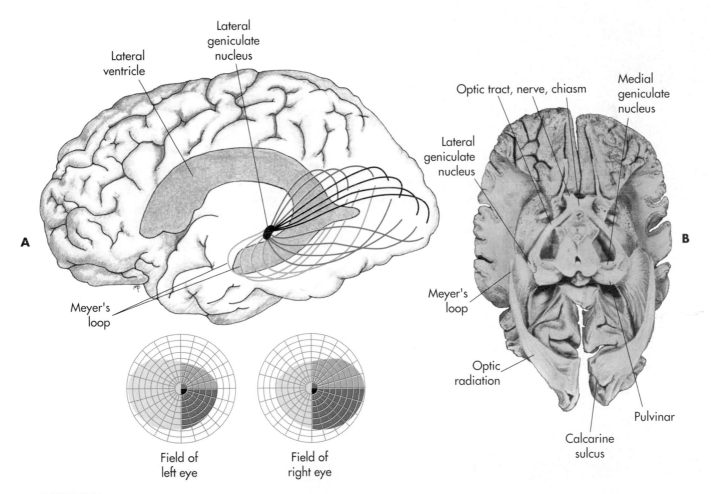

FIGURE 17-24
Two views of the optic radiation. **A,** Schematic illustration of the course of geniculocalcarine fibers as they loop over the lateral aspect of the lateral ventricle and then turn posteriorly to end in the banks of the calcarine sulcus on the medial surface of the hemisphere; note that the fibers representing inferior visual fields end in the upper bank, fibers representing superior visual fields end in the lower bank, and fibers representing the macula end most posteriorly. (See Figure 17-29 for additional information about the mapping of visual fields.) **B,** Inferior aspect of a brain dissected to show the entire visual pathway from optic nerve to striate cortex. (**B** from Ludwig E, Klingler J: *Atlas cerebri humani,* Boston, 1956, Little, Brown & Co.)

posterior and inferior horns of the ventricle. Fibers representing superior *visual* quadrants (i.e., those representing inferior *retinal* quadrants) loop out into the temporal lobe **(Meyer's loop)** before turning posteriorly. As a result, temporal lobe damage can somewhat surprisingly produce a visual deficit.

A retinotopic organization is maintained in the optic radiation. Fibers representing inferior visual fields are most superior, whereas those representing superior visual fields loop farthest out into the temporal lobe. Macular fibers occupy a broad middle area. The visual pathway is more dispersed in the optic radiation than elsewhere, and indi-

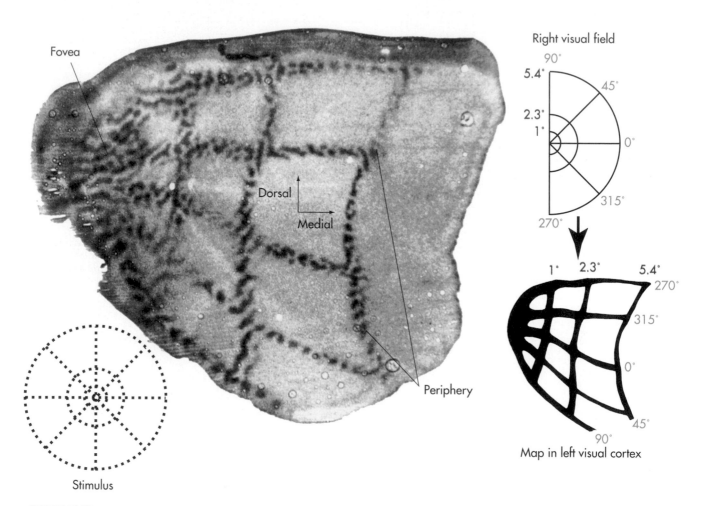

Fovea

Dorsal

Medial

Periphery

Stimulus

Right visual field

90°
5.4°
2.3°   45°
1°
0°
315°
270°

1°   2.3°   5.4°
270°
315°
0°
45°
90°

Map in left visual cortex

FIGURE 17-25

A remarkable, direct demonstration of the precise mapping of the visual field in the visual cortex of a monkey. The stimulus was an array of dashed rings and lines on a gray background; during the experiment, the black and white segments reversed in contrast (the black segments turned white, and vice versa) at a frequency of 3 Hz. While the monkey watched the stimulus with one eye open, the animal was injected with ^{14}C-2-deoxyglucose, a radioactive analog of glucose that is taken up by active neurons and phosphorylated into a metabolite that cannot leave the cell. Subsequent autoradiography of a tangential section through the left visual cortex revealed a distorted but precise map of the right half of the stimulus; each dark area corresponds to a small group of neurons that receive input from a particular small area of the visual field, primarily via the eye that was open during the experiment. The overall change in shape of the visual field by the time it is represented in striate cortex is diagrammed in the lower right part of the figure. Note that the line segments in the cortical map get progressively thicker in moving toward the left part of the map, even though the stimulus lines were the same width everywhere. This is a reflection of the progressively greater amount of cortex devoted to processing foveal information. [From Tootell RBH et al: Functional anatomy of macaque striate cortex. II. Retinotopic organization, *J Neurosci* 8:1531, 1988.]

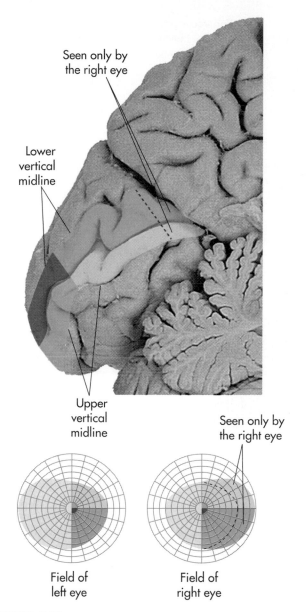

Seen only by
the right eye

Lower
vertical
midline

Upper
vertical
midline

Seen only by
the right eye

Field of
left eye

Field of
right eye

FIGURE 17-26
The map of the right visual field (of both eyes) in primary visual cortex of the left occipital lobe. The foveal representation extends a short distance beyond the medial surface of the occipital lobe, onto the occipital pole. There is considerably more primary visual cortex than it appears from this view; most is actually in the walls of the deep calcarine sulcus. (Modified from Nolte J, Angevine JB Jr: *The human brain in photographs and diagrams,* St. Louis, 1995, Mosby.)

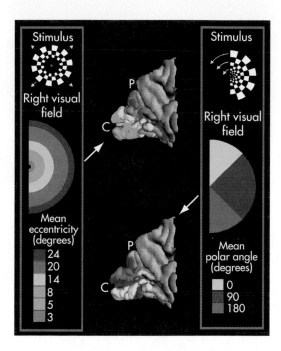

FIGURE 17-27
Retinotopic mapping of the right visual fields in the left occipital lobe, revealed by fMRI as a subject watched an expanding checkered annulus (upper image) or a rotating checkered stimulus (lower image). As indicated in Figure 17-26, the fovea is represented most posteriorly, and inferior visual fields most superiorly. Repeated colors farther from the calcarine sulcus are the beginnings of additional retinotopic maps in extrastriate cortex. *C,* Calcarine sulcus; *P,* parietooccipital sulcus. (From DeYoe EA et al: Mapping striate and extrastriate visual areas in human cerebral cortex, *Proc Natl Acad Sci* 93:2382, 1996.)

vidual fibers still carry information from only one eye, so damage here typically results in deficits that are overlapping but not identical for the two eyes.

The visual pathway ends retinotopically in the cortex above and below the calcarine sulcus (**area 17;** this numerical nomenclature, with which the cerebral cortex is divided into a series of areas called **Brodmann's areas,** is discussed in Chapter 22). Inferior visual fields project to the cortex above the calcarine sulcus and superior fields to the cortex below the sulcus. The macula is represented

more posteriorly and peripheral fields more anteriorly (Figures 17-25 to 17-27). Numerous myelinated fibers ramify within this cortex in a discrete layer that can be seen as a thin, white stripe (the **line of Gennari**) with the naked eye (Figure 17-28). Hence primary visual cortex is also called **striate cortex.**

The striate cortex parallels the calcarine sulcus and extends for a short distance onto the posterior surface of the occipital lobe. It is surrounded by **area 18,** which in turn is surrounded by **area 19,** the two together comprising almost all the rest of the occipital lobe. Areas 18 and 19, together with related parts of the temporal and parietal lobes, are commonly referred to as **visual association cortex** or **extrastriate cortex** and are heavily interconnected with area 17. The parvocellular and magnocellular systems, as described later in this chapter, follow separate though interrelated routes through striate and extrastriate cortex.

Damage in the Visual Pathway Results in Predictable Deficits

Visual fields are tested by moving a small object in from the periphery until the patient, with one eye covered, reports seeing it. By repeating this for many different di-

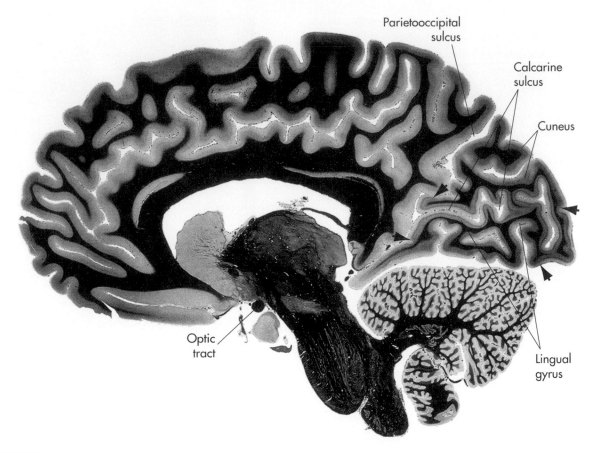

Parietooccipital
sulcus

Calcarine
sulcus

Cuneus

Lingual
gyrus

Optic
tract

FIGURE 17-28
A parasagittal section, stained for myelin, showing the stripe of myelinated fibers for which striate cortex received its name. The stripe ends abruptly *(arrows)* at the area 17–area 18 junction. Note that striate cortex extends a short distance beyond the medial surface of the occipital lobe, onto the occipital pole.

rections of approach, a chart of the visual field can be made (Figure 17-29). Each eye can normally see a surprising 90° from the visual axis in a temporal direction (because of refraction by the cornea), but the field is less extensive in other directions because of obstruction by the nose, eyebrows, and cheeks. The area of overlap of the two visual fields is the area in which binocular vision is possible.

Deficits resulting from damage to various parts of the visual pathway are named according to certain conventions. Most important, visual defects are always named according to the visual field loss and not according to the area of the retina that is nonfunctional. Because the retinal image is inverted and reversed, damage to temporal areas of the retina causes nasal field losses, and damage to superior areas of the retina causes inferior field losses. The combining form "-anopia" (or "-anopsia") is used to denote loss of one or more quadrants of a visual field; **hemianopia** would refer to loss of half of a visual field, **quadrantanopia** to loss of one quarter of a visual field. Finally, the term **homonymous** denotes a condition in which the visual field losses are similar for both eyes, and **heteronymous** denotes a condition in which the two eyes have nonoverlapping field losses. Homonymous losses may

be **congruous** (essentially identical) or overlapping but **noncongruous.**

Using this terminology, it is possible to name the deficits resulting from damage at most locations in the visual pathway (Figure 17-30); some of the names are quite spectacular. A lesion of one optic nerve causes blindness of that eye. Damage in the central region of the optic chiasm, affecting the crossing fibers, causes a heteronymous hemianopia (in this case, a **bitemporal hemianopia;** Figure 17-31, *A*). This can result from midline pressure exerted by a tumor of the pituitary, which lies close to the chiasm (see Figure 3-15). Lateral pressure on one side of the chiasm, affecting the noncrossing fibers on that side, would cause an ipsilateral **nasal hemianopia.** This occasionally results from an aneurysm of the internal carotid artery, which lies adjacent to the chiasm (see Figure 6-3). In the rare event of aneurysms of both internal carotid arteries, a **binasal hemianopia** could result. Destruction of one optic tract would interrupt all the fibers carrying information from the contralateral visual fields, causing a contralateral **homonymous hemianopia.**

Damage to the optic radiation can cause complete hemianopia (Figure 17-31, *B*) but is rarely this extensive; quadrantic or sector deficits are more often the result. For example, a large destructive lesion of the left temporal lobe, interrupting the fibers of Meyer's loop (which represent inferior retinal quadrants), would produce a **right homonymous superior quadrantanopia.** Lesions in either the optic radiation or visual cortex leave the pupillary light reflex undisturbed, as would be predicted from the anatomical pathways involved in this reflex (Figure 17-36).

In cases of massive damage to the visual cortex of one occipital lobe (e.g., after occlusion of one posterior cerebral artery), a contralateral homonymous hemianopia would be the expected result. In fact, it is frequently observed clinically that vision is preserved over much of the fovea. This phenomenon is called **macular** (or **foveal) sparing,** and its existence, extent, and basis have been a topic of debate for many years. Much or all of its origin probably lies in the disproportionately large representation of the fovea in the striate cortex; even very large cortical lesions may leave part of the foveal region undamaged. In addition, the distributions of the middle and posterior cerebral arteries overlap near the occipital pole. Therefore even total occlusion of the posterior cerebral artery allows for supply of part of the foveal region by the middle cerebral artery.

Some Fibers of the Optic Tract Terminate in the Superior Colliculus, Accessory Optic Nuclei, and Hypothalamus

The common vertebrate plan of central visual connections includes not only a projection from the retina to the lateral geniculate nucleus (or its equivalent), but also a projection to the superior colliculus (or its equivalent). In lower vertebrates the collicular (or tectal) pathway is the more important, but in primates it is much less so. Nevertheless, the major inputs to the primate superior colliculus are still visual: one arising in the retina and the second in the striate cortex. The retinal input consists of a substantial number of fibers in each optic tract that bypass the lateral geniculate nucleus, pass over the medial geniculate nucleus in a bundle called the **brachium of the superior colliculus** (or **superior brachium**) (see Figure 24-9), and terminate retinotopically in the superior colliculus and in the nearby **pretectal area** (described later) and other **accessory optic nuclei.** Some of these fibers are collaterals of axons that also terminate in the lateral geniculate nucleus, but most arise from separate subpopulations of ganglion cells. The cortical input consists of cells in area 17 that project to the superior colliculus (again via its brachium) and end in a pattern that coincides with the retinotopic map in the colliculus.

In addition to visual inputs, the superior colliculus receives (1) somatosensory inputs (sometimes referred to as the **spinotectal** or **spinomesencephalic tract**), many of them collaterals of fibers in somatosensory pathways ascending to the thalamus; (2) auditory inputs, chiefly by

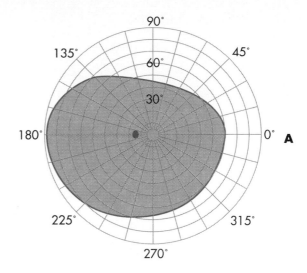

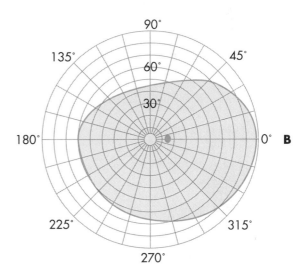

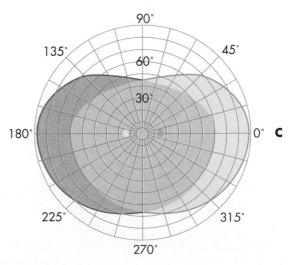

FIGURE 17-29

Normal visual field of the left eye **(A),** the right eye **(B),** and both eyes superimposed **(C).** The blind spot of each eye is indicated in a darker color in **A** and **B.** The view is the patient's view of the charts on which the fields are being recorded.

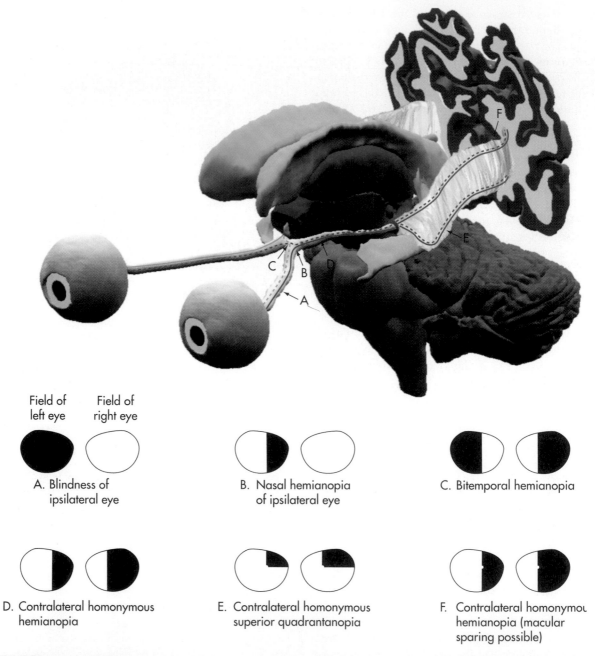

Field of   Field of
left eye   right eye

A. Blindness of
   ipsilateral eye

B. Nasal hemianopia
   of ipsilateral eye

C. Bitemporal hemianopia

D. Contralateral homonymous
   hemianopia

E. Contralateral homonymous
   superior quadrantanopia

F. Contralateral homonymous
   hemianopia (macular
   sparing possible)

FIGURE 17-30
Visual field deficits caused by lesions at various points along the visual pathway. *A,* Destruction of one optic nerve causes blindness of the eye
in which that nerve arises. *B,* Damage to one side of the optic chiasm destroys the noncrossing fibers from the ipsilateral eye; these fibers arise
in the temporal retina, so a nasal hemianopia of the ipsilateral eye results. *C,* Pressure on the middle of the optic chiasm, typically from a pituitary tumor, destroys the crossing fibers from both eyes, causing a bitemporal hemianopia (one type of heteronymous hemianopia). *D,* Destruction of one optic tract causes contralateral homonymous hemianopia. *E,* Damage to one temporal lobe could destroy part of the optic
radiation, specifically the fibers representing the contralateral superior quadrant of each visual field; because the optic radiation is rather spread
out at this point, some fibers are likely to be spared, for example, in this case the macular fibers remain intact. *F,* Massive damage to one occipital lobe (such as might be caused by occlusion of one posterior cerebral artery) causes contralateral homonymous hemianopia; the macular representation is quite large, and some of it is likely to survive, resulting in macular sparing.

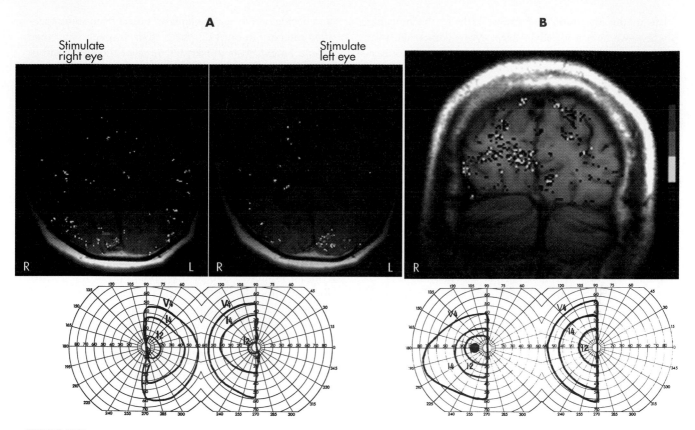

FIGURE 17-31

Visual field deficits demonstrated by fMRI and visual field mapping. In both cases, areas of intact vision were outlined three times, using progressively brighter or larger stimuli (V4 is 256 times larger than I4; I4 is 10 times brighter than I2). **A,** A 46-year-old man with a history of pulmonary tuberculosis developed a sellar tuberculoma that compressed his optic chiasm, resulting in bitemporal hemianopia. Monocular visual stimulation activated only the ipsilateral visual cortex because of damage to crossing fibers in the optic chiasm. **B,** A 58-year-old man had a stroke involving his left optic radiation, resulting in right homonymous hemianopia. Even though visual cortex appeared structurally normal bilaterally, visual stimulation of both eyes activated only his right visual cortex. (**A** from Miki A, Nakajima T et al: Detection of visual dysfunction in optic atrophy by functional magnetic resonance imaging during monocular visual stimulation, *Am J Ophthalmol* 122:404, 1996. **B** from Miki A, Nakajima T et al: Functional magnetic resonance imaging in homonymous hemianopia, *Am J Ophthalmol* 121:258, 1996.)

way of projections from the inferior colliculus; and (3) additional inputs from other areas of the cortex.

Efferent connections of the superior colliculus include projections to the reticular formation, the inferior colliculus, and the cervical spinal cord (the **tectospinal tract**). Of interest with respect to the visual system, the superior colliculus also projects to the posterior thalamus, notably to the lateral geniculate nucleus and the pulvinar. The pulvinar, in turn, projects to cortical areas 18 and 19, areas of visual association cortex.

The function of the human superior colliculus is poorly understood. It is presumed to play a role in certain reflexes, such as orienting the head to visual (or other) stimuli, and in certain kinds of eye movements. However, no known clinical condition in humans can be attributed specifically to damage to the superior colliculus. On the other hand, monkeys have been shown, with careful training, to have considerable visual capacity after extensive lesions of the striate cortex, particularly when dealing with moving stimuli. In a few rare cases of selective damage to the striate cortex, humans too have been found to have

residual visual capacities that are strange and paradoxical: for example, despite having no conscious awareness of visual stimuli in the "blind" portions of their visual fields, they may be able to point to such stimuli quite accurately. There are a number of alternatives for the anatomical basis for this residual visual capacity; an example is the pathway to areas 18 and 19 via the superior colliculus and pulvinar. The relative importance of the various possible pathways is poorly understood at present, as is the function of these paths in the intact nervous system.

Photic input is involved in many neuroendocrine functions, so one might expect that there would be projections from the retina to the hypothalamus. It has now been shown directly that such fibers exist in a variety of mammals (including primates like us); these fibers end in a small hypothalamic nucleus above the optic chiasm called the **suprachiasmatic nucleus** (see Figure 23-4). Many of our physical functions wax and wane with a 24-hour rhythm (**circadian rhythm,** from the Latin words *circa* and *diem* meaning "about a day"). For example, our body temperature rises and falls about a degree, being highest late in the afternoon and lowest early in the morning, when we are normally asleep. Many other circadian rhythms are known, involving such things as hormone secretion, eating, drinking, alertness, and excretion of various electrolytes. If no information about day length is available (as in the case of an animal living in constant light or constant darkness), the cycles of these rhythms become a little longer than 24 hours. This implies that one or more "clocks" exist within our bodies, that left to their own devices these clocks have a period of slightly more than 24 hours, and that under normal circumstances information about day length **entrains** the clocks to a period of 24 hours (see Figure 23-5). There is now considerable evidence that the suprachiasmatic nucleus of the hypothalamus is a "master clock" for the timing of many (but not all) circadian rhythms and that direct retinal input to the suprachiasmatic nucleus provides the information for entraining these rhythms to a 24-hour cycle.

PRIMARY VISUAL CORTEX SORTS VISUAL INFORMATION AND DISTRIBUTES IT TO OTHER CORTICAL AREAS

Receptive fields of cells in the lateral geniculate nucleus are generally similar to those of ganglion cells. The contrast detection mechanism is somewhat more efficient, so that uniform illumination causes less response than in the case of ganglion cells. Things change in striate cortex, where incoming visual information is dissected into its component elements (e.g., orientation, color, depth, and motion) and distributed to a multitude of specialized extrastriate areas for further processing. This simultaneous, parallel processing in multiple cortical areas is a common strategy in the CNS, thought to contribute to the speed of things such as visual perception, which is extraordinary. We can, for example, analyze a large, complex visual scene

and decide whether it contains an object from some specified category in only 150 msec. This is much faster than would be expected if every element of the scene had to be analyzed sequentially by our relatively slow neurons.

Visual Cortex Has a Columnar Organization

Striate cortex is an array of repeated, modular collections of neurons occupying the cortex under each square millimeter of cortical surface. (Most or all neocortical areas, as described in Chapter 22, have a related modular organization.) Each module is an assembly of smaller **columns,** in which most or all of the neurons have similar physiological properties (Figure 17-32). For example, all the neurons in one 50 μm × 500 μm slab of cortex might respond best to stimuli received by the ipsilateral eye, with similar contrast properties and in overlapping parts of the visual field. Neurons in an adjacent 50 μm × 500 μm slab might have the same properties except for a preference for stimuli received by the contralateral eye. Collectively, the columns making up one module analyze all aspects of the visual information arriving from discrete areas of the visual field. Modules in the foveal part of the retinotopic map analyze very small areas; modules in the peripheral part analyze areas hundreds of times larger. This means that many more modules are required for the foveal part of the field, partially accounting for its large size in the retinotopic map (Figure 17-26).

The receptive fields of contrast-sensitive cortical neurons are more complicated than those of ganglion cells or lateral geniculate neurons, and names such as "simple," "complex," and "hypercomplex" have been coined to describe them. Simple cells respond best either to a dark bar on a light background or to a light bar on a dark background; uniform illumination has essentially no effect. In addition, the bar must be oriented at a particular angle. It has been hypothesized that the receptive fields of simple cells result from the convergence of a large number of

---

FIGURE 17-32

Organization of the primary visual cortex. **A,** Area 17 is made up of a series of modules, each accounting for about 1 mm² of cortical surface area. Each module receives information from one area of the contralateral visual field—a very small area for foveal parts of the field, a larger area for peripheral parts. As indicated in the schematic illustration on the right, modules are composed of small slabs in which the neurons throughout most of the depth of the cortex respond best to stimuli with a specific orientation and conveyed from one eye or the other. Collectively, the small slabs (orientation columns) cover all possible orientations. The half of the slabs in one module that prefer input from one eye constitute an ocular dominance column. Interspersed among the orientation columns are cylindrical assemblies of cells that are not sensitive to the orientation of a stimulus, but rather to its spectral properties. (The diagram is highly schematic. Orientation columns, for example, are not regular geometric slabs but rather more like a pinwheel array of wedges. In addition, other properties such as motion and depth are also mapped in a systematically distributed way in each module.) **B-D,** Direct demonstration of ocular dominance columns in monkey visual cortex. **B,** Autoradiograph of a section through the visual cortex of a monkey whose ipsilateral eye had been injected with a radioactive amino acid 2 weeks before sectioning. The amino acid was taken up by the ganglion cells of that eye, transported to the lateral geniculate nucleus (presumably after being packaged into proteins), taken up by geniculate cells, and then transported to the visual cortex. Ocular dominance columns for the injected eye show up as light areas in layer IV (where the optic radiation terminates) in this autoradiograph seen with darkfield optics; the interspersed dark areas are ocular dominance columns for the contralateral eye. **C,** Reconstruction of the ocular dominance columns (seen as though one were looking down on the cortical surface) shows that the columns are really more or less parallel slabs. **D,** Fingerprint of a human index finger to the same scale as **C.** (Diagram in **A** based on Livingstone MS, Hubel DH: Anatomy and physiology of a color system in the primate visual cortex, *J Neurosci* 4:309, 1984. **B-D** from Hubel DH, Wiesel TN: Functional architecture of macaque monkey visual cortex, *Proc R Soc Lond* B198: 1, 1977.)

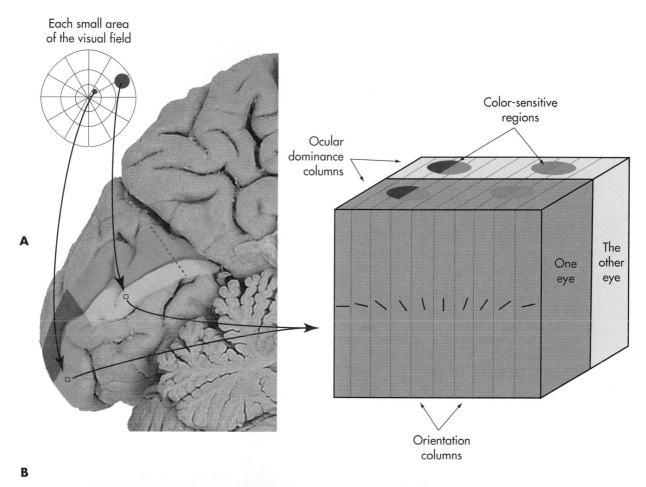

A

Each small area
of the visual field

Ocular
dominance
columns

Color-sensitive
regions

One
eye

The
other
eye

Orientation
columns

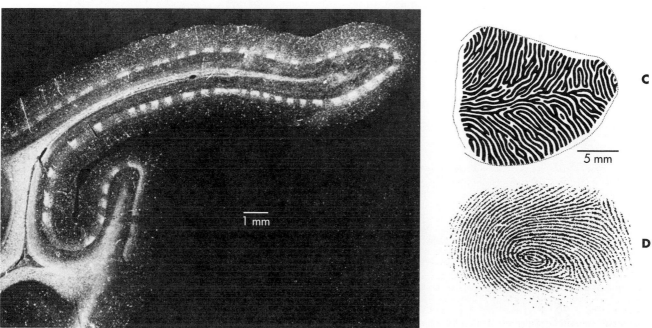

B

1 mm

C

5 mm

D

geniculate axons onto a single cortical neuron; if the receptive fields of these axons fell along a straight line, a bar-shaped receptive field with flanking antagonistic areas could result. Complex and hypercomplex cells respond best to edges, bars, and corners and have particular orientation and movement properties. Many of their properties, like those of the simple cells, could be explained by the convergence of simpler neurons onto a single cell.

Visual Information Is Distributed in Dorsal and Ventral Streams

This account of visual processing is obviously highly simplified. It is selective as well in that data dealing with color vision and binocular interactions have not been discussed. It is known, for example, that many cells in the primate visual system have wavelength-specific properties and that there are cortical neurons that are sensitive to the location of an object in three-dimensional space as well as to its size and shape. Aspects such as color and depth are processed in parallel with form and movement. These various qualities begin to be sorted out in the division of the lateral geniculate into parvocellular and magnocellular layers. The sorting continues as a partially separate—

partially interconnected sequence of projections of the parvocellular and magnocellular systems through striate and extrastriate cortex. Although the details are incompletely understood, and the independence of the two systems is far from total, in general the parvocellular system (color, detailed form) projects to more ventral portions of extrastriate cortex and the magnocellular system (location, movement) to more dorsal portions (Figure 17-33). One consequence is that damage to particular regions of extrastriate cortex can cause selective deficits in only some visual capabilities, such the ability to distinguish colors, motion, or even something as specific as the identity of faces (Box 17-1).

EARLY EXPERIENCE HAS PERMANENT EFFECTS ON THE VISUAL SYSTEM

The visual system has provided a unique opportunity to study the extent to which connections within the CNS are genetically determined and unchangeable and the extent to which they can be influenced by the environment.

Recordings from neurons in the visual cortex of newborn cats and monkeys never previously exposed to light

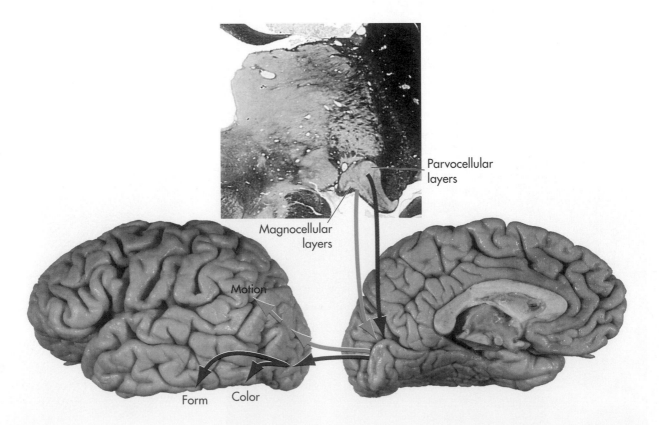

FIGURE 17-33
Schematic indication of the distribution of higher-order visual processing among different cortical areas. The actual distribution system is far more complex than illustrated here; for example, dozens of separate visual areas, related to each other by literally hundreds of sets of interconnections, have been described in primate cortex. However, in a very general sense there is a superior stream of connections (dominated by the magnocellular system) concerned with the location and motion of objects and an inferior stream of connections (dominated by the parvocellular system) concerned with the form and color of objects.

Box 17-1   Selective Loss of Some Visual Capabilities

Damage in posterior parts of the brain commonly affects either the optic radiations or striate cortex, affecting all function in parts of the visual field (Figure 17-30). In a few rare cases, however, patients have incurred bilateral damage to particular regions of extrastriate cortex, sparing the primary visual cortex. Their visual fields were more or less intact, but they had selective visual deficits that illustrate strikingly the functional specialization of different parts of extrastriate cortex. Two such cases are reviewed here.

MOTION BLINDNESS

As a result of a superior sagittal sinus thrombosis, a 43-year-old woman suffered bilateral infarcts of lateral parts of the parietal, occipital, and posterior temporal lobes, including the area shown in Figure 17-34. Visual fields, color vision, depth perception, and reading were unaffected. Her abilities to perceive moving sound sources or somatosensory stimuli moving across her skin were also unaffected, but she complained of a persisting deficit in perceiving visual motion:

> "She had difficulty, for example, in pouring tea or coffee into a cup because the fluid appeared to be frozen, like a glacier. In addition, she could not stop pouring at the right time since she was unable to perceive the movement in the cup (or a pot) when the fluid rose. Furthermore the patient complained of difficulties in following a dialogue because she could not see the movements of the face and, especially, the mouth of the speaker. In a room where more than two other people were walking she felt very insecure and unwell, and usually left the room immediately, because 'people were suddenly here or there but I have not seen them moving.' The patient experienced the same problem but to an even more marked extent in crowded streets or places, which she therefore avoided as much as possible. She could not cross the street because of her inability to judge the speed of a car, but she could identify the car itself without difficulty. 'When I'm looking at the car first, it seems far away. But then, when I want to cross the road, suddenly the car is very near.' She gradually learned to 'estimate' the distance of moving vehicles by means of the sound becoming louder." ★

COLOR BLINDNESS AND PROSOPAGNOSIA

A 51-year-old man experienced the abrupt onset one evening of headache and confusion. He did not lose consciousness, but subsequently remembered nothing that oc- curred during the next 12 hours. He was taken home, helped to bed, and when he awoke the next morning he became aware of several visual deficits. He had bilateral loss of parts of his foveal visual fields above the horizontal meridian and an incomplete left superior homonymous quadrantanopia (Figure 17-35, A). He also had some difficulty recognizing where he was if only using vision, but his most striking deficits were an inability to recognize colors (achromatopsia) or faces (prosopagnosia). The patient described these problems six months later:

> "Everything appears in various shades of grey. My shirts all look dirty and I can't tell one of them from the other. I have no idea which tie to wear...I have difficulty in recognizing certain kinds of food on my plate, until I have tasted or smelled them. I can tell peas or bananas by their size and shape. An omelette, however, looks like a piece of meat and when I open a jar I never know if I'll find jam or pickles in it!...[When trying to identify faces] I can see the eyes, nose, and mouth quite clearly but they just don't add up. They all seem chalked in, like on a blackboard. I have to tell by the clothes or voice whether it is a man or woman, as the faces are all neutral...The hair may help a lot, or if there is a moustache...I cannot recognize people in photographs, not even myself. At the club I saw someone strange staring at me and asked the steward who it was. You'll laugh at me. I'd been looking at myself in a mirror...I later went to London and visited several cinemas and theatres. I couldn't make head or tail of the plots. I never knew who was who."†

He also had trouble distinguishing different animals, especially in photographs, although not as much trouble as he had with faces. He was nevertheless able to identify common objects with ease (as long as color was not a major factor), and his form, motion, and depth perception were preserved. An angiogram indicated partial occlusion of the right posterior cerebral artery. This presumably resulted in damage to visual cortex below the right calcarine sulcus, accounting for the deficits in the left visual fields. However, the smaller deficits in the right visual field imply damage to inferior parts of the left occipital lobe as well. Subsequent similar cases with CT or MRI verification of the lesion sites make it seem likely that this patient had bilateral damage in the lingual and occipitotemporal gyri, including the extrastriate areas indicated in Figure 17-35, B.

★From Zihl J, von Cramon D, Mai N: Selective disturbance of movement vision after bilateral brain damage, *Brain* 106:313, 1983.
†From Pallis CA: Impaired identification of faces and places with agnosia for colours: report of a case due to cerebral embolism, *J Neurol Neurosurg Psychiat* 18:218, 1955.

reveal that the basic properties of these neurons are similar to those of adults. This indicates that the wiring pattern of the visual system is, to a great extent, genetically determined and does not depend on visual input for its formation.

If, however, one eye of a newborn animal is covered for the first few months of its life, that eye will be permanently blind (in a perceptual sense) when uncovered. At the same time, cortical neurons are found to respond only to stimulation of the eye that had not been covered. This appears to be primarily the result of the replacement of "idle" synapses by connections reflecting activity in the noncovered eye.

This effect of covering an eye is specific to the first few months of life, and no deficit results if it occurs later. Also it is not simply a result of the eye not being

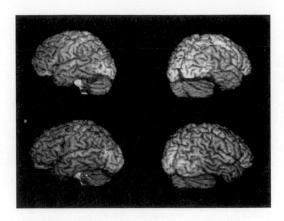

FIGURE 17-34

Combined PET/MRI images demonstrating the cortical areas activated as subjects watched moving visual stimuli (vs. stationary stimuli); each row of two images is from a different subject. (From Watson JDG et al: Area V5 of the human brain: evidence from a combined study using positron emission tomography and magnetic resonance imaging, *Cerebral Cortex* 3:79, 1993.)

exposed to light. If the eye is covered with translucent rather than opaque material so that the retina is exposed to light but not patterns, the same functional blindness results. This is consistent with the fact that normal cortical neurons respond as poorly to diffuse illumination as they do to no illumination at all. This also corresponds to the finding that infantile cataracts (and even more subtle defects) in humans can result in permanent blindness (called **amblyopia**), unless they are corrected at a very early age.

REFLEX CIRCUITS ADJUST THE SIZE OF THE PUPIL AND THE FOCAL LENGTH OF THE LENS

Modern cameras have autoexposure and autofocus mechanisms; reflex connections beginning with the optic nerve subserve similar functions for the eye.

Illumination of Either Retina Causes Both Pupils to Constrict

Light directed into one eye causes both pupils to constrict. The response of the pupil of the illuminated eye is called the **direct pupillary light reflex,** whereas that of the other eye is called the **consensual pupillary light reflex.** The afferent limb of the reflex arc consists of optic tract axons that enter the brachium of the superior colliculus and terminate in the **pretectal area,** which is directly rostral to the superior colliculus at the junction between midbrain and diencephalon. Pretectal neurons project bilaterally to the Edinger-Westphal nucleus, with fibers crossing both through the posterior commissure and through the periaqueductal gray ventral to the aqueduct (Figure 17-36). Axons of cells in the Edinger-Westphal nucleus travel in the

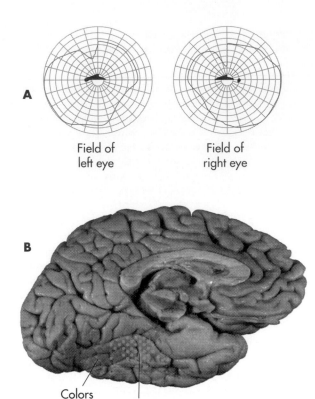

Field of left eye   Field of right eye

FIGURE 17-35

A case of achromatopsia and prosopagnosia. **A,** The patient's visual fields. Areas where vision was lost completely are black, and remaining intact parts of the visual fields are outlined. **B,** Cortical areas likely to have been damaged in this patient (in addition to inferior parts of striate cortex). (**A** redrawn from Pallis CA: Impaired identification of faces and places with agnosia for colours: report of a case due to cerebral embolism, *J Neurol Neurosurg Psychiat* 18:218, 1955.)

third nerve as preganglionic parasympathetic fibers to the ciliary ganglion, where they synapse. Postganglionic fibers in the short ciliary nerves complete the reflex arc, synapsing on the smooth muscle cells of the pupillary sphincter.

Because one optic tract contains axons from ganglion cells in both eyes and because each pretectal area projects bilaterally to the Edinger-Westphal nucleus, light directed into one eye causes the same amount of activity in the Edinger-Westphal nucleus on each side. This is the basis of the consensual light reflex. The result is that both pupils are ordinarily the same size, even if one eye is closed or only one eye is illuminated.

The pathways of the pupillary light reflex are utilized clinically in a procedure known as the **swinging flashlight test** for damage to one retina or optic nerve (Figure 17-36). With the patient seated in a dimly lit room, a light source is quickly moved back and forth from one eye to the other while the examiner observes the behavior of each pupil in turn. For example, assume the right optic nerve is damaged. When the left eye is illuminated, both pupils will constrict. When the right eye is illuminated, the light reflex arc will be less effectively activated, and both pupils will dilate. Therefore when the light is moved from the left eye to the

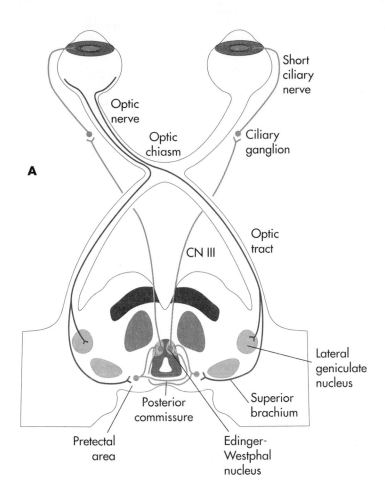

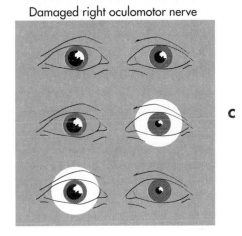

FIGURE 17-36
A, Pathway of the pupillary light reflex. For the sake of simplicity, crossing fibers from one pretectal area to the contralateral Edinger-Westphal nucleus are shown as passing only through the posterior commissure. In fact, some also cross ventral to the aqueduct. **B** and **C,** Pupillary consequences of damage to one optic nerve or one oculomotor nerve, respectively. In each, the upper images show the relative sizes of the pupils in the dark, and the middle and lower images show the expected responses to illumination of the left or right eye. Note that in switching illumination from the left eye to the right eye in **B,** the right pupil dilates in a seemingly paradoxical fashion. This is the basis of the swinging flashlight test. (The right pupil in **C** is *always* dilated, and moving the illumination to the right eye causes no change.) (**A** modified from Nolte J: Iris and pupil. In Records RE, editor: *Physiology of the human eye and visual system,* New York, 1979, Harper & Row.)

right, the right pupil will dilate in a seemingly paradoxical fashion, indicating damage to the right retina or optic nerve.

Both Eyes Accommodate for Near Vision

When visual attention is directed to a nearby object, three things happen in a reflex manner: (1) **convergence** of the two eyes, so the image of the object falls on both foveas; (2) contraction of the ciliary muscle and a resultant thickening of the lens (accommodation), so the image of the object is in focus on the retina; and (3) pupillary constriction, which improves the optical performance of the eye by reducing certain types of aberration and by increasing its depth of focus★ (Figure 17-37).

★Hence there are conflicting effects of pupillary constriction, which makes things *more* easily visible by improving the optical performance of the eye but *less* easily visible by reducing the amount of light reaching the retina. The CNS automatically figures out and implements the pupil size that is the best compromise for a given target distance and level of illumination.

Unlike the pupillary light reflex, the **near reflex** requires the participation of the cerebral cortex. The pathway involved is poorly understood but is generally considered to follow the normal visual pathway to the striate cortex, project to the visual association cortex, and go from there to the superior colliculus and/or pretectal area (Figure 17-38). Impulses are then relayed to the oculomotor nucleus, stimulating medial rectus motor neurons and preganglionic parasympathetic neurons of the Edinger-Westphal nucleus.

Although the same preganglionic parasympathetic fibers are thought to mediate the pupillary constriction of both the light reflex and the near reflex, these two types of constriction can nevertheless be dissociated in certain pathological conditions. An **Argyll Robertson pupil** refers to a condition (usually bilateral and a manifestation of neurosyphilis) in which the pupil constricts during the near reflex but not in response to light. The site of the lesion involved is not known with certainty, but it is often

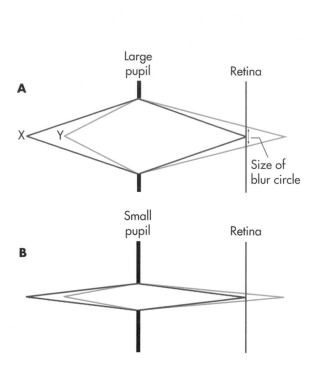

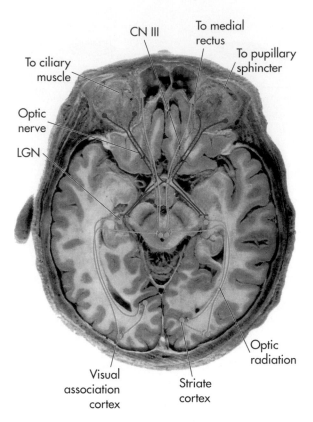

FIGURE 17-37
Effect of pupil size on depth of focus. **A,** When the eye is focused on objects at distance *X* and the pupil is large, the image of a point at distance *Y* will be out of focus and smeared out over a relatively large area. A smaller pupil **(B)** results in a smaller blur-circle for a point at distance *Y*; objects over a greater range of distances are now in acceptable focus.

FIGURE 17-38
Pathway of the near reflex. Although the efferent projections from the occipital lobe to the oculomotor nucleus are usually spoken of as arising in visual association cortex, the exact site of origin is not known with certainty. (Section courtesy Dr. John T. Willson, University of Colorado Health Sciences Center.)

assumed to be in that portion of the pretectal area subserving the light reflex.

SUGGESTED READINGS

Albright TD, Desimone R, Gross CG: Columnar organization of directionally selective cells in visual area MT of the macaque, *J Neurophysiol* 51:16, 1984.

Allison T et al: Electrophysiological studies of color processing in human visual cortex, *Electroencephalogr Clin Neurophysiol* 88:343, 1993.

Baylor D: How photons start vision, *Proc Natl Acad Sci* 93:560, 1996.

Bender MB, Bodis-Wollner I: Visual dysfunction in optic tract lesions, *Ann Neurol* 3:187, 1978. *Clinical observations of nonidentical visual losses in the two eyes, or of selective deficits of only some visual functions, after optic tract damage.*

Clarke S, Miklossy J: Occipital cortex in man: organization of callosal connections, related myelo- and cytoarchitecture, and putative boundaries of functional visual areas, *J Comp Neurol* 298:188, 1990.

Curcio CA et al: Human photoreceptor topography, *J Comp Neurol* 292:497, 1990.

Dacey DM: Circuitry for color coding in the primate retina, *Proc Natl Acad Sci* 93:582, 1996.

Dowling JE: *The retina: an approachable part of the brain,* Cambridge, 1987, The Belknap Press of Harvard University Press.

Haxby JV et al: Face encoding and recognition in the human brain, *Proc Natl Acad Sci* 93:922, 1996.

Holmes G: The organization of the visual cortex in man, *Proc R Soc Lond* B132:348, 1945.

Horton JC, Hoyt WF: The representation of the visual field in human striate cortex: a revision of the classic Holmes map, *Arch Ophthalmol* 109:816, 1991.

Hoyt WF, Luis O: The primate chiasm, *Arch Ophthalmol* 70:69, 1963.

Hubel DH, Wiesel TN: Functional architecture of macaque monkey visual cortex, *Proc R Soc Lond* B198:1, 1977. *A detailed discussion of the elegant experiments on the primate visual system done by these two investigators over the previous 20 years.*

Humphrey NK, Weiskrantz L: Vision in monkeys after removal of the striate cortex, *Nature* 215:595, 1967.

Ishikawa S, Sakiya H, Kondo Y: The center for controlling the near reflex in the midbrain of the monkey: a double labelling study, *Brain Res* 519:217, 1990.

Jampel RS: Representation of the near-response on the cerebral cortex of the macaque, *Am J Ophthalmol* 48:573, 1959.

Kafka MS: Central nervous system control of mammalian circadian rhythms, *Fed Proc* 42:2782, 1982. *The introduction to a series of articles on this topic.*

Kanizsa G: Subjective contours, *Sci Am* 234(4):48, 1976.

Kolb H: The architecture of functional neural circuits in the vertebrate retina, *Invest Ophthalmol* 35:2385, 1994.

Koutalos Y, Yau K-W: Regulation of sensitivity in vertebrate rod photoreceptors by calcium, *Trends Neurosci* 19:73, 1996.

Kupfer C: The projection of the macula in the lateral geniculate nucleus in man, *Am J Ophthalmoml* 54:597, 1962.

Livingstone M, Hubel D: Segregation of form, color, movement, and depth: anatomy, physiology, and perception, *Science* 240:740, 1988. *An intriguing summary pointing out some striking correlations between the basic properties of visual system neurons and the ways in which we perceive things visually.*

Loewenfeld IE: *The pupil: anatomy, physiology, and clinical applications,* Detroit, 1993, Wayne State University Press. *An encyclopedic review of the vast literature on pupils and irises.*

Magoun HW et al: The afferent path of the pupillary light reflex in the monkey, *Brain* 59:234, 1936.

Mills SL, Massey SC: Differential properties of two gap junctional pathways made by AII amacrine cells, *Nature* 377:734, 1995. *A partial unraveling of the ways in which rod signals piggyback on cone pathways at different light intensities.*

Mohler CW, Wurtz RH: Role of striate cortex and superior colliculus in visual guidance of saccadic eye movements in monkeys, *J Neurophysiol* 40:74, 1977.

Moore RY: Retinohypothalamic projection in mammals: a comparative study, *Brain Res* 49:403, 1973.

Nguyen-Legros J: Fine structure of the pigment epithelium in the vertebrate retina, *Int Rev Cytol* (Suppl) 7:287, 1978.

Nordby K: Vision in a complete achromat: a personal account. In Hess RF, Sharpe LT, Nordby K, editors: *Night vision: basic, clinical and applied aspects,* Cambridge, 1990, Cambridge University Press. *Rarely, someone is born with a complete absence of cones. As this personal description indicates, color blindness is only one of the consequences.*

Pearlman AL, Birch J, Meadows JC: Cerebral color blindness: an acquired defect in hue discrimination, *Ann Neurol* 5:253, 1979. *One example of the notion that the primary visual cortex and visual association cortex are not like a screen on which the retinal image is projected; rather, a number of different subareas deal selectively with different aspects of the visual world.*

Perry VH, Cowey A: Retinal ganglion cells that project to the superior colliculus and pretectum in the macaque monkey, *Neuroscience* 12:1125, 1984.

Pollack JG, Hickey TL: The distribution of retinocollicular axon terminals in rhesus monkey, *J Comp Neurol* 185:587, 1979.

Puce A et al: Face-sensitive regions in human extrastriate cortex studied by functional MRI, *J Neurophysiol* 74:1192, 1995.

Ramachandran VS: Blind spots, *Sci Am* 266(5):86, 1992. *Games you can play with your blind spot.*

Rao-Mirotznik R et al: Mammalian rod terminal: architecture of a binary synapse, *Neuron* 14:561, 1995. *An interesting review of the synaptic specializations involved in passing along information about the absorption of single photons.*

Reese BE, Cowey A: Fibre organization of the monkey optic tract. I. Segregation of functionally distinct optic axons. II. Noncongruent representation of the two half-retinae, *J Comp Neurol* 295:385 and 401, 1990.

Rodieck RW, Watanabe M: Survey of the morphology of macaque retinal ganglion cells that project to the pretectum, superior colliculus, and parvicellular laminae of the lateral geniculate nucleus, *J Comp Neurol* 338:289, 1993.

Schiller PH, Sandell JH, Maunsell JHR: Functions of the ON and OFF channels of the visual system, *Nature* 322:824, 1986.

Schneider GE: Two visual systems, *Science* 163:895, 1969. *Differential effects of collicular and cortical damage on a hamster's visual capabilities.*

Schwartz WJ, Gainer H: Suprachiasmatic nucleus: use of ^{14}C-labeled deoxyglucose uptake as a functional marker, *Science* 197:1089, 1977.

Sherman SM, Koch C: The control of retinogeniculate transmission in the mammalian lateral geniculate nucleus, *Exp Brain Res* 63:1, 1986. *The lateral geniculate has an important role in regulating the access of visual information to the cerebral cortex.*

Sherman SM, Spear PD: Organization of visual pathways in normal and visually deprived cats, *Physiol Rev* 62:738, 1982.

Stein J, Walsh V: To see but not to read; the magnocellular theory of dyslexia, *Trends Neurosci* 20:147, 1997. *A review of the evidence that an abnormality in the visual channel specialized for the analysis of rapidly changing stimuli could underlie dyslexia.*

Tanaka, K: Inferotemporal cortex and object vision, *Ann Rev Neurosci* 16:109, 1996.

Tassinari G et al: Magno- and parvocellular pathways are segregated in the human optic tract, *NeuroReport* 5:1425, 1994.

Thorpe S, Fize D, Marlot C: Speed of processing in the human visual system, *Nature* 381:520, 1996. *Clever experiments showing how quickly we can extract significant features from complex visual scenes.*

Tootell RBH et al: Functional anatomy of macaque striate cortex. II. Retinotopic organization, *J Neurosci* 8:1531, 1988.

Walls GL: *The vertebrate eye and its adaptive radiation,* New York, 1967, Hafner Publishing Company. *A monumental, fascinating book describing the myriad variations of every part of the eye that adapt different species to their environments.*

Wässle H, Boycott BB: Functional architecture of the mammalian retina, *Physiol Rev* 71:447, 1991.

Wässle H et al: The rod pathway of the macaque monkey retina: identification of AII-amacrine cells with antibodies against calretinin, *J Comp Neurol* 361:537, 1995.

Weiskrantz L et al: Visual capacity in the hemianopic field following a restricted cortical ablation, *Brain* 97:709, 1974. *Remarkable account of the visual capabilities remaining in one individual after known selective damage to his striate cortex.*

Wilson JR: Circuitry of the dorsal lateral geniculate nucleus in the cat and monkey, *Anat Embryol* 147:1, 1993.

Wilson ME, Cragg BG: Projections from the lateral geniculate nucleus in the cat and monkey, *J Anat* 101:677, 1967.

Wong-Riley MTT: Connections between the pulvinar nucleus and the prestriate cortex in the squirrel monkey as revealed by peroxidase histochemistry and autoradiography, *Brain Res* 134:249, 1977.

Zeki S: *A vision of the brain,* London, 1993, Blackwell. *A well-written overview of central visual processing, with an emphasis on the history of ideas, clinical observations, and experiments regarding the localization of different aspects of visual function.*

Zihl J, von Cramon D, Mai N: Selective disturbance of movement vision after bilateral brain damage, *Brain* 106:313, 1983. *Another example of the apparent parcellation of visual cortical areas into regions dealing with particular aspects of a visual stimulus.*

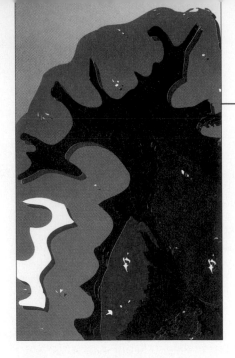

OVERVIEW OF MOTOR SYSTEMS

Each of us has fewer than 1 million motor neurons with which to control muscles. Without them, we would be completely unable to communicate with the outside world. With them, however, we are capable of an enormous range of complex activities, from automatic and semiautomatic movements such as postural adjustments to the characteristically human movements involved in speaking and writing. The ways in which a wide variety of neural structures interact to make these activities possible is the topic of Chapters 18 to 20.

EACH LOWER MOTOR NEURON INNERVATES A GROUP OF MUSCLE FIBERS, FORMING A MOTOR UNIT

Lower motor neurons, the target of CNS pathways and connections involved in motor control, are arranged in the spinal cord and brainstem in groups corresponding to individual muscles (see Figure 10-8). The axons of lower motor neurons leave the CNS in ventral roots (or motor roots of cranial nerves) and divide into terminal branches widely distributed in their target muscles. Each branch ends at the single neuromuscular junction of a muscle fiber (see Figure 8-10). The combination of one motor neuron and all the muscle fibers it innervates is referred to as a **motor unit.** Motor units vary tremendously in size, in a way that makes functional sense: the size of the motor units in a given muscle is related to the degree of fine control involved in the use of that muscle. Thus there may be only 2 or 3 muscle fibers in a motor unit in the stapedius, 10 in an extraocular muscle, 100 in a hand muscle, and 1000 in a large antigravity muscle such as the gastrocnemius (Figure 18-1). Even within a single muscle, however, there is a range of motor units varying in size and functional properties, as described shortly.

Lower Motor Neurons Are Arranged Systematically

Just as there are systematic maps in sensory pathways (see Figure 10-20) and in cortical areas (e.g., see Figures 3-28 and 17-26), so too is there a systematic arrangement of clusters of motor neurons. In the anterior horn of the spinal cord, for example, motor neurons for axial muscles are located medial to those for more distal muscles, and those for flexors are dorsal to those for extensors (Figure 18-2). This axial-distal mapping corresponds to the arrangement of descending pathways, some of which are important for postural adjustments of axial muscles, others for the control of distal muscles (Figure 18-6).

There are Three Kinds of Muscle Fibers and Three Kinds of Motor Units

Most muscles are called upon to contract for different purposes. The gastrocnemius, for example, must contract weakly but for long periods as we stand upright, more strongly during running (which most of us cannot sustain for nearly as long as standing), and very strongly

but very briefly in a jump. Corresponding to these requirements, there are three kinds of skeletal muscle fibers that form the substrate for three different types of motor unit (Figure 18-3). **Red** fibers are thin, contain abundant mitochondria, contract weakly and slowly, but are able to sustain contractions for long periods of time. **White** fibers are larger, contain relatively few mitochondria, and contract in brief, powerful twitches. **Intermediate** fibers, as the name implies, have properties somewhere in between those of red and white fibers. Most muscles contain all three fiber types, but in proportions that vary depending on the principal function of a given muscle.★

All the muscle fibers in a motor unit are of a single type, with the result that there are three types of motor unit (Figure 18-3). The smallest alpha motor neurons innervate red fibers, the largest innervate white fibers, and alpha motor neurons of intermediate size innervate intermediate fibers. The properties of each motor unit type can be predicted from the properties of the muscle fibers: type **S** (*slow-twitch*) motor units produce small amounts of force for prolonged periods, type **FF** (*fast-twitch, fatigable*) units produce large amounts of force for brief periods of time, and type **FR** (*fast-twitch, fatigue-resistant*) produce moderate amounts of force that can be sustained for moderate amounts of time (Figure 18-3).

★In domestic fowl, for example, that do a lot of standing and running but little flying, dark meat is muscle with many red fibers and white meat is muscle with many white fibers.

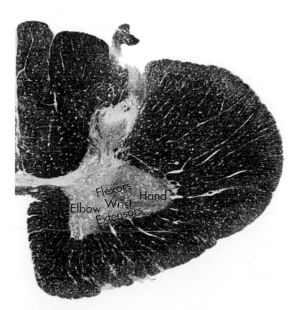

FIGURE 18-2

Arrangement of motor neurons at C8. The large number of motor neurons for distal muscles accounts for the lateral expansion of the anterior horn at this level.

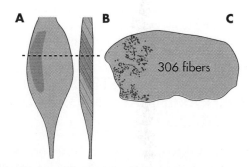

FIGURE 18-1

The muscle fibers of a single motor unit (type FR) in cat gastrocnemius. The general location of the group of fibers is indicated by shading on a drawing of the whole muscle **(A)** and a longitudinal section through the muscle **(B). C,** A cross section of the muscle; each muscle fiber in the motor unit is indicated by a dot. (Redrawn from Burke RE, Tsairis P: Anatomy and innervation ratios in motor units of cat gastrocnemius, *J Physiol* 234:749, 1973.)

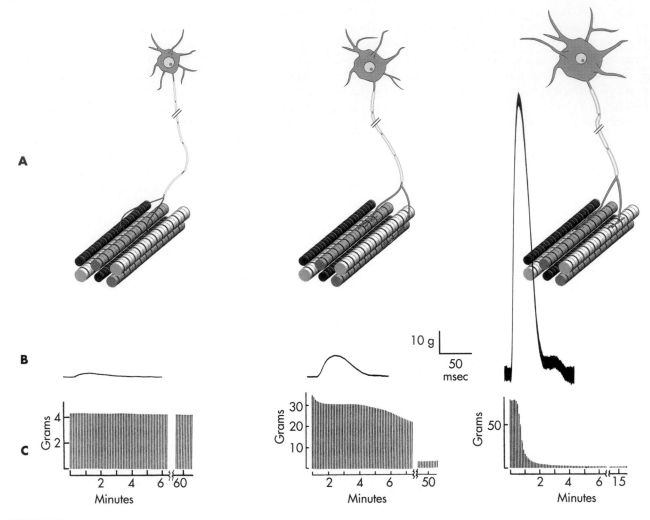

FIGURE 18-3

S *(first column)*, FR *(second column)*, and FF *(third column)* motor units of cat gastrocnemius, showing the anatomical components **(A)**, twitch response to a single stimulus **(B)**, and responses to a series of stimuli **(C)** for each. The same time and force scale applies to all three twitches in **B**. (**B** and **C** modified from Burke RE et al: Physiological types and histochemical profiles in motor units of the cat gastrocnemius, *J Physiol* 234:723, 1973.)

Motor Units Are Recruited in Order of Size

The association of different muscle fiber types with motor neurons of different sizes is the basis of an elegantly simple mechanism for grading the force of muscle contraction. If two neurons have the same density of channels in their surface membranes, the smaller of the two neurons will have fewer total channels and a greater resistance to transmembrane current flow. Hence a given amount of synaptic current will cause a greater membrane potential change in the smaller neuron, making the smaller neuron more easily excitable. As the synaptic drive reaching the anterior horn increases, motor neurons reach threshold in order of increasing size (the **size principle**). S units are recruited first and as they fire faster and faster, FR units are added. As the FR units increase their firing rate, FF units are added. This is just what is required to smoothly increase the force of muscle contraction, beginning with small increases from the background level of tone and

ending with brief maximal contractions (Figure 18-4). The elegant part is that it happens automatically, in all movements, simply by virtue of the increasing size of the motor neurons in the three types of motor unit.

MOTOR CONTROL SYSTEMS INVOLVE BOTH HIERARCHICAL AND PARALLEL CONNECTIONS

The inputs that determine the level of activity of lower motor neurons may be very broadly divided into three overlapping classes (Figure 18-5):

1. Built-in patterns of neural connections.
2. Descending pathways that modulate the activity of motor neurons; these effects may be direct or they may be indirect by way of influences on built-in neural subsystems. Collectively, the neurons that

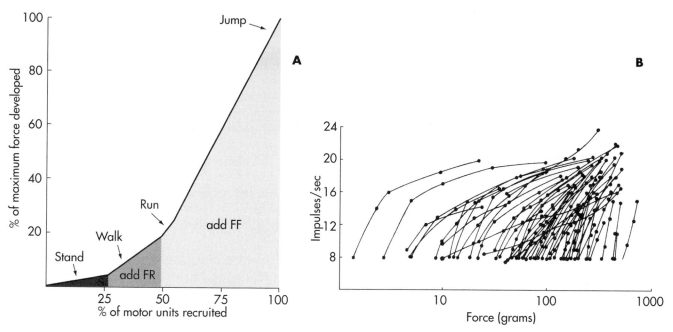

FIGURE 18-4

Recruitment of motor units in order of size. **A,** Graphic indication of the buildup of force in cat gastrocnemius during normal activities as motor units are recruited in order of size. **B,** Firing rates of 60 motor units in a human forearm muscle (extensor digitorum) during isometric contraction of increasing force; each line represents a single motor unit. Force production increases by individual units firing more rapidly and, simultaneously, by additional units being recruited. Note that the force scale is logarithmic, and later-recruited units provide greater increments of force. (**A** modified from Walmsley B, Hodgson JA, Burke RE: Forces produced by medial gastrocnemius and soleus muscles during locomotion in freely moving cats, *J Neurophysiol* 41:1203, 1978. **B** from Monster AW, Chan H: Isometric force production by motor units of extensor digitorum communis muscle in man, *J Neurophysiol* 40:1432, 1977.)

give rise to these descending pathways are **upper motor neurons.**

3. Higher centers that influence the activity of descending pathways.

Damage to either upper or lower motor neurons causes weakness, each with its own distinctive set of accompanying symptoms and signs. Damage to higher centers also causes distinctive movement abnormalities (e.g., inappropriate movements, incoordination, difficulty initiating movement), but is not accompanied by substantial weakness.

Reflex and Motor Program Connections Provide Some of the Inputs to Lower Motor Neurons

The stretch reflex is an obvious and simple example of a built-in pattern of neural connections that controls, to some extent, the activity of motor neurons. Stretching a muscle stimulates its muscle spindles, whose afferent fibers end on motor neurons that in turn cause the muscle to contract (see Figure 10-9). Other reflexes, such as the flexor reflex (see Figures 10-11 and 10-13), are more complex and involve a number of muscles and spinal segments. Finally, there are networks of interneurons in the brainstem and spinal cord that can act as pattern generators for rhythmic movements such as breathing and walking. Although some of the same interneurons that are involved in reflexes may also be part of the circuitry of these

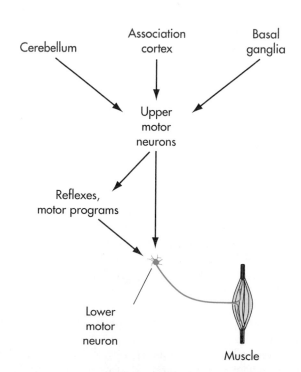

FIGURE 18-5

Schematic overview of motor control components. The association cortex, basal ganglia, and cerebellum play vital roles in the choice, design, and monitoring of movement, but have no direct effect on either lower motor neurons or strength.

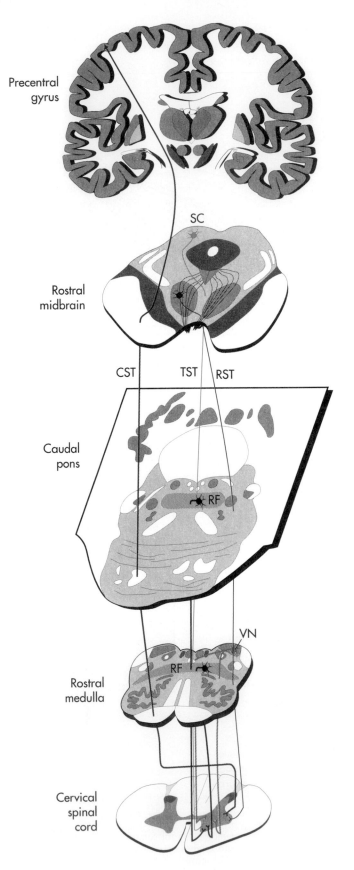

Precentral gyrus

SC

Rostral midbrain

CST   TST   RST

Caudal pons

RF

VN

RF

Rostral medulla

Cervical spinal cord

central programs (as they are often called), these programs are more than simply a stringing together of reflexes, each one triggering the next. One indication is that the principal features of central programs can persist in the absence of afferent input. As an extreme example, the spinal cord of a lamprey (a primitive, jawless fish) can be kept alive in a dish for several days. Such a spinal cord, completely isolated from the rest of the lamprey, can exhibit in its ventral roots oscillating bursts of action potentials that in an intact animal would produce rhythmic, coordinated swimming movements. Upper motor neurons and higher centers harness the basic elements of these central programs and adapt them as necessary, for example modifying a stepping cycle to avoid an obstacle.

Upper Motor Neurons Control Lower Motor Neurons Both Directly and Indirectly

Upper motor neurons, neurons whose axons descend to the spinal cord (and to cranial nerve motor nuclei) to affect the activity of lower motor neurons, are located in both the cerebral cortex and the brainstem. The descending pathways involved, most of which have already been mentioned, are summarized in Figure 18-6. The **vestibulospinal tracts** (see Figure 14-26) are important mediators of postural adjustments and head movements. The **corticospinal tract** (see Figure 10-22) classically has been considered the principal mediator of voluntary movement although, as discussed in this chapter, its real role is not so clear these days. The **reticulospinal tracts** (see Figure 11-16) and, to a lesser extent, the **rubrospinal tract** are the principal alternate routes for the mediation of voluntary movement. The rubrospinal tract originates in the red nucleus, crosses to the other side of the midbrain, descends in the lateral part of the brainstem tegmentum, and travels through the lateral funiculus of the spinal cord in company with the lateral corticospinal tract. The rubrospinal tract of humans is quite small, and the reticulospinal tracts are the major alternate route to the spinal cord. A **tectospinal tract** has also been described, descending from the superior colliculus through the contralateral anterior funiculus to cervical levels of the spinal cord. It is assumed to be important in reflex turning of the head in response to visual and perhaps other stimuli, but little is actually known of its function in humans.

The lateral corticospinal and rubrospinal tracts terminate in lateral parts of the anterior horn, where they in-

FIGURE 18-6

Principal locations and projections of upper motor neurons. Only one corticospinal fiber is indicated and is shown crossing the midline to join the lateral corticospinal tract. However, some corticospinal fibers, mostly headed for lower motor neurons for axial muscles, do not cross in the pyramidal decussation and join the anterior corticospinal tract. *CST*, Corticospinal tract; *RF*, reticular formation; *RST*, rubrospinal tract; *SC*, superior colliculus; *TST*, tectospinal tract; *VN*, vestibular nuclei.

fluence motor neurons for distal muscles. All the others terminate primarily in more medial parts of the anterior horn, where they influence the motor neurons for axial muscles important in postural adjustments.

Association Cortex, the Cerebellum, and the Basal Ganglia Modulate Motor Cortex

Even though corticospinal, rubrospinal, reticulospinal, and vestibulospinal fibers are able to influence motor neurons and their local connections, this still does not explain how a voluntary movement is made. At the present time we are able to say very little about the nature of the little person within the CNS who pulls the strings when we decide to move. We can, however, specify some of the structures and connections that must be involved in the sense that damage to these structures and connections results in defective movements. In addition to the portions of the CNS already mentioned, these structures include the basal ganglia, the cerebellum, some areas of association cortex, and portions of the thalamus. The basal ganglia and the cerebellum are the subjects of Chapters 19 and 20, but the general way in which the various components of the motor system are interconnected is briefly discussed here. Cortical association areas are discussed in Chapter 22.

In one sense, the components of the motor system are organized hierarchically, as though association cortex "decides" that a movement is called for, premotor areas of the cortex devise a plan for the movement and pass this information on to the motor cortex, which then issues commands to motor neurons either directly or indirectly by way of nuclei and interneurons of the brainstem and spinal cord. In another sense the components of the motor system are organized in parallel, much as in the case of sensory pathways; messages are conveyed to motor neurons not only from motor cortex but also from premotor areas themselves (Figure 18-12). The basal ganglia and cerebellum are involved in various aspects of planning and monitoring movements but have no outputs of their own to the spinal cord. Rather, they act primarily by affecting motor and premotor cortex (Figure 18-7).

This is an extremely simplified overview of the central motor apparatus and omits a number of important details. Some of these details are mentioned in this and the next two chapters, whereas others are beyond the scope of this book. For example, no mention has been made of the role of sensory input to this system. Such input is clearly involved because we are easily able to make appropriate modifications in the walking program to accommodate an increased load, such as a backpack, or modifications in the running program to accommodate the sight of an impending brick wall. A variety of pathological conditions reflect motor deficits resulting from sensory losses. One example already cited is the ataxia resulting from damage to the posterior columns. We can

make simple movements involving single joints or basic rhythms fairly accurately without sensory feedback, but not more complex movements (Figure 18-8) or corrections in response to perturbations.

THE CORTICOSPINAL TRACT HAS MULTIPLE ORIGINS AND TERMINATIONS

During the nineteenth century it was discovered that electrical stimulation of certain areas of the mammalian cerebral cortex causes movements of the contralateral side of the body. In humans the area with the lowest threshold for this effect lies in the precentral gyrus (Figure 18-9) and so this area has come to be called the **primary motor cortex.** Subsequent work showed that there is a distorted mapping of the body in the primary motor cortex (Figure 18-10), so stimulation of restricted cortical areas causes contraction of small groups of muscles or even single muscles. The **somatotopic** map is not as precise as Figure 3-28 seems to indicate—different body parts overlap and interdigitate with one another—but it is distorted in such a way that the parts of the body capable of intricate movements (such as the fingers and lips) have disproportionately large representations. The **motor homunculus** is similar in this way to the sensory homunculus in the somatosensory cortex of the postcentral gyrus, and this corresponds to (among other things) the notion that detailed sensory information is required for fine motor control.[*]

It was also known in the previous century that the primary motor cortex contains giant pyramidal cells called **Betz cells,** whose axons descend to the spinal cord through the medullary pyramids; it was further known that cerebral lesions that destroy either motor cortex and adjoining areas, or the posterior limb of the internal capsule as the axons of Betz cells pass through it, cause contralateral spastic paralysis. Therefore it became accepted neurological thinking that the corticospinal tract (1) consists exclusively of large axons, (2) originates in the precentral gyrus, (3) proceeds exclusively to the spinal cord, (4) is necessary for voluntary movement, and (5) is a tract whose destruction results in spastic paralysis. However, it has gradually become apparent that this traditional description is incorrect in almost every way.

Corticospinal Axons Arise in Multiple Cortical Areas

The large (up to 22 μm) axons of Betz cells are included in the corticospinal tract, but they account for only about 3% of the tract's 1 million fibers. The vast majority of cor-

---

[*]Other species have maps distorted in different but appropriate ways. For example, nearly two thirds of the fibers leaving an elephant's motor cortex are bound for its facial motor nucleus, reflecting an elephant's fine control over trunk movements; only one third of the fibers reach the spinal cord.

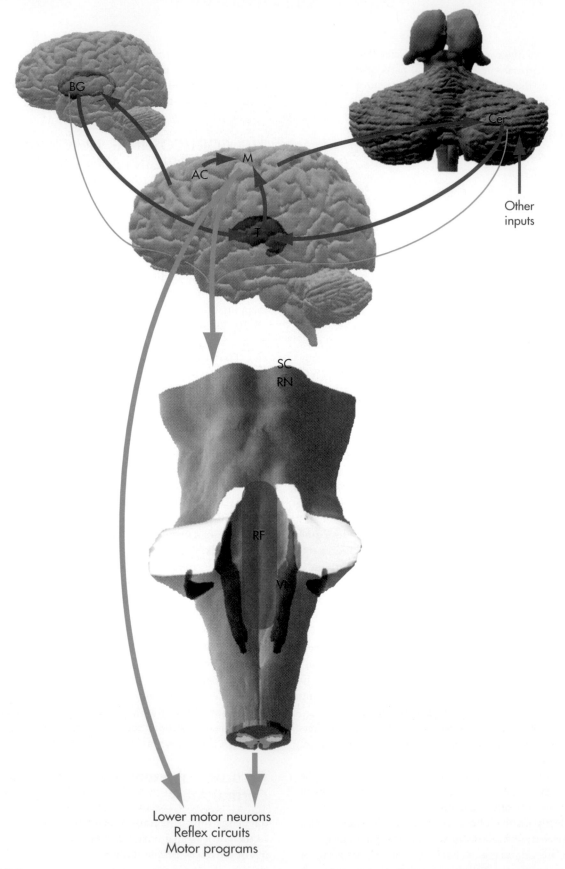

FIGURE 18-7

Major components and schematic connections involved in motor control. The cerebellum and basal ganglia participate in movement control primarily by influencing the output from cerebral cortex to the brainstem and spinal cord. (These connections are discussed in greater detail in Chapters 19 and 20.) Each also has additional outputs to brainstem nuclei (minor for the basal ganglia, more substantial for the cerebellum). The basal ganglia receive inputs primarily from the cerebral cortex, as well as from other parts of the basal ganglia system. The cerebellum, in contrast, receives large quantities of sensory information from noncortical sources. *AC,* Association (e.g., prefrontal) cortex; *BG,* basal ganglia; *Cer,* cerebellum; *M,* motor areas of cortex (primary motor, premotor, and supplementary motor areas; see Figure 18-10); *RF,* reticular formation; *RN,* red nucleus; *SC,* superior colliculus; *VN,* vestibular nuclei.

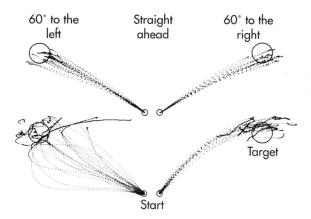

60° to the
left

Straight
ahead

60° to the
right

Target

Start

FIGURE 18-8

Ataxia caused by a somatosensory deficit. A normal subject *(upper records)* and a patient *(lower records)* with a peripheral neuropathy that selectively affected large-diameter sensory fibers used a computer mouse held in the right hand to move a cursor from a starting point to a target. The position of the mouse was digitized every 20 msec, producing a dotted-line record of hand movement. The subjects could see the position of the target and the cursor on the computer screen, but not the mouse or the right hand holding it. The normal subject made the movements smoothly and accurately in either direction. The patient was inaccurate and somewhat irregular when moving to the right and had much more trouble when moving to the left, because this was a more complex movement of the right hand across the midline. [From Gordon J, Ghilardi MF, Ghez C: Impairments of reaching movements in patients without proprioception. I. Spatial errors, *J Neurophysiol* 73:347, 1995.]

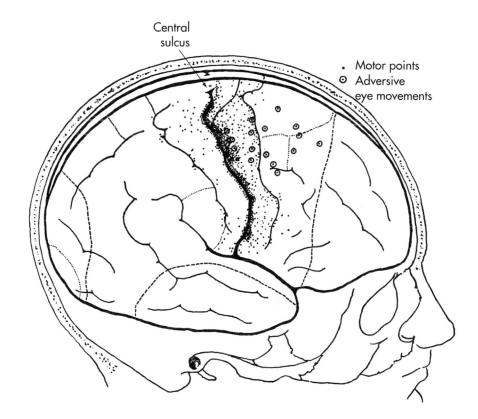

Central
sulcus

• Motor points
⊙ Adversive
   eye movements

FIGURE 18-9

Composite diagram of the locations that yielded discrete movements when stimulated with a very weak electrical current in a series of conscious human patients during the course of neurosurgical procedures. Note that most of the sensitive points lie on the precentral gyrus, particularly near the central sulcus, but a significant number are on the postcentral gyrus and a few are anterior to the precentral gyrus. [From Penfield, W, Boldrey E: Somatic motor and sensory representation in the cerebral cortex of man as studied by electrical stimulation, *Brain* 60:389, 1937.]

ticospinal fibers are much smaller, in the 1- to 4- μm range. Whether the small fibers have a role different from that of the larger fibers is not known.

Betz cells reside specifically in primary motor cortex, but only about a third of the corticospinal fibers originate in this cortical area. The remainder come from adjacent frontal motor areas and from the parietal lobe, particularly the somatosensory cortex of the postcentral gyrus. In view of this fact, many investigators now refer to the cortical complex on both sides of the central sulcus as the **sensorimotor cortex.** Hence primary motor cortex is neither the

only source of corticospinal fibers nor the only cortical area involved in motor control. There are also maps of the body in the **premotor cortex** directly anterior to primary motor cortex and in the **supplementary motor area,** located on the medial surface of the hemisphere just anterior to the representation of the foot in primary motor cortex (Figure 18-11). (Much as in the case of the mosaic of visual association areas mentioned in Chapter 17, the premotor and supplementary motor areas are actually complexes of smaller areas. The supplementary motor area, for example, actually contains four separate and distinct motor areas, two

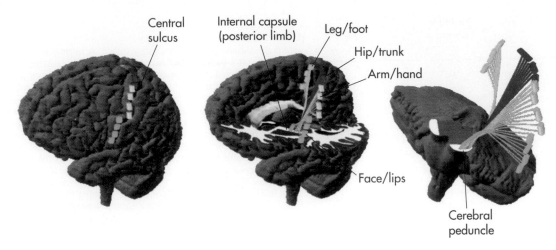

FIGURE 18-10
Course of corticospinal axons through the internal capsule and into the cerebral peduncle. Only those from the precentral gyrus are shown, but axons from the premotor and supplementary motor areas traverse the same region of the internal capsule. (From Sundsten JW et al: *Interactive brain atlas*, Seattle, 1994, University of Washington School of Medicine.)

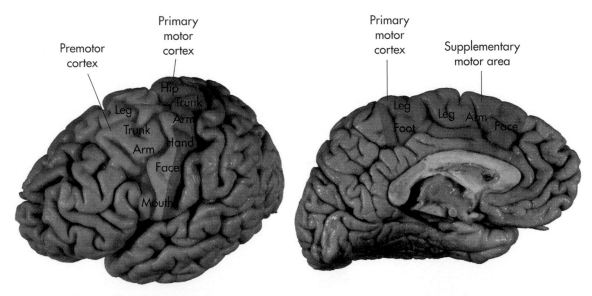

FIGURE 18-11
Location, extent, and somatotopic arrangement in motor areas of cerebral cortex. The indicated maps in premotor and supplementary motor areas are at best approximate; each of these includes multiple subareas, each with its own map, and not all are in register with each other.

in the superior frontal gyrus and two in the banks of the cingulate sulcus.) The premotor and supplementary motor areas provide another third of the corticospinal tract, and both also project to primary motor cortex (Figure 18-12).

Movements can be elicited by electrically stimulating the premotor and supplementary motor areas, but more current is required than in the case of primary motor cortex. In addition, the movements are more complex. Stimulating the premotor cortex may cause turning of the trunk to the opposite side or movement of the entire contralateral arm. Stimulating the supplementary motor area can cause bilateral movements, vocalizations, or the arrest of speech. Some of the movements elicited by stimulating premotor and supplementary motor cortex arise via direct

connections and others via primary motor cortex. For example, hand movements can no longer be produced by stimulation of the supplementary motor area after primary motor cortex has been removed, whereas trunk movements are unaffected. However, these two cortical areas are more than simply additional sources of motor command signals. Although the details are far from clear, they probably have distinctive roles in the planning and production of movement. Premotor cortex may have a special role in movements guided by external stimuli, such as reaching for a seen object. The supplementary motor area may be more important in planning complex, internally generated movements; blood flow increases in this area even if a movement is mentally rehearsed but not actually per-

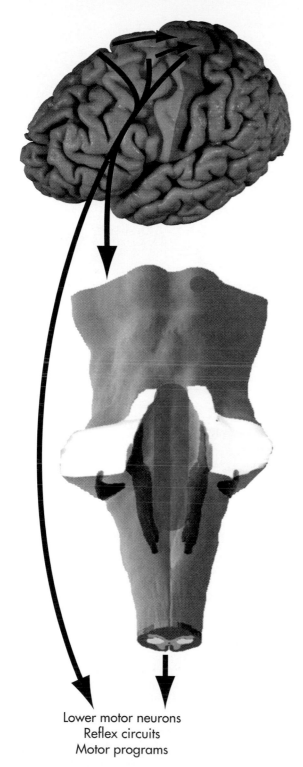

Lower motor neurons
Reflex circuits
Motor programs

FIGURE 18-12
Projection of premotor and supplementary motor areas to primary motor cortex, and of all three motor areas to the brainstem and spinal cord.

formed (Figure 18-13). The existence of multiple motor areas, each with its own access to lower motor neurons, is consistent with the observation that cortical damage sometimes causes inability to move in some circumstances but not in others (Figure 18-14).

Motor Cortex Projects to Both the Spinal Cord and the Brainstem

Corticospinal fibers, as their name implies, end in the spinal cord. However, in their course from cortex to cord they give rise to large numbers of collaterals that end in a wide variety of locations, including the basal ganglia, the thalamus, the reticular formation, and various sensory nuclei such as the posterior column nuclei. Even within the spinal cord some end in the posterior horn, others end in the intermediate gray matter, and a minority end directly on alpha and gamma motor neurons. These numerous connections make it seem unlikely that the corticospinal tract has a single, easily specified function. The projections to sensory nuclei, for example, might serve to compensate somehow for the altered afferent activity to be caused by an impending movement.

The corticospinal tract does, of course, have a major effect on motor neurons as well, both directly and indirectly by way of interneurons. In general, both alpha and gamma motor neurons are affected similarly. The utility of this **alpha-gamma coactivation** can be seen in Figure 9-13. If only the alpha motor neurons were activated, during the resulting contraction the muscle spindles would be "de-stretched" and hence inactive. Stretch reflexes thus would be inoperative and unable to help compensate for sudden changes in load during the movement. Activating the gamma motor neurons as well serves to maintain spindle sensitivity throughout the movement.

Corticospinal input is essential for only some movements

Studies in which both medullary pyramids of monkeys were carefully and selectively severed have demonstrated that after an initial period of flaccid paralysis, surprisingly little chronic motor deficit results from a total loss of corticospinal function. In moving about their cages, these animals are virtually indistinguishable from normal monkeys. The only behaviorally obvious deficit is a permanent inability to use their fingers individually (e.g., picking up a small object between thumb and forefinger). This corresponds to the evolution of corticospinal connections, which in most animals reach interneurons in the posterior horn and intermediate gray matter but not lower motor neurons. The lower motor neurons of primates capable of individual finger movements, in contrast, are contacted directly by corticospinal endings (Figure 18-15). Loss of such finger movements is certainly serious for creatures who use their hands as much and as skillfully as many primates do, but nevertheless it falls far short of being a generalized weakness or paralysis of voluntary movements.

If lesions of medial portions of the medullary reticular formation are added to the corticospinal lesion, a severe and permanent disability of the axial muscles results. Conversely, if lesions of the lateral portions of the medullary

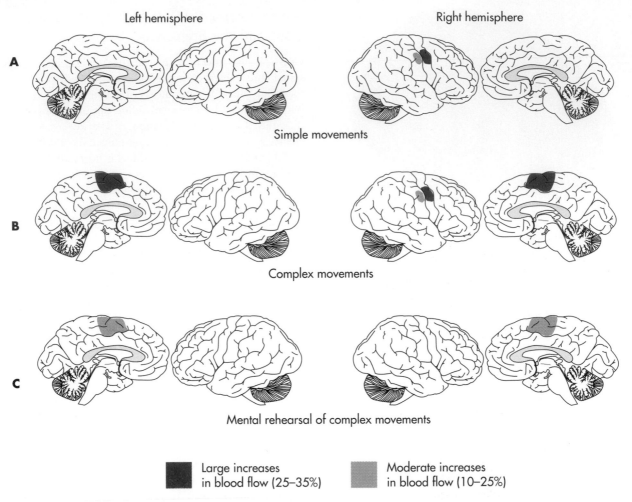

Left hemisphere   Right hemisphere

A

Simple movements

B

Complex movements

C

Mental rehearsal of complex movements

Large increases   Moderate increases
in blood flow (25–35%)   in blood flow (10–25%)

FIGURE 18-13
Changes in cerebral blood flow during real or imagined movements; in this illustration all movements involve the left hand. In **A**, the subject repeatedly flexes the left index finger, compressing a spring. Blood flow to primary motor cortex increases on the right; blood flow also increases in the corresponding part of the right postcentral gyrus, presumably because of the somatosensory input created by the repeated flexions. In **B** the subject rapidly touches each finger of the left hand to the left thumb; now blood flow also increases *bilaterally* in the supplementary motor area. In **C** the subject mentally rehearses the complex movement in **B** but does not actually perform it; blood flow increases only in the supplementary motor area (still bilaterally). (Modified from Roland PE et al: Supplementary motor area and other cortical areas in organization of voluntary movements in man, *J Neurophysiol* 43:118, 1980.)

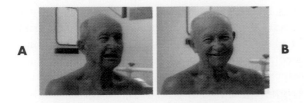

A   B

FIGURE 18-14
Selective weakness of lower facial muscles after cortical damage. This patient had suffered a stroke that resulted in weakness of his left hand (not shown) and the left side of his face. When he tried to bare his teeth on request (**A**), weakness of left lower facial muscles was apparent. However, when told a joke he smiled almost symmetrically (**B**).

reticular formation are added to the corticospinal lesion, a severe and permanent disability of independent use of the arms (including, of course, the fingers) results. Evidently the reticulospinal and/or rubrospinal tracts can compensate for the role normally played by the corticospinal tract in most aspects of voluntary movement.

Naturally occurring lesions in humans are seldom as neatly restricted as those in the monkeys just mentioned, and comparable cases of humans with selective damage to the pyramids are rare. However, there once was a neurosurgical procedure (whose rationale is explained in the next chapter) in which the corticospinal tract was cut in the cerebral peduncle. In these cases, the results were quite similar to those encountered with pyramid-sectioned monkeys, and relatively little chronic deficit resulted. Se-

Squirrel monkey

Cebus monkey

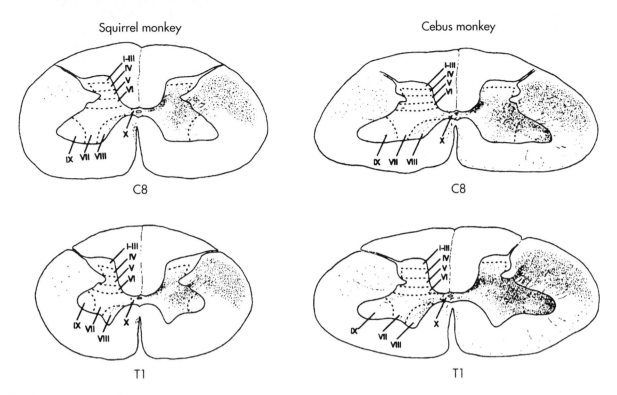

FIGURE 18-15
Terminations of corticospinal axons (labeled by axoplasmic transport of a marker) in two species of monkey, one that does not use individual finger movements (squirrel monkey) and one that does (cebus monkey). In both species there is a broad band of corticospinal terminals in the intermediate gray, but only in the cebus monkey are there terminals in the lateral extension of the anterior horn, where finger motor neurons live. (From Bortoff GA, Strick PL: Corticospinal terminations in two new-world primates: further evidence that corticomotoneuronal connections provide part of the neural substrate for manual dexterity, *J Neurosci* 13:5105, 1993.)

lective damage to the medullary pyramids of humans also causes less pronounced weakness and spasticity than does damage to motor areas of the cortex. (How much less is still being debated, in large part because so few cases have been reported.) The reason for the apparent discrepancy can be seen in Figure 18-6. Damage to a medullary pyramid affects a select group of fibers, the final portions of certain axons just before they reach the spinal cord. In contrast, damage to motor/premotor/supplementary motor cortex or to the internal capsule affects not only corticospinal fibers but also projections from the cortex to the thalamus, basal ganglia, reticular formation, and other structures. Furthermore, even if it were possible to selectively damage only corticospinal fibers in the internal capsule, they would be affected before they gave off their many collaterals rather than after (as in the case of damage to the pyramid). Which part of this additional damage is responsible for the appearance of spasticity is not known with certainty, but the loss of certain projections from the premotor cortex to the reticular formation, and consequent reticulospinal dysfunction, is a likely cause.

The **pyramidal tract** received its name historically from the medullary pyramids and, like many other historically named neural structures, has now come to mean different things to different people. For some, it has the functional meaning of the combination of the corticospinal

and corticobulbar tracts, with the emphasis on the fibers that more or less directly affect motor neurons. For others, it retains the historical-anatomical meaning and is the collection of fibers in the medullary pyramids. For still others, it means the collection of neurons whose destruction results in the clinically observed **pyramidal tract syndrome** (discussed shortly). People are sometimes misled into thinking that all three of these meanings refer to the same collection of fibers, but a major point of this section has been that they do not. Hence selective destruction of the medullary pyramids, though rare, is perverse enough not to cause a full-blown pyramidal tract syndrome. Also, many corticospinal and corticobulbar fibers have no particular effect on motor neurons but instead modulate transmission through ascending pathways.

Upper motor neuron damage causes a distinctive syndrome

The most common cause of motor problems clinically attributed to the pyramidal system is a cerebrovascular accident involving the motor and premotor cortex or the posterior limb of the internal capsule. Immediately after the stroke a period of flaccid paralysis ensues, analogous to spinal shock. After a period of days to weeks, tone and reflexes return and increase, and the situation resolves into

spastic hemiplegia or **hemiparesis.**★ Tone is increased because stretch reflexes are increased in a velocity-dependent fashion (Figure 18-16), so that when a muscle is stretched rapidly (as by an examiner forcibly flexing the patient's leg), its resistance to further stretch increases greatly. (Slow stretch meets less resistance.) At some point this increased resistance suddenly melts away, and the limb collapses in flexion (or extension, if the arm is forcibly extended). This sudden collapse is called the **clasp-knife effect** and is usually attributed to inhibition of motor neurons by reflex connections of Golgi tendon organs (see Figure 10-10); inhibitory effects of other muscle receptors are also likely to be important. Sudden stretch of a muscle may lead to **clonus,** a rapid series of rhythmic contractions maintained for the duration of the stretch. Increased tone is especially pronounced in the flexors of the arm and fingers and in the extensors of the leg, contributing to the typical hemiparetic stance and gait. This combination of hyperreflexia and hypertonia is spasticity. In addition, certain normal reflexes disappear and some abnormal reflexes appear. The best known of the latter is Babinski's sign. Interestingly, Babinski's sign is normally seen in human infants before the corticospinal tract is fully myelinated and functional and is also seen after selective damage to the corticospinal tract in the cerebral peduncle or pyramid.

Some voluntary movement eventually returns, again in a characteristic pattern. Proximal muscles recover more

───────────────────────────────

★Hemiplegia (from the Greek –*plegia,* meaning "stroke"), strictly speaking, means total paralysis on one side. Because some voluntary movement returns after injury to the motor cortex or internal capsule, the condition is actually a hemiparesis (from the Greek *paresis,* meaning "slackening"), indicating weakness or partial paralysis.

than distal muscles, and movements of the fingers are the most severely and permanently affected. Skilled movements recover less than do coarser movements of entire limbs, suggesting that a major role of the corticospinal tract is to increase the speed and dexterity of movements whose basic characteristics can be generated by other descending pathways.

There Are Upper Motor Neurons for Cranial Nerve Motor Nuclei

Some corticospinal fibers, as we have seen, end directly on spinal motor neurons, whereas the rest end in the posterior horn, in the intermediate gray matter, or on interneurons of the anterior horn. Those not ending directly on motor neurons have a variety of effects, ranging from regulating the access of information to ascending pathways to affecting the activity of motor neurons via interneurons. In a similar manner, other fibers leave the cerebral cortex, descend through the internal capsule (immediately anterior to the corticospinal tract), and end in the brainstem on cells of sensory relay nuclei, of the reticular formation, and of motor nuclei of some cranial nerves. Strictly speaking, this entire collection of fibers is the **corticobulbar tract.**★ However, in common usage the term "corticobulbar tract" is often used to refer selectively to those fibers that affect the motor neurons of cranial nerves (Figure 18-17). As in the spinal cord, some of these corticobulbar fibers end directly on motor neurons, but most act through interneurons of the reticular forma-

───────────────────────────────

★*Bulb* is an old term for the medulla or, by extension, for the entire brainstem.

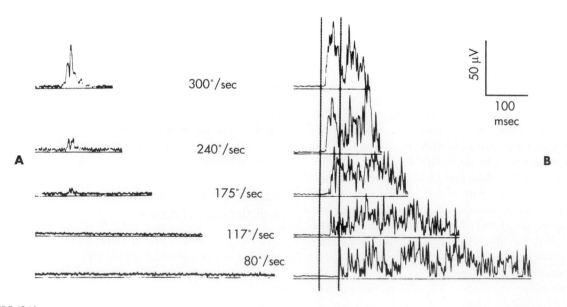

FIGURE 18-16

Biceps EMG records from a normal (**A**) and a spastic (**B**) subject in response to a 30° extension at the rates indicated. (From Thilmann AF, Fellows SJ, Garms E: The mechanism of spastic muscle hypertonus. Variation in reflex gain over the time course of spasticity, *Brain* 114:233, 1991.)

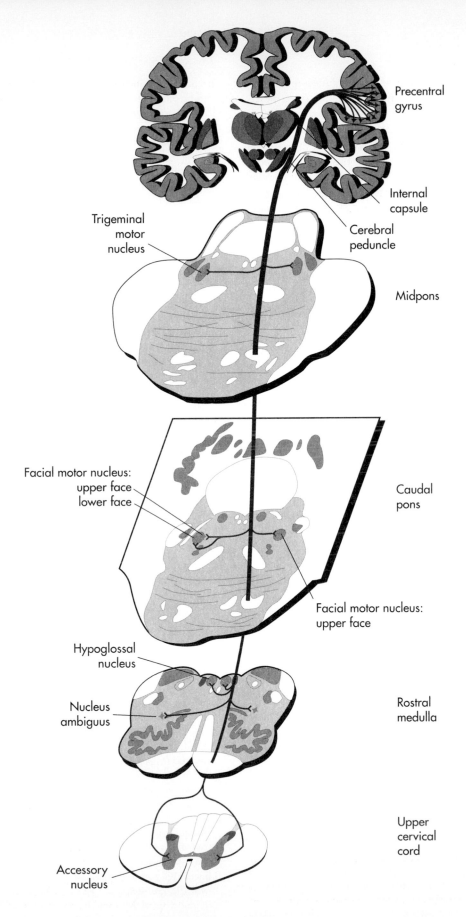

Precentral
gyrus

Internal
capsule

Cerebral
peduncle

Trigeminal
motor
nucleus

Midpons

Facial motor nucleus:
upper face
lower face

Caudal
pons

Facial motor nucleus:
upper face

Hypoglossal
nucleus

Nucleus
ambiguus

Rostral
medulla

Upper
cervical
cord

Accessory
nucleus

FIGURE 18-17
Corticobulbar pathway (except for cranial nerves III, IV, and VI). Three simplifications were used to keep the diagram manageable. First, corticobulbar fibers are shown ending directly on motor neurons, but most actually end on interneurons in the reticular formation. Second, corticobulbar fibers are shown with an equal bilateral distribution to the trigeminal, hypoglossal, and accessory nuclei. The trigeminal and hypoglossal nuclei and the trapezius motor neurons of the accessory nucleus often receive a preponderance of crossed fibers. Finally, all corticobulbar fibers are shown accompanying the corticospinal tract, whereas many actually leave this tract at various levels caudal to the cerebral peduncle and pursue a variety of aberrant courses through the brainstem.

tion. The oculomotor, trochlear, and abducens nuclei receive no direct corticobulbar fibers; there are other peculiarities about the innervation of these nuclei, so they are treated separately in Chapter 21. Thus the following discussion pertains to the trigeminal, facial, and hypoglossal motor nuclei, nucleus ambiguus, and the spinal accessory nucleus.

In general, these nuclei receive a bilateral corticobulbar innervation. The fibers originate from the face portion of the motor cortex and from other areas of the frontal and parietal lobes as well. They accompany the corticospinal tract almost to the level of the nucleus they influence. Here they part company with the corticospinal tract and end in the appropriate motor nucleus on both sides or in the adjacent reticular formation. The major exception to this general pattern is in the case of the facial motor nucleus. As mentioned in Chapter 12, motor neurons to the lower facial muscles are innervated mainly by contralateral cortex, whereas those to upper facial muscles are bilaterally innervated. The result is that an individual with unilateral corticobulbar damage (as in a lesion of one cerebral peduncle) would be unable to smile or bare the teeth symmetrically or puff out the contralateral cheek; however, the ability to blink and wrinkle the forehead on both sides would remain. In addition, even though the hypoglossal and trigeminal motor nuclei and those neurons of the spinal accessory nucleus that innervate the trapezius receive some input from the cortex of both hemispheres, the input from the contralateral side predominates (to a degree that varies from one individual to another). Hence after damage to the motor cortex, internal capsule, or cerebral peduncle on one side, there may be slight (and typically transient) weakness of the contralateral trapezius and masseter and the contralateral side of the tongue.*

SUGGESTED READINGS

Balagura S, Katz RG: Undecussated innervation to the sternocleidomastoid muscle: a reinstatement, *Ann Neurol* 7:84, 1980.

Brinkman J, Kuypers HGJM: Cerebral control of contralateral and ipsilateral arm, hand and finger movements in the split-brain rhesus monkey, *Brain* 96:653, 1973. *Complex but interesting experiments whose results indicate that each cerebral hemisphere can exercise some control over the movements of both arms but not the fingers of both hands.*

Brodal A: Self-observations and neuro-anatomical considerations after a stroke, *Brain* 96:675, 1973. *A fascinating account by an eminent neuroanatomist of a stroke suffered by him and the pattern of his recovery. Such an individual is able to provide information about motor control and other cerebral functions that is probably impossible to obtain in any other way.*

Bucy P, Keplinger JE, Siqueira EB: Destruction of the "pyramidal tract" in man, *J Neurosurg* 21:385, 1964.

Cruccu G, Fornarelli M, Manfredi M: Impairment of masticatory function in hemiplegia, *Neurol* 38:301, 1988.

Davidoff RA: The pyramidal tract, *Neurol* 40:332, 1990.

Dum RP, Strick PL: The corticospinal system: a structural framework for the central control of movement. In Rowell LB, Shepherd JT, editors: *Exercise: regulation and integration of multiple systems (handbook of physiology, section 12)*, New York, 1996, Oxford University Press.

Gerloff C et al: Stimulation over the human supplementary motor area interferes with the organization of future elements in complex motor sequences, *Brain* 120:1587, 1997.

Gilman S, Lieberman JS, Marco LA: Spinal mechanisms underlying the effects of unilateral ablation of areas 4 and 6 in monkeys, *Brain* 97:49, 1974. *How are motor and premotor cortex related to the mechanism of spasticity?*

Grillner S: Neurobiological bases of rhythmic motor acts in vertebrates, *Science* 228:143, 1985. *A brief review of central pattern generators.*

Grillner S, Wallén P: Central pattern generators for locomotion, with special reference to vertebrates, *Ann Rev Neurosci* 8:233, 1985.

Kleinschmidt A, Nitschke MF, Frahm J: Somatotopy in the human motor cortex hand area: a high-resolution functional MRI study, *Eur J Neurosci* 9:2178, 1997.

Kuypers HGJM: Corticobulbar connexions to the pons and lower brain-stem in man, *Brain* 81:364, 1958.

Laplane D et al: Clinical consequences of corticectomies involving the supplementary motor area in man, *J Neurol Sci* 34:301, 1977.

Lawrence DG, Hopkins DA: The development of motor control in the rhesus monkey: evidence concerning the role of corticomotoneuronal connections, *Brain* 99:235, 1966.

Lawrence DG, Kuypers HGJM: The functional organization of the motor system in the monkey. I. The effects of bilateral pyramidal lesions. II. The effects of lesions of the descending brain-stem pathways, *Brain* 91:1 and 15, 1968. *Two classic papers on the chronic effects of selective corticospinal lesions in primates, including information about which other descending pathways are able to compensate for loss of the corticospinal tract.*

Libet B: Unconscious cerebral initiative and the role of conscious will in voluntary action, *Behav Brain Sci* 8:529, 1985. *Under certain conditions, electrical changes related to voluntary movement appear to start in the brain **before** a person is aware of having decided to move. This paper and the commentaries that follow it discuss these experiments, their validity, and their philosophical implications.*

Lüders HO, editor: *Supplementary sensorimotor area (Adv Neurol, vol 70)*, Philadelphia, 1996, Lippincott-Raven.

Luppino G et al: Multiple representations of body movements in mesial area 6 and the adjacent cingulate cortex: an intracortical microstimulation study in the macaque monkey, *J Comp Neurol* 311:463, 1991. *In additional to the supplementary motor area, the medial surface of the hemisphere contains two additional regions from which movements can be elicited.*

---

*Corticobulbar innervation of sternocleidomastoid motor neurons is still a matter of debate. It is observed clinically that motor cortex damage is frequently followed by weakness of turning the head toward the side *contralateral* to the lesion, implying that one cerebral hemisphere projects to motor neurons for the *ipsilateral* sternocleidomastoid. However, electrical studies indicate that corticobulbar fibers for this muscle are distributed bilaterally with a contralateral preponderance. The apparent discrepancy may involve the role of other muscles, such as neck muscles and the platysma, in head turning.

Mushiake H, Inase M, Tanji J: Neuronal activity in the primate premotor, supplementary, and precentral motor cortex during visually guided and internally determined sequential movements, *J Neurophysiol* 66:705, 1991. *Electrophysiological evidence that the supplementary motor area is more involved in movements repeated from memory, and premotor cortex more involved in movements that follow sensory cues.*

Nathan PW, Smith MC: The rubrospinal and central tegmental tracts in man, *Brain* 105:223, 1982.

Nathan PW, Smith MC, Deacon P: The corticospinal tracts in man: course and location of fibres at different segmental levels, *Brain* 113:303, 1990.

Okano K, Tanji J: Neuronal activities in the primate motor fields of the agranular frontal cortex preceding visually triggered and self-paced movement, *Exp Brain Res* 66:155, 1987. *Description of a population of neurons in the supplementary motor area that change their firing rate many hundreds of milliseconds before a voluntary movement begins.*

Polit A, Bizzi E: Processes controlling arm movements in monkeys, *Science* 201:1235, 1978. *An article dealing with the motor abilities of a monkey receiving no afferent input from one arm.*

Ralston DD, Ralston HJ III: The terminations of corticospinal tract axons in the macaque monkey, *J Comp Neurol* 242:325, 1985.

Russell JR, DeMyer W: The quantitative cortical origin of pyramidal axons of *Macaca rhesus, Neurology* 11:96, 1961.

Thaler D et al: The functions of the medial premotor cortex. I. Simple learned movements, *Exp Brain Res* 102:445, 1995.

Thompson ML, Thickbroom GW, Mastaglia FL: Corticomotor representation of the sternocleidomastoid muscle, *Brain* 120:245, 1997.

Urban PP et al: The course of cortico-hypoglossal projections in the human brainstem: functional testing using transcranial magnetic stimulation, *Brain* 119:1031, 1996.

Wise SP et al: Premotor and parietal cortex: corticocortical connectivity and combinatorial computations, *Ann Rev Neurosci* 20:25, 1997.

Yousry TA et al: Localization of the motor hand area to a knob on the precentral gyrus: a new landmark, *Brain* 120:141, 1997.

Zilles K et al: Mapping of human and macaque sensorimotor areas by integrating architectonic, transmitter receptor, MRI and PET data, *J Anat* 187:515, 1995.

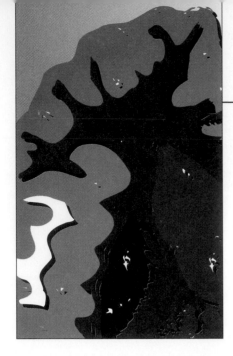

BASAL GANGLIA

In 1817 James Parkinson, an English country physician, published a brief monograph entitled *An Essay on the Shaking Palsy,* in which he described the symptoms of several individuals who had the disease that now bears his name. Parkinsonian patients, as described in more detail later in this chapter, are characterized by tremor, generally increased muscle tone, and difficulty in initiating voluntary movements (which are unusually slow once begun). Disorders of this sort, whose signs typically include involuntary movements and generalized alterations in muscle tone, have come to be associated with damage to the basal ganglia. They are often referred to as **extrapyramidal disorders,** although as explained in the previous chapter, such terminology can be somewhat misleading; for example, many of the involuntary movements are actually effected through the corticospinal tract.

THE BASAL GANGLIA INCLUDE FIVE MAJOR NUCLEI

The term *basal ganglia* originally referred to all the masses of gray matter buried within the cerebrum and thus included the **putamen, caudate nucleus, globus pallidus,** amygdala, claustrum, and occasionally even the thalamus (Figures 19-1 and 19-2). However, it is now used to refer to those structures whose damage causes "extrapyramidal" syndromes. This list of structures includes at least one brainstem nucleus but excludes some nuclei buried within the cerebrum. Thus the amygdala, claustrum, and thalamus are no longer spoken of as basal ganglia because the amygdala is part of the limbic system,*

---

*However, as discussed briefly in this chapter and in Chapter 23, there are connections between the limbic system and the basal ganglia, including projections from the amygdala to the striatum.

the claustrum has a largely unknown function, and the thalamus is part of a multitude of different pathways. Use of the term *basal ganglia* still varies, but most people mean the combination of caudate nucleus, putamen, globus pallidus, **subthalamic nucleus,** and **substantia nigra** (both **compact** and **reticular** parts; see Figure 11-21).

Various names are applied to different combinations of members of the basal ganglia (Figure 19-3). The putamen and globus pallidus together comprise the **lenticular** or **lentiform nucleus** (from the Latin word for "lentil"). The caudate nucleus and putamen have a common embryological origin, identical histological appearances, and similar connections. One indication of their common origin is the bridges of gray matter growing across the internal capsule between them, giving this region a striped appearance in many planes of section (Figure 19-4); hence the caudate nucleus and putamen together are referred to as the **striatum.**

These assorted names give rise to prefixes and suffixes that are used to describe fibers coming from or going to different members of the basal ganglia. *Strio-* and *-striate* are used for the striatum; thus *striopallidal* fibers go from the caudate nucleus or putamen to the globus pallidus, and *corticostriate* fibers go from the cerebral cortex to the caudate nucleus or putamen. The globus pallidus is also called the **pallidum,** so *pallidothalamic* fibers go from the globus pallidus to the thalamus. *Nigroreticular* fibers go from the substantia nigra to the reticular formation.

The Striatum and Globus Pallidus Are the Major Forebrain Components of the Basal Ganglia

The lenticular nucleus is shaped somewhat like a wedge cut from a sphere (Figures 19-1 and 19-2). The putamen (from the Latin for "husk"), which is approximately coex-

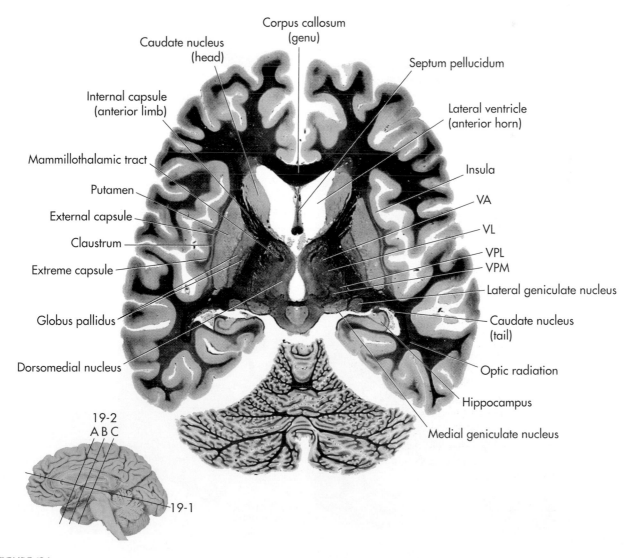

FIGURE 19-1
Basal ganglia and surrounding structures as seen in an approximately horizontal section. The inset shows the planes of section used in Figures 19-1 and 19-2. [Modified from Nolte J, Angevine JB Jr: *The human brain in photographs and diagrams,* St. Louis, 1995, Mosby.]

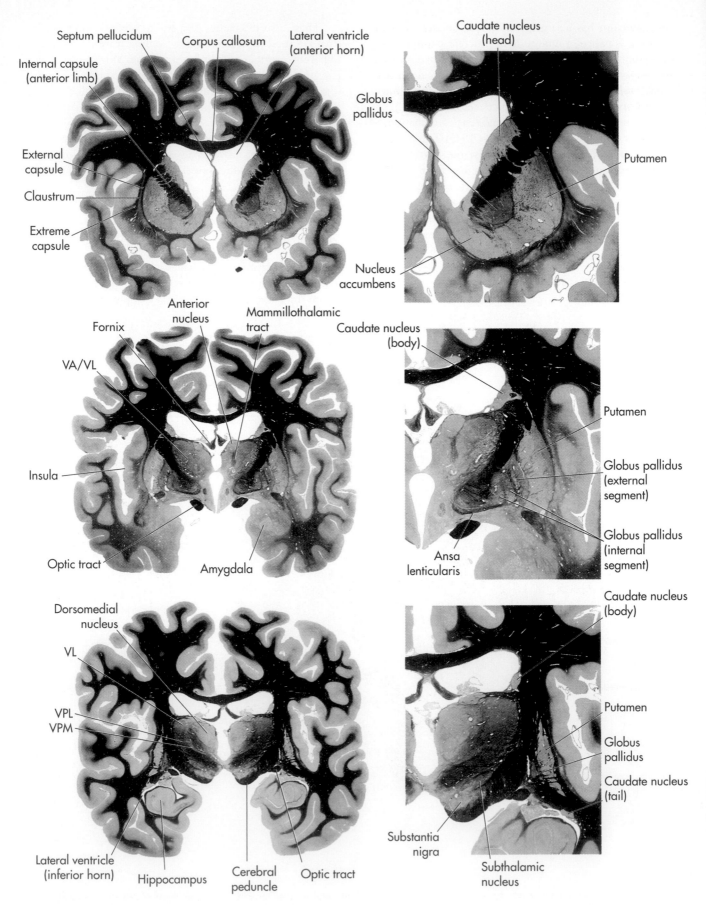

FIGURE 19-2
Basal ganglia and surrounding structures as seen in coronal sections.

tensive with the insula, forms the outermost portion of this wedge. It is separated from the more medial globus pallidus by a thin **lateral medullary lamina** of myelinated fibers. The globus pallidus is itself divided into **internal** and **external** (or **medial** and **lateral**) portions by a **medial medullary lamina.** In unstained sections through the lenticular nucleus, the globus pallidus has a distinctively pale appearance as a result of the large number of myelinated fibers that traverse it, terminate in it, and originate in it. (In myelin-stained sections such as those shown in Figures 19-1 and 19-2, it is therefore relatively dark.)

The caudate nucleus starts out embryologically from the same mass of cells that gives rise to the putamen. In the course of development, the caudate nucleus remains in the wall of the lateral ventricle and grows around with it in a C-shaped course. The caudate nucleus (Latin for "nucleus with a tail") of the adult has an enlarged **head** that bulges into the anterior horn, a **body** that forms the lateral wall of the body of the ventricle, and a slender **tail** that borders on the inferior horn (Figures 19-1, 19-2, and 19-5). The caudate nucleus and putamen retain their embryological continuity just above the orbital surface of the frontal lobe, where the head of the caudate appears to be

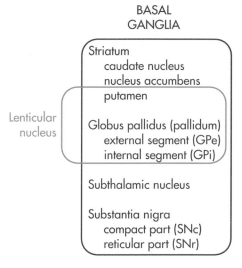

FIGURE 19-3
Terminology associated with the basal ganglia.

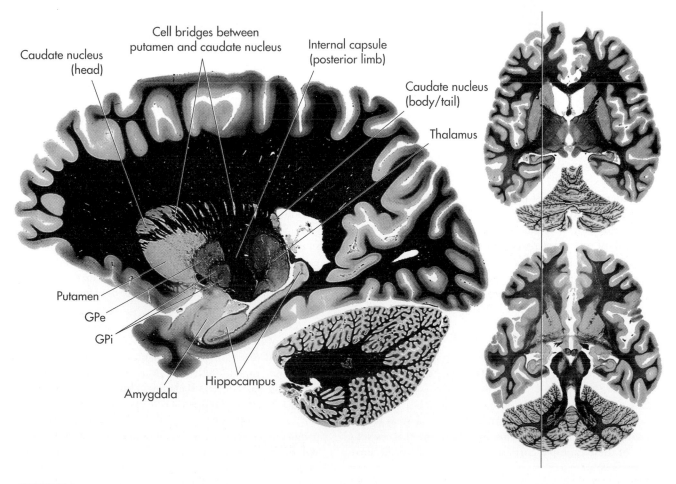

FIGURE 19-4
Parasagittal section showing how the striatum got its name. (Modified from Nolte J, Angevine JB Jr: *The human brain in photographs and diagrams,* St. Louis, 1995, Mosby.)

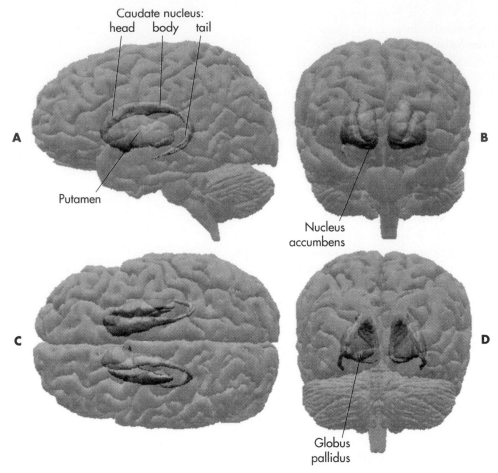

Caudate nucleus:
head   body   tail

A

Putamen

B

Nucleus
accumbens

C

D

Globus
pallidus

FIGURE 19-5
Three-dimensional reconstruction of the lenticular and caudate nuclei inside a translucent CNS, seen from the left (**A**), front (**B**), above (**C**), and behind (**D**).

continuous with the anterior part of the putamen. This region of continuity is the **nucleus accumbens,*** which (together with adjacent parts of the caudate nucleus, putamen, and base of the forebrain) forms a separate striatal division called the **ventral striatum.** In the temporal lobe, the tail of the caudate nucleus is continuous with the amygdala, which in turn is continuous with the putamen (see Figure 24-5), but these physical continuities are of no apparent functional significance.

BASAL GANGLIA CIRCUITRY INVOLVES MULTIPLE PARALLEL LOOPS THAT MODULATE CORTICAL OUTPUT

The principal circuit of the basal ganglia is a loop that starts with projections from multiple cortical areas to the basal ganglia and then returns, by way of the thalamus, to one of these multiple cortical areas (Figure 19-6, *A*). Pro-

---

*Named historically for its physical location. Its original name was **nucleus accumbens septi**—literally, "the nucleus leaning against the septum"—because the region of apparent fusion of the putamen and caudate nucleus appears to lean up against the base of the septum pellucidum (Figure 19-2).

jections from the cortex reach the striatum, which in this sense is the principal input element of the basal ganglia. Outputs leave from the internal segment of the globus pallidus and the reticular part of the substantia nigra (GPi/SNr). There are multiple versions of this loop, all similar in principle but each utilizing different cortical areas and a distinctive portion of the striatum and globus pallidus; each includes a frontal or limbic area among the cortical input areas, and each returns to a frontal or limbic area.

Axons leaving the striatum, globus pallidus, and reticular part of the substantia nigra use GABA as a neurotransmitter and make inhibitory synapses on their targets. Pallidal and nigral (SNr) neurons are tonically active, inhibiting parts of the thalamus. This is the key to basal ganglia function (Figure 19-6, *B*) because GPi/SNr neurons provide the final output from the basal ganglia. Basal ganglia processes that excite some of these output neurons will further inhibit the parts of the thalamus to which the neurons project. Conversely, inhibition of some of these output neurons will **disinhibit** the thalamus (i.e., release some parts of the thalamus from inhibition). Because thalamocortical connections are excitatory, GPi/SNr neurons are in a position to facilitate or suppress cortical activity.

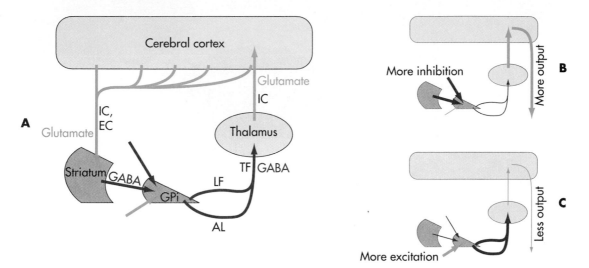

FIGURE 19-6

The principal circuit involving the basal ganglia. **A,** A schematic diagram showing the general elements of this circuit. The loop starts in multiple cortical areas and ends in one of these areas in the frontal lobe or limbic cortex. The bundles through which the fibers of this circuit travel are indicated by abbreviations: *AL,* Ansa lenticularis; *EC,* external capsule; *IC,* internal capsule; *LF,* lenticular fasciculus; *TF,* thalamic fasciculus. Excitatory connections are in *green,* inhibitory connections are in *red.* Particular cortical areas project to particular parts of the striatum, which is the input nucleus of the basal ganglia. Outputs of the striatum are inhibitory, some ending in the internal segment of the globus pallidus, which (together with the reticular part of the substantia nigra [not indicated]) provides the inhibitory output from the basal ganglia to the thalamus. The balance of inhibitory and excitatory inputs to GPi/SNr determines the amount and pattern of inhibition of the thalamus. **B,** A preponderance of inhibitory inputs to GPi/SNr will disinhibit the thalamus and facilitate cortical output. **C,** A preponderance of excitatory inputs to GPi/SNr will inhibit the thalamus and suppress cortical output.

The major circuit through which the basal ganglia participate in the control of movement provides one example of such a loop (Figure 19-7, *A*). The striatum and globus pallidus form by far the largest part of the basal ganglia, yet they have no way to affect motor neurons directly (see Figure 18-7). Thus the only way the basal ganglia can play a role in the control of movement is by somehow influencing one or more of the descending pathways mentioned in the previous chapter. They do so primarily by affecting the activity of motor areas of the cerebral cortex. Somatosensory and motor areas project to a portion of the striatum (mostly putamen), which in turn projects by way of the globus pallidus to VL/VA; the circuit is completed by projections from VL/VA back to motor areas of the cortex. Other basal ganglia loops use their own distinctive portions of the striatum, globus pallidus, thalamus, and cerebral cortex. Collectively the loops roughly correspond to the putamen, caudate nucleus, and ventral striatum, which receive inputs from motor/somatosensory cortex, association cortex, and limbic areas, respectively (Figure 19-7, *B*).

Most of the remaining connections of the basal ganglia, described a little later in this chapter, fall into three categories: interconnections of the compact part of the substantia nigra (SNc) with the striatum (Figure 19-8, *A*), interconnections of the subthalamic nucleus with the globus pallidus (Figure 19-8, *B*), and interconnections of thalamic intralaminar nuclei with the striatum and globus pallidus. In the account that follows, only the best-documented connections of the basal ganglia are described. Although the precise function of most of these connections is un-

known, there has been enough recent progress that we can not only consider the consequences of damage to some of these connections, but also begin to speculate about their normal functions.

The Cerebral Cortex, Substantia Nigra, and Thalamus Project to the Striatum

The caudate nucleus, putamen, and ventral striatum receive inputs from the cerebral cortex, the substantia nigra (SNc), and the intralaminar nuclei of the thalamus (Figure 19-9). The cortical input is by far the most massive of the three. These fibers originate in all areas of the cortex, pass through the internal and external capsules, and end in a roughly topographical pattern in the striatum. The projection from the motor and somatosensory cortex thus goes mostly to the putamen. The caudate nucleus, as it curves around with the ventricular system, receives most of the projections from association areas; as the size and location of the head of the caudate might imply, the projection is particularly heavy from prefrontal cortex. Finally, the ventral striatum receives inputs not only from limbic cortex, but also from the hippocampus and amygdala. Thus the basal ganglia are constantly informed about most aspects of cortical function. The substantia nigra projects to all areas of the striatum in a point-to-point fashion by way of very fine axons that use dopamine as their neurotransmitter. Destruction of this **nigrostriatal** pathway is the major factor causing Parkinson's disease (Figure 19-18). Finally, the intralaminar nuclei, especially the centromedian and parafascicular nuclei, project to the striatum. Many of

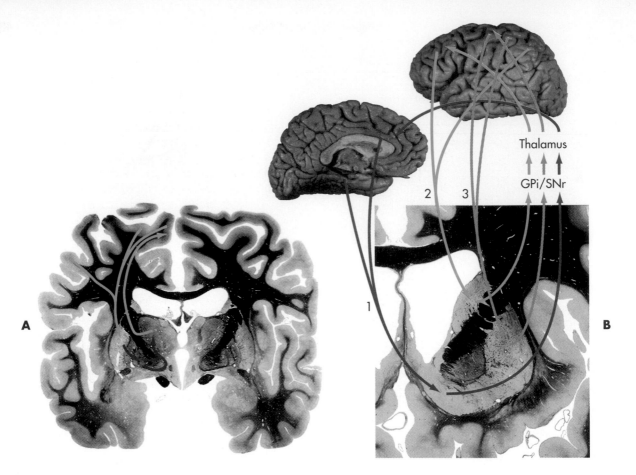

FIGURE 19-7

Parallel loops through the basal ganglia. **A,** The principal circuit involving the basal ganglia, projected onto the coronal section shown in Figure 19-2, B. At this level, near the central sulcus, the circuit primarily involves sensory and motor cortex on either side of the central sulcus, the putamen, and motor areas of cortex. These connections are mostly uncrossed, but there is some bilaterality (not shown). Excitatory connections are in *green,* inhibitory connections are in *red.* **B,** The three general categories of parallel loops, with inputs directed to the putamen *(3),* caudate nucleus *(2),* and ventral striatum *(1).*

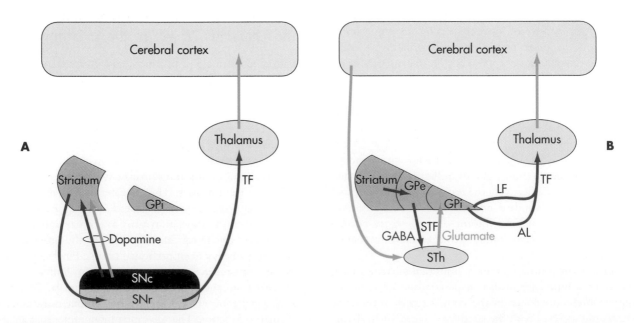

FIGURE 19-8

Two additional basal ganglia circuits of importance. Excitatory connections are in *green,* inhibitory connections are in *red.* **A,** The substantia nigra is interconnected with the striatum. As described further in the text, the pigmented, compact part of the substantia nigra *(SNc)* projects to the striatum, exciting some striatal neurons and inhibiting others; the striatum projects to the reticular part of the substantia nigra *(SNr),* which, like GPi, projects to the thalamus via the thalamic fasciculus *(TF).* **B,** The subthalamic nucleus receives inputs from the cerebral cortex and also is reciprocally connected with the globus pallidus. As described further in the text, this allows a substantial degree of subthalamic control over pallidal output. Abbreviations for fiber bundles: *AL,* Ansa lenticularis; *LF,* lenticular fasciculus; *STF,* subthalamic fasciculus; *TF,* thalamic fasciculus. A basal ganglia loop involving the centromedian and parafascicular nuclei of the thalamus is also prominent anatomically, but was omitted from these schematic diagrams because its functional significance is unclear.

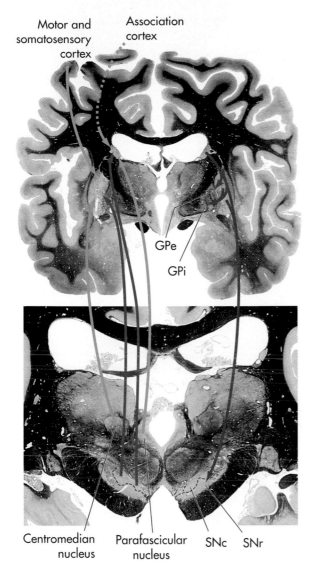

Motor and somatosensory cortex

Association cortex

GPe

GPi

Centromedian nucleus   Parafascicular nucleus   SNc   SNr

FIGURE 19-9
Connections of the striatum (putamen and caudate nucleus; ventral striatum not indicated). Afferents to the striatum are on the left, efferents from the striatum are on the right. Excitatory connections are in *green*, inhibitory connections are in *red*. (Inputs from SNc are shown in a third color because they excite some striatal neurons and inhibit others.) Projections from association cortex to the caudate nucleus are represented by a dashed line because for the most part they arise from cortical areas not in this plane of section.

these same fibers, as mentioned in Chapter 16, have collateral branches that end in the cerebral cortex. This **thalamostriate** pathway is particularly well developed in primates, but very little is known of its function. As described later in this chapter, various clinical findings can be associated with damage to different parts of the basal ganglia and their connections; however, there are no particular symptoms that we can ascribe to malfunction of the intralaminar nuclei→basal ganglia→intralaminar nuclei loop.

The caudate nucleus and putamen are cytologically uniform, and it was thought for a time that they were functionally uniform as well. However, it is now known

that they are divided into discrete patches, or **striosomes,** embedded in a background **matrix,** both compartments having distinctive types of connections and types of neurotransmitters (Figure 19-10). It seems likely that the striosomes and matrix fit together in some as yet undefined modular way to form striatal functional units.

In addition, the putamen, caudate nucleus, and ventral striatum, by virtue of their participation in different basal ganglia loops, have somewhat different functions. The putamen receives most of the inputs from motor and somatosensory areas of cortex and projects by way of the globus pallidus and thalamus to the motor, premotor, and supplementary motor areas. Corresponding to this, individual neurons in the putamen fire in conjunction with particular movements or positions, and stimulation of small areas of the putamen causes discrete movements. Thus the putamen is probably centrally involved in most of the motor functions of the basal ganglia. The caudate nucleus, in contrast, receives most of its inputs from association areas of cortex and projects by way of the globus pallidus and thalamus mostly to prefrontal areas. Few caudate neurons respond to movements or positions. Thus the caudate nucleus is involved more prominently in cognitive functions and less directly in movement (Box 19-1). The limbic connections of the ventral striatum indicate its probable role in the initiation of drive-related behavior (see Figure 23-23).

The Striatum Projects to the Globus Pallidus and Substantia Nigra

Striatal efferents collect into numerous bundles of myelinated fibers that converge on the globus pallidus. Most of them are striopallidal fibers; some terminate in the internal segment of the globus pallidus, others in the external segment. Still others pass through the globus pallidus and reach the substantia nigra.

The Globus Pallidus and Substantia Nigra Provide the Output From the Basal Ganglia

Afferents to both segments of the globus pallidus arise in the striatum and the subthalamic nucleus (Figure 19-12). As Figure 19-13 shows, the subthalamic nucleus is located right across the internal capsule from the globus pallidus. The small bundles of fibers that cross the internal capsule and interconnect these two nuclei are collectively called the **subthalamic fasciculus.**

Although the two segments of the globus pallidus have similar inputs, their efferents are separate and distinct (Figure 19-12). The external segment projects through the subthalamic fasciculus to the subthalamic nucleus, as well as to other sites such as the internal segment of the globus pallidus. The internal pallidal segment projects mainly to the thalamus through two collections of fibers. One collection, the **lenticular fasciculus,** runs directly through

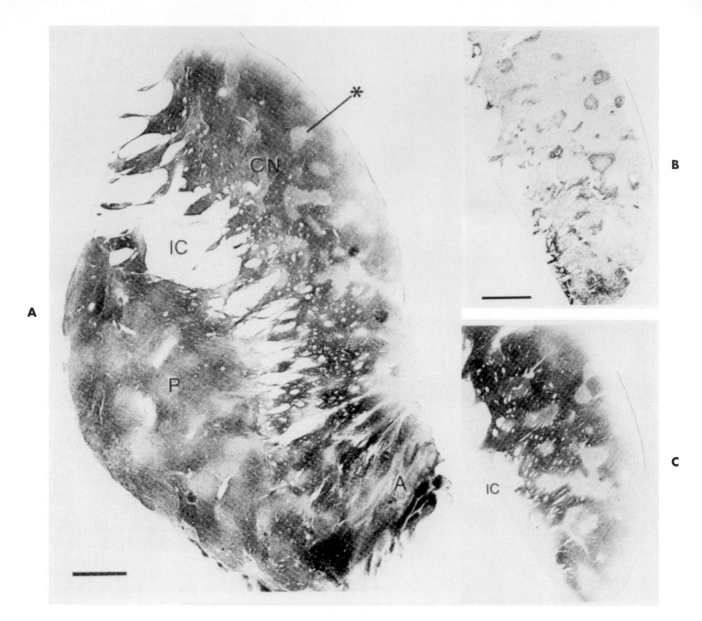

FIGURE 19-10

Chemical compartmentalization of the striatum. **A,** A coronal section through a human putamen *(P)* and caudate nucleus *(CN)*, separated by the anterior limb of the internal capsule *(IC)*. The area of fusion of the caudate and putamen is called *nucleus accumbens (A)* and has limbic connections. Histochemical staining for the enzyme acetylcholinesterase (AChE) was applied to the section, revealing that the striatum is made up of an AChE-rich background (matrix) with embedded AChE-poor regions (one indicated by an asterisk). The AChE-poor regions are about 300 to 600 μm wide and are often referred to as *striosomes*. Scale mark = 3 mm. Matrix and striosome regions have a number of other chemical differences. An example is shown in **B** and **C**, two adjacent coronal sections through the head of a human caudate nucleus. The section in **B** was stained immunocytochemically for enkephalin; the section in **C** was stained for AChE. High enkephalin levels are found precisely in the striosomes, especially around their peripheries. Scale mark = 3 mm. [From Graybiel AM: Neurochemically specified subsystems in the basal ganglia. In *Functions of the basal ganglia*, Ciba Foundation Symposium 107, London, 1984, Pitman.]

Box 19-1   A Case of Bilateral Damage to the Caudate Nucleus

Damage in the basal ganglia is usually associated with movement disorders, as in Parkinson's disease. However, the loop from association cortex, through the caudate nucleus, and ultimately back to prefrontal association cortex implies that caudate damage would result in findings related to those that occur after prefrontal damage (see Chapter 22). Several cases consistent with this idea have been reported, none more striking than the case of a 25-year-old woman who incurred extensive bilateral damage to the head of the caudate nucleus (Figure 19-11).

> Prior to the onset of her illness she had been a high school honor student, was employed full-time, had been living independently, and was engaged to be married. From February to

March of 1983 she suffered from daily headaches with occasional nausea and vomiting. In April she disappeared for 3 days. When found, she had undergone a dramatic personality change manifested by alterations in affect, motivation, cognition, and self-care. . . Her abnormal behaviors included vulgarity, impulsiveness, easy frustration, violent outbursts, hypersomnia, enuresis, indifference, wandering, increased appetite, polydipsia, hypersexuality, minor criminal behavior including shoplifting and exposing herself, and poor hygiene. . . . [A year later] the patient had married and divorced, continued to be unemployed, and had little improvement in behavior. Two psychiatric hospitalizations and treatment with a variety of major tranquilizers were not beneficial.*

*From Richfield EK, Twyman R, Berent S: Neurological syndrome following bilateral damage to the head of the caudate nuclei, *Ann Neurol* 22:768, 1987.

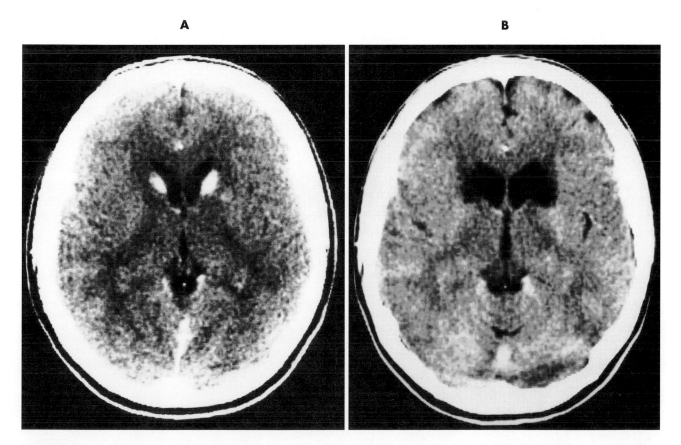

A   **B**

FIGURE 19-11

Contrast-enhanced CT scans immediately after the patient's 3-day disappearance (**A**) and 8 months later (**B**). Contrast enhancement, indicative of pathology and blood-brain barrier breakdown, was seen in the head of the caudate nucleus bilaterally in the early scan. Eight months later, these areas were about the same density as CSF, as though the heads of the caudate nuclei had degenerated. The cause of the pathology was never determined. (From Richfield EK, Twyman R, Berent S: Neurological syndrome following bilateral damage to the head of the caudate nuclei, *Ann Neurol* 22:768, 1987.)

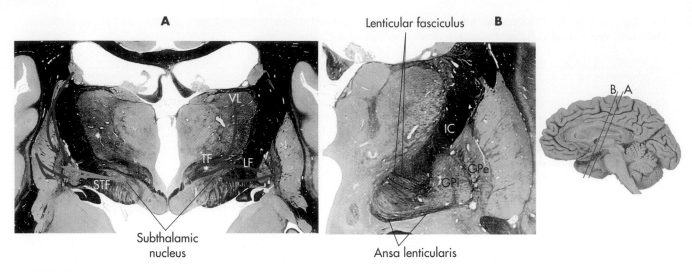

FIGURE 19-12

A, Connections of the globus pallidus; afferents to the globus pallidus on the left, efferents from the globus pallidus on the right. Excitatory connections are in *green*, inhibitory connections are in *red*. Plane of section shown in the inset to the right. Efferents to the centromedian and parafascicular nuclei are not indicated because these nuclei are posterior to this level. **B,** Enlargement of part of the section in Figure 19-2, *B,* showing fibers of the lenticular fasciculus passing through the internal capsule *(IC)* and the ansa lenticularis hooking around it.*, Zona incerta. Other abbreviations for fiber bundles: *LF,* Lenticular fasciculus; *STF,* subthalamic fasciculus; *TF,* thalamic fasciculus.

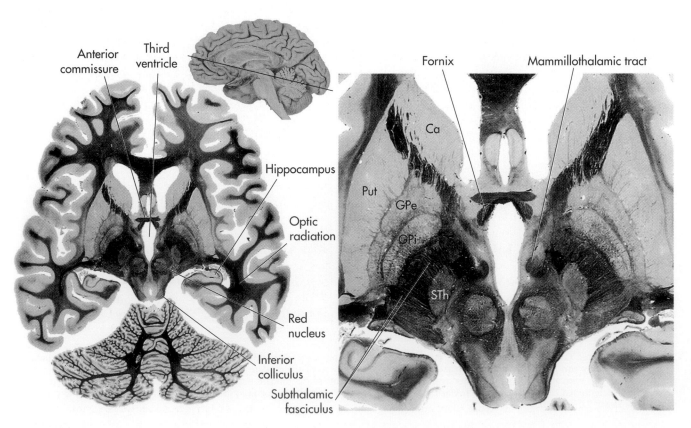

FIGURE 19-13

The subthalamic fasciculus as seen in a horizontal section. *Subthalamic fasciculus* is a collective term for the small bundles of fibers that pass through the internal capsule interconnecting the subthalamic nucleus *(STh)* and the globus pallidus *(GPe, GPi). Ca,* Head of the caudate nucleus; *Put,* putamen. [Modified from Nolte J, Angevine JB Jr: *The human brain in photographs and diagrams,* St. Louis, 1995, Mosby.]

the internal capsule and then passes medially as a sheet of fibers between the subthalamic nucleus and the zona incerta (Figure 19-12). At the medial edge of the zona incerta, the lenticular fasciculus makes a hairpin turn in a lateral and dorsal direction and enters the thalamus. The second collection loops around the medial edge of the internal capsule as the **ansa lenticularis** (the Latin word *ansa* means "loop") (Figures 19-2 and 19-12); it joins the lenticular fasciculus in the **thalamic fasciculus,**★ which then enters the thalamus. The thalamic fasciculus terminates in a variety of thalamic nuclei. Fibers related to movement control end in VL/VA, those related to the caudate nucleus and prefrontal cortex end in the dorsomedial nucleus and in part of VA, and others end in the centromedian and parafascicular nuclei. The VL/VA and dorsomedial nuclei then project to frontal cortex, thus completing the principal circuit through the basal ganglia (Figure 19-6).

A few fibers leave the ansa lenticularis and lenticular fasciculus to end in the habenula, the substantia nigra, the superior colliculus, and in a portion of the midbrain tegmentum that in turn projects to the reticular formation. However, their numbers are meager compared with the major outputs to the thalamus and subthalamic nucleus.

The Subthalamic Nucleus Is Part of an Indirect Pathway Through the Basal Ganglia

The subthalamic nucleus provides a powerful excitatory input to GPi/SNr neurons, and is thereby thought to play a major role in determining the pattern of inhibitory output from the basal ganglia. Major inputs to the subthalamic nucleus (Figure 19-14, *A*) arise in the external segment of the globus pallidus (GPe) and in the cerebral cortex (especially motor cortex). Although subthalamic connections are actually considerably more widespread than this, and the determinants of subthalamic output are not fully understood, this nucleus is usually considered to occupy a pivotal position in an **indirect pathway** (Figure 19-14, *B*) through the basal ganglia (in contrast to the cortex→striatum→GPi/SNr→ thalamus→cortex **direct pathway**). Because the direct and indirect pathways have opposite effects on GPi/SNr neurons (Figure 19-19), the balance of activity in these two pathways may facilitate some cortical outputs while simultaneously suppressing others.

Part of the Substantia Nigra Modulates the Output of the Striatum

The region referred to as the *substantia nigra* actually has two parts, a dorsal compact part containing closely packed, pigmented neurons and a reticular part nearer the cerebral peduncle containing more loosely packed neurons, most of which are nonpigmented. These correspond to two distinctly different ways in which the substantia nigra participates in the circuitry of the basal ganglia (Figures 19-8, *A* and 19-15).

The reticular part of the substantia nigra resembles in many respects a displaced portion of the internal segment of the globus pallidus. Like GPi, the reticular part of the substantia nigra receives inputs from the striatum and the subthalamic nucleus, and projects to VL/VA and the dorsomedial nucleus of the thalamus. It is in fact a more important route for information from the caudate nucleus to reach the thalamus than is the globus pallidus. In addition, projections from the reticular part of the substantia nigra to the superior colliculus and the reticular formation have been described. The connection with the superior colliculus is one route through which the basal ganglia participate in the control of eye movements.

The pigmented neurons of the compact part of the substantia nigra, which use dopamine as their neurotransmitter, project in a precisely organized topographic fashion to the caudate nucleus, putamen, and ventral striatum. These dopaminergic endings in the striatum ultimately modulate the output from the globus pallidus (Figure 19-19). Defects in this influence can result in movement disorders (putamen connections) and presumably in cognitive deficits as well (caudate connections). Comparable dopaminergic projections to the ventral striatum arise mainly in the ventral tegmental area and have been implicated in such limbic functions as responses to novel or rewarding stimuli (see Figure 23-23).

PENETRATING BRANCHES FROM THE CIRCLE OF WILLIS SUPPLY THE BASAL GANGLIA

Like other deep structures located superior to the circle of Willis, the basal ganglia receive their blood supply from small ganglionic or penetrating branches of arteries in and adjacent to the circle. One would therefore expect the substantia nigra and subthalamic nucleus, located just below the posterior thalamus (Figure 19-2, *C*), to be supplied by branches from posterior portions of the circle of Willis. The striatum and globus pallidus are mostly anterior to this level (Figure 19-1), and so their supply should come from more anterior portions of the circle. Hence the substantia nigra and subthalamic nucleus are mainly supplied by penetrating branches of the posterior cerebral and posterior communicating arteries, the striatum by penetrating branches of the middle cerebral artery (also referred to as **lateral striate** or **lenticulostriate arteries**), and the globus pallidus by the anterior choroidal artery (see Figure 6-20). Branches of the anterior cerebral artery help supply the striatum in the vicinity of the nucleus accumbens and the head of the caudate nucleus; one

---

★This complex bundle also includes cerebellar output fibers described in the next chapter.

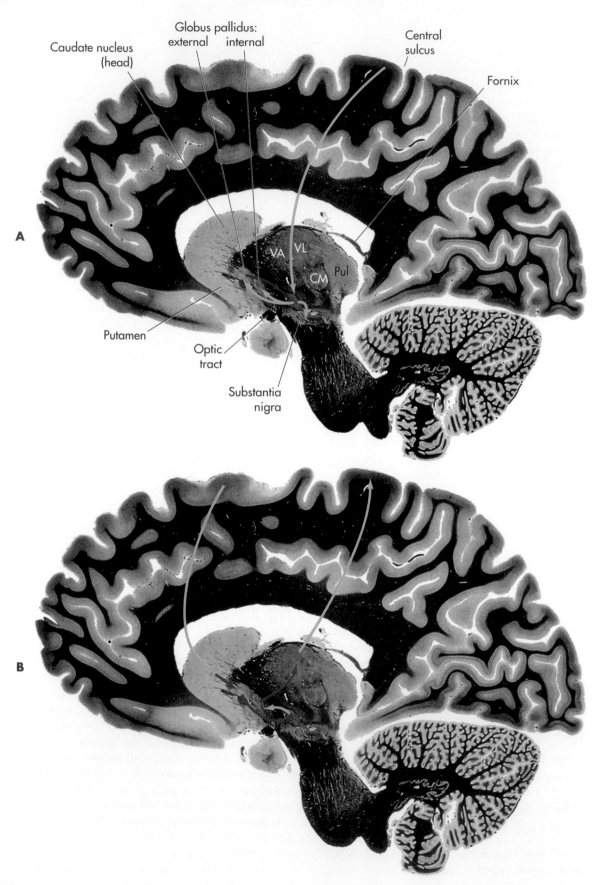

FIGURE 19-14
Major connections of the subthalamic nucleus, as seen in a parasagittal section. Excitatory connections are in *green*, inhibitory connections are in *red*. **A,** Inputs and outputs. *CM,* Centromedian nucleus; *Pul,* pulvinar; *VA* and *VL,* ventral anterior and ventral lateral nuclei. **B,** The indirect pathway involving the subthalamic nucleus: cortex→striatum→GPe→subthalamic nucleus→GPi→thalamus→cortex. [Modified from Nolte J, Angevine JB Jr: *The human brain in photographs and diagrams,* St. Louis, 1995, Mosby.]

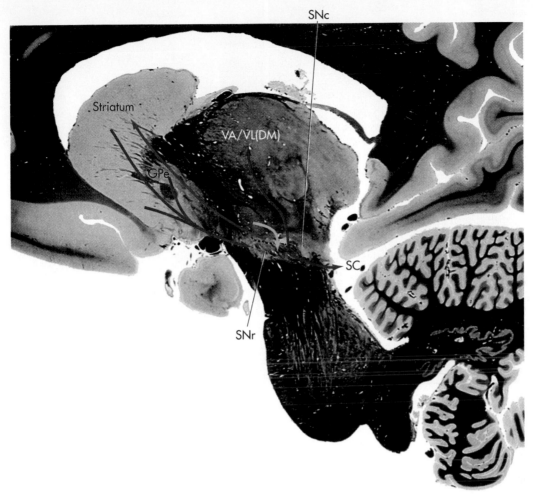

FIGURE 19-15
Major connections of the substantia nigra, as seen in an enlarged version of the same parasagittal section shown in Figure 19-14. Excitatory connections are in *green*, inhibitory connections are in *red*. (Outputs from SNc are shown in a third color because they excite some striatal neurons and inhibit others.) *DM,* Dorsomedial nucleus (indicated parenthetically because it is not actually present this far from the midline); *GPe,* external segment of the globus pallidus; *SC,* superior colliculus (also not present this far from the midline); *SNc* and *SNr,* compact and reticular parts of the substantia nigra; *VA* and *VL,* ventral anterior and ventral lateral nuclei. (Modified from Nolte J, Angevine JB Jr: *The human brain in photographs and diagrams,* St. Louis, 1995, Mosby.)

of these may be a particularly large branch referred to as the **medial striate artery** (of Heubner).

MANY BASAL GANGLIA DISORDERS RESULT IN ABNORMALITIES OF MOVEMENT

Involuntary movements and disturbances of muscle tone figure prominently in the best-known disorders involving the basal ganglia. The involuntary movements are customarily subdivided into tremors and states of **chorea, athetosis,** and **ballismus.** The disturbances of tone may be such that tone is increased in flexors and extensors generally (as in the rigidity of Parkinson's disease), or in only some muscles so that the patient's body is bent or twisted into an abnormal, relatively fixed posture. The latter condition is called **dystonia.** In still other cases, tone may be decreased.

Patients with chorea (from the Greek word for "dance") exhibit a series of nearly continuous rapid movements of the face, tongue, or limbs (usually the distal portions of the limbs). The movements often resemble fragments of normal voluntary movements. **Huntington's disease** (formerly called **Huntington's chorea**) is a hereditary disorder characterized by neuronal degeneration that is particularly severe in the striatum, especially in the caudate nucleus (Figure 19-16), and to a lesser extent affects neurons in the cerebral cortex and elsewhere. Typically symptoms first appear between the ages of 30 and 50 as some combination of involuntary choreiform movements and alterations of mood or cognitive function. The movements slowly become more pronounced, and this symptom is followed by or accompanied by gradually worsening dementia and personality changes. The chorea is presumably caused by striatal degeneration, and the dementia by some combination of caudate and cortical degeneration. This is a particularly nasty disease because it is

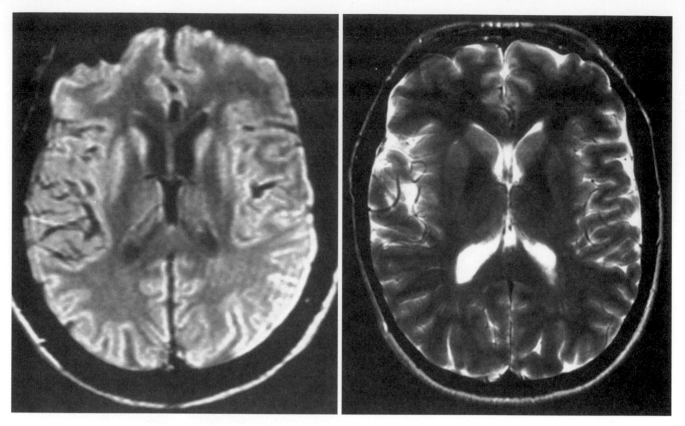

FIGURE 19-16

Horizontal MRIs of a 29-year-old man with Huntington's disease (**A**) and of a normal individual (**B**). Notice how much smaller the caudate nucleus and putamen are in **A**, and how the anterior horn of the lateral ventricle has expanded to take up the volume vacated by the caudate nucleus. (**A** courtesy Dr. Erwin B. Montgomery, Jr., The University of Arizona College of Medicine. **B** courtesy Dr. Roger Bird, St. Joseph's Hospital, Phoenix.)

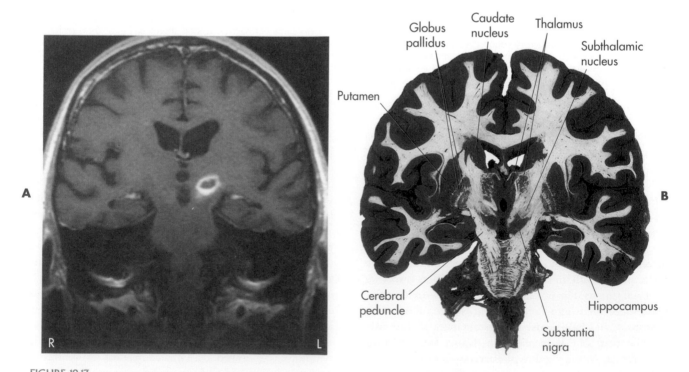

FIGURE 19-17

Hemiballismus. **A**, A 65-year-old HIV-positive man developed, over the course of several months, "unintentional, forceful flinging movements of his right arm and leg." Contrast-enhanced coronal MRI revealed a rim-enhancing mass (an appearance characteristic of an abscess) in the location of the subthalamic nucleus (compare to **B**). The involuntary movements resolved after several weeks of antitoxoplasmosis treatment. **B**, A coronal slice of a normal brain, in approximately the same plane as **A**. (**A** from Provenzale JM, Schwarzschild MA: Hemiballismus, *AJNR Am J Neuroradiol* 15:1377, 1994. **B** prepared by Pamela Eller, University of Colorado Health Sciences Center.)

inherited as an autosomal dominant, but is usually not manifested until after individuals are old enough to have started families. The defective gene has been localized to the short arm of chromosome 4, and tests are now available to determine if a potential victim is indeed a carrier and will develop the disease. Hence it is also possible to determine whether half of the children of an individual at risk are likely to be affected.

Athetosis (from a Greek word meaning "without position") is characterized by slow, writhing movements, most pronounced in the hands and fingers, so that a patient may be unable to keep the affected limb in a fixed position (hence the name "athetosis"). The responsible lesion seems to be in the striatum. All intermediate forms between chorea and athetosis are seen, and questionable cases are often referred to as **choreoathetosis.** No one knows why a particular lesion in the striatum should induce one state rather than the other.

Hemiballismus (ballismus comes from a Greek word meaning "jumping about") is one of the most dramatic of the disorders of the basal ganglia. Its most prominent characteristic is wild flailing movements of one arm and leg. The responsible lesion is in the contralateral subthalamic nucleus (Figure 19-17). Hemiballismus is most often seen in older people, having been caused by a stroke involving a small ganglionic branch of the posterior cerebral artery. The reason movements are seen contralateral to the lesion is apparent from Figure 19-14: each subthalamic nucleus is related by way of GPi/SNr and VL/VA primarily to the ipsilateral motor cortex, which in turn is concerned with movements of the contralateral side of the body.

Parkinson's disease (Figure 19-18) is the most common and best-known disease involving the basal ganglia. The symptoms are variable in relative severity and onset, but they usually include tremor, rigidity, and difficulty in moving. The tremor is a **resting tremor,** characteristically involving the hands in a "pill-rolling" movement; it diminishes during voluntary movement and increases during emotional stress. The **rigidity** is caused by increased tone in all muscles, although strength is nearly normal and reflexes are not particularly affected. The rigidity may be uniform throughout the range of movements imposed by an examiner (called **plastic** or **lead-pipe rigidity**), or it may be interrupted by a series of brief relaxations (called **cog-wheel rigidity**). Thus parkinsonian rigidity is quite distinct from spasticity; in spastic patients muscle tone is increased selectively in the extensors of the leg and the flexors of the arm and can be overcome in the clasp-knife reaction, and stretch reflexes are hyperactive. Finally, the difficulty in moving (**bradykinesia,** or slow movements; **hypokinesia,** or few movements) is shown by such things as decreased blinking, an expressionless face, and the absence of the arm movements normally associated with walking. Bradykinesia and hypokinesia are fundamental deficits; they are not simply the result of rigidity because

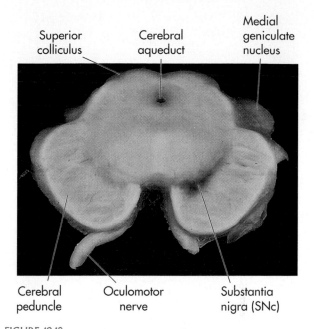

FIGURE 19-18
The midbrain of a patient with Parkinson's disease, showing loss of pigmentation in the compact part of the substantia nigra, more pronounced on the right side. (Courtesy Dr. Naomi Rance, The University of Arizona College of Medicine.)

patients whose rigidity is not pronounced can nevertheless have great difficulty moving.

Anatomical and Neurochemical Properties of the Basal Ganglia Suggest Effective Treatments for Disorders

Many disorders of the basal ganglia include striking positive signs (e.g., tremor, rigidity, and ballistic movements), in which motor neurons are made to fire when they should not; they may also include negative signs as well (e.g., hypokinesia), in which motor neurons cannot easily be made to fire by their owner. Recent advances in our knowledge of the anatomy and physiology of the basal ganglia now allow some tentative explanations of these clinical observations.

Each small portion of the internal segment of the globus pallidus has an inhibitory influence on the restricted portion of the thalamus to which it projects. Thalamocortical projections are excitatory. Hence changes in the activity of a small portion of the globus pallidus cause inverse changes in the activity of a corresponding small cortical area. Thus the basal ganglia may function by facilitating activity in some cortical areas and suppressing activity in others. One recent model proposes that the direct cortex→striatum→GPi/SNr→thalamus→cortex loop facilitates selected cortical activity (Figure 19-19, *A*), while activity in the indirect loop involving the subthalamic nucleus suppresses other cortical activity (Figure 19-19, *B*). A further implication is that decreased activity of neurons in the subthalamic nucleus should cause disor-

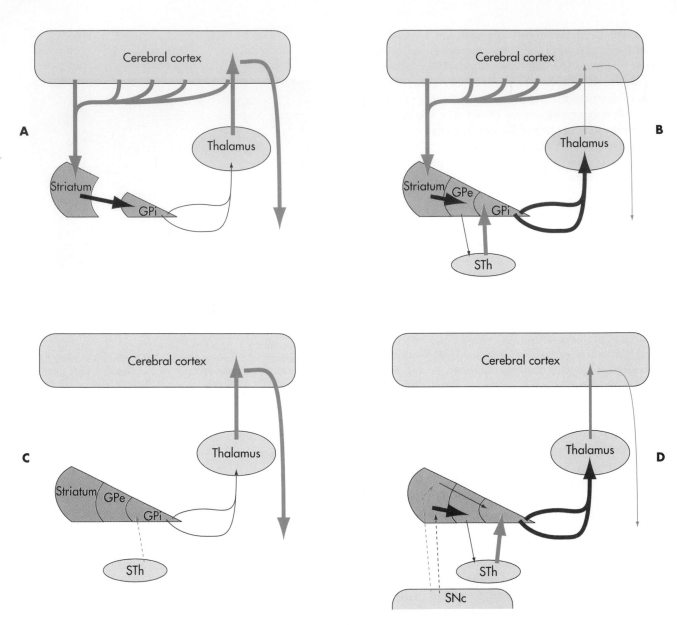

FIGURE 19-19

Some of the excitatory *(green)* and inhibitory *(red)* interactions in the basal ganglia, with an indication of how they may function together to affect cortical output in health and disease. This is by no means a complete depiction of all such interactions in the basal ganglia, but it does provide an illustration of how alteration of single elements could unbalance the entire system. The level of activity in each pathway is roughly indicated by the thickness of a line; dashed lines indicate projections that have been lost. **A,** The effect of the direct pathway through the basal ganglia in a normal individual. The striatum inhibits GPi (and SNr, which is not indicated), thus disinhibiting the thalamus. This allows the thalamus to facilitate certain cortical outputs. **B,** The effect of the indirect pathway, utilizing the subthalamic nucleus, in a normal individual. In this case, diminished output from the external pallidal segment (GPe) leads indirectly to increased inhibition of the thalamus and to diminished cortical output. Acting together, the direct and indirect pathways (**A** and **B**) could facilitate activity in some cortical areas while inhibiting activity in others. **C,** Loss of excitatory subthalamic projections would disinhibit the thalamus, in turn leading to a failure to suppress some cortical outputs, which could manifest itself as involuntary movements (as in hemiballismus). **D,** The striatal neurons projecting into the direct and indirect pathways have different dopamine receptors; dopamine excites the former and inhibits the latter. In Parkinson's disease, loss of dopaminergic neurons from the compact part of the substantia nigra (SNc) causes decreased activity in the direct pathway and increased activity in the indirect pathway, both of which enhance the output of GPi/SNr. The resulting inhibition of the thalamus causes a diminished cortical output that could underlie bradykinesia and hypokinesia.

ders that include many involuntary movements (hyperkinetic disorders), whereas increased activity of subthalamic neurons should cause hypokinetic disorders. Many of the clinical observations described earlier are consistent with this. The involuntary movements of hemiballismus result from direct damage to the contralateral subthalamic nucleus (Figure 19-19, *C*). Removal of the dopaminergic in-

put to the striatum, as in Parkinson's disease and its accompanying hypokinesia, results in increased subthalamic activity (Figure 19-19, *D*).

James Parkinson remarked in his original description on a patient whose tremors disappeared on one side after suffering a stroke. This seems consistent with the idea that altered activity in the cortex→basal ganglia→cortex loop underlies these movement disorders, and it was reasoned some time ago that surgical intervention in some part of the loop might alleviate some symptoms. Because the globus pallidus affects motor areas of the cortex by way of the VL/VA complex, logical sites for surgical destruction might seem to be GPi or VL/VA.

Somewhat astoundingly, this turns out to be partially effective. Stereotactic lesions in the VL/VA region (**thalamotomy;** VL is the principal target) or, more commonly, in the internal segment of the globus pallidus (**pallidotomy**) are reasonably successful in relieving the tremor and rigidity of parkinsonism, the flailing movements of hemiballismus, and some (but not all) other involuntary movements and abnormalities of tone. Carefully placed lesions can even improve negative signs such as hypokinesia. In the case of hemiballismus, the excessive activity of the basal ganglia is apparently expressed primarily through the corticospinal tract. This tract has been sectioned in the cerebral peduncle in a few humans (on the side contralateral to the ballistic movements) for the relief of hemiballismus. The involuntary movements were permanently abolished, and a transient, flaccid paralysis ensued on the side contralateral to the surgery; however, as explained in the previous chapter, there were rather limited long-term deficits.

Considering the proximity of VL/VA and GPi to structures such as the internal capsule, such surgery has always been a last resort, and other forms of treatment have long been sought. Postmortem examination of the brains of patients with parkinsonism indicated that damage is most consistently evident in the substantia nigra (Figure 19-18), reflecting degeneration of the pigmented nigral cells that normally manufacture dopamine and transport it to the striatum. It was therefore reasoned that if the dopamine could somehow be replaced, the symptoms might be ameliorated. Because dopamine does not cross the blood-brain barrier, it is necessary to administer L-dopa (levodopa), a precursor of dopamine that does cross the barrier.

Although this form of therapy has been a great help for many patients, it also has a number of shortcomings. Therefore other therapeutic approaches continue to be sought. One promising area of current research has been attempts to replace degenerated nigral cells. Because the CNS is largely isolated from the immune system, rejection of implanted tissue is not as great a concern as in other organs, and dopaminergic cells from human fetal midbrains (and even the midbrains of other mammals) have been successfully implanted into the striatum of a small number of parkinsonian patients. The extent to which such implants can mimic a patient's original substantia nigra, and the long-term efficacy of such treatment, are not yet known.

Additional avenues of research in basal ganglia disorders have been opened by the recent development of a primate model of Parkinson's disease. In the early 1980s several young individuals with what appeared to be severe Parkinson's disease were found to have injected themselves with a "synthetic heroin," which turned out to be meperidine contaminated with a compound called *MPTP* (1-methyl-4-phenyl-1,2,3,6-tetrahydropyridine). It was quickly found that MPTP is selectively toxic to dopaminergic neurons of the primate substantia nigra. This not only made certain types of controlled experiments more feasible, but also lent additional credence to the idea that some as yet unidentified environmental agent plays a major role in most cases of Parkinson's disease.

The basal ganglia have proved to be a treasure trove of chemically coded neural subsystems. The dopaminergic projection from the substantia nigra to the striatum is one example, but there are many others. The many common features of the various syndromes caused by damage to diverse parts of the basal ganglia give rise to the concept of these neural structures as forming a finely tuned system in which malfunction of any part can throw the whole system out of balance. The study of the balancing mechanisms in neurochemical terms is currently an active area of research. Thus a decrease in dopamine levels in the striatum causes parkinsonian symptoms. This can occur naturally (in Parkinson's disease) or as a side effect of drugs that act as dopamine antagonists (such as the phenothiazines used for psychiatric disorders). In contrast, increased levels of dopamine in the striatum, as in parkinsonian patients who receive too much L-dopa, can cause choreiform and athetoid movements, as though the system were now tilted in the opposite direction.

SUGGESTED READINGS

Alexander L: The vascular supply of the striopallidum, *Res Publ Assoc Res Nerv Ment Dis* 21:77, 1942.

Alexander GE, DeLong MR: Microstimulation of the primate neostriatum. II. Somatotopic organization of striatal microexcitable zones and their relation to neuronal response properties, *J Neurophysiol* 53:1417, 1985.

Alexander GE, DeLong MR, Strick PL: Parallel organization of functionally segregated circuits linking basal ganglia and cortex, *Ann Rev Neurosci* 9:357, 1986.

Alheid GF, Heimer L, Switzer RC III: Basal ganglia. In Paxinos G, editor: *The human nervous system,* San Diego, 1990, Academic Press.

Bergman H, Wichmann T, DeLong MR: Reversal of experimental parkinsonism by lesions of the subthalamic nucleus, *Science* 249:1436, 1990. *Recent work emphasizing the critical role of the subthalamic nucleus in the movement abnormalities seen in multiple basal ganglia disorders, including Parkinson's disease.*

Carpenter MB: Athetosis and the basal ganglia: review of the literature and study of forty-two cases, *Arch Neurol Psychiatry* 63:875, 1950.

Chesselet M-F, Delfs JM: Basal ganglia and movement disorders: an update, *Trends Neurosci* 19:417, 1996. *Every year it gets a little more complicated.*

Cummings JL: Frontal-subcortical circuits and human behavior, *Arch Neurol* 50:873, 1993. *A recent review of the involvement of basal ganglia damage in cognitive and behavioral disorders.*

Denian JM, Menetrey A, Charpier S: The lamellar organization of the rat substantia nigra pars reticulata: segregated patterns of striatal afferents and relationship to the topography of corticostriatal projections, *Neurosci* 73:761, 1996.

Dick JPR et al: Simple and complex movements in a patient with infarction of the supplementary motor area, *Movement Disorders* 1:255, 1986. *Clinical evidence bearing on the relationship between the putamen and the supplementary motor area.*

van Domburg PHMF, ten Donkelaar HJ: The human substantia nigra and ventral tegmental area: a neuroanatomical study with notes on aging and aging diseases, *Adv Anat Embryol Cell Biol* 121:1, 1991.

Flowers K: Some frequency response characteristics of parkinsonism on pursuit tracking, *Brain* 101:19, 1978.

Flowers K: Lack of prediction in the motor behavior of parkinsonism, *Brain* 101:35, 1978.

Gage FH, Fisher LJ: Intracerebral grafting: a tool for the neurobiologist, *Neuron* 6:1, 1991.

Goldman PS, Nauta WJH: An intricately patterned prefronto-caudate projection in the rhesus monkey, *J Comp Neurol* 171:369, 1977. *Early results indicating that the traditional view of the striatum as a uniformly organized structure is an oversimplification.*

Graybiel AM, Ragsdale CW Jr: Histochemically distinct compartments in the striatum of human, monkey, and cat demonstrated by acetylthiocholinesterase staining, *Proc Natl Acad Sci* 75:5723, 1978. *Additional results, complementary to those of Goldman and Nauta, indicating that the striatum is a jigsaw puzzle in terms of both connections and neurotransmitters.*

Guridi J, Lozano AM: A brief history of pallidotomy, *Neurosurg* 41:1169, 1997.

Holt DJ, Graybiel AM, Saper CB: Neurochemical architecture of the human striatum, *J Comp Neurol* 384:1, 1997.

Hopkins DA, Niesser LW: Substantia nigra projections to the reticular formation, superior colliculus and central gray in the rat, cat and monkey, *Neurosci Lett* 2:253, 1976.

Hore J, Meyer-Lohmann J, Brooks VB: Basal ganglia cooling disables learned arm movements of monkeys in the absence of visual guidance, *Science* 195:584, 1977. *Some exciting work bearing on the possible role of the basal ganglia in the formulation of voluntary movements.*

Kemp JM, Powell TPS: The connexions of the striatum and globus pallidus: synthesis and speculation, *Philos Trans R Soc Lond* B262:441, 1971. *An early hypothesis of basal ganglia connectivity, before the multiple parallel loops were found.*

Kopin IJ, Markey SP: MPTP toxicity: implications for research in Parkinson's disease, *Ann Rev Neurosci* 11:81, 1988.

Langston JW et al: Chronic parkinsonism in humans due to a product of meperidine-analog synthesis, *Science* 219:979, 1983. *One of the original descriptions of MPTP-induced parkinsonism.*

Laplane D et al: Clinical consequences of corticectomies involving the supplementary motor area in man, *J Neurol Sci* 34:301, 1977.

Lindvall O et al: Grafts of fetal dopamine neurons survive and improve motor function in Parkinson's disease, *Science* 247:574, 1990.

Marsden CD, Obeso JA: The functions of the basal ganglia and the paradox of stereotaxic surgery in Parkinson's disease, *Brain* 117:877, 1994. *The paradox lies in trying to explain why damage to the globus pallidus or VA/VL does not impair movement further.*

Martin JP: *The basal ganglia and posture,* Tunbridge Wells, UK, 1967, Pitman Medical Publishing.

Middleton FA, Strick PL: Anatomical evidence for cerebellar and basal ganglia involvement in higher cortical function, *Science* 266:458, 1994.

Middleton FA, Strick PL: The temporal lobe is a target of output from the basal ganglia, *Proc Natl Acad Sci* 93:8683, 1996. *Initial evidence that basal ganglia influences may reach areas of association cortex outside the frontal lobe.*

Obeso JA et al, editors: *The basal ganglia and new surgical approaches for Parkinson's disease (Adv Neurol vol 74),* Philadelphia, 1997, Lippincott-Raven. *Includes a number of concise, current reviews of different aspects of basal ganglia anatomy, connections, and pathophysiology.*

Ohye C, Kimura M, McKenzie JS, editors: *The basal ganglia V (Adv Behav Biol vol 47),* New York, 1996, Plenum Press.

Parent A, Hazrati L-N: Functional anatomy of the basal ganglia. I. The cortico-basal ganglia-thalamo-cortical loop. II. The place of subthalamic nucleus and external pallidum in basal ganglia circuitry, *Brain Res Rev* 20:91, 128, 1995.

Rinne JO et al: Dementia in Parkinson's disease is related to neuronal loss in the medial substantia nigra, *Ann Neurol* 26:47, 1989. *Additional evidence about the role of the basal ganglia in cognitive functions—the medial part of the substantia nigra is preferentially connected to the caudate nucleus.*

Sadikot AF, Parent A, Franois C: The centre médian and parafascicular thalamic nuclei project respectively to the sensorimotor and associative-limbic striatal territories in the squirrel monkey, *Brain Res* 510:161, 1990.

Selemon LD, Goldman-Rakic PS: Longitudinal topography and interdigitation of corticostriatal projections in the rhesus monkey, *J Neurosci* 5:776, 1985.

Shink E et al: The subthalamic nucleus and the external pallidum: two tightly interconnected structures that control the output of the basal ganglia in the monkey, *Neurosci* 73:335, 1996.

Smith Y, Parent A: Differential connections of caudate nucleus and putamen in the squirrel monkey *(Saimiri sciureus), Neurosci* 18:347, 1986.

Smith Y, Hazrati L-N, Parent A: Efferent projections of the subthalamic nucleus in the squirrel monkey as studied by the PHA-L anterograde tracing method, *J Comp Neurol* 294:306, 1990.

Spokes EGS: Neurochemical alterations in Huntington's chorea: a study of post-mortem brain tissue, *Brain* 103:179, 1980.

Tetrud JW, Langston JW: The effect of deprenyl (Selegiline) on the natural history of Parkinson's disease, *Science* 245:519, 1989. *An important recent advance in the treatment of Parkinson's disease—a pharmacological strategy, suggested by studies of the mechanism of MPTP toxicity, that may slow the degenerative process in the substantia nigra.*

Whittier JR: Ballism and the subthalamic nucleus (nucleus hypothalamicus; corpus Luysi): review of the literature and study of thirty cases, *Arch Neurol Psychiatry* 58:672, 1947.

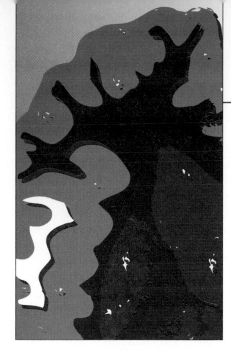

CEREBELLUM

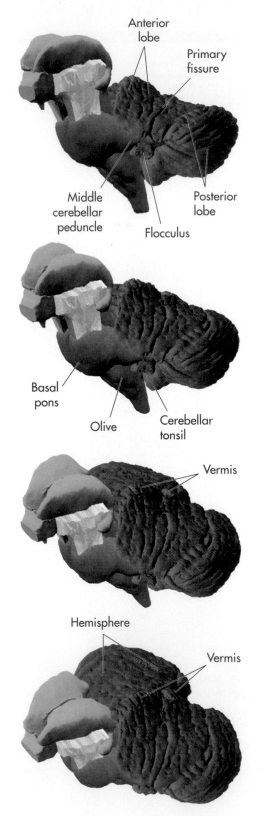

Anterior
lobe

Primary
fissure

Middle
cerebellar
peduncle

Flocculus

Posterior
lobe

Basal
pons

Olive

Cerebellar
tonsil

Vermis

Hemisphere

Vermis

FIGURE 20-1
Three-dimensional reconstructions of the cerebellum, brainstem, and
diencephalon.

Cerebellum literally means "little brain," and in a real
sense it is, containing as many neurons as all the rest
of the CNS. This semidetached mass of neural tissue covers most of the posterior surface of the brainstem, anchored there by three pairs of fiber bundles called **cerebellar peduncles.** Sensory inputs of virtually every
description find their way to the uniquely structured
cortex of the cerebellum, which in turn projects (via a set
of **deep cerebellar nuclei**) to various sites in the
brainstem and thalamus. Although the cerebellum is extensively concerned with the processing of sensory information, and although it has few ways to influence motor
neurons directly, it is considered part of the motor system
because cerebellar damage results in abnormalities of
equilibrium, postural control, and coordination of voluntary movements.

THE CEREBELLUM CAN BE DIVIDED INTO TRANSVERSE AND LONGITUDINAL ZONES

The outside of the cerebellum has a banded appearance,
as though its surface were folded like an accordion (Figures 20-1 and 20-2). This folding is a successful device for
increasing the cerebellar surface area; if the cortex could
be unfolded into a flat sheet, it would be over 1 meter
long (Figure 20-3). Deep **fissures,** most easily seen in
sagittal sections (Figure 20-2, *D*), indent the cerebellar
surface. Smaller fissures indent the walls of these deep fissures, with the result that the entire cerebellar surface is
made up of cortical ridges called **folia,**★ most of which
are transversely oriented; prominent fissures are the basis
of common systems of dividing the cerebellum into
lobes and **lobules.** Beneath the cortex is a mass of white
matter, the **medullary center** of the cerebellum, which
is composed of fibers going to or coming from the cerebellar cortex.

Transverse Fissures Divide the Cerebellum Into Lobes

The first fissure to appear during development is the **posterolateral fissure,** which separates the **flocculonodular lobe** from the **body of the cerebellum (corpus
cerebelli).** In humans, the body of the cerebellum is by
far the larger of the two, and the posterolateral fissure is so
deep that the **flocculus** of each side is almost pinched off
from the rest of the cerebellum (Figures 20-1 and 20-2).
The **primary fissure,** a prominent landmark in mid-

★The white matter of the cerebellum has a treelike appearance in sagittal sections (Figure 20-2, *D*), and so was named *arbor vitae* ("tree of life")
by early anatomists. In a continuation of the tree analogy, each of the cortical folds on the surface of the arbor vitae is called a **folium** (Latin for
"leaf," as in foliage).

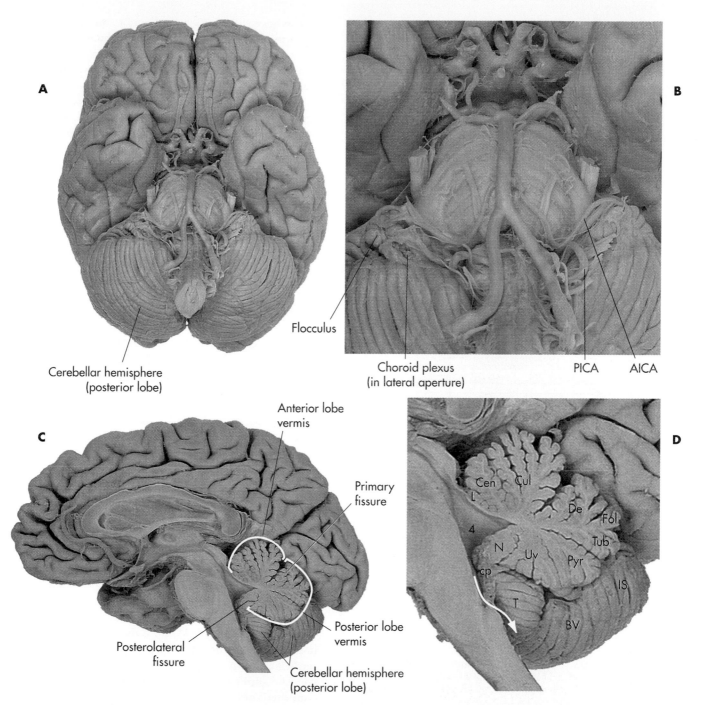

FIGURE 20-2
Gross anatomy of the cerebellum. **A,** Inferior surface, enlarged in **B.** *AICA,* Anterior inferior cerebellar artery; *PICA,* posterior inferior cerebellar artery. **C** (enlarged in **D**), Medial surface of a hemisected cerebellum, demonstrating the depth of many of the cerebellar fissures and the way in which the fissures divide the vermis into a number of lobules. The same fissures continue laterally and divide up the cerebellar hemispheres. The *arrow* passes through the median aperture of the fourth ventricle and into cisterna magna. Abbreviations for lobules of the vermis (see also Figure 20-4): *Cen,* Central lobule; *Cul,* culmen; *De,* declive; *Fol,* folium; *L,* lingula; *N,* nodulus; *Pyr,* pyramis; *Tub,* tuber; *Uv,* uvula. Other abbreviations: *4,* Fourth ventricle; *BV,* biventral lobule; *cp,* choroid plexus (in the roof of the fourth ventricle); *IS,* inferior semilunar lobule; *T,* tonsil. (Modified from Nolte J, Angevine JB Jr: *The human brain in photographs and diagrams,* St. Louis, 1995, Mosby.)

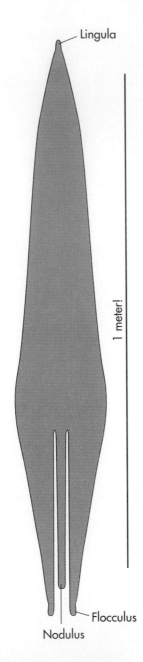

Lingula

1 meter!

Flocculus

Nodulus

FIGURE 20-3
What the human cerebellar cortex would look like if it could be peeled off the surface of the cerebellum and laid out as a flat sheet. (Redrawn from Braitenberg V, Atwood RP: Morphological observations on the cerebellar cortex, *J Comp Neurol* 109:1, 1958.)

sagittal sections of the cerebellum, subdivides the body of the cerebellum into **anterior** and **posterior lobes** (Figures 20-1 and 20-2).

Functional Connections Divide the Cerebellum Into Longitudinal Zones

The cerebellum may also be subdivided into longitudinal zones, perpendicular to the fissures, which cut across the anterior, posterior, and flocculonodular lobes (Figure 20-4, *A*). The most medial zone, straddling the midline, is the

vermis (from the Latin for "worm"). On either side of the vermis is a large **cerebellar hemisphere.** Each hemisphere is subdivided into a medial longitudinal strip adjacent to the vermis, called the **intermediate** or **paravermal zone,** and a larger, more lateral portion. The vermis is fairly clearly set off from the hemispheres on the inferior surface of the cerebellum (Figure 20-5), but other longitudinal lines of separation are not as obvious from the outside (e.g., Figure 20-1). The demarcation into longitudinal zones is based on patterns of connections and on the functional differences that result, as described shortly; cerebellar cortex has the same structure everywhere and is smoothly continuous from one hemisphere across the midline to the other. The fissures that carve the cerebellum into lobules and folia are also continuous across the midline, so each transverse wedge of cerebellum has a vermal portion and a more lateral portion. Thus the **nodulus** is the vermal portion of the flocculonodular lobe and continues laterally into the flocculus. The **tonsils** are the hemispheric portions just across the posterolateral fissure from the flocculi; appropriately enough, their vermal continuation is the **uvula.** An additional assortment of exotic names is applied to the lobules and the vermal areas of the corpus cerebelli (Figures 20-2, *D* and 20-4), and a Roman numeral system is used as well for the vermis, but for the most part these names and numbers are of limited utility in clinical settings.★

Three Peduncles Convey the Input and Output of Each Half of the Cerebellum

The cerebellum is attached to the brainstem by three substantial peduncles on each side (Figures 20-5 and 20-6). The **inferior cerebellar peduncle** (or **restiform** ["ropelike"] **body†)** (Figure 20-6, *A*; see also Figures 11-9 and 11-10) is composed mainly of afferents to the cerebellum from the spinal cord and brainstem. The **middle cerebellar peduncle** (or **brachium pontis**) (Figure 20-6, *B*; see also Figure 11-10) is the largest of the three. It is composed virtually exclusively of afferents to the cerebellum from the pontine nuclei of the contralateral side. The **superior cerebellar peduncle** (or **brachium conjunctivum‡**) (Figure 20-6, *C*; see also Figures 11-10

★One exception is the tonsil. Because this is the part of the cerebellum adjacent to the foramen magnum, expanding masses in the posterior fossa can cause tonsillar herniation and compression of the medulla (Figure 4-19, *D*).

†There is a bit of a logical inconsistency in using the terms *inferior cerebellar peduncle* and *restiform body* interchangeably. The **juxtarestiform body,** carrying vestibular traffic to and from the cerebellum, is also part of the inferior cerebellar peduncle. In common usage, the logical inconsistency is often ignored.

‡A similar logical inconsistency exists in using the terms *superior cerebellar peduncle* and *brachium conjunctivum* synonymously. Brachium conjunctivum refers specifically to the large mass of cerebellar efferents bound mostly for the red nucleus and thalamus, whereas the total superior cerebellar peduncle also includes a few cerebellar afferents such as those of the anterior spinocerebellar tract.

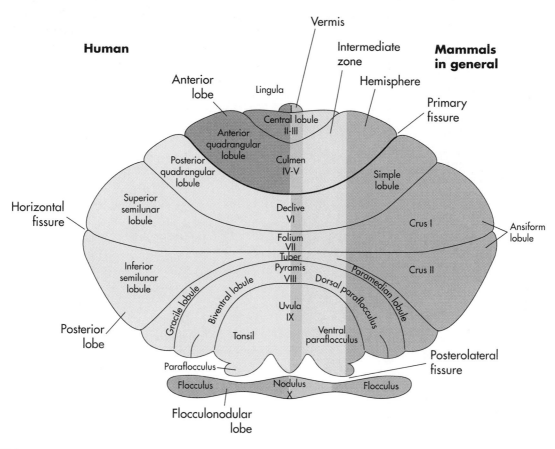

FIGURE 20-4

Cerebellar terminology on a schematic cerebellum projected as though the cerebellum were flattened out with its vermis now in one plane (compare with Figure 20-1). The general division into transversely oriented lobes is indicated on the left side of the diagram and the division into longitudinal zones is on the right. Also indicated is terminology for the various subdivisions of the vermis (including Roman numerals) and lobules of the hemispheres. On the left side of the diagram are terms classically used for the human cerebellum. On the right side are terms from comparative anatomy used more frequently in describing the cerebella of experimental animals. (Modified from Larsell O: *Anatomy of the nervous system*, ed 2, New York, 1951, Appleton-Century-Crofts.)

to 11-14) contains the major efferent pathways from the cerebellum.

Deep Nuclei Are Embedded in the Cerebellar White Matter

A series of **deep cerebellar nuclei** is buried in the medullary center of each side of the cerebellum (Figure 20-7). The most lateral is the **dentate nucleus,** a crumpled sheet of cells that looks strikingly like the inferior olivary nucleus. Most of the fibers in the superior cerebellar peduncle originate from the dentate nucleus and emerge from its medially facing mouth, or **hilus** (Figure 20-6, *C*). Medial to the dentate nucleus are the **emboliform nucleus** and the **globose nucleus.** In most nonhuman cerebella, the equivalent cells form a single nuclear mass called the **interposed nucleus** (or **nucleus interpositus**), and so even in human neuroanatomy the term *interposed nucleus* is often used for the combination of the emboliform and globose nuclei. Finally, the most medial of the deep cerebellar nuclei is the **fastigial nucleus.**

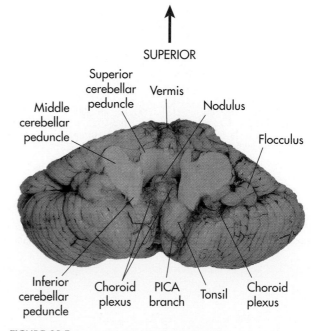

FIGURE 20-5

Ventral surface of a cerebellum that had been removed from the brainstem by severing the cerebellar peduncles. The view is as if one were looking up from the floor of the fourth ventricle toward its roof.

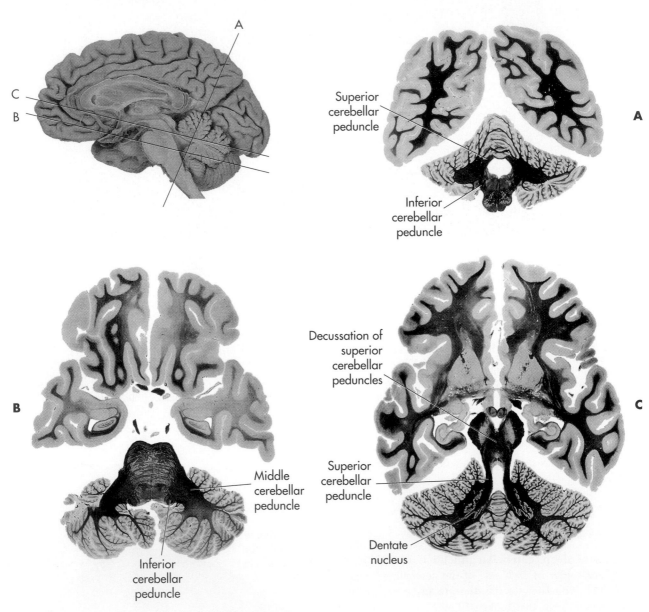

FIGURE 20-6
Cerebellar peduncles as seen in coronal and horizontal sections. **A,** Coronal section showing the inferior cerebellar peduncle as it turns dorsally and enters the cerebellum. **B,** Horizontal section showing the middle cerebellar peduncle connecting the cerebellum and basal pons. **C,** Horizontal section slightly superior to **B,** showing the superior cerebellar peduncles leaving the cerebellum, entering the brainstem, and decussating in the midbrain. (Inset and **C** modified from Nolte J, Angevine JB Jr: *The human brain in photographs and diagrams*, St. Louis, 1995, Mosby.)

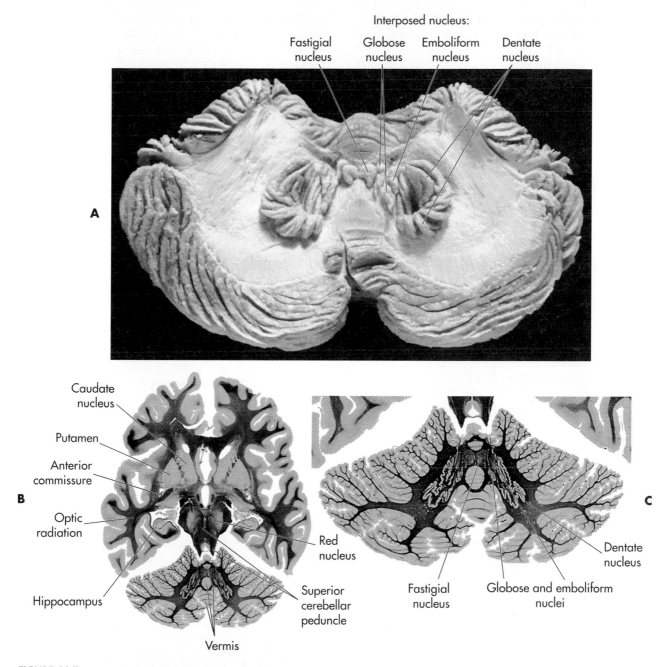

Interposed nucleus:

Fastigial nucleus Globose nucleus Emboliform nucleus Dentate nucleus

A

Caudate nucleus
Putamen
Anterior commissure
Optic radiation
B
Hippocampus
Vermis
Red nucleus
Superior cerebellar peduncle
C
Dentate nucleus
Fastigial nucleus
Globose and emboliform nuclei

FIGURE 20-7
Deep cerebellar nuclei. **A,** A beautiful dissection demonstrating the deep nuclei of a human cerebellum. **B,** The deep nuclei as seen in a horizontal section (enlarged in **C**). (**A** from Gluhbegovic N: Three-dimensional appearance and topographical relationships of the cerebellar nuclear complex of man: a microdissectional study, *J Anat* 137:396, 1983.)

ALL PARTS OF THE CEREBELLUM SHARE COMMON ORGANIZATIONAL PRINCIPLES

Cerebellar cortex has a systematic, strikingly regular organization (Figures 20-9 and 20-10), and the cerebellum as a whole has a straightforward organization (Figure 20-8): inputs arrive at the cerebellar cortex, the cortex works its magic and projects to the deep nuclei, and the deep nuclei provide the cerebellar output. The uniformity of this organization suggests that all regions

of the cerebellum perform the same fundamental operation, and that distinctive inputs and outputs of different regions allow the cerebellum to be involved in different neural functions.

Inputs Reach the Cerebellar Cortex as Mossy and Climbing Fibers

The cortex of the cerebellum has a uniform and fairly simple three-layered structure (Figure 20-9). The most superficial layer is the **molecular layer,** consisting mainly of the axons and dendrites of various cerebellar neurons. Deep to the molecular layer is a single layer of large neurons called **Purkinje cells.** Finally, adjacent to the medullary center is the **granular layer,** composed mainly of small **granule cells** arranged in a stratum many cells thick. The molecular and granular layers also contain characteristic types of interneurons (Figures 20-10 and 20-14, *B*), but the fundamental circuitry of the cerebellar cortex can be described in terms of Purkinje cells, granule cells, and the afferents to the cortex (Figures 20-10 and 20-14, *A*).

Purkinje cells are the only neurons whose axons leave the cerebellar cortex. They are, in addition, among the most anatomically distinctive neurons to be found in the nervous system. Each Purkinje cell has an intricate, extensive dendritic tree (see Figure 1-4, *A*) that is flattened out in a plane perpendicular to the long axis of the folium in which it resides (Figure 20-10). Each granule cell (Figure 20-11) sends its axon into the molecular layer, where it bifurcates to form a fine, unmyelinated **parallel fiber** (Figure 20-12) that extends for about 5 mm along the long axis of the folium. In its course, each parallel fiber passes through and synapses on the dendritic trees of a succession of Purkinje cells (as many as 500 of them). Each of us is estimated to have an incredible 10^{10} or more granule cells, and each of our 15 million Purkinje cells receives synapses from perhaps 10^5 of them.

There are two sets of afferent fibers to the cerebellar cortex: **climbing fibers** and **mossy fibers.** A single climbing fiber ends directly on each Purkinje cell, winding around the proximal portions of its dendrites like ivy climbing a trellis (Figure 20-13). All of these climbing fibers arise in the contralateral inferior olivary nucleus. By elimination, then, all the rest of the afferents to the cerebellar cortex are mossy fibers. Mossy fibers end on the dendrites of granule cells, so this is an indirect route to the Purkinje cells (mossy fiber→granule cell→parallel fiber →Purkinje cell).

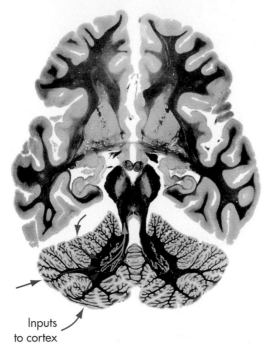

Inputs
to cortex

FIGURE 20-8
The fundamental organization of the cerebellum: inputs→cerebellar cortex→deep nuclei→output targets.

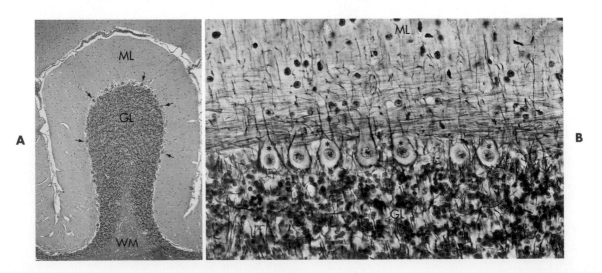

FIGURE 20-9
Light micrographs of cerebellar cortex. **A,** Cross section of a single folium from a human cerebellum (stained with hematoxylin and eosin). The molecular layer *(ML)* adjacent to the pial surface of the cerebellum contains relatively few neurons and is the main site of synaptic interactions between cerebellar interneurons and Purkinje cells. The granular layer *(GL),* adjacent to the central white matter *(WM)* of the cerebellum, contains the tightly packed cell bodies of tiny granule cells (Figure 20-11). Between the molecular and granular layers is a single layer of large Purkinje cells *(arrows).* **B,** Higher-magnification view of the Purkinje cell layer of monkey cerebellar cortex (Bodian silver stain), showing the large cell bodies (*) of these neurons surrounded by silver-stained processes of cerebellar interneurons. Purkinje cell dendrites project into the molecular layer *(ML),* where they are contacted by parallel fibers, whose parent axons arise in the granular layer *(GL).* (Courtesy Dr. Nathaniel T. McMullen, Department of Cell Biology and Anatomy, The University of Arizona College of Medicine.)

FIGURE 20-10

Composite drawings of Golgi-stained cerebellar neurons, from sections cut in three nearly orthogonal planes. **A,** A transverse section cut perpendicular to the long axis of a folium, showing mossy fibers, climbing fibers, and the major neuronal cell types of the cerebellar cortex. The elements of the principal circuit through the cerebellar cortex (Figure 20-14, *A*) can be seen clearly. Other cell types in the cerebellar cortex: **Basket cells,** whose dendrites spread out in the molecular layer and whose axons branch to enclose the cell bodies of a series of Purkinje cells; **stellate cells,** whose axons and dendrites all ramify in the molecular layer; and **Golgi cells,** whose dendrites spread out in the molecular layer and whose axons end on granule cell dendrites. **B,** A section parallel to the long axis of a folium, cut at an oblique angle so that it passes through the molecular layer on the right and the Purkinje cell layer on the left. This view demonstrates how the parallel fibers and the flattened dendritic trees of Purkinje cells are oriented perpendicular to each other. **C,** Another section parallel to the long axis of a folium, this time perpendicular to its surface to demonstrate the layers of the cerebellar cortex. [Modified from Ramón y Cajal S: *Histologie du système nerveux de l'homme et des vertébrés*, Paris, 1909, 1911, Maloine.]

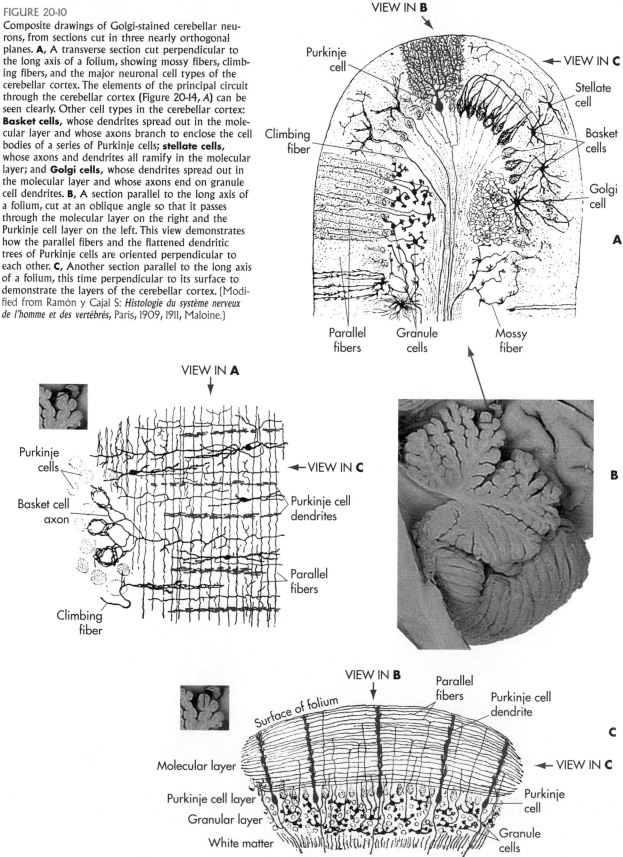

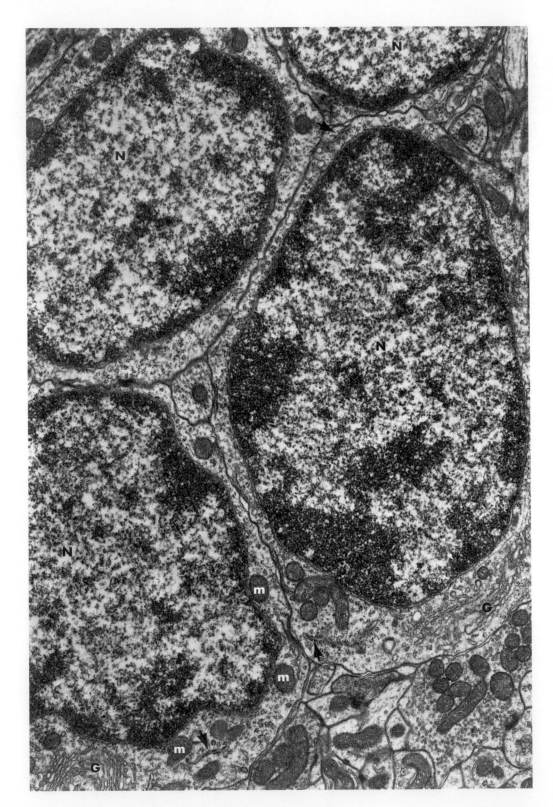

FIGURE 20-11
Granule cells of rat cerebellar cortex. These neurons are so small that each cell body is occupied almost entirely by the nucleus *(N)*. However, the scanty cytoplasm contains typical organelles such as mitochondria *(M)*, Golgi cisternae *(G)*, and tiny Nissl bodies *(arrows)*. Each neuron is only about 5 μm in diameter, meaning that a row of 5000 of them would be only an inch long. (From Pannese E: *Neurocytology: fine structure of neurons, nerve processes, and neuroglial cells*, New York, 1994, Thieme Medical Publishers, Inc.)

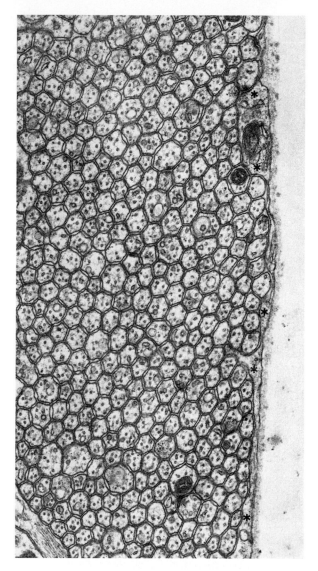

FIGURE 20-12

Regular array of parallel fibers in the molecular layer of rat cerebellar cortex (plane as in Figure 20-10, *A*). Only a thin glial covering (*) separates some parallel fibers from the surface of the cerebellum. Despite the tiny size of these unmyelinated axons (about 0.2 μm in diameter), each contains the usual microtubules and neurofilaments. (From Pannese E: *Neurocytology: fine structure of neurons, nerve processes, and neuroglial cells*, New York, 1994, Thieme Medical Publishers, Inc.)

Cerebellar Cortex Projects to the Deep Nuclei

Although Purkinje cell axons are the only route out of the cerebellar cortex, few of them leave the cerebellum itself. Rather, they project to the deep nuclei, which in turn give rise to the cerebellar output. However, it has become clear in recent years that the deep nuclei are not just simple relay stations; they have a more intricate relationship with the cerebellar cortex than had been realized previously (Figure 20-14, *C*). For example, climbing fibers and many mossy fibers send collateral branches to the deep nuclei. It has

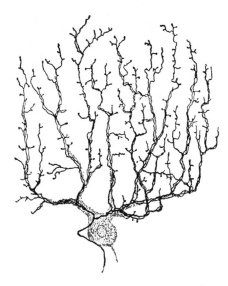

FIGURE 20-13

A drawing of a Golgi-stained climbing fiber, demonstrating the origin of its name as it climbs up the dendritic tree of a Purkinje cell (shown in color). (Modified from Ramón y Cajal S: *Histologie du système nerveux de l'homme et des vertébrés*, Paris, 1909, 1911, Maloine.)

been suggested that these inputs provide a tonic excitatory drive to neurons of the deep nuclei, and that inhibitory projections from Purkinje cells then modulate the firing rates of these neurons. Furthermore, in addition to giving rise to axons that leave the cerebellum, the deep nuclei project back to the same areas of cerebellar cortex from which they receive Purkinje axons. The functional implications of these additional connections are not fully understood, but they make it less surprising that the consequences of cerebellar damage are much more severe and long-lasting when the deep nuclei are included in the lesion.

One Side of the Cerebellum Affects the Ipsilateral Side of the Body

There are many crossings of the midline in the various circuits interconnecting the cerebellum and other parts of the CNS, primarily reflecting the fact that one cerebral hemisphere controls skeletal muscle of the contralateral limbs but one half of the cerebellum influences movements of the ipsilateral limbs (see Figures 3-31 and 20-21). Hence, for example, pontine nuclei receive inputs from the ipsilateral cerebral cortex and project to the contralateral half of the cerebellum (Figure 20-16), and one half of the cerebellum projects to the contralateral thalamus (Figure 20-19).

Details of Connections Differ Among Zones

The cerebellum is involved in equilibrium, in muscle tone and postural control, and in the coordination of voluntary movements; thus it would seem reasonable for it to receive vestibular, spinal, and cerebral cortical inputs. This is indeed the case, and even though the cerebellar cortex has the

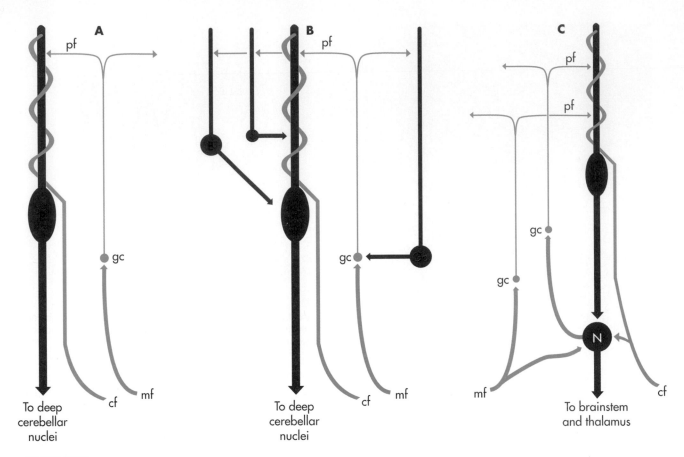

FIGURE 20-14
Connections of neurons in cerebellar cortex. Inhibitory connections are shown in *red*, excitatory in *green* (projections of the deep nuclei are shown in *blue* because most are excitatory but some are inhibitory). **A,** Schematic diagram of the principal circuit through the cerebellar cortex. Climbing fibers *(cf)* reach Purkinje cells *(P)* directly and mossy fibers *(mf)* reach them indirectly by way of granule cells *(gc)* and parallel fibers *(pf)*. **B,** Additional interconnections in cerebellar cortex. One striking thing about the cerebellar cortex is the large amount of inhibition used in processing there: the mossy fiber–granule cell inputs and the climbing fiber inputs are excitatory, but everything else is inhibitory. Golgi cells *(Go)* make inhibitory feedback connections onto granule cells. Basket cells *(B)* and stellate cells *(S)* make inhibitory synapses on the cell bodies and dendrites, respectively, of Purkinje cells. Finally, all synapses of Purkinje cells, as far as we know, are inhibitory. **C,** Schematic diagram of general interconnections of cerebellar cortex and deep cerebellar nuclei. Climbing fibers and many mossy fibers send collaterals to cells of deep nuclei *(N)* before continuing to cerebellar cortex, where climbing fibers end directly on Purkinje cells and mossy fibers influence Purkinje cells indirectly through granule cell→parallel fiber pathway. Purkinje cells in turn end on cells of deep nuclei, and deep nuclei send mossy fibers to cortex as well as massive numbers of fibers to extracerebellar sites in the brainstem and thalamus. (Modified from Thach WT: Cerebellar output: properties, synthesis and uses, *Brain Res* 40:89, 1972.)

same anatomical appearance everywhere, different areas are concerned with particular functions. The flocculonodular lobe and part of the uvula receive vestibular inputs, and so this area is referred to as the **vestibulocerebellum.** Most of the vermal and paravermal regions (except for the nodulus and uvula) receive spinal inputs and so are called the **spinocerebellum.** Projections from the cerebral cortex (via relays in the pontine nuclei) form the single major input to lateral parts of the cerebellar hemispheres, so the lateral hemispheres are sometimes referred to as the **cerebrocerebellum** or the **neocerebellum.**★ There is a cer-

tain amount of overlap of these functional divisions in terms of connections. For example, the spinocerebellum receives afferents from pontine nuclei, and parts of it receive vestibular afferents as well.

Different areas of the cerebellar cortex are preferentially related not only to particular inputs but also to particular deep nuclei. The dentate nucleus receives projections mainly from the lateral parts of the cerebellar hemispheres, the interposed nucleus from the paravermal cortex, and the fastigial nucleus from the vermis (Figure 20–15).

CEREBELLAR CORTEX RECEIVES MULTIPLE INPUTS

The cerebellar cortex receives some of its complement of mossy fibers from the deep cerebellar nuclei; the remaining mossy fibers carry information from three principal

---

★Many authors use the terms *archicerebellum, paleocerebellum,* and *neocerebellum* synonymously with *vestibulocerebellum, spinocerebellum,* and *cerebrocerebellum* in reference to what is thought to be the phylogenetic sequence of development of these different cerebellar areas. Unfortunately, different authors use these terms in slightly different ways. Vestibulocerebellum, spinocerebellum, and neocerebellum, as defined here, seem to be the most common usage of the terminology at present.

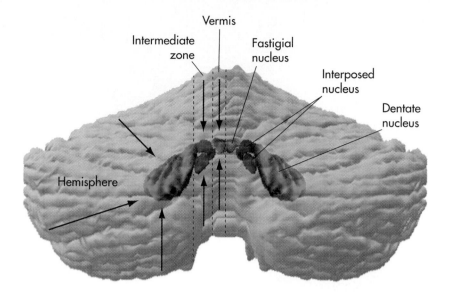

FIGURE 20-15

Projections from cerebellar cortex to deep cerebellar nuclei. The cortex is generally divided into three longitudinal zones that project in a me-dial-to-lateral sequence to the fastigial, interposed, and dentate nuclei. Superimposed on this is a projection (not shown) from the vermis and flocculonodular lobe directly to the vestibular nuclei.

extracerebellar sources (Figure 20-16): (1) the vestibular nerve and nuclei, (2) the spinal cord, and (3) the cerebral cortex (via pontine nuclei). The climbing fiber input to the cerebellar cortex, as mentioned previously, arises in the inferior olivary nucleus.

Vestibular Inputs Reach the Flocculus and Vermis

Some primary vestibular afferents enter the cerebellum through the juxtarestiform body (see Figure 15-6) and end as mossy fibers in the nodulus and uvula. A larger number of secondary fibers, arising in the vestibular nuclei, follow the same course to the flocculonodular lobe and most of the vermis, bilaterally.

The Spinal Cord Projects to the Vermis and Intermediate Zone

A great deal of somatosensory information (principally from various mechanoreceptors of the skin, muscles, and joints) reaches the vermal and paravermal cortex. Some of it reaches the cerebellum directly via the spinocerebellar tracts and the cuneocerebellar tract (see Figure 10-21). Some arrives indirectly by way of the reticular formation (remember that several reticular nuclei of the medulla and pons project to the cerebellum). Not surprisingly, similar information from the head also reaches the cerebellum from the trigeminal system. All the trigeminal nuclei participate in this projection to some extent, but the bulk of it arises in the rostral two thirds of the spinal nucleus (interpolar and oral nuclei). The anterior spinocerebellar tract travels in the superior cerebellar peduncle, but all the rest of the somatosensory input from both body and head traverses the inferior cerebellar peduncle (Table 20-1).

Electrophysiological studies have shown that this projection ends somatotopically in a peculiar and interesting way. Each part of the body is mapped three times onto the cerebellar cortex, once ipsilaterally in a pattern mostly contained in the anterior lobe (Figure 20-17) and again with some bilateral representation in the posterior lobe. In each of the three somatotopic maps, the head is nearest the primary fissure and the trunk is adjacent to the midline. The mapping is not nearly as precise as in the sensory and motor areas of the cerebral cortex. Adjacent small areas of cerebellar cortex may contain representations of noncontiguous areas of the body, in a pattern sometimes referred to as **fractured somatotopy.**

Cerebral Cortex Projects to the Cerebellum by Way of Pontine Nuclei

You may recall that the basis pedunculi of each cerebral peduncle is considerably larger than a medullary pyramid. One basis pedunculi contains about 21 million fibers, of which only about 1 million continue on into the ipsilateral pyramid. Some of the remaining 20 million fibers are bound for the reticular formation or for the motor nuclei of cranial nerves, but the vast majority end in ipsilateral pontine nuclei. The pontine nuclei of one side contain about 12 million cells that project through the middle cerebellar peduncle to virtually all parts of the cerebellar cortex.★ Almost all of these fibers cross the midline in the basal pons and end in the contralateral half of the cerebellum; indeed, the pathway is usually treated as entirely crossed. However, a few fibers (particularly some of those destined for the vermis) end ipsilaterally.

★Pontocerebellar input to the flocculonodular lobe is sparse, and the nodulus may receive none at all.

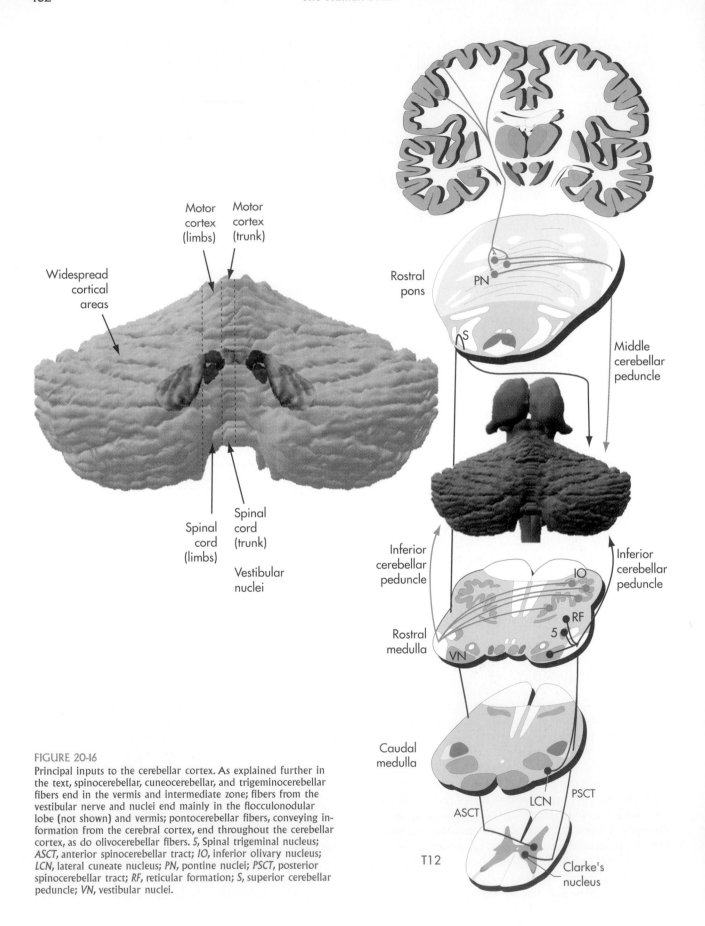

FIGURE 20-16

Principal inputs to the cerebellar cortex. As explained further in the text, spinocerebellar, cuneocerebellar, and trigeminocerebellar fibers end in the vermis and intermediate zone; fibers from the vestibular nerve and nuclei end mainly in the flocculonodular lobe (not shown) and vermis; pontocerebellar fibers, conveying information from the cerebral cortex, end throughout the cerebellar cortex, as do olivocerebellar fibers. *5,* Spinal trigeminal nucleus; *ASCT,* anterior spinocerebellar tract; *IO,* inferior olivary nucleus; *LCN,* lateral cuneate nucleus; *PN,* pontine nuclei; *PSCT,* posterior spinocerebellar tract; *RF,* reticular formation; *S,* superior cerebellar peduncle; *VN,* vestibular nuclei.

Table 20-1 Inputs to Cerebellar Cortex*

Tract	Origin	Termination	Peduncle
Anterior spinocerebellar	Contralateral spinal cord	Vermis and intermediate zone, mostly ipsilateral to origin (recrosses in cerebellum)	Superior
Posterior spinocerebellar	Clarke's nucleus	Vermis and intermediate zone, mostly ipsilateral	Inferior
Cuneocerebellar	Lateral cuneate nucleus	Vermis and intermediate zone, mostly ipsilateral	Inferior
Vestibulocerebellar†	Vestibular ganglion	Ipsilateral nodulus and uvula	Inferior (juxtarestiform body)
Vestibulocerebellar‡	Vestibular nuclei	Flocculus, nodulus and vermis, bilaterally	Inferior (juxtarestiform body)
Reticulocerebellar	Lateral, paramedian, reticular tegmental nuclei	Mainly vermis and intermediate zone, mostly ipsilateral	Inferior and middle§
Trigemino-cerebellar	Spinal and main sensory nuclei (V)	Vermis and intermediate zone, mostly ipsilateral	Inferior
Olivocerebellar	Inferior olivary, accessory olivary nuclei	All contralateral areas	Inferior
Pontocerebellar	Pontine nuclei	All contralateral areas‖; some to ipsilateral vermis	Middle

*Not including inputs from the deep cerebellar nuclei or modulatory inputs from places such as the raphe nuclei and locus ceruleus.
†Primary afferents.
‡Second-order fibers.
§The reticular tegmental nucleus projects through the middle cerebellar peduncle.
‖ With the possible exception of the nodulus.

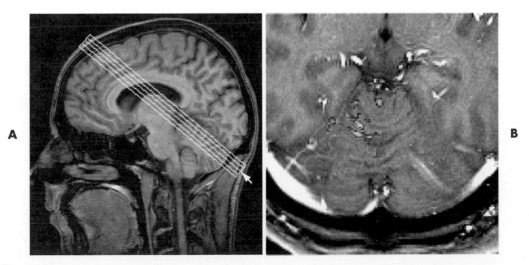

FIGURE 20-17
Demonstration of somatotopy in the anterior lobe of a human subject demonstrated by functional MRI. **A,** The planes of section used in this study, parallel to the peak of the tentorium cerebelli and the superior surface of the anterior lobe. The plane of section in **B** is indicated by an arrow. **B,** Areas of increased blood flow during repeated flexion and extension of the ipsilateral hand *(red/orange)* or foot *(blue).* (From Nitschke et al: Somatotopic motor representation in the human anterior cerebellum: a high-resolution functional MRI study, *Brain* 119:1023, 1996.)

The corticopontocerebellar pathway is therefore a mammoth one, dwarfing the corticospinal tract by comparison. Several areas of the cerebral cortex project to the pontine nuclei (Figure 20-18), but contributions from the vicinity of the central sulcus predominate (i.e., from the motor and premotor cortex and from somatosensory cortex and adjacent parts of the parietal lobe). There are projections from other parts of the cortex, such as visual, limbic, and association areas, but these are not as heavy as the others just mentioned. The vermis and intermediate zone

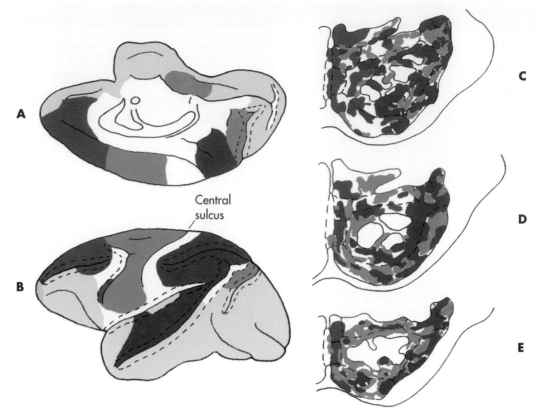

FIGURE 20-18

Diagram illustrating the distribution within the basal pons of the rhesus monkey of projections derived from association cortices in the prefrontal *(purple)*, posterior parietal *(blue)*, temporal *(red)*, and parastriate and parahippocampal regions *(orange)*, and from motor, premotor, and supplementary motor areas *(green)*. The medial **(A)** and lateral **(B)** surfaces of the cerebral hemisphere are shown at the left, and sections through the basal pons in the rostral pons **(C)**, midpons **(D)**, and caudal pons **(E)** are shown on the right. Areas in white depict cortical regions that project to the pons, but details regarding the terminations are incomplete; note that this includes limbic areas such as the cingulate gyrus. Cortical areas shown in yellow are not currently thought to have pontine projections. There is a complex mosaic of terminations in the pons, with each cerebral region having preferential sites of pontine terminations. There is considerable interdigitation of the terminations, but almost no overlap. [Modified from the cover figure accompanying Schmahmann JD: From movement to thought: anatomic substrates of the cerebellar contribution to cognitive processing, *Hum Brain Mapping* 4:174, 1996.]

preferentially receive their cortical input from the motor cortex of the precentral gyrus, and the pathway is somatotopically organized so that the pontocerebellar fibers end in the same pattern as do those carrying information from the spinal cord. The lateral parts of the cerebellar hemispheres, in contrast, receive most of their cortical input from premotor, somatosensory, and association areas of the cerebral cortex.

Climbing Fibers Arise in the Inferior Olivary Nucleus

The inferior olivary nucleus (actually a complex of a **principal** and two **accessory** olivary nuclei) is unique among structures providing afferents to the cerebellum. All olivary efferents emerge medially, enter the contralateral inferior cerebellar peduncle, and blanket the entire contralateral cerebellar cortex with climbing fibers.

The information these climbing fibers convey comes from diverse sources, including the spinal cord, the red nucleus, the cerebral cortex, and the cerebellum itself. Fibers

from the ipsilateral red nucleus, forming the bulk of the central tegmental tract, are the numerically most important olivary input. Spinal inputs, all crossed, reach the inferior olivary complex both directly (via **spinoolivary** fibers) and indirectly (through relays in the posterior column nuclei). A few fibers from the cerebral cortex of both sides, mostly from motor cortex, also reach the olive. Finally, there is a topographically highly organized projection from the contralateral dentate and interposed nuclei to the inferior olivary complex (Figure 20-19).

A structure with these sorts of connections would be expected to play an important role in cerebellar function. This appears to be the case because selective destruction of the inferior olive in experimental animals has acute effects similar to those of destruction of the entire contralateral half of the cerebellum (described shortly). However, selective olivary destruction is exceedingly rare in human pathology. Damage in this part of the brainstem is likely to affect the nearby pyramid or inferior cerebellar peduncle as well, and it becomes difficult to sort out those symptoms for which olivary damage is responsible.

Visual and Auditory Information Reaches the Cerebellum

Electrophysiological studies have also shown that responses to visual and auditory stimuli can be recorded from the vermis, approximately midway along its length (i.e., in the same general area that receives somatosensory information from the head). Visual information reaches this part of the cerebellum from a particular subset of pontine nuclei (in the dorsolateral part of the basal pons), which in turn receive it from visual cortical areas and the superior colliculus. Auditory information probably reaches pontine nuclei from auditory cortical areas and the inferior colliculus. The reticular tegmental nucleus projects visual information to the flocculus, where it is used in the control of eye movements.

EACH LONGITUDINAL ZONE HAS A DISTINCTIVE OUTPUT

The output of the cerebellar cortex is entirely in the form of the axons of Purkinje cells. Some of these, arising in the flocculonodular lobe and in parts of the vermis of both anterior and posterior lobes as well, leave the cerebellum via the juxtarestiform body and end in the vestibular nuclei. This then provides the only reasonably direct access the cerebellar cortex has to motor neurons of the spinal cord (via the vestibulospinal tracts); all other Purkinje axons end in the deep cerebellar nuclei. They do so in an orderly medial-to-lateral way: the vermis projects to the fastigial nucleus, the paravermal or intermediate zone projects to the interposed nucleus, and the lateral hemisphere projects to the dentate nucleus (Figure 20-15).

Most neurons of the deep nuclei use glutamate as a neurotransmitter and make excitatory synapses on neurons they contact. However, the projection from the deep nuclei to the inferior olivary nucleus arises from a separate population of inhibitory neurons that use GABA as their transmitter. The output connections of the fastigial nucleus are distinctive, whereas those of the dentate and interposed nuclei are similar to each other. In addition to the connections described in the next three sections, all the deep nuclei project back to the cerebellar cortex.

The Vermis Projects to the Fastigial Nucleus

The fastigial output is directed primarily to the brainstem, ending in the vestibular nuclei of both sides and in the reticular formation, mainly contralaterally (Figure 20-19). Fibers that end ipsilaterally go right out through the juxtarestiform body. Those bound for contralateral targets cross the midline within the cerebellum, loop over the superior cerebellar peduncle as the **uncinate fasciculus** (or **hook bundle**), and descend through the contralateral juxtarestiform body. A few fibers also project to the con-

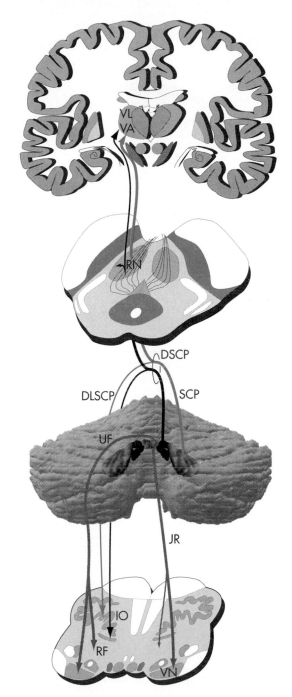

FIGURE 20-19
Principal efferent connections of the deep cerebellar nuclei. The fastigial nucleus projects bilaterally to the vestibular nuclei and the reticular formation; a few fibers (not shown) reach the contralateral VL/VA complex. The interposed nucleus (globose + emboliform) projects heavily to the red nucleus and less heavily to the VL/VA complex; the dentate nucleus does just the opposite. Both the interposed and dentate nuclei also send fibers to the contralateral inferior olivary complex and reticular formation. *DLSCP*, Descending limb of the superior cerebellar peduncle; *DSCP*, decussation of the superior cerebellar peduncle; *IO*, inferior olivary nucleus; *JR*, juxtarestiform body; *RF*, reticular formation; *RN*, red nucleus; *SCP*, superior cerebellar peduncle; *UF*, uncinate fasciculus; *VL/VA*, ventral lateral and ventral anterior nuclei of the thalamus; *VN*, vestibular nuclei.

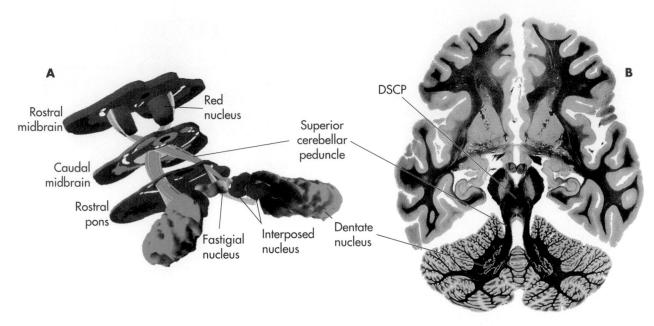

FIGURE 20-20
Origin and course of the superior cerebellar peduncle, as seen in a three-dimensional reconstruction (**A**) and a horizontal section (**B**). *DSCP,* Decussation of the superior cerebellar peduncles. (**B** modified from Nolte J, Angevine JB Jr: *The human brain in photographs and diagrams,* St. Louis, 1995, Mosby.)

tralateral VL/VA complex of the thalamus and to the contralateral cervical spinal cord.

The Intermediate and Lateral Zones Project to the Interposed and Dentate Nuclei

The major output from the cerebellum is the brachium conjunctivum, which arises in the dentate and interposed nuclei and leaves the cerebellum as the bulk of the superior cerebellar peduncle. This peduncle joins the brainstem in the rostral pons (see Figures 11-12 and 20-6, *C*); at this level some fibers turn caudally as the **descending limb of the superior cerebellar peduncle** and end in the reticular formation and the inferior olivary nucleus (Figure 20-19). Most of the fibers, however, continue rostrally, decussate in the midbrain (Figure 20-20; see also Figures 11-10 to 11-14), and reach the red nucleus, where many of the fibers from the interposed nucleus and a minority of the dentate fibers terminate. The remaining fibers pass through or around the red nucleus, join the thalamic fasciculus, and end in the VL/VA complex of the thalamus. The projections of these two cerebellar nuclei therefore differ mainly in emphasis. The interposed nucleus preferentially influences the red nucleus, whereas the dentate nucleus preferentially influences the thalamus. The dentate and interposed nuclei project to separate but interdigitated groups of cells in the thalamus. From these thalamic cells, dentate information is conveyed to motor and premotor cortex, whereas information from the interposed nucleus is conveyed selectively to the limb areas of motor cortex (Figure 20-21).

PATTERNS OF CONNECTIONS INDICATE THE FUNCTIONS OF LONGITUDINAL ZONES

The cerebellum is a great delight for anatomists and physiologists because of its uniform, precisely organized cortex and its well-worked-out connections. It is also something of an embarrassment because in the final analysis we do not understand much about how it works; the nature of the fundamental operation performed similarly all over the cerebellum is not yet understood. However, characteristic motor disorders and no significant sensory deficit* follow cerebellar damage. Based on the nature of these motor disabilities (detailed in the next section) and on the anatomy and physiology of different parts of the cerebellum, some general comments about function can be made.

The Lateral Hemispheres Are Involved in Planning Movements

The lateral hemispheres form the largest part of the human cerebellum. The major neural circuit in which they are involved is the great loop from several areas of the cerebral cortex to the cerebellum and back to the motor and pre-

---

*"I have, however, examined every modality of sensation in many cases [of cerebellar damage] but have never found disturbances of any form...No matter how irregular the movements may be, or how far the affected limb deviates from the point to which it should be moved, the patient always has a full and accurate recognition of its position in space." (From Holmes G: The symptoms of acute cerebellar injuries due to gunshot injuries, *Brain* 40:461, 1917.)

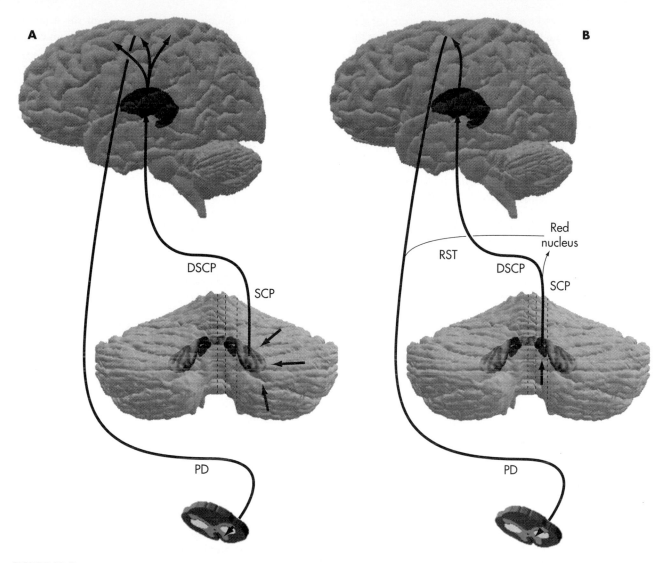

FIGURE 20-21

The principal output circuits through which the cerebellar hemispheres and intermediate zone influence movement. **A,** The hemispheres receive input via the pontine nuclei from widespread areas of cerebral cortex (not shown) and then, via the dentate nucleus, superior cerebellar peduncle *(SCP),* and VL/VA, influence the output of motor and premotor cortex. Notice that this cerebellar output crosses the midline in the decussation of the superior cerebellar peduncles *(DSCP)* and that the output from motor and premotor cortex recrosses the midline in the pyramidal decussation *(PD).* The result is that one cerebellar hemisphere affects the ipsilateral side of the spinal cord and brainstem. **B,** Output connections of the intermediate zone are similar in many respects to hemispheric circuitry, but in this case only the limb areas of motor cortex are affected; premotor cortex is not involved. However, the red nucleus and rubrospinal tract *(RST)* are also called into play. Here again there are compensating decussations: cerebellar output fibers cross in the decussation of the superior cerebellar peduncles *(DCSP)* and rubrospinal fibers cross on their way to the spinal cord. The few fastigial fibers that reach VL/VA behave in a similar manner, but their information is relayed to the trunk area of motor cortex.

motor cortex (Figure 20-21, *A*). This circuitry suggests that the cerebellar hemispheres could be involved somehow in the planning of movements, acting by influencing the output of motor cortex. Consistent with this notion, it has been found that most neurons in the dentate nucleus change their firing rates before voluntary movements occur, and indeed many of them change firing rates even before activity in motor cortex changes. (This is not to say that voluntary movements are *initiated* in the cerebellum, because in anticipation of a movement, various areas of cerebral association cortex become active long before the dentate nucleus does.) Thus the currently most prevalent

hypothesis about the function of the lateral hemisphere–dentate nucleus portion of the cerebellum is that it participates in the planning and programming of voluntary movements, particularly learned, skillful movements that become more rapid, precise, and automatic with practice. This is consistent with the clinical observation that although a great deal of compensation may take place after cerebellar injury, deficits in skilled learned movements (e.g., piano playing) may be permanent. Note that the connections between cerebral and cerebellar hemispheres are crossed (Figure 20-21, *A*). This means that, for example, the left side of the cerebellum is related to motor cortex on the right. Because the right motor cortex controls the left side of the body, it would be expected (and is observed) that the symptoms of unilateral cerebellar damage are found on the ipsilateral side of the body.

The Intermediate Zone Is Involved in Adjusting Limb Movements

The major inputs to the intermediate or paravermal cortex are superimposed, somatotopically arranged projections from the motor cortex and spinal cord (Figure 20-16). The major output of this part of the cerebellum is via the interposed nucleus to the red nucleus and also back to the motor cortex (through VL/VA, Figure 20-21, B). Thus the intermediate cerebellum can influence spinal cord motor neurons through the corticospinal tract and also through the rubrospinal pathway. This led to the hypothesis that the intermediate zone of the cerebellum compares the commands emanating from motor cortex (it receives this information via pontine nuclei) with the actual position and velocity of the moving part (it receives this information via spinocerebellar and similar tracts), and then, by way of the interposed nucleus, issues correcting signals. This is consistent with the observation that most neurons of the interposed nucleus have firing rates related to voluntary movements, but unlike those of dentate neurons their rates tend to change *during* rather than *before* movement. Note that here again a given side of the cerebellum winds up affecting ipsilateral motor neurons (e.g., left side of cerebellum→right thalamus→right motor cortex→left side of spinal cord).

The Vermis Is Involved in Postural Adjustments

The vermis includes the representation of the trunk conveyed by the spinocerebellar tracts. Its major outputs reach the vestibular nuclei and the reticular formation both through the fastigial nucleus and through direct projections to the vestibular nuclei. The vestibulospinal and reticulospinal tracts then influence spinal motor neurons. Because this part of the cerebellum has so little effect on more rostral levels of the CNS, it seems reasonable that it should be most concerned with the regulation of posture and of stereotyped movements that are programmed in the brainstem and spinal cord. For example, the cerebellum-vestibulospinal pathway has been shown to be partly responsible for rhythmic modulation of the basic pattern of walking movements generated in the spinal cord.

The Flocculus and Vermis Are Involved in Eye Movements

The principal connections of the flocculonodular lobe are with the vestibular nerve and nuclei, implying that it should have something to do with the maintenance of equilibrium. As discussed in the next section, this is indeed the case, and damage to this part of the cerebellum causes a general disequilibrium and vertigo (one of the few situations in which cerebellar damage causes perceptual changes), as though some controls had been removed from the vestibular nuclei. In addition, the flocculus has a special role in the coordination of slow eye movements (see Chapter 21), which is not surprising in view of the involvement of the vestibular nuclei in eye movements. Deciding how to track a moving target visually is not as easy as it sounds because a target's image moves across the retina if the target moves, if the eyes move, or if the head moves. Some Purkinje cells in the flocculus receive all three kinds of information, make the appropriate computations, and reflect true target velocity in their output.

The Cerebellum Is Involved in Motor Learning

We usually think of learning in terms of facts and concepts, although we also learn in terms of becoming more skillful in various kinds of movements. A common example is agility with hands and feet in playing a piano; another is the skillful shots in handball that can be developed over time. Evidence is accumulating that the cerebellum plays a special role in at least some forms of motor learning (Figure 20-22). Two well-studied examples are described in this section.

The vestibuloocular reflex was mentioned briefly in Chapter 14 (see Figure 14-28). This reflex occurs during head movement, moving the eyes the same amount as the head but in the opposite direction. That is, the gain of the reflex is one: every degree of head movement elicits a degree of compensating eye movement. The result is that the direction of gaze stays constant, and the visual world remains stable. The basic circuitry of the reflex is a simple three-neuron chain. The afferent limb is formed by vestibular primary afferents. These synapse on cells of the vestibular nuclei, which in turn project to the motor neurons of extraocular muscles. If the optics of the eye were to change (e.g., if a person started to wear glasses), a reflex gain of one might no longer be appropriate, and it has been found that the vestibuloocular reflex arc is remarkably adaptable to changes in visual input. As an extreme example, if an experimental animal or a person wears reversing prisms, so that eye or head movement in one direction causes apparent movement in the opposite direction, an unaltered vestibuloocular reflex would be counterproductive. However, if the prisms are worn continuously as the subject moves about, the gain of the reflex slowly changes until by the end of a day or so it actually reverses direction. When the prisms are removed, the gain of the reflex slowly reverts to its usual state. Removal of the flocculus, or removal of a particular area of the inferior olivary nucleus, prevents these adaptive changes in the gain of the vestibuloocular reflex.

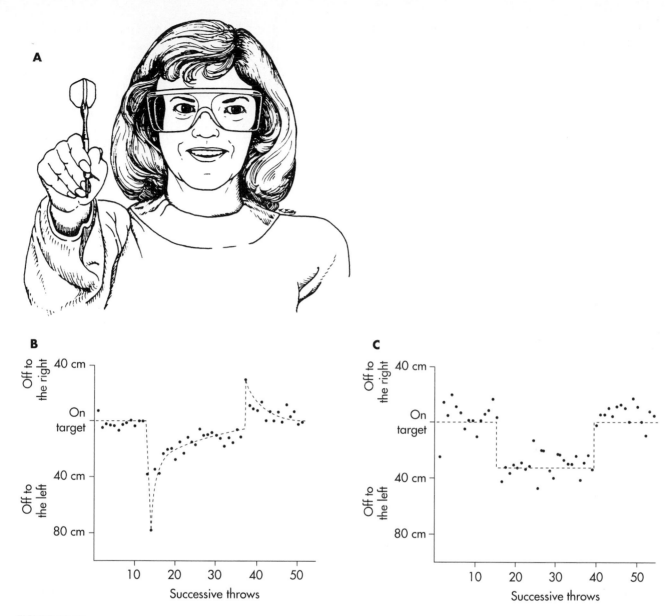

FIGURE 20-22

An example of the involvement of the cerebellum in motor learning, in this case learning to alter dart-throwing technique while wearing prisms that displace images to one side. **A,** The experimental arrangement. The subject is wearing spectacles containing prisms that bend the path of light 15° to the right. The effects of the prisms can be seen by the apparent displacement of the part of her face behind the spectacles and by the deviation of her eyes 15° to her left; she is actually looking directly at you, but must deviate her eyes to compensate for the prisms. **B,** The effects of prism spectacles on the dart-throwing ability of a normal subject. When the spectacles are first put on, the subject's throws become wide to the left. After a little practice the throws become reasonably accurate again, and at this point the thrower would look like the subject in **A,** with gaze deviated to one side but the dart aimed straight ahead. When the spectacles are removed, throws deviate to the right but then quickly become accurate again. **C,** The effects of prism spectacles on the dart-throwing ability of a patient with degenerative disease of the inferior olivary nuclei. In this case there is no compensation for the prism spectacles, and throws are wide to the left for as long as the spectacles are worn. (Redrawn from Thach WT, Goodkin HP, Keating JG: The cerebellum and the adaptive coordination of movement, *Annu Rev Neurosci* 15:403, 1992.)

Some forms of conditioned responses also depend on the cerebellum. The best-studied example is a conditioned blink response. A puff of air directed at a rabbit's cornea elicits a reflex blink. If the puff of air is regularly preceded by a sound, then after a while the sound by itself elicits the same blink. Removal of a particular small area of the interposed nucleus abolishes the conditioned response of the ipsilateral eye, even though the reflex response to the

air puff, as well as the conditioned response of the contralateral eye, is unaffected. Lesions of the inferior olivary nucleus prevent acquisition of the conditioned response by the contralateral eye of an unconditioned animal. If the response was acquired before the olivary lesion, it slowly fades after the lesion, as though the inferior olivary nucleus is required to establish and sustain the conditioned response.

The exact locations of the modifiable synapses underlying these long-term changes are not yet known with certainty. However, it seems possible that similar changes may underlie the acquisition of skilled, voluntary movements in general.

The Cerebellum May Be Involved in Cognitive Functions

Despite the fact that most corticopontine neurons reside in motor or somatosensory cortex, there are also many in limbic and association areas (Figure 20-18). This is consistent with scattered clinical reports that cerebellar damage or malformation can be associated with a variety of cognitive or behavioral disturbances. Just as the basal ganglia had traditionally been associated primarily with movement and are now thought to have broader functions, so too is the possible role of the cerebellum in nonmotor functions receiving increasing attention. It has been suggested that connections between the lateral cerebellum and association cortex may be involved in cognition, and that connections between the medial cerebellum and limbic cortex (as well as cerebellum-hypothalamus interconnections) may play a role in affective and autonomic functions.

CLINICAL SYNDROMES CORRESPOND TO FUNCTIONAL ZONES

Despite the fact that the cerebellum is functionally divided into longitudinal vermal-intermediate-hemispheric zones, syndromes referable to individual zones are rarely seen clinically. To destroy only the intermediate zone on one side, for example, a lesion would need to extend from the superior surface of the cerebellum near the midbrain to the inferior surface of the cerebellum overlying the medulla. The lesion would also need to extend into the depths of the cerebellar fissures. It is extremely unlikely that this could happen without damaging other parts of the cerebellum and possibly parts of the brainstem. As a result, what is typically seen clinically are problems referable to the flocculonodular lobe, the vermis, or one or both sides of the body of the cerebellum as a whole.

Midline Damage Causes Postural Instability

The malnutrition often accompanying chronic alcoholism causes a degeneration of the cerebellar cortex that tends to start at the anterior end of the anterior lobe and spread backwards. A great deal of the anterior lobe is occupied by vermis and paravermis (Figure 20-4), and the legs are represented most anteriorly (Figure 20-17). The result is a syndrome (called the **anterior lobe syndrome**) in which the legs are primarily affected, and the most prominent symptom is a broad-based, staggering gait, similar in

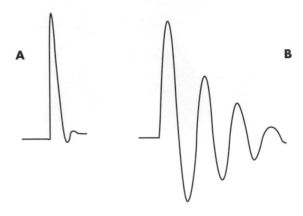

FIGURE 20-23
Reflex changes accompanying cerebellar damage. **A,** Tracing of limb movement during a knee-jerk reflex in a normal subject. Note that the brief reflex limb movement is followed by a small secondary movement that dies out quickly; even the small secondary movement is frequently missing in normal subjects. **B,** Tracing of a knee-jerk reflex of the right leg in a patient who had sustained right-sided cerebellar damage 8 years previously. Note the poorly damped oscillation after the reflex response. (Redrawn from Holmes G: The symptoms of acute cerebellar injuries due to gunshot injuries, *Brain* 40:461, 1917.)

many ways to that seen after damage to the flocculonodular lobe. In the anterior lobe syndrome, however, there is a general incoordination, or **ataxia,** (Greek for "lack of order") of leg movements, even when the trunk is supported.

Lateral Damage Causes Limb Ataxia

Most of the cerebellum is made up of the lateral hemispheres, and with a few exceptions such as the one just mentioned, this is the region most heavily damaged in lesions of the body of the cerebellum. The result is called the **neocerebellar syndrome,** which is characterized by a variable combination of changes in muscle tone, reflexes, and the coordination of voluntary movements, all ipsilateral to the side of the lesion.

Widespread decreases in muscle tone **(hypotonia)** may occur with small lesions, so that the limbs offer little resistance to passive movement and muscles feel abnormally soft and flaccid. Stretch reflexes are often reduced **(hyporeflexia),** and as a result of the hypotonia a limb may swing back and forth after a reflex contraction **(pendular reflexes,** Figure 20-23).

Most prominent, however, is a lack of coordination of voluntary movements. This is caused by a fundamental deficit in the timing of movements and the regulation of their rates. As shown in Figure 20-24, voluntary movements take longer than usual to initiate, and there are problems in stopping them or changing their direction. This is manifest in a number of different ways: patients are likely to overshoot or undershoot targets **(dysmetria),** corrective movements when the patient nears a target have the appearance of a tremor **(intention tremor),** and

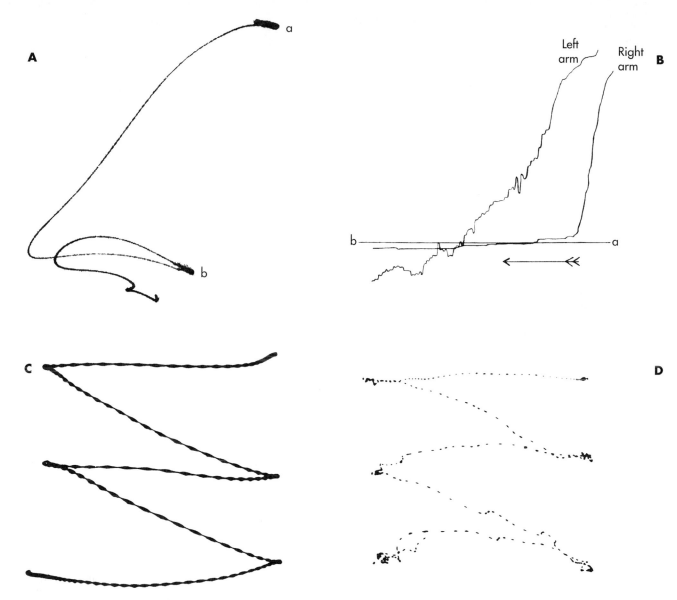

FIGURE 20-24

Movements made by patients with cerebellar lesions (all involving one or both hemispheres), recorded by the simple but ingenious technique of photographing a light bulb attached to the patient's finger (**A, C,** and **D**) or by recording the movement on a revolving drum (**B**). **A,** A patient attempts to touch his nose (at *b*) with the tip of his finger, starting from point *a* above his head; the movement has two distinct parts to it instead of being a smooth, continuous sweep (decomposition of movement), and the patient misjudges the range (dysmetria), striking his nose and then making irregular corrective movements. **B,** A patient with left-sided cerebellar damage attempts to stretch two similar springs and then keep them stretched to the level of the line *ab*; time progresses from right to left in this record. The normal right arm moves promptly and accurately, but the left arm starts slowly, moves slowly, makes many small corrective movements, overshoots the line, and is then unable to maintain a constant stretch. **C** and **D,** A patient with right-sided cerebellar damage moves each hand back and forth between a series of small targets; the light attached to his fingertip was flashing at a constant rate, so the separation between spots is a measure of finger velocity. The left hand (**C**) performs smoothly and accurately, but the right hand (**D**) moves at varying speeds and has particular difficulty stopping and changing direction. [From Holmes G: The cerebellum of man, *Brain* 62:1, 1939.]

rapid alternating movements, such as repeatedly pronating and supinating the forearm, may be especially difficult **(dysdiadochokinesia).** Note that the intention tremor of cerebellar disease is quite different from the resting tremor seen in disorders of the basal ganglia, partly because it is seen *during* voluntary movements and partly because it is not so rhythmic or regular. When complex movements involving more than one joint are performed, the timing of different parts may be defective in different

ways, leading to **decomposition of movement** (Figure 20-24, *A*). The complex movements used in speaking may be affected in this way, in which case the normal flow and rhythm of speech is disrupted; successive syllables may emerge slowly and separated from each other **(scanning speech).**

In view of current notions of the function of the cerebellar hemispheres in the programming of skilled voluntary movements, it is important to note again that the neocerebellar syndrome is not accompanied by any sensory deficits. Gordon Holmes (a famous British neurologist) described a patient who had incurred damage to his right cerebellar hemisphere and who said, "The movements of my left arm are done subconsciously, but I have to think out each movement of the right arm. I come to a dead stop in turning and have to think before I start again."

Damage to the Flocculus Affects Eye Movements

The nodulus sits on the roof of the caudal part of the fourth ventricle. Tumors called *medulloblastomas* occasionally arise in the roof of the ventricle, usually in young children, and are the most common cause of damage to the flocculonodular lobe. Affected individuals have a general loss of equilibrium—they sway from side to side when standing; walk with a staggering, wide-based gait; and tend to fall over. The basic mechanisms used in moving the limbs are unaffected, so that when the trunk is supported (e.g., when lying in bed), movements of the arms and legs are normal. In contrast to the findings after damage to the cerebellar hemispheres, there is no tremor, and both reflexes and muscle tone remain normal. A variety of eye movement difficulties may also be seen, such as problems with pursuit eye movements, with maintaining eccentric gaze, or with making accurate voluntary eye movements (see Chapter 21). However, eye movement disorders may be found after damage to other cerebellar regions as well. As a further consequence of these tumors, the lateral and median apertures of the fourth ventricle may be squeezed shut, with ensuing noncommunicating hydrocephalus.

SUGGESTED READINGS

Aas J-E: Subcortical projections to the pontine nuclei in the cat, *J Comp Neurol* 282:331, 1989.

Angevine JB Jr, Mancall EL, Yakovlev PI: *The human cerebellum: an atlas of gross topography in serial sections,* Boston, 1961, Little, Brown & Co. *A review of various systems of cerebellar nomenclature and terminology together with a collection of beautiful sections cut in several different planes.*

Asanuma C, Thach WT, Jones EG: Distribution of cerebellar terminations and their relation to other afferent terminations in the ventral lateral thalamic region of the monkey, *Brain Res Rev* 5:237, 1983.

Bloedel JR, Dichgans J, Precht W: *Cerebellar functions,* Berlin, 1985, Springer-Verlag.

Brecha N, Karten HJ: Accessory optic projections upon oculomotor nuclei and vestibulocerebellum, *Science* 203:913, 1979. *A route by which visual information used in guiding eye movements reaches the cerebellum.*

Carpenter MB, Batton RR III: Connections of the fastigial nucleus in the cat and monkey, *Exp Brain Res Suppl* 6:250, 1982.

Chan-Palay V: *Cerebellar dentate nucleus: organization, cytology, and transmitters,* New York, 1977, Springer-Verlag.

Courville J, de Montigny C, Lamarre Y: *The inferior olivary nucleus,* New York, 1980, Raven Press.

Demer JL, Robinson DA: Effects of reversible lesions and stimulation of olivocerebellar system on vestibuloocular reflex plasticity, *J Neurophysiol* 47:1084, 1982.

Desmond JE et al: Lobular patterns of cerebellar activation in verbal working-memory and finger-tapping tasks as revealed by functional MRI, *J Neurosci* 17:9675, 1997.

Fiez JA et al: Impaired non-motor learning and error detection associated with cerebellar damage: a single case study, *Brain* 115:155, 1992. *A particularly well-studied case of cognitive changes after cerebellar damage.*

Flumerfelt BA, Otabe S, Courville J: Distinct projections to the red nucleus from the dentate and interposed nuclei in the monkey, *Brain Res* 50:408, 1973.

Glickstein M: Cerebellar agenesis, *Brain* 117:1209, 1994. *It is sometimes claimed that individuals with congenital absence of the cerebellum have normal or near-normal motor functions. This paper argues that published studies indicate "cerebellar agenesis is always associated with profound motor deficits."*

Glickstein M, Yeo C: The cerebellum and motor learning, *J Cog Neurosci* 2:69, 1990. *A brief but enjoyable review of the history of theories about cerebellar function and of recent evidence that it is important for motor learning.*

Gould BB, Graybiel AM: Afferents to the cerebellar cortex in the cat: evidence for an intrinsic pathway leading from the deep nuclei to the cortex, *Brain Res* 110:601, 1976.

Grant G, Xu Q: Routes of entry into the cerebellum of spinocerebellar axons from the lower part of the spinal cord: an experimental study in the cat, *Exp Brain Res* 72:543, 1988.

Haines DE, May PJ, Dietrichs E: Neuronal connections between the cerebellar nuclei and hypothalamus in *Macaca fascicularis, J Comp Neurol* 299:106, 1990.

Harvey RJ, Napper RMA: Quantitative studies on the mammalian cerebellum, *Prog Neurobiol* 36:437, 1991.

Herrup K, Kuermerle B: The compartmentalization of the cerebellum, *Ann Rev Neurosci* 20:61, 1997. *The beginnings of a molecular basis for the medial-lateral and anterior-posterior subdivisions of the cerebellum.*

Holmes G: The cerebellum of man, *Brain* 62:1, 1939. *Still the all-time great description of the neocerebellar syndrome in man and the source of the striking illustrations used in Figure 20-24.*

Ikeda M: Projections from the spinal and the principal sensory nuclei of the trigeminal nerve to the cerebellar cortex in the cat, as studied by retrograde transport of horseradish peroxidase, *J Comp Neurol* 184:57, 1979.

Ito M: *The cerebellum and neural control,* New York, 1984, Raven Press.

Kalil K: Projections of the cerebellar and dorsal column nuclei upon the inferior olive in the rhesus monkey: an autoradiographic study, *J Comp Neurol* 188:43, 1979.

Keele SW, Ivry R: Does the cerebellum provide a common computation for diverse tasks? A timing hypothesis, *Ann NY Acad Sci* 608:179, 1990. *A broad hypothesis, proposing that the cerebellum comes into play whenever there is a need for accurate computations involving time—whether for timing movements or for judging durations or velocities.*

Langer T et al: Afferents to the flocculus of the cerebellum in the rhesus macaque as revealed by retrograde transport of horseradish peroxidase, *J Comp Neurol* 235:1, 1985.

Langer T et al: Floccular efferents in the rhesus macaque as revealed by autoradiography and horseradish peroxidase, *J Comp Neurol* 235:26, 1985.

Larsell O, Jansen J: *The comparative anatomy and histology of the cerebellum: the human cerebellum, cerebellar connections, and the cerebellar cortex,* Minneapolis, 1972, University of Minnesota Press.

Lechtenberg R, Gilman S: Speech disorders in cerebellar disease, *Ann Neurol* 3:285, 1978. *Cerebellar speech disorders are often considered to be caused by damage to the vermis, but this report presents an alternative view.*

Marinković S et al: The anatomical basis for the cerebellar infarcts, *Surg Neurol* 44:450, 1995. *A recent review of the blood supply of the cerebellum.*

Martin TA et al: Throwing while looking through prisms. I. Focal olivocerebellar lesions impair adaptation. II. Specificity and storage of multiple gaze-throw calibrations, *Brain* 119:1183 and 1199, 1996.

Massion J, Rispal-Padel L: Spatial organization of the cerebello-thalamo-cortical pathway, *Brain Res* 40:61, 1972.

McCormick DA, Steinmetz JE, Thompson RF: Lesions of the inferior olivary complex cause extinction of the classically conditioned eyeblink response, *Brain Res* 359:120, 1985.

Mercier BE, Legg CR, Glickstein M: Basal ganglia and cerebellum receive different somatosensory information, *Proc Nat Acad Sci* 87:4388, 1990.

Meyer-Lohmann J, Hore J, Brooks VB: Cerebellar participation in generation of prompt arm movements, *J Neurophysiol* 40:1038, 1977. *What happens to voluntary movements when one dentate nucleus is temporarily disabled.*

Middleton FA, Strick PL: Dentate output channels: motor and cognitive components. In De Zeeuw CI, Strata P, Voogd J, editors: *The cerebellum: from structure to control* (*Prog Brain Res* vol 114), Amsterdam, 1997, Elsevier.

Mihailoff GA: Cerebellar nuclear projections from the basilar pontine nuclei and nucleus reticularis tegmenti pontis as demonstrated with PHA-L tracing in the rat, *J Comp Neurol* 330:130, 1993.

Murphy MG, O'Leary JL: Neurological deficit in cats with lesions of the olivocerebellar system, *Arch Neurol* 24:145, 1971.

Orlovsky GN: Activity of vestibulospinal neurons during locomotion, *Brain Res* 46:85, 1972. *The activity is rhythmically modulated, and the modulation disappears after cerebellar lesions.*

Palay SL, Chan-Palay V: *Cerebellar cortex: cytology and organization,* New York, 1974, Springer-Verlag. *A beautiful book, full of Golgi-stained cells and electron micrographs.*

Papka M, Ivry RB, Woodruff-Pak DS: Selective disruption of eyeblink classical conditioning by concurrent tapping, *NeuroReport* 6:1493, 1995. *Clever experiments suggesting that you can use multiple memory systems simultaneously, but only for one task each.*

Parenti R et al: The projections of the lateral reticular nucleus to the deep cerebellar nuclei: an experimental analysis in the rat, *Eur J Neurosci* 8:2157, 1996.

Payne JN: The cerebellar nucleo-cortical projection in the rat studied by the retrograde fluorescent double-labelling method, *Brain Res* 271:141, 1983.

Raymond JL, Lisberger SG, Mauk MD: The cerebellum: a neuronal learning machine? *Science* 272:1126, 1996.

Sanes JN, Dimitrov B, Hallet M: Motor learning in patients with cerebellar dysfunction, *Brain* 113:103, 1990.

Schmahmann JD: From movement to thought: anatomic substrates of the cerebellar contribution to cognitive processing, *Hum Brain Mapping* 4:174, 1996.

Schwarz C, Schmitz Y: Projection from the cerebellar lateral nucleus to precerebellar nuclei in the mossy fiber pathway is glutamatergic: a study combining anterograde tracing with immunogold labeling in the rat, *J Comp Neurol* 381:320, 1997.

Shepherd GM: *The synaptic organization of the brain,* ed 4, New York, 1998, Oxford University Press. *A nice, readable book about a number of areas of the CNS; Chapter 7 covers the cerebellum.*

Snider RS: Recent contributions to the anatomy and physiology of the cerebellum, *Arch Neurol Psychiatry* 64:196, 1950. *A summary of the electrophysiologically determined mapping of the cerebral cortex and the body surface onto the cerebellar cortex.*

Sugihara I, Wu H, Shinoda Y: Morphology of axon collaterals of single climbing fibers in the deep cerebellar nuclei of the rat, *Neurosci Lett* 217:33, 1996.

Thach WT: Timing of activity in cerebellar dentate nucleus and cerebral motor cortex during prompt volitional movement, *Brain Res* 88:233, 1975.

Thompson RF: The neurobiology of learning and memory, *Science* 233:941, 1986. *A review by one of the principal investigators of the role of the cerebellum in classical conditioning.*

Tolbert DL, Bantli H, Bloedel JR: Organizational features of the cat and monkey cerebellar nucleocortical projection, *J Comp Neurol* 182:39, 1978.

Victor M, Adams RD, Mancall EL: A restricted form of cerebellar cortical degeneration occurring in alcoholic patients, *Arch Neurol* 1:578, 1959.

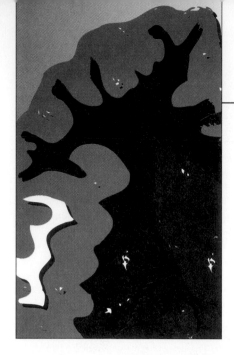

CONTROL OF EYE MOVEMENTS

Photoreceptors are sensitive but slow, and all animals have mechanisms to prevent images of interest from moving across the retina too quickly to be analyzed. (Dredging up the camera analogy from Chapter 17, our eyes behave in many respects like cameras with a shutter speed of about 1/10 of a second.) In addition, we have good spatial acuity for only a small area of central vision (see Figure 17-17). Finally, effective binocular vision requires precise alignment of the two eyes.

Our eyes do a fairly remarkable job of tracking (or moving to look at) various objects as the objects and/or we move about in three-dimensional space. Throughout this process the two eyes stay aligned with each other to a high degree of accuracy. Two general types of movement are involved: (1) **conjugate movements,** in which the two eyes move the same amount in the same direction, as in visually tracking an object that moves about at a fixed distance from us, and (2) **vergence movements,** in which the two eyes

move in opposite directions, as in the **convergence** that occurs when we look at a nearby object. Normally, conjugate and vergence movements are smoothly integrated with one another so that images of the outside world fall on the two retinas in proper registration. The CNS circuits that control eye movements for these various purposes have many properties in common with those described in the last three chapters for the control of other skeletal muscles—upper motor neurons, lower motor neurons, and interactions with the basal ganglia and cerebellum.

SIX EXTRAOCULAR MUSCLES MOVE THE EYE IN THE ORBIT

Six small **extraocular muscles** (Figure 21-1) rotate each eye in its orbit, like a ball in a socket. Four **rectus** muscles (**medial, lateral, superior,** and **inferior**) originate from

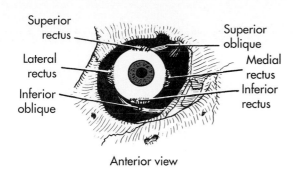

Anterior view

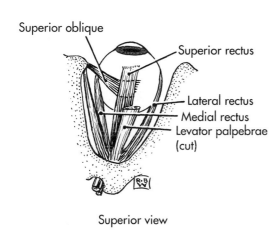

Superior view

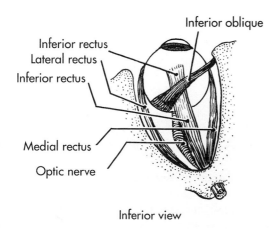

Inferior view

FIGURE 21-1
Anterior, superior, and inferior views of the extraocular muscles of the right eye. (From von Noorden GK: *Atlas of strabismus*, ed 4, St. Louis, 1983, Mosby.)

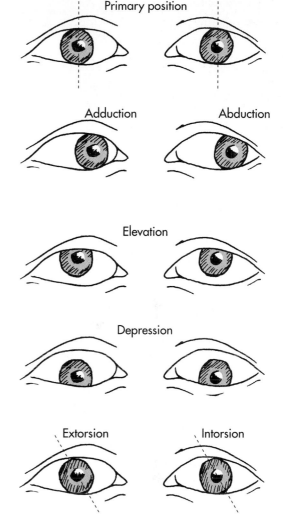

FIGURE 21-2
Terminology for eye movements around different axes.

rior oblique originates near the common tendinous ring, from the sphenoid bone at the back of the orbit, but takes a most unusual course in reaching the eye. Near the front of the orbit, the superior oblique tendon passes through a fibrous loop (the **trochlea★**) attached to the frontal bone, turns posteriorly and laterally, and inserts in the sclera of the posterior half of the eye. The **inferior oblique** originates anteriorly and medially from the floor of the orbit, passes across the inferior surface of the eye, and inserts posteriorly.

Different patterns of contraction of the six extraocular muscles rotate the eye horizontally **(adduction, abduction),** vertically **(elevation, depression),** or around the anterior-posterior axis **(extorsion, intorsion)** (Figure 21-2).

a common tendinous ring (annulus of Zinn) in the back of the orbit and insert *anteriorly* in the sclera, 5 to 8 mm from the limbus (Figure 21-3). Two **oblique** muscles, as the name implies, pass obliquely over the surface of the eye and insert in the sclera of its *posterior* half. The **supe-**

★*Trochlea*, from which the fourth cranial nerve derives its name, is Greek for "pulley."

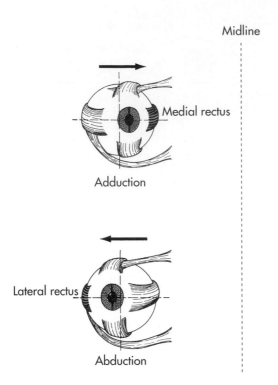

FIGURE 21-3
Actions of the medial and lateral recti of the right eye. (Modified from Moses RA, editor: *Adler's physiology of the eye,* ed 5, St. Louis, 1970, Mosby.)

The Medial and Lateral Recti Adduct and Abduct the Eye

The medial and lateral recti are situated in a horizontal plane, so contractions of these muscles rotate the eye around a vertical axis. This makes their actions straightforward (Figure 21-3)—the medial rectus adducts and the lateral rectus abducts the eye.

The Superior and Inferior Recti and the Obliques Have More Complex Actions

The actions of the superior and inferior recti and the obliques are not quite so straightforward, because the anatomical axis of the orbit is deviated about 23° laterally from the visual axis of the eye (Figure 21-4). The result, as indicated for the superior rectus and superior oblique in Figure 21-5 but equally true for the inferior rectus and inferior oblique, is that when one of these muscles contracts the eye rotates around an axis that is neither vertical nor transverse nor anterior-posterior. Rather, each of these four muscles has one principal action and weaker additional actions (Figure 21-6).

Many extraocular muscle actions are neglected in this chapter to keep things reasonably simple. Torsional move-

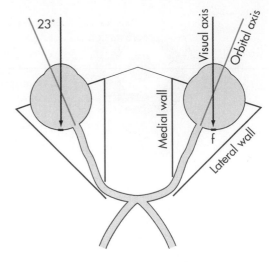

FIGURE 21-4
Relative orientations of the eyes and orbits. The eye, when focused for far vision, points more or less straight ahead so that images land on the fovea (*f*). Because the lateral wall of each orbit is oriented about 45° from the sagittal plane, the axis of the orbit, along which the superior and inferior recti pull, is oriented about 23° from the visual axis.

ments are not discussed,★ and adduction, abduction, elevation, and depression are treated as the result of contraction of one of the rectus muscles. However, eye movements actually involve coordinated changes in the activity of all six extraocular muscles (Table 21-1), some contracting and some relaxing in response to changing levels of input from the oculomotor, trochlear, and abducens nuclei (see Figures 12-3 to 12-5). For example, adduction involves simultaneous contraction of the medial, superior, and inferior recti and relaxation of the lateral rectus and the superior and inferior obliques; the intorsion and extorsion of the superior and inferior recti cancel each other.

THERE ARE FAST AND SLOW CONJUGATE EYE MOVEMENTS

Conjugate movements serve two general purposes—to move an object's image onto the fovea and then to keep it there. We use fast eye movements called **saccades** (from a French word meaning "a pull on the reins") to redirect gaze so an image falls on the fovea. These are brief, rapid movements of the kind we use to move our eyes voluntarily in any given direction, and the same

---

★We tend not to think much about torsional movements, but if you tilt your head to one side, both of your eyes counterrotate in partial compensation. Tilts like this do not disturb images on the fovea too much, so torsional movements are less important for us than for more lateral-eyed animals.

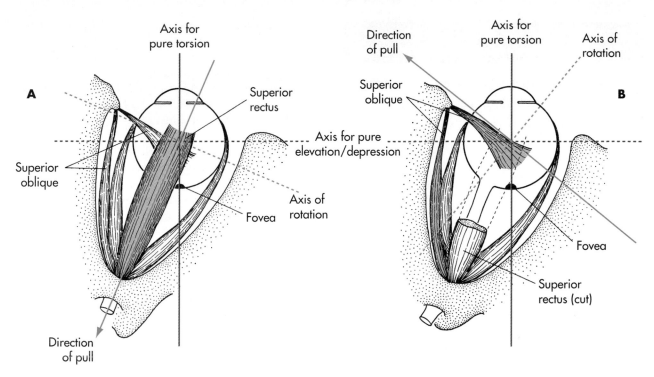

FIGURE 21-5
Directions of pull and axes of rotation of the right superior rectus **(A)** and superior oblique **(B)**, relative to the axes of rotation for pure torsion or pure elevation/depression. [Modified from Moses RA, editor: *Adler's physiology of the eye*, ed 5, St. Louis, 1970, Mosby.]

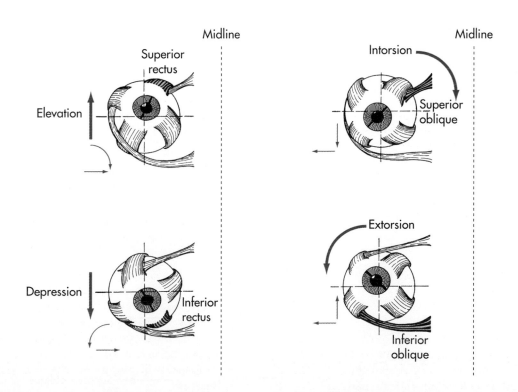

FIGURE 21-6
Actions of the right superior and inferior recti and obliques. Each has a primary action *(large arrow)* and two secondary actions *(small arrows)* when starting from primary position. The actions are determined both by the direction of insertion of a muscle's tendon and by the position of the insertion. For example, the superior rectus and superior oblique both insert on the superior surface of the globe. However, the superior rectus inserts anteriorly and pulls posteriorly, so it elevates the eye. In contrast, the superior oblique inserts posteriorly and pulls in part anteriorly (Figure 21-5), so part of its action is depression. [Modified from Moses RA, editor: *Adler's physiology of the eye*, ed 5, St. Louis, 1970, Mosby.]

Table 21-1 Extraocular Muscles Contributing to Movements Around Different Axes

Movement	Principal muscle	Other muscles contributing
Adduction	Medial rectus	Superior rectus Inferior rectus
Abduction	Lateral rectus	Superior oblique Inferior oblique
Elevation	Superior rectus	Inferior oblique
Depression	Inferior rectus	Superior oblique
Extorsion	Inferior oblique	Inferior rectus
Intorsion	Superior oblique	Superior rectus

Box 21-1 Smooth Eye Movements Usually Require a Target Moving Across the Retina

It comes as a surprise to most that with the head stationary we can only move our eyes smoothly when we are tracking a slowly moving object. This is easily demonstrated, however. Watch someone's eyes as he or she tries to move them slowly and smoothly while there is nothing to track, or concentrate on your own eyes while you try to do the same thing. In either case the result will be the same: a series of rapid, jerky movements (Figure 21-7, *A* and *B*). Some individuals can learn to have voluntary control of smooth tracking movements, but under normal circumstances and for most people, this is usually impossible. Interestingly enough, real moving stimuli in other sensory modalities provide an adequate stimulus for some smooth movements. For example, many people can use smooth eye movements to track their own index finger as it moves back and forth in the dark (Figure 21-7, *C*), even though they would be unable to use such eye movements to track an imaginary moving finger. Similarly, smooth eye movements can be used to track a moving sound source in the dark.

neural machinery is used to generate the fast phase of nystagmus. We use different kinds of smooth, slower eye movements to keep an image on the fovea, corresponding to the fact that an image could move on the retina if we moved or if the object moved. The **vestibuloocular reflex** (see Figures 14-27 and 14-28) compensates for head movements, supplemented in this function by **optokinetic** movements (see Figure 14-29, *A*); for large head movements, these smooth eye movements become the slow phase of nystagmus. **Smooth pursuit movements** are used to track a visual stimulus that is itself moving. Without special training, we are unable to move our eyes smoothly unless an image threatens to leave the fovea (Box 21-1).

A network of neural structures in both the brainstem and the cerebral hemispheres is involved in the initiation and coordination of conjugate eye movements (Figure 21-8). Basically it involves reflex connections and motor programs for these eye movements, located in the brain-

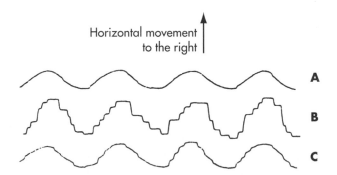

FIGURE 21-7

Recordings of the horizontal eye movements of a normal subject in an otherwise dark room as he tracked an LED moving back and forth (**A**), tried to imagine an LED moving back and forth and track it with his eyes (**B**), and tried to follow the position of his finger as he moved his arm back and forth in the dark (**C**); upward deflections indicate movement to the right. Movements with the somatosensory assist are much smoother than those with only an imaginary target. You can approximate this experiment yourself by closing your eyes and concentrating on how they move as you try to track an imaginary target or your own moving finger. (From Hasiba M et al: Non-visually induced smooth pursuit eye movements using sinusoidal target motion, *Acta Otolaryngol Suppl* 525:158, 1996.)

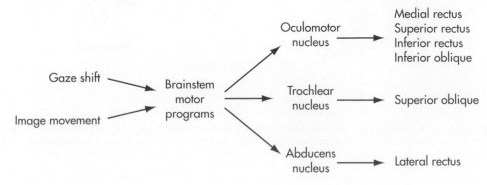

FIGURE 21-8
Schematic overview of eye movement control systems.

stem, together with cerebral and cerebellar centers that are able to trigger or modulate these brainstem mechanisms. No corticobulbar fibers reach the abducens, trochlear, or oculomotor nuclei directly (Figures 21-11 and 21-14).

Fast, Ballistic Eye Movements Get Images Onto the Fovea

Saccades and the fast phases of nystagmus are extremely rapid, reaching velocities of 700°/sec (Figure 21-9). This is too fast for the visual system to provide useful feedback★ under most circumstances, and fast eye movements generally behave as though the CNS computes the size of the required movement in advance (which takes about 200 msec), initiates the movement, and makes no corrections during its course. Preprogrammed movements such as this are referred to as *ballistic.*

Motor programs for saccades are located in the pons and midbrain

Moving an eye at 700°/sec to a target requires a brief, strong contraction of one or more extraocular muscles, followed by a weaker, sustained contraction to keep the eye in its new position. This is accomplished by motor programs whose circuitry resides in the brainstem: appropriate patterns of excitation are provided to motor neurons in the abducens, trochlear, or oculomotor nuclei by specialized areas of the pontine and mesencephalic reticular formation.

The neural machinery for generating rapid horizontal movements is located in the medial reticular formation of the pons near the abducens nucleus, a region commonly referred to by the logical but cumbersome name **paramedian pontine reticular formation (PPRF).** Signals from this region project to the abducens nucleus, with each PPRF directing movements to the ipsilateral side (Figure 21-11). The machinery for rapid vertical movements is located in the reticular formation of the rostral midbrain (in a region called the **rostral interstitial nucleus of the MLF**). Upward and downward movements depend on slightly different areas of this part of the reticular formation. One of the common early effects of pineal tumors is paralysis of upward gaze (together with disturbances of convergence). Downward gaze is usually affected only later or when lesions are situated more deeply in the mesencephalic tegmentum. Both upward and downward gaze seem to be represented bilaterally in the midbrain, as unilateral lesions do not cause paralysis of vertical movements.

★We do not have a sensation of blurred vision during these fast eye movements (even though images move across the retina very rapidly) because the CNS suppresses or ignores visual input during these brief periods.

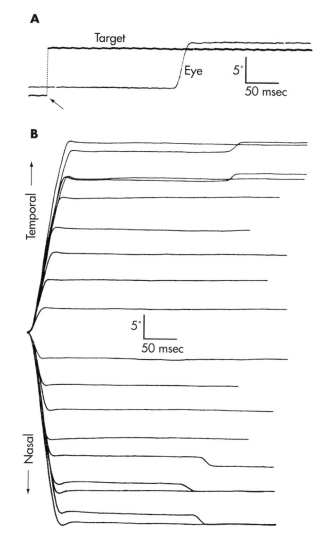

FIGURE 21-9

Time course of saccades, shown in recordings of the horizontal eye movements of a monkey trained to make gaze shifts (with head stationary) to follow a target that makes occasional jumps in position; upward deflections indicate movement to the right. **A,** After a target jump *(arrow)* the monkey makes a rapid (about 580°/sec) saccade to its new position after a latency of about 200 msec. **B,** Larger and larger target jumps elicit saccades of increasing duration and peak velocity. Saccades in response to the largest target jumps are often a little too small and are followed by a corrective saccade, after an additional 200 to 250 msec latency. (From Fuchs AF: Saccadic and smooth pursuit eye movements in the monkey, *J Physiol* 191:609, 1967.)

The frontal eye fields and superior colliculus trigger saccades to the contralateral side

Saccades are the eye movements we use routinely to explore the world visually during activities as varied as scanning scenes and pictures (Figure 21-10) and reading. Cortical control of saccades parallels that of other voluntary movements, with an equivalent of primary motor cortex and contributions from other cortical areas.

The **frontal eye field,** located in the posterior portion of the middle frontal gyrus just in front of the representa-

A   **B**

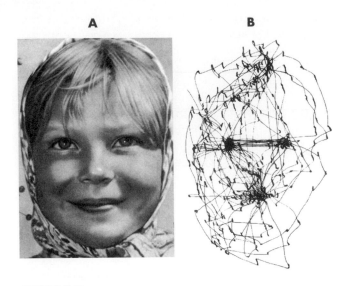

FIGURE 21-10

Using saccades to scan visual scenes. **A,** A photograph called "Girl from Volga," which a subject was asked to look at for 2 minutes. **B,** Recordings of eye position during this 2-minute period. Thin lines represent saccades between points of fixation, which center around parts of the face of greatest visual interest. The subject has no conscious sensation of making these saccades and of having brief periods of blurred vision. Rather, the CNS ignores inputs during the saccades and combines the visual inputs during the periods of fixation into a single, unified visual perception. (From Yarbus AL: *Eye movements and vision,* New York, 1967, Plenum Press.)

tion of the face in the precentral gyrus (Figure 21-11), is prominently involved in the initiation of saccades. Stimulation here causes horizontal or oblique conjugate movements to the contralateral side, mediated in part by direct projections to the PPRF and in part by projections to the superior colliculus, which in turn projects to the PPRF. Part of the supplementary motor area and part of the parietal lobe also participate in the initiation of saccades, both through connections with the frontal eye field and through direct projections to the brainstem. Stimulation of these areas also elicits saccades and, as in the case of other voluntary movements, it is assumed that each of these cortical areas has a distinctive role. The parietal eye field may be especially involved in more automatic saccades to things that appear in the periphery, and the supplementary eye field in sequences of multiple saccades.

Damage to the frontal eye field of one hemisphere causes inability to look voluntarily to the contralateral side. It can easily be shown, however, that the appropriate muscles are not paralyzed, because other movements, such as those of the vestibuloocular reflex, remain intact. Vertical eye movements are not impaired after a unilateral lesion, and even the deficit in horizontal movements is transitory, with recovery usually occurring in a matter of days. The relative roles of increased activity of the superior colliculus, other cortical areas, and the contralateral frontal eye field in this recovery of function are unclear. However, combined damage to the frontal eye fields and superior colliculi causes a severe and long-lasting deficit in the ability to generate saccades.

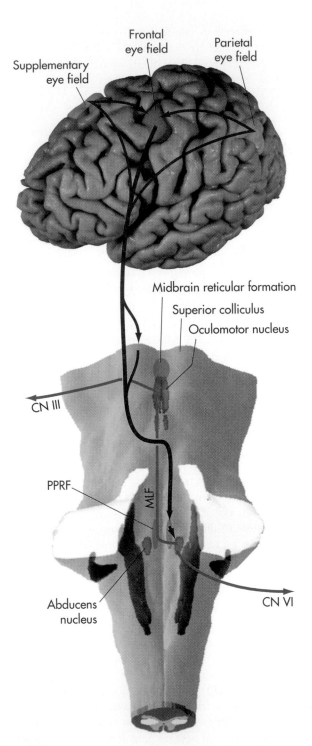

FIGURE 21-11

Cortical areas and brainstem circuitry concerned with generating saccades to the right. The part of the supplementary motor area involved with eye movements is sometimes referred to separately as the **supplementary eye field.**

Slow, Guided Eye Movements Keep Images on the Fovea

The eye movements used to keep images from moving off the fovea are slower than saccades—typically up to about 100°/sec, rather than 700°/sec—slow enough to utilize continuous feedback from the vestibular and visual systems to regulate their speed and duration. As noted earlier, images move on the retina if you move or if some part of the outside world moves. These often happen simultaneously (think about playing any sport that involves a ball), and we have smoothly integrated mechanisms, all funneling through the vestibular nuclei, for dealing with both.

Vestibuloocular and optokinetic movements compensate for head movement

One of the greatest threats to stability of images on the retina is the constant head movement that occurs as creatures walk, run, or swim through their environments, and all jawed vertebrates use essentially similar mechanisms to deal with this. Head movement not only stimulates the semicircular canals and otolithic organs, but also causes the image of the outside world to begin sweeping across the retina; both sets of sensory signals are used to generate compensatory eye movements.

The semicircular canals developed in parallel with the extraocular muscles (Box 21-2) and form the afferent limb of the vestibuloocular reflex (VOR) (see Figures 14-27 and 14-28). As described in Chapter 14, this is a three-neuron reflex arc★ that generates compensatory eye movements in the opposite direction from head movements. Primary afferents are in the vestibular gan-

---

★Except for reflex contraction of the medial rectus, which requires an additional interneuron whose cell body is in the abducens nucleus.

Box 21-2 Using the Same VOR for Eyes With Different Orientations

The vestibuloocular system appeared early in vertebrate phylogeny and has not changed much in its essentials. Each semicircular canal is nearly parallel to the plane in which one extraocular muscle of each eye pulls, and increased activity of the semicircular canal selectively excites those two muscles and inhibits their antagonists (Table 21-2). This creates some interesting challenges for the vestibuloocular reflex, because not all animals have their eyes situated in their heads the same way. Consider the example of rotating a lateral-eyed rabbit and a frontal-eyed human about an anterior-posterior axis (i.e., an axis passing through the bridge of the nose and the occiput). For a rotation that moves the left ear downward, the appropriate compensatory eye movements for a rabbit would be elevation of the left eye and depression of the right eye; for a human, the appropriate movements would be torsional—intorsion of the left eye and extorsion of the right. Yet in both, the rotation causes depolarization of hair cells in the left anterior and posterior canals and contraction of the left superior rectus and superior oblique. The remarkable resolution of this apparent conflict lies in the fact that as orbits evolved into different positions, so did the origins and insertions of extraocular muscles (Figure 21-12). The result is that contraction of a rabbit's left superior oblique and superior rectus produces elevation of the left eye; contraction of the same two muscles in a human produces intorsion.

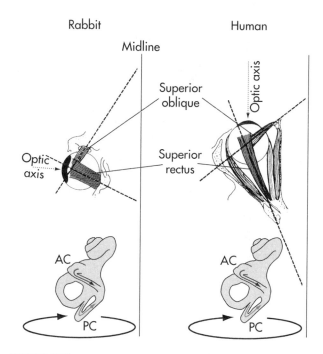

FIGURE 21-12
Effects of the same rotation (rolling to left) on the left eye of a rabbit and a person; the view is as if you were looking down from above on both subjects. The insertion of the rabbit's superior oblique is anterior, so both the superior oblique and superior rectus elevate the eye; the torsions of the two muscles cancel each other. The insertion of the human superior oblique is posterior, so it is a depressor that in this movement cancels the elevation of the superior rectus; both muscles combine to intort the eye. *AC,* Anterior semicircular canal; *PC,* posterior semicircular canal. (Modified from Simpson JI, Graf W: Eye-muscle geometry and compensatory eye movements in lateral-eyed and frontal-eyed animals, *Ann NY Acad Sci* 374:20, 1981.)

Table 21-2 Effects of Increased Activity From Individual Semicircular Canals on Extraocular Muscles

Canal	Excitation (ipsilateral)	Inhibition (ipsilateral)	Excitation (contralateral)	Inhibition (contralateral)
Anterior	Superior rectus	Inferior rectus	Inferior oblique	Superior oblique
Posterior	Superior oblique	Inferior oblique	Inferior rectus	Superior rectus
Horizontal	Medial rectus	Lateral rectus	Lateral rectus	Medial rectus

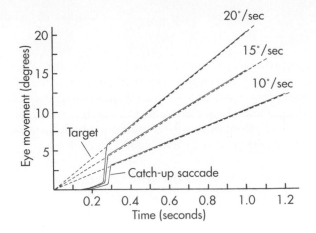

FIGURE 21-13
Time course of smooth pursuit movements, shown in recordings of
the horizontal eye movements of a monkey trained to track (with
head stationary) a target moving at different velocities; upward deflections indicate movement to the right. Smooth pursuit starts
sooner than a saccade could, about 150 msec after target movement
begins, but by then the target has moved off the fovea. The CNS
"knows" this will happen, however, and generates a saccade at about
250 msec that places the target image back on the fovea. (From
Fuchs AF: Saccadic and smooth pursuit eye movements in the monkey,
J Physiol 191:609, 1967.)

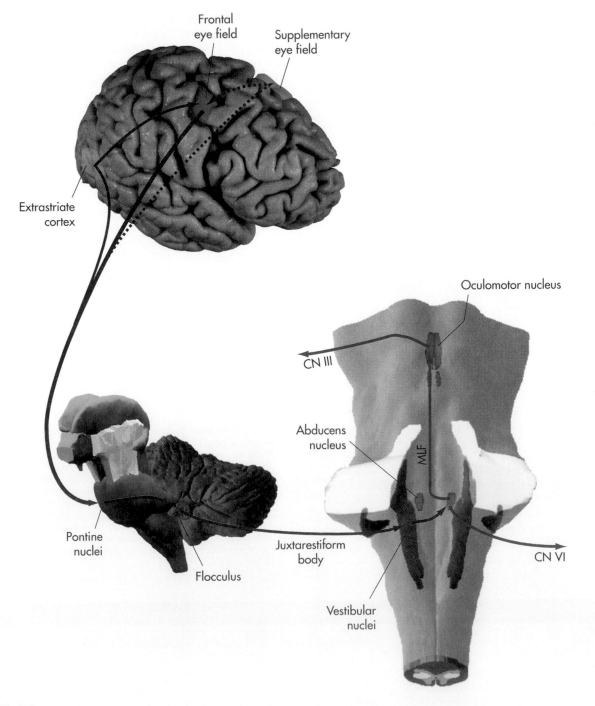

FIGURE 21-14
Cortical areas and other neural circuitry involved in smooth pursuit movements. The involvement of the supplementary eye field is shown
dashed because its role is still uncertain.

glion, interneurons in the vestibular nuclei, and motor neurons in the abducens, trochlear, and oculomotor nuclei. The vestibuloocular reflex, with a latency of only about 15 msec, is the fastest mechanism available for generating compensatory eye movements and is particularly effective at dealing with the high-frequency components of head movements during locomotion. Interactions between the flocculus and the brainstem can cancel part or all of the VOR, allowing combined use of head and eye movements to shift gaze or follow targets.

The vestibuloocular reflex is not so effective with prolonged or low-frequency components of movement, which call into play a complementary system of compensatory optokinetic movements. Motion-sensitive ganglion cells project not only to the lateral geniculate nucleus but also to a series of small **accessory optic nuclei** in the rostral midbrain. These in turn project to the vestibular nuclei, stimulating the same neurons that drive the vestibuloocular reflex and producing eye movements that oppose image movement on the retina. This brainstem optokinetic system is present but rudimentary in humans, having been largely supplanted by cortically driven smooth pursuit movements (which also utilize the vestibular nuclei; see next section).

Smooth pursuit movements compensate for target movement

The development of a fovea adds a requirement for another kind of eye movement, one designed to keep small but interesting images on the fovea even if they are moving relative to the background.★ This is accomplished by smooth pursuit movements (Figures 21-7 and 21-13), which use visual feedback to keep images of moving targets on the fovea. For objects that move too fast to track, or that change speed or direction unpredictably, a combination of saccades and smooth pursuit is used (Figure 21-13).

A probable evolutionary relationship between smooth pursuit movements and VOR cancellation is suggested by the common elements in the neural circuitry used to generate them (Figure 21-14). Both utilize the cerebellum (especially the flocculus) and vestibular nuclei, which makes smooth pursuit the only kind of movement known to require the cerebellum for its generation. Commands for smooth pursuit movements originate in extrastriate areas sensitive to visual motion, which project to the brainstem both directly and indirectly by way of the frontal eye field. Damage to these cortical areas on one side causes pursuit deficits in both directions; however, contrary to the situation for saccades, the deficit is greater when tracking toward the side *ipsilateral* to the damage. A role for the supplementary eye field in smooth pursuit has also been suggested, but data on this point are still fragmentary.

CHANGES IN OBJECT DISTANCE REQUIRE VERGENCE MOVEMENTS

Images of objects moving horizontally or vertically move the same distance across both retinas, providing a signal that can be used to guide conjugate movements. Movements toward or away from the eyes, however, cause images to fall on increasingly disparate parts of the two retinas (Figure 21-15). In addition, because the eye is only well-focused on a particular range of depths for any accommodative state of the lens, the same movements may cause image blurring. Both retinal disparity and accommodation signals are used to guide vergence eye movements.

Little is known of the pathways involved in vergence movements. It is thought that the visual association cortex of the occipital lobe is important, along with projections from there to the midbrain (see Figure 17-38). The pathway ultimately influences the oculomotor nuclei (particularly the motor neurons for the two medial recti), which then converge the eyes. Consistent with this are the observations that damage to the midbrain and occasionally to the occipital lobes interferes with convergence, whereas damage to more caudal portions of the brainstem (including the MLF) does not.

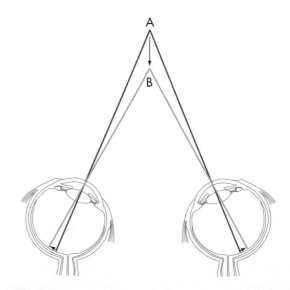

FIGURE 21-15
Retinal disparity created by images at different depths. With the eyes converged so that the image of an object at **A** falls on both foveas, images of objects at other depths, such as **B**, fall on disparate points on the two retinas. This disparity information is used by the CNS to figure out how to change convergence when looking from **A** to **B**.

★"Lateral-eyed afoveate animals are happy prisoners of their VORs. Foveate animals in hot pursuit of a dodging prey could not afford this." (From Robinson DA: The biology of eye movements. In Albert DM, Jakobiec FA, editors: *Principles and practice of ophthalmology*, Philadelphia, 1994, WB Saunders.)

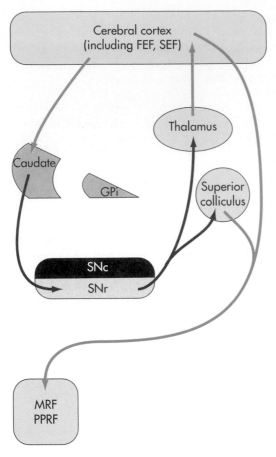

FIGURE 21-16
Basal ganglia connections affecting eye movements. See Chapter 19 for additional details. *FEF*, Frontal eye field; *GPi*, internal segment of the globus pallidus; *MRF*, midbrain reticular formation; *PPRF*, paramedian pontine reticular formation; *SEF*, supplementary eye field; *SNc*, substantia nigra (compact part); *SNr*, substantia nigra (reticular part).

THE BASAL GANGLIA AND CEREBELLUM PARTICIPATE IN EYE MOVEMENT CONTROL

One of the multiple, parallel loops through which the basal ganglia affect cortical output (see Chapter 19) directly influences the production of saccades (Figure 21-16). The input side of the loop originates in the frontal and supplementary eye fields and other cortical areas and projects to the body of the caudate nucleus. The output side involves modulation of the frontal and supplementary eye fields and the superior colliculus by varying levels of inhibition emerging from the substantia nigra (reticular part). Consistent with this pattern of connections, patients with basal ganglia disorders such as Parkinson's and Huntington's diseases exhibit a variety of eye movement abnormalities reminiscent of the abnormalities of other movements. These include involuntary saccades during attempted steady gaze, small saccades, diminished numbers of spontaneous saccades, and slowed smooth pursuit.

The cerebellum plays critical roles in both fast and slow eye movements. Although there is considerable overlap, the vermis is related more to fast movements and the flocculus to slow movements. Some of these roles are comparable to cerebellar involvement in other movements, but others are unique:

1. Parts of the vermis near the horizontal fissure (see Figure 20-4) help regulate the timing of muscle contractions during saccades. Damage here causes dysmetric saccades (Figure 21-17, *A*) comparable to the dysmetric limb movements seen after damage to other parts of the cerebellum (see Figure 20-24).
2. The role of the cerebellum in at least some forms of motor learning was mentioned in Chapter 20. The

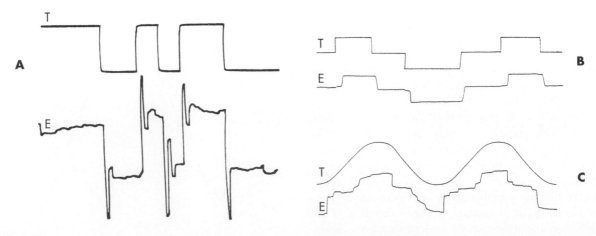

FIGURE 21-17
Abnormalities of eye movements in patients with damage to the cerebellum or its connections. **A,** Horizontal saccades of the right eye of a patient with cerebellar disease that presumably affected the vermis. When trying to shift gaze in response to target steps, saccades are dysmetric and overshoot the target. **B,** Horizontal eye movements of a 73-year-old woman with an infarct in the right basal pons, including the pontine nuclei known to convey visual motion signals to the cerebellum for use in pursuit movements. Saccades were normal **(B)** but smooth pursuit movements **(C)** were nearly absent, mostly replaced by saccades. (**A** from Selhorst JB et al: Disorders in cerebellar ocular motor control. I. Saccadic overshoot dysmetria: an oculographic, control system and clinico-anatomical analysis, *Brain* 99:497, 1976. **B** from Gaymard B et al: Smooth pursuit eye movement deficits after pontine nuclei lesions in humans, *J Neurol Neurosurg Psychiatry* 56:799, 1993.)

flocculus is essential for changing the gain of the vestibuloocular reflex in response to changes affecting the optics of the eye. Similarly the flocculus, sometimes in conjunction with the vermis, underlies plasticity of other eye movements such as saccades. This allows a degree of compensation for such things as changes in strength of an extraocular muscle.

3. As noted earlier in this chapter, pursuit movements are unique in requiring the cerebellum for their very production. Damage to the flocculus causes substantial slowing of pursuit movements, and extensive cerebellar damage results in their total abolition (Figure 21-17, *B* and *C*).

SUGGESTED READINGS

Anderson TJ et al: Cortical control of saccades and fixation in man: a PET study, *Brain* 117:1073, 1994.

Bahill AT, LaRitz T: Why can't batters keep their eye on the ball? *Am Sci* 72:249, 1984.

Bender MB: The oculomotor decussation, *Am J Ophthalmol* 54:591, 1962. *Evidence about the level at which corticobulbar fibers to the PPRF cross the midline.*

Bogousslavsky J, Meienberg O: Eye-movement disorders in brain-stem and cerebellar stroke, *Arch Neurol* 44:141, 1987.

Burr DC, Morrone MC, Ross J: Selective suppression of the magnocellular visual pathway during saccadic eye movements, *Nature* 371:511, 1994.

Büttner-Ennever JA, editor: *Neuroanatomy of the oculomotor system (Rev Oculomotor Res* vol 2), Amsterdam, 1988, Elsevier.

Carpenter RHS: *Movements of the eyes*, ed 2, London, 1988 Pion Limited.

Chen LL, Wise SP: Supplementary eye field contrasted with frontal eye field during acquisition of conditional oculomotor associations, *J Neurophysiol* 73:1122, 1995.

Demer JL et al: Evidence for fibromuscular pulleys of the recti extraocular muscles, *Inv Ophthalmol* 36:1125, 1995.

Erkelen CJ, Steinman RM, Collewijn H: Ocular vergence under natural conditions. II. Gaze shifts between real targets differing in distance and direction, *Proc Roy Soc Lond* B236:441, 1989.

Estanol B, Romero R, Corvera J: Effects of cerebellectomy on eye movements in man, *Arch Neurol* 36:281, 1979.

Gamlin PDR, Yoon K, Zhang H: The role of cerebro-ponto-cerebellar pathways in the control of vergence eye movements, *Eye* 10:167, 1996.

Gottlieb JP, Bruce CJ, MacAvoy MG: Smooth eye movements elicited by microstimulation in the primate frontal eye field, *J Neurophysiol* 69:786, 1993.

Green JP, Newman NJ, Winterkorn JS: Paralysis of downgaze in two patients with clinical-radiologic correlation, *Arch Ophthalmol* 111:219, 1993.

Heide W, Kurzidim K, Kömpf D: Deficits of smooth pursuit eye movements after frontal and parietal lesions, *Brain* 119:1951, 1996.

Künzle H, Akert K: Efferent connections of cortical area 8 (frontal eye field) in *Macaca fascicularis*: a reinvestigation using the autoradiographic technique, *J Comp Neurol* 173:147, 1977.

Leigh RJ, Zee DS: *The neurology of eye movements*, ed 2, Philadelphia, 1991, FA Davis.

Müri RM et al: Location of the human posterior eye field with functional magnetic resonance imaging, *J Neurol Neurosurg Psychiatry* 60:445, 1996.

Optican LM, Zee DS, Chu FC: Adaptive response to ocular muscle weakness in human pursuit and saccadic eye movements, *J Neurophysiol* 54:110, 1985.

Petit L et al: Dissociation of saccade-related and pursuit-related activation in human frontal eye fields as revealed by fMRI, *J Neurophysiol* 77:3386, 1997.

Pierrot-Deseilligny C et al: Saccade deficits after a unilateral lesion affecting the superior colliculus, *J Neurol Neurosurg Psychiatry* 54:1106, 1991.

Pierrot-Deseilligny C et al: Cerebral ocular motor signs, *J Neurol* 244:65, 1997.

Robinson DA: The biology of eye movements. In Albert DM, Jakobiec FA, editors: *Principles and practice of ophthalmology*, Philadelphia, 1994, WB Saunders.

Schiller PH, True SD, Conway JL: Deficits in eye movements following frontal eye-field and superior colliculus ablations, *J Neurophysiol* 44:1175, 1980.

Tian J-R, Lynch JC: Slow and saccadic eye movements evoked by microstimulation in the supplementary eye field of the Cebus monkey, *J Neurophysiol* 74:2204, 1995.

Vahedi K et al: Horizontal eye movement disorders after posterior vermis infarctions, *J Neurol Neurosurg Psychiatry* 58:91, 1995.

Wurtz RH: Vision for the control of movement, *Inv Ophthalmol* 37:2131, 1996. *The role of the superior colliculus in the generation of saccades.*

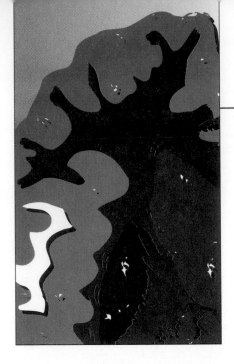

CEREBRAL CORTEX

The cerebral cortex is a sheet of neurons and their interconnections, about 2.5 sq ft in area, that plates the corrugated surface of the cerebral hemispheres in a layer just a few millimeters thick. This thin layer of gray matter is estimated to contain about 25 billion neurons, interconnected by more than 100,000 km of axons, receiving an incredible 3×10^{14} synapses. Figure 22-1 reviews the gross topography of this cortical covering.

One of the more striking changes that has occurred in the course of the evolution of brains in vertebrate animals is the tremendous increase in the relative size of the cerebral hemispheres and the even greater increase in the area of cerebral cortex on their surfaces. One inference drawn from this fact (and one abundantly supported by clinical evidence) is that the cerebral cortex has a great deal to do with the abilities and activities we think of as reaching their highest level of development in humans (or in some cases as existing uniquely in humans). Obvious examples are language and abstract thinking. This is, of course, not the only function of the cerebral cortex; basic aspects of perception, movement, and adaptive response to the outside world also depend on it.

MOST CEREBRAL CORTEX IS NEOCORTEX

Cerebral cortex does not have the same structure everywhere. Almost all the cortex that can be seen from the outside of the brain is of a type called **neocortex,** *neo* referring to the idea that it first appeared fairly late in vertebrate evolution. Reptiles have cerebral cortex, but all of it is of three-layered types that continue in us as **paleocortex** and **archicortex,** named in reference to their supposedly more ancient origins.★ Paleocortex covers some restricted parts of the base of the telencephalon (Figure 22-2), and archicortex comprises the hippocampus. Neocortex has a different structure, described shortly, and develops interposed between the paleocortex and archicortex. Some mammals have relatively little neocortex, but it expands greatly in primates, accounting for more than 90% of the total cortical area of humans. This expansion causes the ap-

---

★Although the pattern of evolution of cerebral cortex continues to be debated, the earliest vertebrates probably had telencephalic regions that, although not cortical in structure, were the forerunners of paleocortex, archicortex, and neocortex. In that sense, one is not "newer" than the others.

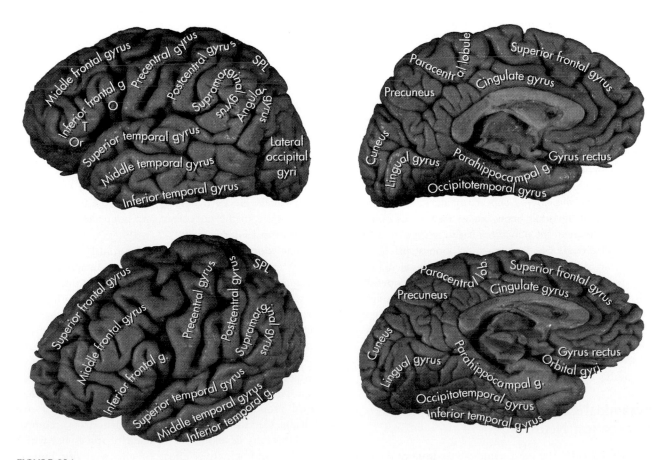

FIGURE 22-1

The major gyri of a human cerebral hemisphere. *O, Or, T,* Opercular, orbital, and triangular parts of the inferior frontal gyrus; *SPL,* superior parietal lobule.

Parahippocampal   Olfactory   Anterior
gyrus   bulb   perforated
                                          substance

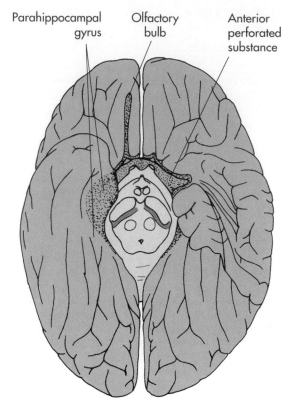

FIGURE 22-2
Inferior surface of the brain, with neocortical and non-neocortical
(stippled) areas of the telencephalon indicated. Note that the vast majority of the cortical surface is neocortex. [Modified from von
Economo C, Koskinas GN: *Die Cytoarchitektonik der Hirnrinde des erwach-
senen Menschen*, Heidelberg, 1925, Julius Springer.]

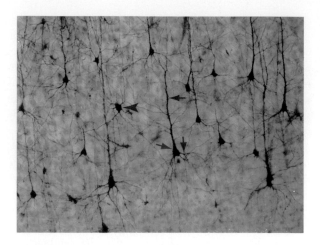

FIGURE 22-3
Golgi-stained cerebral cortex. The cell body *(blue arrow)* and apical
and basal dendrites *(red arrows)* of a pyramidal cell, and the cell body
of a nonpyramidal cell *(red arrowhead)* are indicated. [Courtesy Dr.
Nathaniel T. McMullen, Department of Cell Biology and Anatomy, The
University of Arizona College of Medicine.]

parent rotation of the cerebral hemispheres into their characteristic C shape, with paleocortex and archicortex at the
two ends of the C (see Figure 2-12).

   All neocortical areas go through a period during development in which they have a six-layered structure. As discussed shortly, this layered appearance does not persist in
some areas of the adult brain, but in view of its uniform
early development, the neocortex is also referred to as **ho-
mogenetic cortex** or **isocortex.** In contrast, paleocortex
and archicortex never go through such a six-layered stage
and are referred to collectively as **heterogenetic cortex** or
allocortex (from the Greek word *allo* meaning "other").
The hippocampus is a component of the limbic system (see
Chapter 23), and the paleocortex, which develops in conjunction with the olfactory system (see Chapter 13), is
closely interconnected with limbic structures; the remainder of this chapter deals with the neocortex.

Pyramidal Cells Are the Most Numerous Neocortical Neurons

Pyramidal cells, the most numerous neurons of the neocortex, are named for their shape (Figure 22-3). These cells
have a conical cell body from which a series of spine-stud-
ded dendrites emerge—a long **apical dendrite** that leaves

the "top" of each cell and ascends vertically toward the cortical surface, and a series of **basal dendrites** that emerge
from nearer the base of the cell and spread out horizontally.
Pyramidal cells range in size from 10 μm in diameter all
the way up to the 70- to 100-μm giant pyramidal cells
(Betz cells) of the motor cortex, which are among the
largest neurons in the CNS. Most or all pyramidal cells
have long axons that leave the cortex to reach either other
cortical areas or various subcortical sites, where they make
excitatory (glutamate) synapses. The remaining cortical
neurons are spoken of collectively as **nonpyramidal cells.**
Many are small (in the range of less than 10 μm), multipolar **stellate** (or **granule**) **cells,** but a variety of other types
and sizes have been described (Figure 22-4). With few exceptions, nonpyramidal cells have short axons that do not
leave the cortex and make inhibitory (GABA) synapses on
their targets. Hence pyramidal cells are the principal output neurons of the neocortex, and nonpyramidal cells are
the principal interneurons.

   The **dendritic spines** of pyramidal cells (Figure
22-5) are preferential sites of synaptic contacts and have
been the source of considerable interest and some mystery
as well. They are not merely a device for increasing dendritic surface area because the portions of a dendrite located between spines are sparsely populated with synaptic
contacts. It has been suggested that dendritic spines may
be the sites of synapses that are selectively modified as a
result of learning, because small changes in the geometry
of a spine could cause relatively large changes in its electrical properties and therefore in the efficacy of that
synapse. Certain cases of mental retardation are accompanied by faulty development of dendritic spines, but which
is cause and which is effect (if either) is not known.
Certainly, however, the most remarkable change that
occurs in the cortex after birth is the tremendous expansion of the dendritic trees of its neurons and a parallel

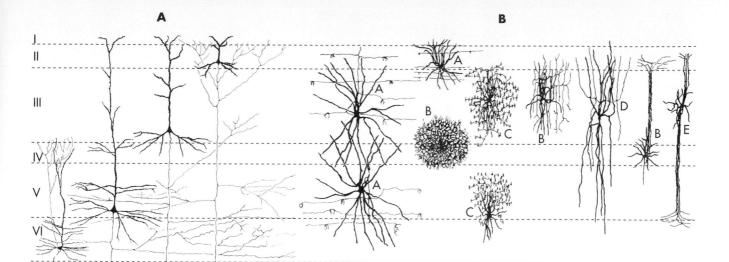

FIGURE 22-4

Neocortical neurons. **A,** Pyramidal neurons in different layers have characteristically different soma sizes and patterns of distribution of axon collaterals. **B,** Nonpyramidal neurons come in a variety of sizes and shapes; many have names attributable to their shapes. Basket cells *(A)* are usually large and make basket-shaped endings that partially surround the cell bodies of pyramidal cells. Other kinds of smaller multipolar cells *(B)* may have elaborate dendritic and axonal arborizations. Chandelier cells *(C)* have vertically oriented synaptic "candles" that end on the initial segments of pyramidal cell axons. Bipolar cells *(D)* have dendrites that both ascend and descend, and double bouquet cells *(E)* have axons that both ascend and descend. [**A** from Jones EG: Identification and classification of intrinsic circuit elements in the neocortex. In Edelman GM, Gall WE, Cowan WM, editors: *Dynamic aspects of neocortical function,* New York, 1984, John Wiley and Sons. **B** from Hendry SHC, Jones EG: Sizes and distributions of intrinsic neurons incorporating tritiated GABA in monkey sensory-motor cortex, *J Neurosci* 1:390, 1991.]

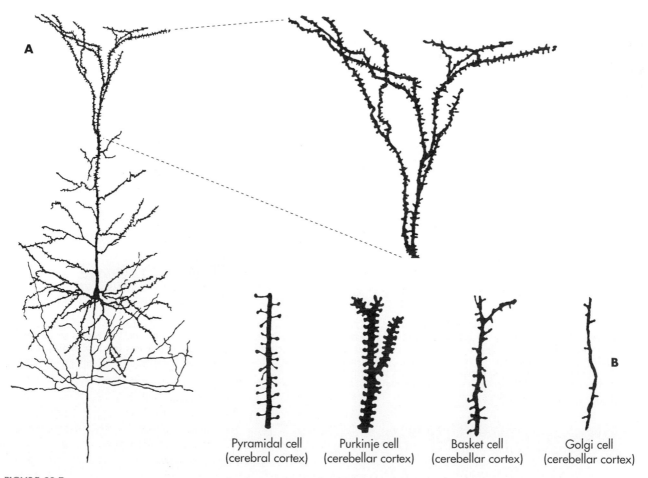

Pyramidal cell
(cerebral cortex)

Purkinje cell
(cerebellar cortex)

Basket cell
(cerebellar cortex)

Golgi cell
(cerebellar cortex)

FIGURE 22-5

Spines on the dendrites of Golgi-stained neurons. **A,** The dendrites of cortical pyramidal cells are studded with spines; these are easily visible on the enlarged portion of the apical dendrite but are also present on the basal dendrites. **B,** Just as different kinds of neurons have characteristic dendritic trees (see Figure 1-4) and arrangements of Nissl bodies (see Figure 1-11), so too do they have distinctive dendritic spines. (Those of cortical pyramidal cells remind people in the Southwest of ocotillo leaves.) [From Ramón y Cajal S: *Histologie du système nerveux de l'homme et des vertébrés,* Paris, 1909, 1911, Maloine.]

Golgi stain   Nissl stain   Weigert stain

I. Molecular layer

II. External
     granular layer

III. External
      pyramidal layer

IV. Internal
     granular layer

V. Internal
    pyramidal layer

VI. Multiform layer

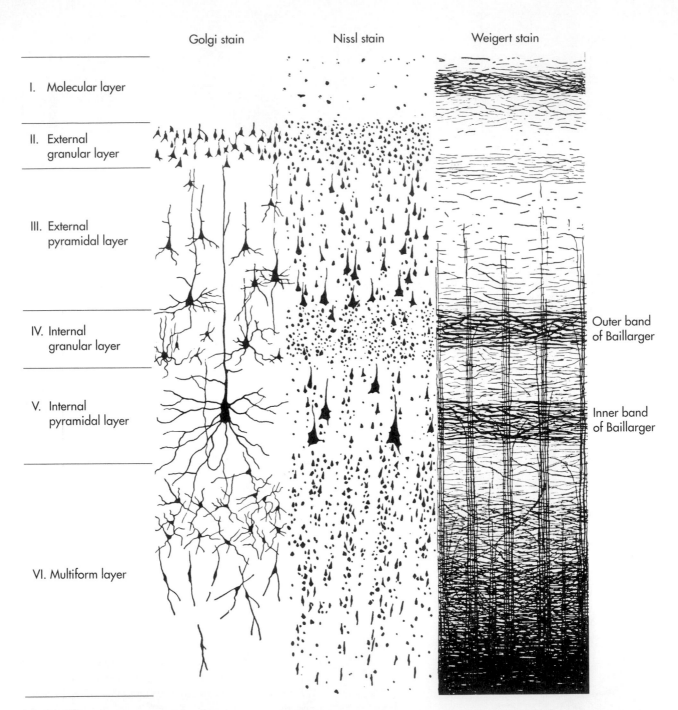

Outer band
of Baillarger

Inner band
of Baillarger

FIGURE 22-6
Cross section of neocortex stained by three different methods; the six cortical layers are indicated. The Golgi stain reveals the shapes of the arborizations of cortical neurons by completely staining a small percentage of them. The Nissl method stains the cell bodies of all neurons, showing their shapes and packing densities. The Weigert method stains myelin, revealing the horizontally oriented bands of Baillarger as well as vertically oriented collections of cortical afferents and efferents. (From Brodmann, K: *VergleichendeLokalisation lehre der Grosshirnrinde in ihren Prinzipien dargestellt auf Grund des Zellenbaues*, Leipzig, 1909, JA Barth.)

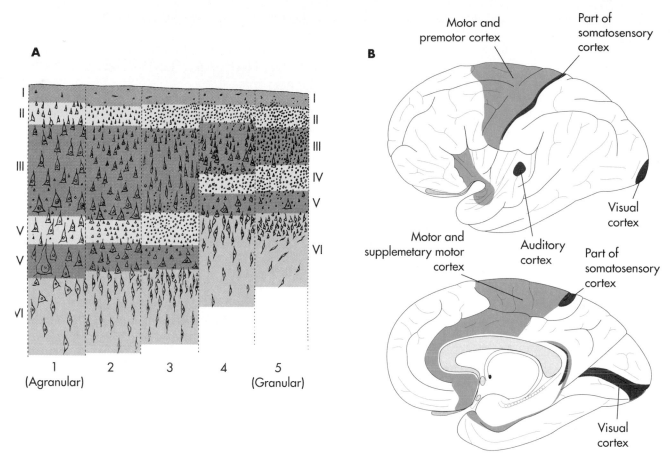

FIGURE 22-7

A, Different types of neocortex. At the two extremes are the heterotypical cortices: agranular cortex dominated by large pyramidal cells and granular cortex (koniocortex) dominated by small cells. Areas with intermediate structures in which six layers can be discerned are homotypical and were divided into three types by von Economo: *2,* frontal type; *3,* parietal type; *4,* polar type; **B,** Distribution of heterotypical cortex. The lateral view, above, is drawn as though the lateral sulcus had been pried open, exposing the insula. Agranular cortex is found primarily in motor areas, granular cortex primarily in sensory areas (compare with Figure 22-15). (Modified from von Economo C: *The cytoarchitectonics of the human cerebral cortex,* Oxford, 1929, Oxford University Press.)

increase in the numbers of dendritic spines. It should be noted that spines are not unique to cortical pyramidal cells; they are also found on the dendrites of some other neurons, such as Purkinje cells (see Figures 8-15 and 22-5, *B*) and many striatal neurons.

Neocortex Has Six Layers

The cells of the neocortex are arranged in a series of six layers, more apparent in some areas than in others. Most superficial is a cell-poor **molecular layer,** and deepest is the **polymorphic** (or **multiform**) **layer,** which is populated largely by fusiform-shaped modified pyramidal cells. In between these two are four layers alternately populated mostly by small cells or mostly by large pyramidal cells. The layers are commonly designated by Roman numerals and by names, as indicated in Figure 22-6.

Myelin staining reveals vertically oriented bundles of cortical afferents and efferents, as well as horizontal bands through which these fibers and intracortical axons spread (Figure 22-6). Two particularly prominent horizontal

bands are contained in layers IV and V and are called, respectively, the **outer** and **inner bands of Baillarger.**

The six neocortical cell layers are not equally prominent everywhere. Areas that give rise to many long axons (for example, the motor cortex) would be expected to have numerous large pyramidal cells, and this is indeed the case (Figure 22-7). In these areas, nonpyramidal cells appear minor by comparison, and layers II through V are dominated by large pyramidal cells to the extent that individual layers are no longer obvious. Because of the apparent lack of stellate (granule) cells, such cortex is called **agranular.** In contrast, primary sensory areas project mainly to adjacent cortical areas and do not give rise to many long axons. They have a corresponding dearth of large pyramidal cells; here too, layers II through V look like one continuous layer, but in this case they are dominated by small cells (both pyramidal and nonpyramidal; Figure 22-7). Such cortex is therefore called **granular cortex** or **koniocortex** (from the Greek word *konia* meaning "dust," referring to the numerous tiny cells). There is a continuum of structural types ranging between thick

(4.5 mm) agranular cortex and thin (1.5 mm) granular cortex (Figure 22-7). The intermediate kinds, in which the six neocortical layers can be seen, are called **homotypical** cortices (as opposed to granular and agranular cortices, which are collectively called **heterotypical**).

The differences among cortical areas are to some extent more apparent than real. Beneath a square millimeter of any area of mammalian cortex, whether from a hamster or a human, lies approximately the same number of neurons (roughly 100,000). The only exception is the binocular portion of the primary visual cortex of primates, where the neurons are packed somewhat more densely. About 75% of the neurons in all cortical areas are pyramidal cells. Hence 75% of the neurons in granular cortex are very small pyramidal cells. Different cortical areas have different appearances and functions because of the relative sizes of the cell types, the complexities of their dendritic trees, and the patterns of their connections. This fundamental similarity of all cortical areas is one aspect of the notion, discussed a little later in this chapter, that the cere-

bral cortex may be a large array of small, repeated functional units.

Different Neocortical Layers Have Distinctive Connections

Afferents to the cortex can come from only two general places: other cortical areas or subcortical sites. Afferents from other cortical sites, which are discussed at various points in this chapter, may arise in the same hemisphere **(association fibers)** or in the contralateral hemisphere **(commissural fibers).** The single major subcortical source of afferents is the thalamus, and its pattern of projections was described in Chapter 16. Other subcortical sites, such as the locus ceruleus and other chemically coded nuclei, also provide some afferents to the cortex (see Chapter 11).

These various types of incoming fibers ramify within the cortex in different patterns (Figure 22-8). For example, specific thalamic afferents end in a dense arborization

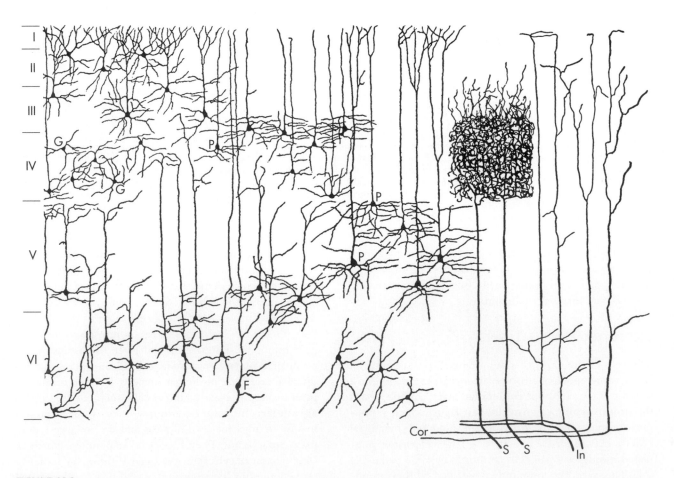

FIGURE 22-8
Types of cortical neurons as seen in Golgi-stained cerebral cortex from a mouse; main types of cortical afferents shown on the right. Cells: *F*, fusiform-shaped modified pyramidal cells; *G*, granule (stellate) cells; *P*, pyramidal cells. Afferents: *Cor*, association fibers from other cortical areas; *In*, fibers from intralaminar thalamic nuclei; *S*, fibers from specific thalamic nuclei. Note the strongly vertical orientation of many cortical elements. [From Lorente de Nó R: Cerebral cortex: architecture, intracortical connections, motor projections. In Fulton JF: *Physiology of the nervous system*, ed 3, Oxford, 1949, Oxford University Press.]

located primarily in layer IV*; fibers from other thalamic nuclei and from other cortical areas ascend vertically and terminate diffusely along their course in distinctive patterns, for example, those from intralaminar nuclei mostly in layer VI, and those from other cortical areas mostly in layers II and III.

Efferents from the cortex, like afferents to it, must be connected either with other cortical areas or with subcortical sites. Efferents to subcortical sites have been mentioned in various places throughout this book. Most of them descend through the internal capsule along a pathway that (for some) continues through the cerebral peduncle, the basal pons, and the medullary pyramids, finally reaching the spinal cord. Along this pathway many other structures are contacted, including (but by no means limited to) the caudate nucleus and putamen, the thalamus, the superior colliculus, the red nucleus, the reticular formation, motor neurons of cranial and spinal nerves, and various sensory nuclei of the brainstem and spinal cord. Some corticostriate fibers travel through the external capsule. Just as afferents to the cortex have a distinctive laminar pattern of termination, so do efferents from the cortex have a laminar pattern of origin. Although there is substantial overlap, layer III is the major source of corticocortical fibers, layer V of corticostriate fibers and fibers to the brainstem and spinal cord, and layer VI of corticothalamic fibers.

---

*Because the line of Gennari in the striate cortex represents a particularly large outer band of Baillarger and is located in layer IV, it is often assumed that it represents the massive projection from the lateral geniculate nucleus to the striate cortex. However, cutting all the afferents to the striate cortex does not cause the line of Gennari to disappear. Hence it is thought to be a collection of intracortical axons, although the details of its structure and function are unknown.

The corpus callosum and anterior commissure interconnect the two cerebral hemispheres

Most efferents to the cortex of the contralateral hemisphere pass through the **corpus callosum,** as described later in this chapter (Figure 22-22). Those interconnecting parts of the temporal lobes (particularly the middle and inferior temporal gyri) traverse the **anterior commissure,** along with crossing fibers from the anterior olfactory nucleus (see Figures 13-15 and 13-16).

Association bundles interconnect areas within each cerebral hemisphere

Efferents to ipsilateral cortical areas come in all lengths, from very short ones that never leave the cortex, to U-shaped fibers that dip under one sulcus to reach the next gyrus, and to longer association fibers that travel to a different lobe. The longer fibers collect into reasonably well-defined bundles (Figure 22-9) that can be found by gross dissection (Figure 22-10). The most prominent of these association bundles are the **superior longitudinal fasciculus,** the **superior** and **inferior occipitofrontal fasciculi,** and the **cingulum.** The superior longitudinal fasciculus (also called the **arcuate fasciculus**) sweeps along in a great arc above the insula from the frontal lobe to posterior portions of the hemisphere, where it fans out among the parietal, occipital, and temporal lobes. The superior occipitofrontal fasciculus, as its name implies, runs between the frontal and occipital lobes parallel to the corpus callosum for much of its course. Within the hemisphere, the superior occipitofrontal fasciculus is located between the corpus callosum and the caudate nucleus, and so it is also called the **subcallosal bundle.** The inferior occipitofrontal fasciculus passes below the insula from the frontal lobe through the temporal lobe and back to the

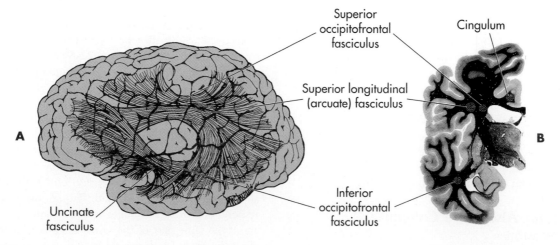

FIGURE 22-9
Long association bundles interconnecting cortical areas. **A,** Major bundles projected onto a lateral view of a cerebral hemisphere. **B,** Position of association bundles in a coronal section through one cerebral hemisphere.

Superior longitudinal
(arcuate) fasciculus

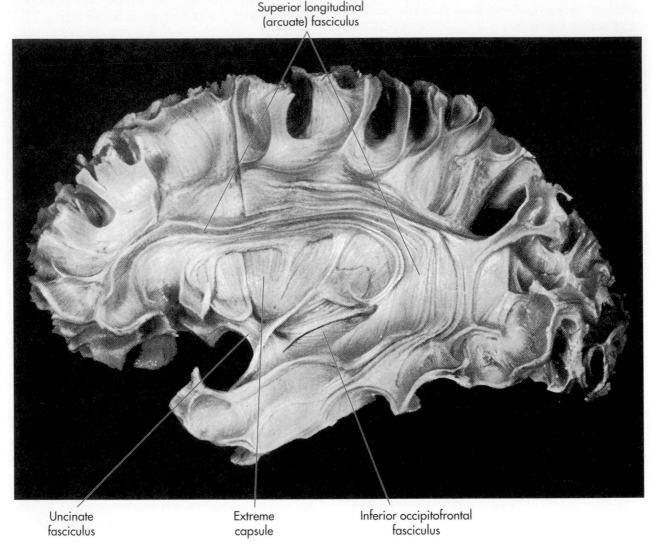

Uncinate
fasciculus

Extreme
capsule

Inferior occipitofrontal
fasciculus

FIGURE 22-10
Some long association bundles as seen in a partially dissected left cerebral hemisphere. (From Ludwig E, Klingler J: *Atlas cerebri humani*, Boston, 1956, Little, Brown & Co.)

occipital lobe. Its fibers fan out at both ends of the fasciculus, and those that hook around the margin of the lateral sulcus to interconnect the orbital cortex and anterior temporal cortex are often considered separately as the **uncinate fasciculus** (from the Latin *uncus* meaning "hook"). Finally, the cingulum courses within the cingulate gyrus and continues around within the parahippocampal gyrus to nearly complete a circle. None of these association bundles should be thought of as a discrete, point-to-point pathway from one place to another; rather, fibers enter and leave each all along its course.

Neocortex Also Has a Columnar Organization

In spite of the fact that the cortex is horizontally laminated, one gets the strong impression that there is also a vertical organization ("vertical" meaning perpendicular to

the surface). Apical dendrites of pyramidal cells have vertical courses, as do afferents to the cortex and the axons of some intracortical cells (Figure 22-8); even the cell bodies of cortical neurons often look as though they are arranged in vertical columns (Figure 22-6). Both physiological and anatomical studies have shown that this is not just an illusion. If an electrode is slowly advanced through the somatosensory cortex along a path perpendicular to the cortical surface, all the cells encountered are found to respond with about the same latency to the same type of stimulus delivered to about the same region of the body. Similarly all the cells along a vertical path through the visual cortex respond best to bars or edges with the same orientation in about the same part of the visual field (see Figure 17-32, *A*); if the electrode is moved 50 μm or so across the surface of the cortex, cells with a different preferred stimulus orientation are encountered. Furthermore, each cell along such a vertical path responds better to stimulation of one eye than to stimulation of the other eye; cells in a nearby vertical region may have not only a different preferred stimulus orientation but also a different preferred eye. The picture that has emerged is of the organization of the cortex into vertical slabs or columns, each 50 to 500 μm wide, in which some parameter (e.g., stimulus orientation) is constant for all cells. Vertical slabs of different types (e.g., stimulus orientation or ocular dominance) intersect one another in patterns that are still not fully understood.

This kind of columnar organization probably reflects a general strategy used in the construction of neocortex. For most areas this is currently impossible to test physiologically because we cannot define the "best" stimulus for the cells in most parts of the cortex. However, some anatomical tracing techniques make it possible to visualize the columns (see Figure 17-32, *B*), and there are indications that columnar organization is widespread. For example, in at least some cortical areas afferents from the thalamus, from other ipsilateral cortical areas, and from contralateral cortical areas each end in vertical slabs separated by slabs that do not receive that particular kind of input.

NEOCORTICAL AREAS ARE SPECIALIZED FOR DIFFERENT FUNCTIONS

Just as there has been a long controversy about whether the nature of a stimulus is signaled by the type of peripheral receptor that is activated or by the pattern of activity in many receptors, so too has there been a controversy about localization of function in the cerebral cortex. At one extreme have been those who maintain (in a kind of phrenology moved inward) that particular patches of cortex are the unique sites of particular functions. At the other extreme have been those who maintain that large areas of cortex form uniform fields in which functions are not localized and that complex activities depend on the amount of such cortex that is intact, not on the particular areas. As is often the case, the truth appears to lie somewhere in between. Consider the "simple" visual examination of an object, for example. This involves analysis of its size, shape, color, movement, and position in space; correlation of that object with objects seen in the past; cross-correlation of the appearance of the object with its sound, smell, and other properties; and decision making about whether, for instance, to run away or to grab it. Not surprisingly, large expanses of cortex are involved in even simple activities such as this, and performance of complex tasks can be impaired by damage to widely separated cortical areas. Nevertheless, many years of clinical experience have shown that reasonably predictable deficits are found after damage at various cerebral sites. This could mean that a given function actually is localized in a particular area, that the area performs one crucial step in the function, or that the area facilitates the activity of one or more other structures. Whichever is the case, the consistent association of some deficits with certain areas of damage provides a useful diagnostic tool, and we often speak as though functions are localized to specific cortical areas.

Different Neocortical Areas Have Subtly Different Structures

Seeing that various cortical areas are structurally distinct from one another in fairly obvious ways (e.g., granular versus agranular cortex, or striate versus extrastriate cortex [see Figure 17-28]), a number of anatomists have sought to map the cortex in terms of these differences and often of considerably more subtle differences. One mapping system whose terminology has come into widespread use is that devised by Brodmann (Figure 22-11), who divided the cortex of each hemisphere into 52 areas. The boundaries between many of these areas are not precise, as they often grade into each other by degrees. In addition, as noted previously, the correlation of functions with specific anatomical areas is not nearly as precise as once was hoped. Nevertheless, many of the areas described by Brodmann correspond remarkably well to areas defined by other measures of connection or function, and so many of the numbers proposed by him are commonly used for reference purposes (Table 22-1).

Although each of us has roughly the same total amount of cerebral cortex, there are surprisingly large variations in the sizes of particular areas. The areas of visual, somatosensory, and motor cortex may vary by a factor of 2 to 3 among normal individuals. Because the total area is constant, someone with a larger than average visual cortex presumably has other areas that are smaller than average. Whether these differences in areas are correlated with differences among individuals in various skills and functional capacities is not known.★

There Are Sensory, Motor, Association, and Limbic Areas

The neocortex of each cerebral hemisphere is traditionally considered as made up of **primary sensory areas** (receiving inputs from thalamic sensory relay nuclei), a **primary motor area** (giving rise to much of the pyramidal tract), **association areas,** and **limbic areas.** In this view the somatosensory cortex occupies the postcentral gyrus, the visual cortex the banks of the calcarine sulcus, the auditory cortex a small part of the superior temporal gyrus, and the motor cortex the precentral gyrus. These areas are

---

★Mark Twain apparently alluded to this possibility: "I never could keep a promise. I do not blame myself for this weakness, because the fault must lie in my physical organization. It is likely that such a liberal amount of space was given to the organ which enables me to make promises that the organ which should enable me to keep them was crowded out." (From Twain M: *The innocents abroad*, New York, 1869, Charles L Webster. Recounted in Harvey PH, Krebs JR: Comparing brains, *Science* 249:140, 1990.)

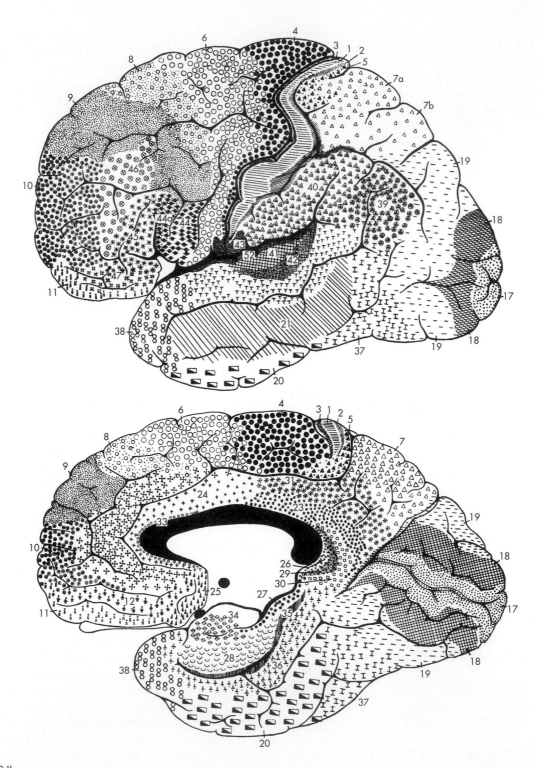

FIGURE 22-11
Brodmann's anatomically defined areas of the human cerebral cortex (see Table 22-I). [From Brodmann K: *Vergleichende Lokalisation lehre der Grosshirnrinde in ihren Prinzipien dargestellt auf Grund des Zellenbaues*, Leipzig, 1909, JA Barth.]

Table 22-1   Selected Brodmann's Areas

Lobe	Number	Location	Other names
Frontal	4	Precentral gyrus, paracentral lobule	Primary motor area; M1
	6	Superior and middle frontal gyri, precentral gyrus	Premotor area, supplementary motor area
	44, 45	Opercular and triangular parts of inferior frontal gyrus	Broca's area (on the left)
Parietal	3, 1, 2	Postcentral gyrus, paracentral lobule	Primary somatosensory area; S1
	5, 7	Superior parietal lobule	Somatosensory association area
	39	Inferior parietal lobule	Angular gyrus
	40	Inferior parietal lobule	Supramarginal gyrus
Occipital	17	Banks of calcarine sulcus	Primary visual area; V1
	18, 19	Surrounding 17	Visual association area; V2, V3, V4, V5
Temporal	41	Superior temporal gyrus	Primary auditory area; A1
	42	Superior temporal gyrus	Auditory association area; A2
	22	Superior temporal gyrus	Auditory association area; posterior portion = Wernicke's area

Box 22-1   Star-Nosed Moles, Revisited

Star-nosed moles (see Box 9-1) have an elaborate array of 11 appendages, or rays, surrounding each nostril that are used for somatosensory exploration of their environment. Corresponding to the behavioral importance of these rays, more than 50% of the mole's somatosensory cortex is used to process information from them (Figure 22-12). Further details of the somatosensory map, although not apparent in Figure 22-12, also make functional sense. The moles move their noses around as they travel through their tunnels, contacting objects more or less at random with the rays. If contact is made by one of the first 10 rays, the animal reorients its nose so that the object can be explored in more detail by ray 11, a small ventrally directed ray just above the mouth. If the object feels like it might be good to eat, it gets gobbled up. Interestingly, ray 11 has fewer Eimer's organs (see Figure 9-11) than almost any other ray, but each of these ray-11 organs has four times more cortical space devoted to it than do the organs from other rays. This behavior pattern and cortical organization has been likened to the way we detect a visual target in the periphery and then point our foveas at it.

characterized by a topographical organization in which the body surface, the range of audible frequencies, or the outside world is mapped onto the cortical surface (see Figures 3-28, 14-18, and 17-26). The maps are distorted (Box 22-1) so that highly discriminating or finely controlled items have a disproportionately large representation (e.g., the fovea in the visual cortex or the fingers in the motor and somatosensory cortex).

These primary areas come to occupy relatively less and less of the cortical surface over the course of mammalian evolution (Figure 22-13), and most of the human neocortex is of the association variety. Association cortex in turn is commonly divided into two broad types. The areas adjacent to a primary area are typically **unimodal association areas,** devoted to an elaboration of the business of that primary area. Thus areas 18 and 19, which surround the primary visual cortex, are part of the **visual association cortex.** Similarly the superior parietal lobule, much of the superior temporal gyrus, and the premotor cortex are involved in somatosensory, auditory, and motor functions, respectively. This still leaves the inferior parietal lobule and large portions of the frontal and temporal lobes. Neurons in these areas typically respond to multiple sensory modalities and may change their response properties under different circumstances. For example, a neuron in the inferior parietal lobule might respond to a visual stimulus but *only* if it was something interesting, such as a cue or a piece of food. These **multimodal** or **heteromodal association areas** are therefore thought to be concerned somehow with high-level intellectual functions.

Although there is a great deal of validity to this broad view of cortical organization, it is also clear that it is a considerable oversimplification in some respects. For one thing, the distinction between primary areas and association areas is not nearly so clear as the traditional formulation implies. One example given in an earlier chapter is the finding that the pyramidal tract originates not just from the classical primary motor cortex but also from other areas, including the somatosensory cortex. As another example, we now know there are *several* separate, distinct, and topographically arranged representations of motor and sensory functions in the cortex. In addition, the

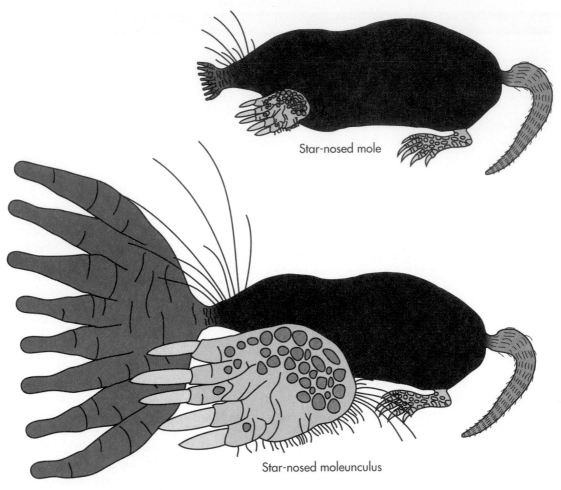

Star-nosed mole

Star-nosed moleunculus

FIGURE 22-12
The actual proportions of a star-nosed mole compared with the proportions of the map of its body surface in somatosensory cortex. (Courtesy Dr. Kenneth C. Catania, Department of Psychology, Vanderbilt University.)

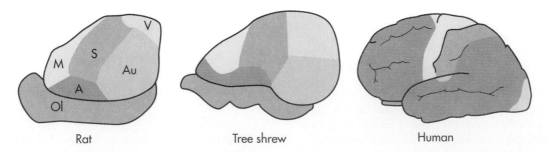

Rat   Tree shrew   Human

FIGURE 22-13
Motor *(M)*, auditory *(Au)*, somatosensory *(S)*, visual *(V)*, olfactory *(Ol)*, and association *(A)* areas of the cerebral hemispheres of three different mammalian species. All three brains are drawn the same size, even though the human brain is far larger than the other two; the relative and absolute increase in the amount of association cortex is apparent. (Modified from Penfield W: Speech, perception and the cortex. In Eccles JC, editor: *Brain and conscious experience*, New York, 1966, Springer-Verlag.)

concepts that primary sensory areas receive all the input (which is then acted on in some more complex fashion by the association cortex) and that motor activity is formulated in association areas and then funnels down to the primary motor area for expression are certainly not completely correct. Monkeys (and humans as well) with ex-

tensive damage to the precentral or postcentral gyrus are not rendered unable to move or to perceive tactile stimuli. They are impaired in these capacities, but the fact that they suffer only a partial disability indicates that other cortical areas play a role as well and that these other areas can function independently of the primary areas, at least to some extent (Figure 22-14).★ The details of the ways in which different areas of the cortex and other parts of the CNS cooperate to produce something like a simple voluntary movement or a simple visual perception are still largely mysterious. The best we can do at present is specify some known cortical connections and the consequences of damage to some cortical areas.

Primary somatosensory cortex is in the parietal lobe

Somatosensory information traveling rostrally in the medial lemniscus and in the spinothalamic and trigeminothalamic tracts relays in VPL and VPM and projects through the posterior limb of the internal capsule mainly to areas 3, 1, and 2. These are three long, parallel strips of cortex that together occupy almost the entire postcentral gyrus; most of area 3 is in the posterior wall of the central sulcus. These areas are not only structurally distinct from one another, but they also differ slightly in their connections; in fact, the body surface is mapped separately in each area in terms of different types of sensory input. Cells in area 3 mostly reflect activity of slowly adapting cutaneous receptors, those in area 1 rapidly adapting cutaneous receptors, and those in area 2 deep receptors such as those of joints. The result is a map in which the progression from tongue to contralateral toe is spread out along an inferior-superior line (see Figure 3-28) and in which sensory modalities are spread out along a much shorter anterior-posterior line. Because this is the most prominent (but not the only) area concerned with somatic sensation, it is often referred to as the **first somatosensory area,** or **S1.** Another parallel strip of cortex (area 3a), located in the depths of the central sulcus between areas 3 and 4, should also be included in S1 because it receives information from muscle receptors. The fact that none of area 3a is exposed at the surface of the brain contributed to the long-held but erroneous notion that muscle receptors have no cortical representation and do not contribute to conscious experience.

A **second somatosensory area (S2)** has also been described; it receives its inputs not only from S1, but also to a lesser extent directly from VPL/VPM. It occupies part of the parietal operculum, and much of it is buried in the lateral sulcus, possibly extending onto the insula (Figure 22-15). S2 is also somatotopically organized but in an order that is the reverse of that in S1; that is, the face areas of both maps are adjacent to one another, and the rest of the S2 map extends into the lateral sulcus. The cells in S2 tend to have bilateral receptive fields so that touching either of two symmetrically placed sites activates them.

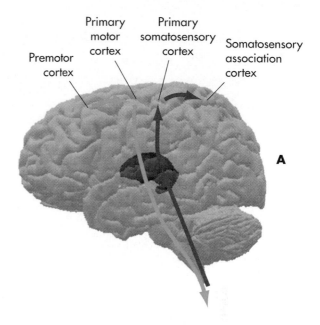

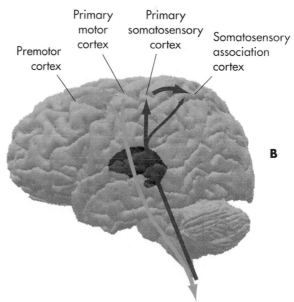

FIGURE 22-14

Cortical connections in sensory and motor systems. The somatosensory system is used as an example in this illustration, but the same principles apply to other sensory systems. **A,** Traditional serial-processing formulation. In this view, all sensory inflow from the thalamus ends in the primary sensory cortex, which then processes the information and passes it on to association areas. Similarly, all motor outflow originates in the primary motor cortex, which receives its inputs from motor association areas such as the premotor area. **B,** Current formulation, in which there is a combination of serial and parallel processing. Sensory inflow from the thalamus is distributed to both primary and association areas. Similarly, motor outflow originates in both primary motor and motor association areas. In both cases, the primary area is of major importance, but association areas have some connections in parallel.

★The extent to which this applies varies in different association areas and in different species. In primates, for example, some portions of the visual and somatosensory association cortex absolutely depend on the primary areas for their continued function, whereas other portions do not.

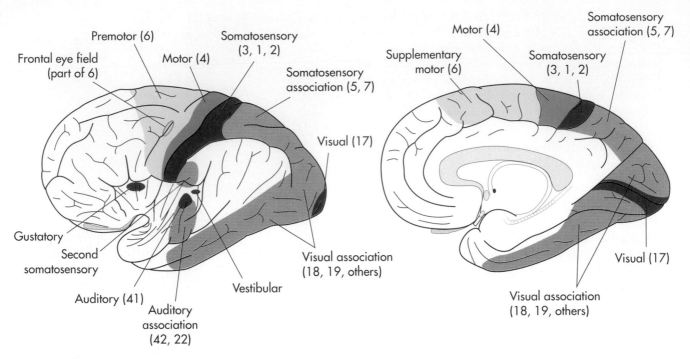

FIGURE 22-15
Summary diagram of some functional areas of the cerebral cortex. The lateral view, as in Figure 22-7, is drawn as though the lateral sulcus had been pried open, exposing the insula. Visual association cortex is particularly extensive in primate brains, occupying not only most of the occipital lobe but also much of the temporal lobe. Many of these various functional areas are associated with one of Brodmann's anatomically defined areas, although sometimes the correspondence is only approximate; commonly used Brodmann numbers are indicated in parentheses. [Modified from von Economo C: *The cytoarchitectonics of the human cerebral cortex,* Oxford, 1929, Oxford University Press.]

Stimulation of the postcentral gyrus in conscious humans produces sensations usually described as tingling or numbness in a contralateral part of the body whose location is related in an orderly way to the site stimulated (see Figure 3-28). The sensations generally do not resemble those caused by natural stimuli such as bending a hair or touching the skin, presumably because electrical stimulation of the cortex is a poor imitation of the pattern of activity set up by natural stimuli. Interestingly, sensations of pain can rarely be elicited from the postcentral gyrus, and the way in which pain is represented in the cerebral cortex continues to be something of a mystery. Large lesions affecting all of the postcentral cortex cause a considerable impairment of the finer aspects of somatic sensation (such as judging the exact location or intensity of a stimulus) and a serious deficit in the sense of position and movement of the affected parts, but such damage does not abolish tactile sensation or sensation of pain. Indeed, on the few occasions when removal of the postcentral cortex was tried as a treatment for intractable pain, the patient's pain was usually relieved only partially and briefly, and this was often followed by a hyperpathic state reminiscent of thalamic pain. On the other hand, small lesions affecting only the part of the postcentral gyrus adjacent to the central sulcus cause not a loss of pain and temperature sensation, but rather difficulty localizing painful stimuli in the somatotopically appropriate part of the body on the contralateral side. Corresponding to this clinical observation, neurons specifically responsive to painful stimuli have been found in the somatosensory cortex of monkeys at about the junction between areas 3 and 1. However, processing of pain information is not the exclusive province of S1. Pain-sensitive neurons have also been found in S2, and functional imaging studies have demonstrated increased blood flow in S1, S2, part of the insula, and anterior cingulate cortex in response to painful stimuli. The relative roles of these four cortical regions in pain perception, and the reasons why large cortical lesions should cause a hyperpathic state, are not yet clear.

Primary visual cortex is in the occipital lobe

The retinotopic projection from the lateral geniculate nucleus to the banks of the calcarine sulcus, conveying information about the contralateral visual field, was described in Chapter 17. This primary visual cortex (called the **striate cortex;** see Figure 17-28) corresponds to area 17 of Brodmann's map. Peripheral parts of the visual field are represented anteriorly, the fovea has a disproportionately large representation located posteriorly, and the vertical meridian is represented along the upper and lower borders of area 17 (see Figure 17-26). Although area 17 looks fairly small on maps such as those in Figures 22-11 and 22-15, it really occupies a substantial amount of the cortical surface and appears small only because most of it forms the walls of the deep calcarine sulcus.

A two-part visual association cortex occupies the rest of the occipital lobe. Area 18 surrounds area 17 and is itself surrounded by area 19. This association cortex receives its visual information both from area 17 and via the superior colliculus-pulvinar pathway. Areas 18 and 19 are themselves complex mosaics of smaller, retinotopically organized areas, one interested in the movements of objects, another in the colors of objects, and still others in other properties. Additional visual association areas occupy much of the temporal lobe (Figure 22-15), reflecting the importance of vision for primates.

The relative roles of primary visual cortex and visual association cortex in human vision are not completely understood. It seems safe to say that the primary area is extremely important because its destruction results in a total or near-total loss of conscious awareness of visual stimuli. A simplified view of its function, then, would be that the primary visual cortex does some initial processing on inputs from the lateral geniculate nucleus (e.g., combining inputs from the two eyes and beginning to analyze depth), then distributes this information to the various subareas of the visual association cortex where motion, color, and other parameters are analyzed more elaborately (see Figure 17-33). If this is true, bilateral lesions of the visual association cortex could conceivably disrupt single aspects of visual function. (Such cases would also be extremely rare because they would need to involve symmetrically placed areas and would need to spare the optic radiations.) As discussed in Chapter 17, a few cases have in fact been reported in which bilateral damage to the inferior surfaces of the occipital lobes caused color-blindness, or in which more lateral damage near the occipital-temporal junction caused motion-blindness.

Primary auditory cortex is in the temporal lobe

The superior surface of the temporal lobe forms one wall of the lateral sulcus. Two **transverse temporal gyri** (of Heschl; see Figure 14-17) cross the posterior part of this surface and form Brodmann's areas 41 and 42. Area 41 is granular cortex (like areas 3 and 17) and receives most of the auditory radiation from the medial geniculate nucleus via the sublenticular part of the internal capsule; thus it serves as the **primary auditory cortex,** or **A1** (Figure 22-16). Just as the body is mapped onto the postcentral gyrus **(somatotopy)** and the retina is mapped onto striate cortex **(retinotopy),** so the spectrum of audible frequencies is mapped onto area 41 **(tonotopy;** see Figure 14-18). Area 42 is adjacent to area 41 and receives auditory information both from area 41 and from the medial geniculate nucleus. This is analogous to the arrangement found in the second somatosensory area (S2), so area 42 is often referred to as **A2.** The cortex surrounding area 41 in monkeys includes at least four different subareas, each with its own tonotopic map. The same is assumed to be true for humans, but the exact details of the arrangement

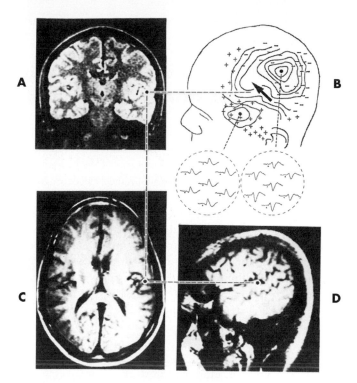

FIGURE 22-16

A striking demonstration of the location of auditory cortex on the superior surface of the superior temporal gyrus in a living human. The current flows associated with nerve impulses are accompanied by fluctuating external magnetic fields. The fields and their fluctuations are tiny, but the changes can be measured using extremely sensitive recording instruments based on special detectors called *superconducting quantum interference devices (SQUIDs)*. Magnetic field changes can then be mapped out using a technique called *magnetoencephalography*. In the study shown here, 1-kHz tone bursts 400 msec in duration were presented to the right ear and the resulting magnetic field changes were mapped out over the left hemisphere **(B)**; some of the actual magnetic field-change recordings are shown in the circular insets. The calculated source of these field changes was then mapped as a dot onto coronal, horizontal, and sagittal magnetic resonance images of the same individual **(A, C, and D,** respectively). [From Yamamoto T et al: Magnetic localization of neuronal activity in the human brain, *Proc Natl Acad Sci USA* 85:8732, 1988.]

of these multiple maps with respect to area 42 are not known. Area 42 is itself flanked by area 22, which forms much of the superior temporal gyrus and is called the **auditory association cortex.**

At levels rostral to the cochlear nuclei, both ears are represented in the auditory pathway of each side of the brain, although the contralateral ear predominates (Chapter 14). As a result, even total destruction of the auditory cortex has relatively little effect. An individual with such damage may have some difficulty localizing sounds on the contralateral side and may have some subtle hearing loss that is greater for the contralateral ear, but the deficits are not nearly comparable in magnitude to those that follow unilateral damage to the somatosensory or visual cortex. On the other hand, if the auditory association cortex of area 22 is damaged in the dominant hemisphere, severe language problems ensue, as discussed later in this chapter.

There are primary gustatory and vestibular areas

Gustatory information, relayed from VPM through the posterior limb of the internal capsule, apparently reaches the frontal operculum and part of the anterior insula. These seem like logical places for gustatory cortex because part is near both the representation of the tongue in the somatosensory cortex and orbital olfactory cortex (see Chapter 13); however, these probable gustatory areas are rarely exposed during surgical procedures, so little direct information is available about them for humans. A few cases have been reported in which stimulation of the frontal operculum or nearby insula caused sensations of taste or in which seizures originating in this vicinity were preceded by an aura that included sensations of taste.

The vestibular area was long thought to be located in the superior temporal gyrus and posterior insula near the auditory cortex (Figure 22-15) because stimulation of this region sometimes produces a sensation of movement or dizziness. However, more recent work on monkeys has shown that there are also cortical projections from the vestibular nerve to the parietal lobe adjacent to the representation of the head in the primary somatosensory cortex. Which of these should be considered primary vestibular cortex is unclear, but in monkeys the insular neurons that respond to vestibular stimuli commonly respond to somatosensory and visual stimuli as well.

The olfactory system is unique in that it does not relay in the thalamus before reaching its primary sensory area, and that the primary olfactory cortex is paleocortical rather than neocortical (see Figure 13-15). Primary olfactory cortex projects both directly and by way of the dorsomedial nucleus to olfactory association cortex on the orbital surface of the frontal lobe (see Figure 13-17).

Most motor areas are in the frontal lobe

Just as the somatosensory, visual, and auditory systems have multiple representations in the cortex, so too are there several areas from which movements can be elicited. The **primary motor cortex** corresponds to Brodmann's area 4, occupying a tapering strip in the precentral gyrus. Area 4 is agranular, the thickest cortex in the brain, and contains a preponderance of large pyramidal cells, including the giant pyramidal cells (Betz cells). In the midnineteenth century, before the motor cortex had been explored electrically, the British neurologist Hughlings Jackson predicted the pattern in which movements are mapped on the precentral gyrus, based on his careful observation of patients with epileptic foci in this area. He noted that such patients typically had seizures that started as a twitching in one part of the body and then spread to other regions on the same side in a sequence that was similar from one patient to another. This sequence corresponds to the now-familiar homunculus for the motor cortex, which is generally parallel to the homunculus found in the somatosensory cortex (Figure 22-17). As might be expected from the distortions of the mo-

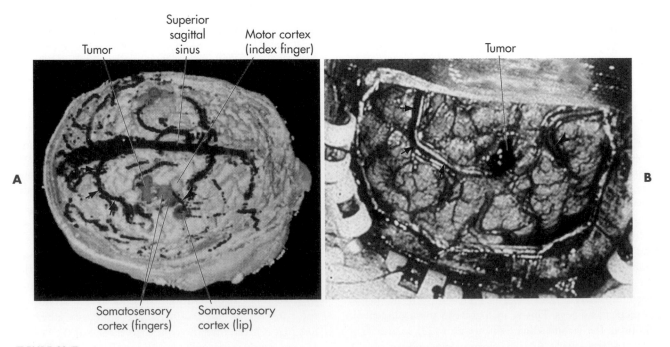

FIGURE 22-17
Use of functional imaging to map cortical areas before neurosurgery. A 56-year-old woman with a history of metastatic breast cancer began to experience tingling and numbness of her left hand and forearm. MRI was combined with magnetic resonance angiography and with magnetoencephalography during finger movements or touching her fingers or lower lip, yielding a detailed map of functional areas, the cortical surface, and cerebral veins (**A**). At surgery (**B**) the correspondence of this map with the actual anatomy was apparent. [From Gallen GC, Bucholz R, Sobel DF: Intracranial neurosurgery guided by functional imaging, *Surg Neurol* 42:523, 1994.]

tor homunculus, Jackson also observed that these seizures were more likely to begin as twitchings of the fingers or lips. Such attacks are still referred to as **jacksonian seizures** and the spread of motor activity as a **jacksonian march.** Stimulation of area 4 in conscious humans causes discrete movements involving one muscle or a small group of muscles (such as flexion of a single finger joint), which the patient is unable to prevent.* The movements are always contralateral to the side stimulated except in movements of the palate, the pharynx, the masseter, and often the tongue (but not the lower face), where the movements are bilateral; this corresponds nicely to the partly crossed–partly uncrossed corticobulbar projection (see Figure 18-17).

Several cortical areas in addition to area 4 give rise to corticospinal fibers and to other cortical efferents that participate in motor control (see Figure 18-12). Among them is area 6, which is also agranular cortex similar to area 4 except that it lacks Betz cells. Movements can be elicited by stimulating area 6 on the lateral surface of the hemisphere (the **premotor area**), but the threshold is slightly higher than in the case of area 4, the movements are slower, and they are more likely to involve larger groups of muscles. Corticospinal fibers also arise in the somatosensory cortex of the postcentral gyrus, and movements can be elicited from this region too, according to a pattern identical to the somatosensory homunculus. Finally, there is a **supplementary motor area** on the medial surface of the hemisphere; it is located anterior to the representation of the foot in the primary motor cortex, in the medial extension of area 6 (Figure 22-15). Stimulation of the supplementary motor area causes movements that are usually described as the assumption of postures and may involve muscles on both sides of the body. For example, there might be a turning of the head and trunk to the contralateral side, accompanied by raising the contralateral arm.

The multiple representation of movements in the cerebral cortex, with a primary area and several other nearby areas, is strikingly similar to the situation with sensory systems. In this case, too, the primary motor area seems to be the most important in terms of the deficits that follow its destruction. Lesions of area 4 cause an initial contralateral flaccid paralysis, which resolves fairly quickly into hemiparesis accompanied by mild spasticity. The paresis is worse for more distal muscles, and its effects are seen most when fine, skilled movements (such as individual finger movements) are attempted. There is disagreement as to the degree of spasticity (or whether there is any at all) after damage that is entirely restricted to area 4, but the spasticity is certainly slight compared with that seen in cases of more widespread cortical damage or of lesions of the internal capsule. Selective damage to area 6 or to the supplementary motor cortex does not produce paralysis or reflex changes, but if such damage accompanies destruction of the primary motor area, full-blown spastic hemiparesis results.

_____

*However, the patient has no sensation of *willing* the movement.

Association Areas Mediate Higher Mental Functions

Humans use language, create visual art and music, and otherwise behave in ways totally or nearly totally beyond the capacities of nonhuman species. Such behavior therefore can be studied only in humans, in contrast to our ability to obtain useful information about basic aspects of motor and sensory systems from experimental animals. Until the recent advent of techniques such as PET scanning and functional MRI (see Figures 6-18 and 6-19) this obviously constrained us to examining the effects of naturally occurring lesions of the brain or the effects of neurosurgical procedures, neither of which is likely to affect single anatomical areas in isolation. Our knowledge of higher mental functions is therefore largely based on clinical case studies, often on small numbers of patients with extremely rare lesions; as a result, it is not very satisfactory from a strictly scientific point of view. Nevertheless, as in the case of motor and sensory cortex, damage to certain cortical areas results in predictable deficits. PET scanning and related techniques, which can demonstrate changes in blood flow and metabolism in active areas of the brain, have begun to provide dramatic advances in our understanding of higher cortical function.

The right and left cerebral hemispheres are specialized for different functions

All the functions discussed thus far have been related equally to both cerebral hemispheres, so that the hemisphere in which a lesion occurs makes a difference only insofar as determining the side of the body on which a deficit is found. In contrast, it has long been known that language deficits are far more likely to occur after damage to the left hemisphere than after damage to the right. Thus it appears that language tends to be lateralized in the human brain, and the hemisphere that is more important for the comprehension and production of language is now commonly called the **dominant hemisphere.** Its mate is of course called the **nondominant hemisphere,** although this is rather chauvinistic terminology because (as will be seen) the so-called nondominant hemisphere is quite superior in some things.

Nearly all right-handed people (about 95%) have dominant left hemispheres. Left-handed people are more likely than right-handers to have dominant right hemispheres or to have some language representation in each hemisphere, but still the majority of left-handers are left-dominant. Thus the side that is dominant is correlated to some extent with handedness, but regardless of whether an individual is left-handed or right-handed, the left hemisphere is more likely to be dominant.

On casual inspection, brains look bilaterally symmetrical, but searches for an anatomical basis for the lateralization of language have revealed that a variety of asymmetries actually exist. As discussed in the next section, certain cortical areas abutting the lateral sulcus are important for linguistic functions, and so the consistent asymmetries found in the vicinity of the lateral sulcus are of great interest in this regard. The part of the superior surface of the superior temporal gyrus located posterior to the primary auditory cortex is called the **planum temporale** (or **temporal plane**) and is, on average, considerably larger on the left than on the right. Because the lateral border of the planum temporale forms part of the lower bank of the lateral sulcus, it stands to reason that the lateral sulcus should extend farther posteriorly on the left than on the right. This too has been found to be the case (Figure 22-18). These asymmetries are present before birth, which seems to indicate that left-hemisphere dominance for language is, at least in part, genetically determined. (This assumes, of course, that the connections of the planum temporale are as predetermined as its size.)

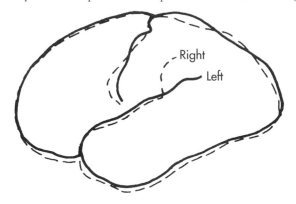

FIGURE 22-18
Typical asymmetry of the two lateral sulci of a single human brain. Both hemispheres were photographed, then one of the photographs was reversed and superimposed on the other. Notice that the left lateral sulcus extends farther posteriorly than does the right, corresponding to the fact that the planum temporale is usually larger on the left. (From Rubens AB, Mahowald MW, Hutton JT: Asymmetry of the lateral (sylvian) fissures in man, *Neurol* 26:620, 1976.)

Language areas border on the lateral sulcus, usually on the left

Stimulation of the part of motor cortex where the mouth is represented causes an inability to speak and at the same time produces involuntary grunts, cries, or other forms of vocalization. This is similar to what happens when any other part of the motor cortex is stimulated: there is a discrete movement during which the patient is powerless to use those muscles for anything else. However, there are two areas whose stimulation on the dominant side causes the patient to cease speaking but not to do something else with the vocal muscles; more strikingly, stimulation of these areas can cause the patient to make linguistic errors or be unable to find appropriate words. The first of these two areas occupies the opercular and triangular parts of the inferior frontal gyrus and is called **Broca's area.** The second area occupies the posterior part of the superior temporal gyrus and much of the inferior parietal lobule. This posterior part of the superior temporal gyrus is called **Wernicke's area;** some authors extend the meaning of the term to include the inferior parietal lobule as well. Because these areas largely surround the lateral sulcus (of Sylvius), they are commonly referred to as the **perisylvian** language zone.

Inability to use language (i.e., loss of the use of or access to the set of symbols that we use to represent concepts) is called **aphasia.** (This is not necessarily the same thing as loss of the ability to communicate. If you were in a foreign country where a different language was spoken, for example, you would still be able to communicate and understand to some extent through things like intonation, mimicry, and gestures.) Aphasia can be divided into two broad types. The first type is associated with damage to Broca's area and underlying parts of the insula (Figure 22-19, *A*). Broca's aphasics produce few words,

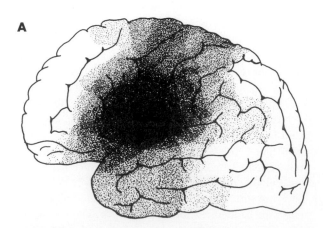
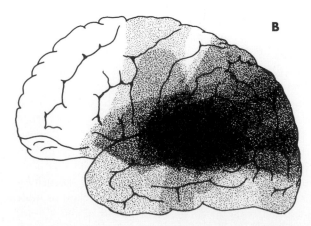

FIGURE 22-19
Sites of damage causing Broca's or Wernicke's aphasia. **A,** The areas infarcted in 14 patients, all diagnosed as suffering from Broca's aphasia, were determined by radioisotope brain scan (which measures leakage from damaged capillaries in an area of infarct). All 14 lesions were then superimposed, indicating a focus of damage in the posterior part of the left inferior frontal gyrus. **B,** The areas infarcted in 13 patients, all diagnosed as suffering from Wernicke's aphasia, were determined by radioisotope brain scan. All 13 lesions were then superimposed, indicating a focus of damage in the posterior part of the left superior temporal gyrus. (From Kertesz A, Lesk D, McCabe P: Isotope localization of infarcts in aphasia, *Arch Neurol* 34:590, © 1977, American Medical Association.)

either written or spoken, and have great difficulty producing them. They tend to leave out all but the most meaningful words in a sentence and to speak or write in a telegraphic manner. In contrast to their difficulties in producing language, Broca's aphasics have relatively less difficulty comprehending it. Broca's aphasia is also called **nonfluent, motor,** or **expressive aphasia.** The second type of aphasia is associated with damage to Wernicke's area (Figure 22-19, *B*). Wernicke's aphasics are able to produce written and spoken words, but the words or the sequences in which they are used are defective in their linguistic content. There may be substitutions of one letter or word for another **(paraphasia),** insertion of new and meaningless words **(neologisms),** or stringing together of words and phrases in an order that conveys little or no meaning **(jargon aphasia).** All of this suggests that such patients have difficulty comprehending whether their own speech makes sense, and indeed Wernicke's aphasics (in contrast to Broca's aphasics) are more deficient in the comprehension of language generally. Because in this condition language can be produced but not understood, Wernicke's aphasia is also called **fluent, sensory,** or **receptive aphasia.**

These two broad types of aphasia are consistent with the notions that Broca's area contains motor programs for the generation of language and Wernicke's area contains mechanisms for the formulation of language. Destruction of Broca's area would then deprive the motor cortex of the instructions needed to generate language, but the muscles involved would be normal in other activities; comprehension of language would be relatively unaffected. Destruction of Wernicke's area would leave Broca's area unchecked so that words could be produced without regard for their meaning. This implies that there must be neural projections from Wernicke's area to Broca's area that would most likely travel in the superior longitudinal (arcuate) fasciculus (Figures 22-9 and 22-10). It could be predicted that selective destruction of these fibers would also leave Broca's area unchecked and would result in a form of fluent aphasia. Cases have been reported (with lesions at the predicted site) in which the patient speaks like a Wernicke's aphasic but has intact comprehension, as Wernicke's area itself is undamaged. This syndrome is called **conduction aphasia.** Destruction of the angular gyrus in the dominant hemisphere causes a type of fluent aphasia in which one major deficit is an inability to name objects **(anomic aphasia).** This has been used to argue that the angular gyrus performs associations between objects and the symbols (such as words) for objects. According to this model, then, the sequence of cerebral events that occurs during the verbal description of a seen object is as follows: visual information reaches the occipital lobe, is processed in various ways in areas 17, 18, and 19, and is projected to the dominant angular gyrus, which associates words with the object and its attributes; the words (or their cerebral representations) are

transferred to Wernicke's area, which assembles them into sentences and activates the appropriate motor programs in Broca's area; these programs in turn activate the motor cortex.

As appealingly simple as such a model is (and as successful as it is in explaining a variety of aphasic disorders), it is certainly an oversimplification, and many investigators would violently disagree with it. For one thing, it requires an extraordinary degree of localization of very complex functions to specific small areas. For another, the types of aphasia just described are really abstractions because they are never seen in pure form. This is partly because naturally occurring lesions are not neatly restricted to one of these areas* and partly because aphasias may not exist in pure form. For example, Broca's aphasics typically have a comprehension deficit for grammatically complex statements; comprehension is only spared *relative* to the severe deficit in production of language. Nevertheless, it is consistently found that within the cortical areas important for language, more anterior lesions result in greater deficits in production of language, and more posterior lesions result in greater deficits in comprehension.

Communication by language involves more than just selecting words and then assembling them according to grammatical rules. Most of the emotional content and part of the linguistic content as well is conveyed by varying emphases. This is true of language generally but especially of spoken language. For example, depending on how they were said, the words "Jack is here" could be a statement of fact or a question; they could convey a feeling of happiness or dread. The rhythmic and more or less musical aspects of speech are called **prosody.** There is clinical evidence that the right hemisphere plays a special role in producing and comprehending the affective aspects of the prosody of speech. The right hemisphere system for generating and comprehending prosody is apparently organized in a fashion analogous to the left hemisphere system for producing and comprehending language. That is, the right inferior frontal gyrus is involved in *producing* prosody and the right posterior temporoparietal region in *comprehending* it. One of the first such patients described was a schoolteacher with right frontal damage who had begun to have difficulty controlling her students because she was unable to convey feelings of anger or authority by voice or gesture (even though the feelings were there). She had **motor aprosodia.** Patients with more posterior lesions on the right may have **sensory aprosodia** and have difficulty comprehending the emotional content of the speech or gestures of others.

---

*Full-blown Broca's aphasia, for example, is apparently always associated with damage not just to Broca's area but also including at least the underlying white matter and the anterior insula. Focal damage restricted to Broca's area causes a relatively mild and short-lived problem with language production.

Parietal association cortex mediates spatial orientation

Neurons in the primary somatosensory or visual cortices respond to easily defined and fairly simple stimuli such as the onset of a light touch at a particular site on the back of the contralateral hand or a bar of light oriented at a specific angle and located in a particular part of the contralateral visual field. However, many of the neurons in the parietal association cortex (areas 5 and 7) of a monkey respond to considerably more complicated stimuli. Some respond to movement of the monkey's hand toward some desirable object (e.g., a piece of food) but not at all to stretch of the muscles or rotation of the joints involved in the movement. Others respond only when the monkey visually fixates an object of interest and then continue to respond as the monkey tracks the object (if it moves). Removal of areas 5 and 7 causes a neglect of the contralateral half of the body; even though the tactile threshold is unchanged, the limbs on that side are used little, and reaching with them is inaccurate.

The consequences of large lesions of the right parietal lobe in humans are similar but more complex than those seen in monkeys.* Such a patient has difficulty with spatial orientation to everything on the left and may completely ignore the halves of objects to the left (Figure 22-20) as well as the left half of his own body. Such a lesion is rarely confined to the parietal lobe and is often ac-

companied by hemiparesis and a hemisensory loss. The patient may deny that anything is wrong with the affected limbs and may even maintain that they are someone else's limbs! In some cases there is a general deficit in spatial orientation that shows up as a difficulty in following maps or in finding locations even in familiar surroundings. Contralateral neglect sometimes, but much less frequently, follows left parietal damage. This may be partly (but not entirely) a result of the fact that left parietal lesions are likely to encroach on Wernicke's area and cause much more prominent aphasic disturbances.

Other deficits that may accompany damage to parietal-occipital-temporal association cortex include peculiar disabilities called **agnosias** and **apraxias.** Agnosia (from the Greek word for "lack of knowledge") means the inability to recognize objects when using a given sense, even though that sense is basically intact. A person with visual agnosia, for example, would be unable to recognize common objects by sight, even though the visual fields were perfectly intact and even though the ability to recognize the same objects using other senses (such as hearing or touch) might be intact. Apraxia (from the Greek word for "lack of action") means an inability to perform an action, even though the muscles required are perfectly sound and able to perform the same action in a different context. An apraxic patient might be unable to touch her nose with her index finger when asked to imitate the examiner's movement, but would be quite capable of doing so spontaneously if her nose itched. There are a multitude of subcategories of agnosias and apraxias and numerous theories about whether some types are based on language deficits, spatial disorientation, or other more basic problems. Some (but not all) agnosias tend to

---

*In this discussion of parietal lobe syndromes, some types of symptoms are related to right-sided damage and others to left-sided damage. It is assumed (but in general not proven) that these sides correspond in a given patient to the sides nondominant and dominant for language, respectively. Certainly this is true in the large majority of patients.

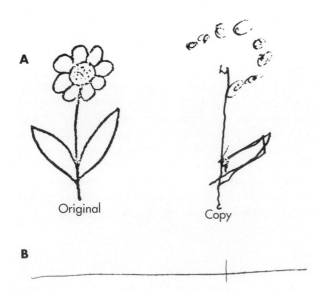

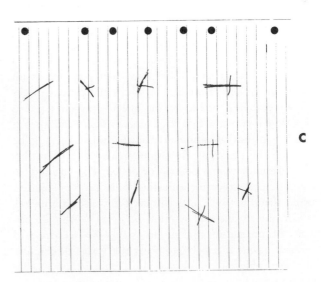

FIGURE 22-20
Neglect of the left half of the world, typically after right parietal damage. Patients were asked to copy a drawing **(A)**, bisect a line **(B)**, or cross all the lines drawn on a sheet of paper **(C)**. [From Heilman KM, Valenstein E, editors: *Clinical neuropsychology,* ed 2, New York, 1985, Oxford University Press.]

be associated with bilateral damage. Apraxia of mouth and face movements often accompanies left frontal lesions and nonfluent aphasia. Apraxia of limb movements often results from inferior parietal damage. However, the exact nature of the apraxia depends on the side and area damaged, and some forms of apraxia can also follow premotor damage.

Prefrontal cortex mediates working memory and decision making

The parts of each frontal lobe anterior to areas 4 and 6 do not cause movements when stimulated and are called **prefrontal cortex.** This part of the brain expanded dramatically during mammalian evolution (Figure 22-13) and now occupies the inside of the distinctive high forehead of humans. An early clue to the role of the prefrontal cortex in human behavior was provided by an unfortunate accident in the nineteenth century. In 1848, Phineas T. Gage, the foreman of a railroad construction crew, was setting a charge of explosives in a hole in rock, using a 13-lb, 3½-foot iron tamping rod. The charge exploded and blew the tamping iron through the front of his head (Figure 22-21), destroying a good deal of his prefrontal cortex. Remarkably, he survived the accident and regained his physical health in a few weeks. However, his personality changed dramatically. Before the accident, he was hardworking, responsible, clever, and thoroughly respectable. After the accident, he seemed to have lost most of his industriousness and his awareness of so-

cial responsibilities.* He wandered aimlessly from job to job, exhibiting himself and his tamping iron in various carnivals, and was tactless and impulsive in his behavior, not particularly concerned about his future or the consequences of his actions.

Various means of separating the prefrontal cortex from the rest of the brain (procedures called **prefrontal lobotomy** or **prefrontal leukotomy**) were used in the first half of the twentieth century as a treatment for certain severe psychoses and other conditions, but these operations have been largely abandoned in favor of therapy with drugs. The procedures were done bilaterally, but similar (though less pronounced) effects were seen after unilateral operations. There was considerable variation from one patient to another, but individuals so treated typically became carefree and often apparently euphoric, which was the beneficial effect sought; someone suffering from intractable pain, for example, would admit that there was no decrease in the pain after a prefrontal leukotomy but

*"The equilibrium or balance, so to speak, between his intellectual faculties and animal propensities, seems to have been destroyed. He is fitful, irreverent, indulging at times in the grossest profanity (which was not previously his custom), manifesting but little deference for his fellows, impatient of restraint or advice when it conflicts with his desires, at times pertinaciously obstinate, yet capricious and vacillating, devising many plans of future operation, which are no sooner arranged than they are abandoned...In this regard his mind was radically changed, so decidedly that his friends and acquaintances said that he was 'no longer Gage.'" (Harlow HM: Recovery from the passage of an iron bar through the head, *Mass Med Soc Publ* 2:327, 1868.)

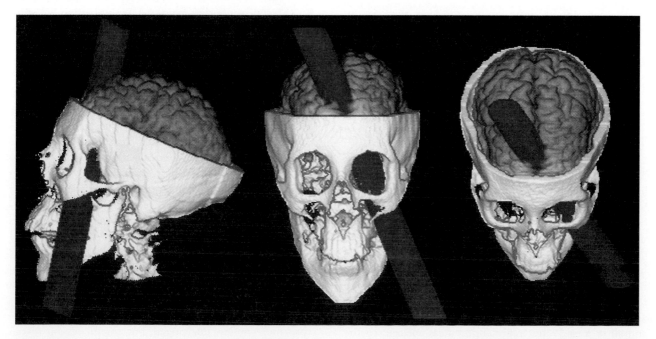

FIGURE 22-21
The probable relationship between Phineas Gage's brain and the tamping iron, based on modern re-examination of his skull and the entry and exit wounds. Orbital and medial prefrontal areas were heavily damaged, but motor cortex, Broca's area, and most dorsolateral prefrontal areas were probably spared. [From the cover illustration accompanying Damasio H et al: The return of Phineas Gage: clues about the brain from the skull of a famous patient, *Science* 264:1102, 1994.]

would no longer be bothered by it. Unfortunately, many also lost some of their capacity to do things for a delayed reward and were inclined not to observe social norms in their behavior; powers of concentration, attention span, initiative, spontaneity, and abstract reasoning all suffered.

There have been protracted debates about whether all aspects of these prefrontal syndromes can be accounted for by defects in one basic type of function. There are extensive interconnections between the entire prefrontal cortex and the dorsomedial nucleus of the thalamus that somehow play an important role in the workings of this cortical area, as shown by the observation that lesions of the dorsomedial nucleus have effects in some ways similar to those of prefrontal leukotomy. On the other hand, there are two broad patterns of prefrontal inputs from other forebrain areas. Dorsal and lateral prefrontal cortex receives massive inputs from somatosensory, visual, and auditory association areas (via the long association bundles mentioned earlier [Figure 22-9]). Many neurons in analogous regions of monkey prefrontal cortex respond to various kinds of stimuli, but respond especially vigorously when the stimulus is gone and the monkey's task is to remember it briefly to receive an award. This is consistent with the idea that dorsal and lateral prefrontal cortex plays a critical role in **working memory,** the ability to keep "in mind" recent events or the moment-to-moment results of mental processing. (A common example of working memory is remembering a telephone number until you have finished keying it in.) Patients with damage in this prefrontal area have problems with planning, solving problems, and maintaining attention. In contrast, orbital and medial cortex receives more inputs from limbic structures such as the amygdala, and patients with damage here are impulsive and have trouble suppressing inappropriate responses and actions. It has been suggested that some psychopathic conditions are a reflection of orbitofrontal dysfunction.

THE CORPUS CALLOSUM UNITES THE TWO CEREBRAL HEMISPHERES

The corpus callosum, which interconnects the two cerebral hemispheres, is by far the largest fiber bundle in the human brain. It contains more than 300 million axons. Most of these fibers interconnect roughly mirror-image sites, but a substantial number end in areas different from those in which they arise, for example, area 17 of one hemisphere projects to areas 18 and 19 of the contralateral hemisphere. Nearly all cortical areas receive commissural fibers (Figure 22-22), with a few notable exceptions such as the hand area of the somatosensory and motor cortex and all of area 17 not representing areas adjacent to the vertical midline. The commissural fibers to and from much of the temporal lobe, particularly the middle and inferior temporal gyri, pass through the anterior commissure.

We all know from common experience that something initially seen in one visual field can be identified if pre-

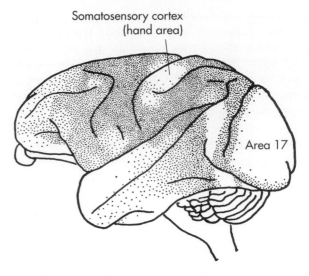

FIGURE 22-22
Distribution of degenerating axon terminals after section of the corpus callosum and anterior commissure in a rhesus monkey. Note that with a few exceptions (e.g., most of the primary visual cortex—exposed here on the lateral surface of the occipital lobe—and the hand area of somatosensory cortex), the cerebral cortex is blanketed with commissural connections. (The hand area of motor cortex also lacks commissural connections, but is not seen in this illustration because the hand area is mostly buried in the central sulcus in monkeys.) (From Myers RE: Phylogenetic studies of commissural connexions. In Ettlinger EG, deReuck AVS, Porter R, editors: *Functions of the corpus callosum,* Edinburgh, 1965, J and A Churchill, Ltd.)

sented later in the contralateral visual field (e.g., we can recognize a picture after it has been reversed left-to-right). The same is true for other sensory modalities such as touch*; similar transfers from one hemisphere to the other can be demonstrated easily in experimental animals. The importance of the corpus callosum for these transfers can be shown dramatically in experiments involving bisection of the optic chiasm of experimental animals. This destroys all fibers crossing from each eye to the contralateral lateral geniculate nucleus, so anything presented to one eye reaches only the ipsilateral cerebral hemisphere. Such animals, despite having bitemporal visual field deficits, continue to show normal transfer of learning from one side to the other. However, if the corpus callosum is also sectioned, the animals no longer show this transfer. It is even possible to train them to give two completely different responses to the same stimulus, depending on which eye sees the stimulus.

Section of the corpus callosum has been used as a treatment of last resort for some human patients suffering from intractable epilepsy to prevent seizures from spreading from one hemisphere to the other. The procedure generally ameliorates the epilepsy, and the patients seem otherwise more or less unchanged, but careful testing reveals

---

*Even though parts of the somatosensory and visual cortices receive no commissural fibers, all areas of the parietal and occipital association cortices do, so each hemisphere has access to data from the contralateral half of the body and the outside world.

some remarkable alterations. Words flashed in the right visual field can be read normally, but words flashed in the left field cannot be read, and the patient denies having seen them. As far as spoken or written responses to visual stimuli are concerned, these "split-brain" patients behave as though they have a left homonymous hemianopia. This is thoroughly consistent with the notion of dominance of the left hemisphere for language, which can organize and execute a spoken or written response; visual stimuli in the left field reach the right hemisphere, which no longer has access to the language areas. However, it is easy to show that the right hemisphere is still quite functional. For example, a picture of some object can be flashed in the left visual field and the patient asked to pick out that object manually from an assortment on a table; this can be done (usually with the left hand), even though the patient denies having seen anything. This is a clear indication that the right hemisphere has some capacity for the comprehension of language and the organization of nonverbal responses.

Continued testing of such patients has yielded some general concepts of hemisphere function that, by and large, confirm and extend the conclusions drawn from studies of patients with unilateral brain damage (Figure 22-23). The left hemisphere in most people appears to be dominant not only for language but also for mathematical ability and the ability to solve problems in a sequential, logical fashion. The right hemisphere seems to be superior in musical skills, in recognition of faces, and in tasks requiring comprehension of spatial relationships; after callosal section, a right-handed patient is likely to be able to draw and copy better with the left hand than with the right hand. Problems are solved in a more comprehensive, holistic fashion by the right hemisphere. As noted previously, the right hemisphere also has some capacity for comprehension of language. The corpus callosum ordinarily welds the two hemispheres together into a unitary consciousness. After section of the corpus callosum, individuals develop close cooperation between their two hemispheres and subtle methods of cross-cuing, but nevertheless each hemisphere appears to have separate conscious experiences, creating a knotty philosophical problem.★

These same studies of split-brain patients also indicate that there is probably somewhat more bilaterality in the connections of somatic sensory and motor pathways than is commonly acknowledged. With time and practice, each hemisphere acquires not only a great deal

of control over ipsilateral proximal muscles but also considerable awareness of stimuli applied to the ipsilateral side of the body.

Disconnection Syndromes Can Result From White Matter Damage

It stands to reason that we could not reach out for a seen object unless visual information could somehow influence the activity of the motor cortex. This has been corroborated experimentally in monkeys: cuts in the parietal lobe that destroy the long association bundles connecting the frontal and occipital lobes interfere with the ability to carry out movements guided by vision in the contralateral visual field. **Disconnection syndromes** similar in principle have been proposed (and in some cases have been shown fairly convincingly) to account for some of the complex disorders that follow cerebral damage in humans.

The classic example of a disconnection syndrome is **pure word blindness,** or **alexia without agraphia.** Patients with this rare condition are able to write (thus no agraphia) but are unable to read (alexia)—even words they have just finished writing; they almost always have a right homonymous hemianopia as well. Alexia without agraphia occasionally follows a stroke that involves the left posterior cerebral artery if it causes destruction of the left visual cortex (hence the hemianopia) and the splenium of the corpus callosum (Figure 22-24). As a result, the language areas (in particular the left angular gyrus) are cut off from all visual input; the destroyed left visual cortex can supply none, and the intact right visual cortex can supply none because the route through the corpus callosum is blocked. Because the language areas are undamaged and still connected to the motor cortex, comprehension of verbal language and production of both verbal and written language are relatively unaffected.

Several other disconnection syndromes have been proposed or demonstrated, and the concept is valuable in terms of understanding some disorders of higher cerebral function. Callosal section represents an ultimate example. Conduction aphasia (discussed earlier), in which Broca's and Wernicke's areas are disconnected from each other, provides another example. Disconnections of language areas from different sensory areas or from motor cortex have been invoked to explain some cases of agnosia or apraxia.

CONSCIOUSNESS AND SLEEP ARE ACTIVE PROCESSES

We all have an intuitive understanding of what consciousness means, but no satisfactory definition for it has yet been devised. Instead we usually settle for a listing of things that are present when consciousness is present; this list usually includes self-awareness, access to memories, and the ability to manipulate abstract ideas and to direct one's attention. Discussing the anatomical basis of con-

★"Everything we have seen so far indicates that the surgery has left these people with two separate minds, that is, two separate spheres of consciousness. What is experienced in the right hemisphere seems to be entirely outside the realm of awareness of the left hemisphere. This mental division has been demonstrated in regard to perception, cognition, volition, learning, and memory. One of the hemispheres, the left, dominant or major hemisphere, has speech and is normally talkative and conversant. The other, the minor hemisphere, however, is mute or dumb, being able to express itself only through nonverbal reactions." (Sperry RW: In Eccles JC, editor: *Brain and conscious experience,* New York, 1966, Springer-Verlag.) Not everyone agrees with Sperry's conclusion.

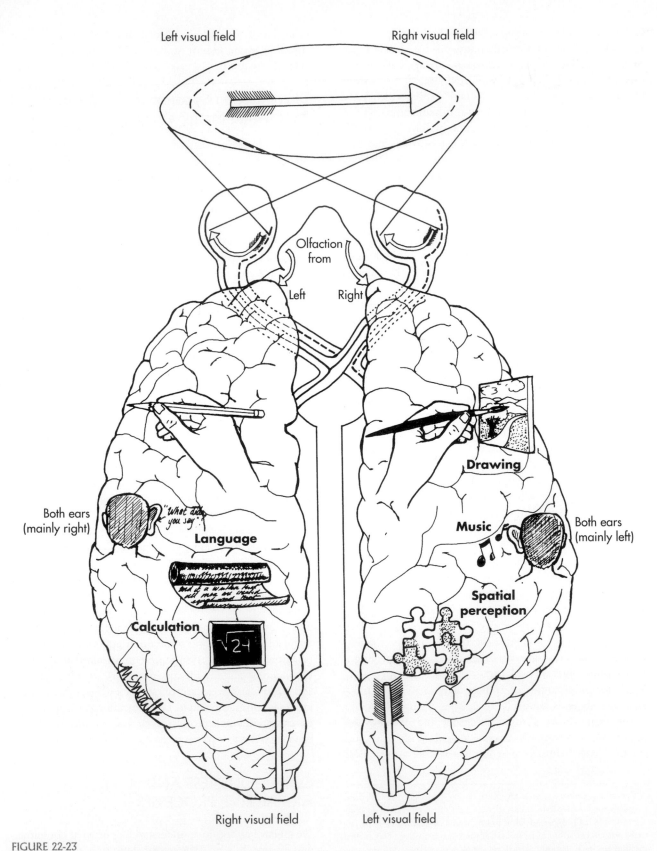

FIGURE 22-23
Schematic illustration of the different functional specializations of two hemispheres as determined from studies of patients after callosal section. (Modified from Sperry RW: Lateral specialization in the surgically separated hemispheres. In Schmitt FO, Worden FG, editors. *The neurosciences: third study program,* Cambridge, Mass, 1974, MIT Press.)

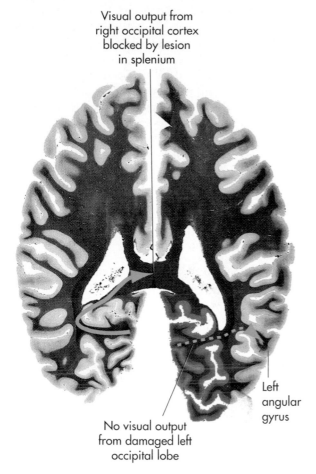

Visual output from
right occipital cortex
blocked by lesion
in splenium

No visual output
from damaged left
occipital lobe

Left
angular
gyrus

FIGURE 22-24
Diagram of a lesion that would cause pure word blindness (alexia without agraphia). Destruction of the left visual cortex prevents information from the right visual field from reaching language areas of the left hemisphere, particularly the left angular gyrus. Destruction of the splenium of the corpus callosum prevents information from the left visual fields from reaching the language areas because the route from the right visual cortex to the left hemisphere is blocked. The language areas themselves are undamaged, so the production of language and the comprehension of speech are intact.

sciousness is also difficult and ultimately probably impossible because a complete description would require a solution to the age-old problem of the physical relationship between mind and brain. However, we can discuss anatomical structures whose well-being is important for the maintenance of consciousness. The first and most important point is that as far as we can tell, consciousness does not "reside" as a single entity in any particular part of the brain but rather arises somehow from interactions among many neural structures. Although the cerebral cortex is undoubtedly essential for many of the attributes associated with consciousness, remarkably large cortical areas can be destroyed without abolishing consciousness, and no single cortical area appears to be crucial for maintaining it. This is not to say that a fully intact cerebral cortex, all by itself, is conscious. As described in Chapter 11, projections from parts of the brainstem (collectively referred to as the *ascending reticular activating system* or *ARAS*)

are essential for maintaining normal cortical function. Cholinergic and other projections from the reticular formation, noradrenergic projections from the locus ceruleus, and serotonergic projections from the raphe nuclei all depolarize thalamic neurons, shifting them toward a tonic mode (see Figure 16-15) in which they are able to transmit information accurately to the cerebral cortex (Figure 22-25, *A*). All of these projections either originate in or traverse the midbrain reticular formation, and bilateral destruction of this area causes coma. (This does not imply that consciousness resides in the reticular formation; your car won't run without a battery, but when it is running, the battery is not the source of power.) Finally, there is good reason to think that other structures, such as the basal ganglia, the hypothalamus, and the thalamic reticular nucleus, participate in the neural interactions whose result is consciousness.

Sleep is a reversible state of unconsciousness that is of great interest, not only because we spend so much time doing it but also because an understanding of the mechanisms of sleep might be expected to have a bearing on the mechanisms of consciousness in general. It was thought for a time that sleep was a passive process reflecting a decreased level of excitation of the ARAS and a consequent "shutting down" of the cerebral cortex. However, it is now apparent that active mechanisms play a major role and that specific neural structures can induce sleep by inhibiting the ARAS.

There Are Two Forms of Sleep

Our sleep is of two different kinds. The first, which includes several stages, is called **slow-wave** (or **synchronized**) sleep, because during it the electroencephalogram (EEG) is dominated by synchronous waves at various low frequencies, principally less than 4 Hz **(delta waves).** The slow waves arise as a result of interactions between cortical neurons and rhythmically bursting thalamic neurons. During slow-wave sleep, muscle tone is somewhat reduced, heart rate and breathing are slowed but steady, and subjects awakened from this state seldom report elaborate dreams. Roughly every 90 to 120 minutes we shift into the second type of sleep, called **desynchronized sleep,** in which thalamic neurons are back in the tonic mode and the EEG is dominated by low-voltage, high-frequency activity that is not organized into obvious waves and is remarkably similar to the activity seen in the waking state. Despite the fact that the EEG looks like that of wakefulness, an individual is harder to awaken from this stage than from slow-wave sleep; as a result, desynchronized sleep is also called **paradoxical sleep.** Desynchronized sleep is a very peculiar state, with several other distinctive properties: there is a nearly complete abolition of muscle tone, and the transmission of impulses over at least some sensory pathways is greatly decreased; blood pressure falls, and heart rate and breathing become erratic; we become

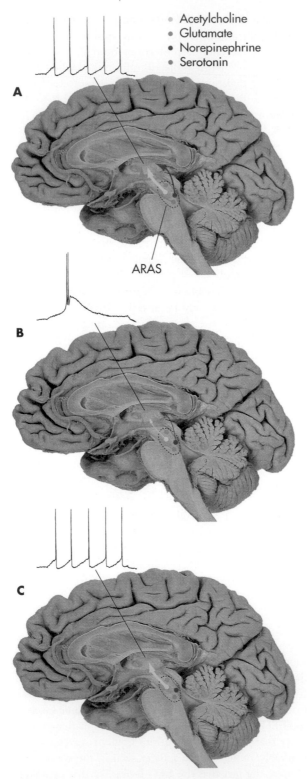

- Acetylcholine
- Glutamate
- Norepinephrine
- Serotonin

A

ARAS

B

C

FIGURE 22-25
Effects of the ascending reticular activating system *(ARAS)* on thalamic function in sleep and wakefulness. During wakefulness **(A)**, multiple inputs from the ARAS depolarize thalamic neurons, shifting them toward tonic mode. During slow-wave sleep **(B)** ARAS activity is suppressed and thalamic neurons switch into burst mode, blocking transmission of detailed information. During REM sleep **(C)**, most ARAS activity is completely suppressed; however, cholinergic activity is as great as during wakefulness, allowing thalamic neurons to remain in tonic mode. (Electrical recordings from Sherman SM, Guillery RW: Functional organization of thalamocortical relays, *J Neurophysiol* 76:1367, 1996.)

lizardlike, in the sense that hypothalamic regulation of body temperature ceases. Superimposed on this background are coincident phasic events. There are bursts of inhibition of motor mechanisms, so the last vestige of muscle tone is eliminated for brief periods. Some twitching movements manage to break through the inhibition, most prominently bursts of rapid eye movements (REMs). The latter phenomenon gives rise to the most commonly used name for desynchronized sleep, which is **REM sleep.** Subjects awakened from REM sleep are likely to report that they were having a visually detailed dream. By most measures the cerebral cortex is in an awake state during REM sleep (Figure 22-25, *C*), but because of the blockade of sensory pathways its activity is internally generated.

Both brainstem and forebrain mechanisms regulate sleep-wake transitions

Many aspects of the anatomical substrate of sleep have been worked out in experimental animals, and the reticular formation figures prominently in these mechanisms (Figure 22-26). Confirmation for humans is difficult to come by because processes that damage the brainstem reticular formation to any great extent are usually fatal. The following account is therefore based mainly on animal studies, but the clinical data available about humans are generally consistent with these results.

The EEG of an animal whose brainstem has been transected in the rostral midbrain shows constant synchronized activity indicative of slow-wave sleep, at least in the acute stages after the operation. This reflects the fact that the ARAS has been disconnected from the forebrain. As long as the reticular formation is still connected to the forebrain (e.g., after a transection of the upper cervical spinal cord), an animal shows all the standard EEG signs of cycling through wakefulness and the various stages of sleep. Some insight into what turns the ARAS off and on is provided by transecting the brainstem at a midpontine level. It might be expected that in such a case the animal would show either normal sleep and wakefulness (if this lesion leaves enough of the reticular formation attached to the forebrain) or constant sleep (if too much of the reticular formation is removed by such a lesion). Instead the animal shows signs of constant wakefulness rostral to the lesion, at least during the acute stages after the operation. This indicates not only that the parts of the ARAS crucial for wakefulness are contained in the midbrain and rostral pons but also that parts of the medullary and caudal pontine reticular formation are responsible for periodically turning the ARAS off and on. The interconnections between the hypothalamic clock for sleep-wake cycles (see Chapter 23) and the caudal brainstem reticular formation are not fully understood, but there are indications that some serotonergic cells of the raphe nuclei are important components. One piece of evidence supporting this concept is the observation that depletion of the brain's sero-

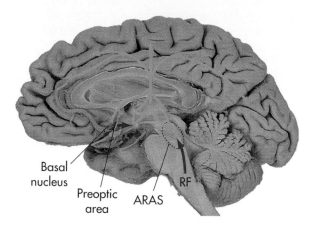

FIGURE 22-26
Summary diagram of the neural structures and connections important for maintenance of the sleep-wake cycle. Wakefulness-promoting structures and connections are shown in green; antagonistic structures and connections, which promote slow-wave sleep, are shown in red. The ascending reticular activating system (ARAS) maintains wakefulness by acting on the cerebral cortex in a generalized manner both directly and through effects on the thalamus. The ARAS is periodically turned off by projections from the medullary and pontine reticular formation (*RF*), inducing sleep. Diencephalic centers are also capable of inducing sleep and wakefulness via arousal-promoting projections from the posterior hypothalamus and basal nucleus and antagonistic projections from the preoptic area. Separate collections of neurons in the pons (not shown) are responsible for triggering periods of REM sleep.

Labels: Basal nucleus, Preoptic area, ARAS, RF

tonin, either by pharmacological techniques or by destruction of the raphe nuclei, causes an insomnia that can be reversed promptly by administration of serotonin. This is not a total explanation, however, because the insomnia partially resolves even if serotonin levels are not restored.

In addition to the brainstem mechanisms that regulate sleep and wakefulness, there is a second system located more rostrally (Figure 22-26). Encephalitic damage to the posterior hypothalamus of humans causes the hypersomnia of sleeping sickness. Stimulation of this area in sleeping animals causes awakening, largely through yet another amine-containing projection to the thalamus and cerebral cortex, this one using **histamine.** (Hence the drowsiness caused by many antihistamines.) Conversely, damage to the general region of the anterior hypothalamus (the preoptic area; see Chapter 23) causes insomnia, and stimulation of this area causes sleep. Finally, the cholinergic projections from the basal nucleus (see Figure 11-24) to the cerebral cortex promote arousal and wakefulness. How these forebrain structures interact with the brainstem mechanisms is not fully known. There are indications that in an intact animal the hypothalamic centers act in part directly on the ARAS to achieve a unified sleep-waking cycle. On the other hand, there are also direct projections from the hypothalamus and basal forebrain to the thalamus and cerebral cortex, and 10 to 15 days after a mesencephalic transection the forebrain once again begins to cycle through the synchronized and desynchronized EEGs of apparent sleep and wakefulness.

Basic machinery for REM sleep is located in the brainstem

The basic anatomical control mechanisms for REM sleep are more localized than are those for slow-wave sleep and are entirely contained in the caudal brainstem. This is shown perhaps most dramatically in the case of a cat with only those parts of its CNS up to the midpons left intact. Such an animal obviously is unable to show EEG signs of sleep and wakefulness, but at periodic intervals throughout the day and night, it does have episodes that include all the parts of REM sleep of which the spinal cord and caudal brainstem are capable. That is, there are periodic spells of decreased muscle tone and twitches of the lateral recti (the only way for REMs to be expressed in this condition).* The timing mechanism for the initiation of REM sleep is thought to be in the caudal pontine reticular formation. This timing mechanism somehow triggers neurons in various parts of the pontine and rostral medullary reticular formation, which mediate the assorted tonic processes and phasic events of REM sleep. Neurons in the vicinity of the locus ceruleus seem to be particularly important for some parts of REM sleep, notably the loss of muscle tone. Cats with bilateral damage just ventral to the locus ceruleus have REM sleep without atonia and appear to "act out" their dreams.

REM sleep normally occurs only in the midst of periods of slow-wave sleep, so it is assumed that the REM sleep mechanisms must ordinarily be primed or triggered by the centers for slow-wave sleep. In some conditions, components of REM sleep may either appear at inappropriate times or not appear when they should. **Narcolepsy** is a disorder characterized by intrusions of elements of REM sleep into periods of wakefulness. Patients have irresistible urges to sleep for brief periods during the day, and enter almost immediately into REM sleep. Even when awake and alert, they may have sudden, brief losses of muscle tone **(cataplexy),** particularly during emotionally charged situations. As they fall asleep at night, narcoleptic patients may have episodes of paralysis or hallucinations while still awake. Conversely, patients (usually older males) with **REM sleep behavioral disorder** flail about in a coordinated way during REM sleep, in a manner consistent with the activities in their dreams.

SUGGESTED READINGS

Ahern GL et al: Right hemisphere advantage for evaluating emotional facial expressions, *Cortex* 27:193, 1991.

Andrews TJ, Halpern SD, Purves D: Correlated size variations in human visual cortex, lateral geniculate nucleus, and optic tract, *J Neurosci* 17:2859, 1997.

Barbas H: Pattern in the laminar origin of corticocortical connections, *J Comp Neurol* 252:415, 1986.

*These REMs in the absence of cerebral hemispheres are one bit of evidence that, whatever the eye movements of REM sleep are, they do not represent "looking-at-a-dream" movements.

Bechara A et al: Dissociation of working memory from decision making within the human prefrontal cortex, *J Neurosci* 18:428, 1998.

Bogousslavsky J: Frontal stroke syndromes, *Eur Neurol* 34:306, 1994.

Bonda E, Frey S, Petrides M: Evidence for a dorso-medial parietal system involved in mental transformations of the body, *J Neurophysiol* 76:2042, 1996. *Imagining your hand in a different orientation causes increased blood flow in parietal association cortex.*

Braun AR et al: Regional cerebral blood flow throughout the sleep-wake cycle: an H$_2$^{15}O PET study, *Brain* 120:1173, 1997.

Brinkman J, Kuypers HGJM: Cerebral control of contralateral and ipsilateral arm, hand and finger movements in the split-brain rhesus monkey, *Brain* 96:653, 1973.

Borbély AA, Tobler I: Endogenous sleep-promoting substances and sleep regulation, *Physiol Rev* 69:605, 1989.

Caramazza A, Hillis AE: Lexical organization of nouns and verbs in the brain, *Nature* 349:788, 1991.

Catania KC, Kaas JH: Somatosensory fovea in the star-nosed mole: behavioral use of the star in relation to innervation patterns and cortical representation, *J Comp Neurol* 387:215, 1997.

Celesia GG: Organization of auditory cortical areas in man, *Brain* 99:403, 1976.

Courtney SM et al: Transient and sustained activity in a distributed neural system for human working memory, *Nature* 386:608, 1997.

Creutzfeldt OD: *Cortex cerebri: performance, structural and functional organization of the cortex,* New York, 1995, Oxford University Press.

Critchley M: *The parietal lobes,* London, 1953, Edward Arnold (Publishers), Ltd. *The classic clinical work on the various syndromes resulting from parietal lesions.*

Damasio AR: Aphasia, *N Engl J Med* 326:531, 1992. *A recent lucid review of the various aphasic syndromes and contemporary notions of their anatomical correlates.*

Damasio H et al: The return of Phineas Gage: clues about the brain from the skull of a famous patient, *Science* 264:1102, 1994.

Douglas R, Martin K: Neocortex. In Shepherd GM, editor: *The synaptic organization of the brain,* ed 4, New York, 1998, Oxford University Press.

Dronkers NF: A new brain region for coordinating speech articulation, *Nature* 384:159, 1996. *Sorting through the anatomical correlates of the various components of Broca's aphasia.*

Feinberg TE, Farah MJ, editors: *Behavioral neurology and neuropsychology,* New York, 1997, McGraw-Hill.

Foote SL, Morrison JH: Extrathalamic modulation of cortical function, *Ann Rev Neurosci* 10:67, 1987.

Frackowiak RSJ et al: *Human brain function,* San Diego, 1997, Academic Press. *A review of methods and findings from the ongoing revolution in functional brain imaging.*

Fuster JM: *The prefrontal cortex,* ed 3, Philadelphia, 1997, Lippincott-Raven.

Galaburda AM et al: Right-left asymmetries in the brain, *Science* 199:852, 1978.

Gazzaniga M: Principles of human brain organization derived from split-brain studies, *Neuron* 14:217, 1995. *A recent review of left hemisphere–right hemisphere specialization and cooperation, by one of the principal workers in this field.*

Geschwind N: Disconnexion syndromes in animals and man. I and II, *Brain* 88:237 and 585, 1965. *A scholarly and influential paper arguing forcefully for the concept of complex syndromes caused by disconnections of various cerebral areas from one another.*

Gironell A, de la Calzada MD, Sagales T: Absence of REM sleep and unaltered non-REM sleep caused by a haematoma in the pontine tegmentum, *J Neurol Neurosurg Psychiatry* 59:195, 1995.

Goldman PS, Nauta WJH: Columnar distribution of cortico-cortical fibers in the frontal association, limbic, and motor cortex of the developing rhesus monkey, *Brain Res* 122:393, 1977. *Pretty pictures.*

Goldman-Rakic PS: Cellular basis of working memory, *Neuron* 14:477, 1995.

Gordon HW, Bogen JE: Hemispheric lateralization of singing after intracarotid sodium amylobarbitone, *J Neurol Neurosurg Psychiatry* 37:727, 1974.

Graff-Radford NR, Welsh K, Godersky J: Callosal apraxia, *Neurol* 37:100, 1987.

Gücer G: The effect of sleep upon the transmission of afferent activity in the somatic afferent system, *Exp Brain Res* 34:287, 1979.

Haaxma R, Kuypers HGJM: Intrahemispheric cortical connexions and visual guidance of hand and finger movements in the rhesus monkey, *Brain* 98:239, 1975. *Direct experimental demonstration of a type of disconnection syndrome.*

Heilman KM et al: The right hemisphere: neuropsychological functions, *J Neurosurg* 64:693, 1986.

Herkenham M: Laminar organization of thalamic projections to the rat neocortex, *Science* 207:532, 1980.

Hobson JA: Sleep and dreaming, *J Neurosci* 10:371, 1990. *An interesting recent review indicating simultaneously how much and how little we know about sleep.*

Jones EG: Neurotransmitters in the cerebral cortex, *J Neurosurg* 65:135, 1986.

Jones EG, Coulter JD, Wise SP: Commissural columns in the sensory-motor cortex of monkeys, *J Comp Neurol* 188:113, 1979.

Jones EG, Powell TPS: An anatomical study of converging sensory pathways within the cerebral cortex of the monkey, *Brain* 93:793, 1970. *A study of the stepwise radiations of auditory, visual, and somatosensory information from the primary receiving areas to parts of the association cortex; done by the straightforward but clever technique of lesioning a primary area, tracing the degenerating fibers, and making lesions where the degeneration terminates.*

Jouandet ML, Gazzaniga MS: Cortical field of origin of the anterior commissure of the rhesus monkey, *Exp Neurol* 66:381, 1979.

Kaas JH: The organization of callosal connections in primates. In Reeves AG, Roberts DW, editors: *Epilepsy and the corpus callosum II,* New York, 1995, Plenum Press.

Kenshalo DR Jr, Isensee O: Responses of primate SI cortical neurons to noxious stimuli, *J Neurophysiol* 50:1479, 1983.

Land EH et al: Colour-generating interactions across the corpus callosum, *Nature* 303:616, 1983. *Clever experiments showing that if the contrast comparisons needed to make decisions about color involve areas that span the vertical midline, then the corpus callosum gets into the act.*

LaPierre D, Braun CMJ, Hodgkins S: Ventral frontal deficits in psychopathy: neuropsychological test findings, *Neuropsych* 33:139, 1995.

LeDoux JE, Wilson DH, Gazzaniga MS: A divided mind: observations on the conscious properties of the separated hemispheres, *Ann Neurol* 2:417, 1977. *An individual with some bilateral language representation may not give the same responses with each hemisphere after section of the corpus callosum.*

Lhermitte F: Human autonomy and the frontal lobes. II. Patient behavior in complex and social situations: the "environmental dependency syndrome," *Ann Neurol* 19:335, 1986. *Quantitative measurement of the effects of prefrontal damage is difficult, but simple observation provides fascinating insights.*

Libet B et al: Subjective referral of the timing for a conscious sensory experience: a functional role for the somatosensory specific projection system in man, *Brain* 102:193, 1979. *How do we decide when a tactile stimulus occurs? Is it at the instant of physical contact, or when the first electrical activity reaches the postcentral gyrus, or after this activity has rattled around the cortex for awhile? A fascinating and provocative paper that addresses this question experimentally.*

Mahowald MW, Schenck CH: Dissociated states of wakefulness and sleep, *Neurol* 42(suppl 6):44, 1992.

McCormick DA, Bal T: Sleep and arousal: thalamocortical mechanisms, *Ann Rev Neurosci* 20:185, 1997.

McKeever WF et al: On language laterality in normal dextrals and sinistrals: results from the Bilateral Object Naming Latency Task, *Neuropsychol* 33:1627, 1995.

Mesulam M-M: Cholinergic pathways and the ascending reticular activating system of the human brain, *Ann NY Acad Sci* 757:169, 1995.

Mountcastle VB: The columnar organization of the neocortex, *Brain* 120:701, 1997.

Mukhametov LM: Sleep in marine mammals, *Exp Brain Res Suppl* 8:227, 1984. *Porpoises appear to have evolved the novel technique of sleeping with one hemisphere at a time.*

Nauta WJH: The problem of the frontal lobe: a reinterpretation, *J Psychiatr Res* 8:167, 1971.

Nieuwenhuys R: The neocortex: an overview of its evolutionary development, structural organization and synaptology, *Anat Embryol* 190:307, 1994.

Northcutt RG, Kaas JH: The emergence and evolution of mammalian neocortex, *Trends Neurosci* 18:373, 1995.

Pakkenberg B, Gundersen HJG: Neocortical neuron number in humans: effect of sex and age, *J Comp Neurol* 384:312, 1997.

Penfield W, Rasmussen T: *The cerebral cortex of man,* New York, 1950, Macmillan, Inc. *A review of the results of cortical stimulations of a large series of patients and of the results of localized cortical excisions from these patients.*

Penfield W, Roberts L: *Speech and brain-mechanisms,* Princeton, NJ, 1959, Princeton University Press.

Posner MI, Raichle ME: The neuroimaging of human brain function, *Proc Natl Acad Sci* 95:763, 1998. *The introduction to a series of 22 papers dealing with multiple aspects of this topic.*

Powell TPS: Certain aspects of the intrinsic organization of the cerebral cortex. In Pompeiano O, Ajmone Marsan C: *Brain mechanisms and perceptual awareness,* IBRO Monograph Series, vol 8, New York, 1981, Raven Press. *A nice review of the evidence concerning uniform organization of the cerebral cortex. Although some of the details may be inaccurate, the general concept appears to be correct.*

Price BH et al: The comportmental learning disabilities of early frontal lobe damage, *Brain* 113:1383, 1990. *An important paper about two patients who had suffered extensive prefrontal damage at an early age, indicating that "In comparison with other types of brain damage which disrupt cognitive development, frontal damage acquired early in life appears to provide the neurological substrate for a special type of learning disability in the realms of insight, foresight, social judgement, empathy, and complex reasoning."*

Purpura DP: Dendritic spine "dysgenesis" and mental retardation, *Science* 186:1126, 1974.

Rechtschaffen A et al: Physiological correlates of prolonged sleep deprivation in rats, *Science* 221:182, 1983.

Rolls ET et al: Emotion-related learning in patients with social and emotional changes associated with frontal lobe damage, *J Neurol Neurosurg Psychiatr* 57:1518, 1994. *"Patients often reported verbally that the contingencies had changed, but were unable to alter their behaviour appropriately. These impairments occurred independently of IQ or verbal memory impairments."*

Ross ED: The aprosodias: functional-anatomic organization of the affective components of language in the right hemisphere, *Arch Neurol* 38:561, 1981.

Russell IS, Ochs S: Localization of a memory trace in one cortical hemisphere and transfer to the other hemisphere, *Brain* 86:37, 1963. *We know that inputs spread to both hemispheres under normal circumstances via the corpus callosum. This interesting paper describes what happens if one hemisphere is temporarily inactivated during acquisition of a memory.*

Sallanon M et al: Long-lasting insomnia induced by preoptic neuron lesions and its transient reversal by muscimol injection into the posterior hypothalamus in the cat, *Neurosci* 32:669, 1989.

Sauerland EK, Harper RM: The human tongue during sleep: electromyographic activity of the genioglossus muscle, *Exp Neurol* 51:160, 1976. *If the muscles of your tongue follow the general pattern and become flaccid during REM sleep, then why don't you get into trouble by inhaling it? Read this and find out.*

Scalaidhe SPÓ, Wilson FAW, Goldman-Rakic PS: Areal segregation of face-processing neurons in prefrontal cortex, *Science* 278:1135, 1997. *Different prefrontal areas for different working memories.*

Scott TR et al: Gustatory responses in the frontal opercular cortex of the alert cynomolgus monkey, *J Neurophysiol* 56:876, 1986.

Shapiro CM et al: Slow-wave sleep: a recovery period after exercise, *Science* 214:1253, 1981. *An old hypothesis about sleep is that we do it as some sort of "restorative" process. Our sleep patterns don't change much after ordinary exercise, but after running a marathon they do.*

Sherin JE et al: Activation of ventrolateral preoptic neurons during sleep, *Science* 271:216, 1996.

Siegel JM: Brainstem mechanisms generating REM sleep. In Kryger MH, Roth T, Dement WC: *Principles and practice of sleep medicine,* ed 2, Philadelphia, 1994, WB Saunders.

Sperry RW: Lateral specialization in the surgically separated hemispheres. In Schmitt FO, Worden FG, editors: *The neurosciences: third study program,* Cambridge, Mass, 1974, The MIT Press. *A general review of results from humans with a sectioned corpus callosum by the principal figure in this type of research.*

Steriade M, McCarley RW: *Brainstem control of wakefulness and sleep,* New York, 1990, Plenum Press.

Steriade M: Brain electrical activity and sensory processing during waking and sleep states. In Kryger MH, Roth T, Dement WC: *Principles and practice of sleep medicine,* ed 2, Philadelphia, 1994, WB Saunders.

Szentagothai J: The neuron network of the cerebral cortex: a functional interpretation, *Proc R Soc Lond* B201:219, 1978.

Talbot JD et al: Multiple representations of pain in human cerebral cortex, *Science* 251:1355, 1991. *PET scanning studies indicating that the perception of pain is accompanied by increased blood flow at least in the contralateral S1, S2, and cingulate gyrus.*

Tang Y, Nyengaard JR: A stereological method for estimating the total length and size of myelin fibers in human brain white matter, *J Neurosci Meth* 73:193, 1997.

Teuber HL: The brain and human behavior. In Held R, Leibowitz HW, Teuber HL, editors: *Handbook of sensory physiology,* vol 8, *Perception,* New York, 1978, Springer-Verlag. *An interesting, scholarly, wide-ranging correlation of deficits and brain damage in humans and experimental animals.*

Türe T, Yaşargil MG, Pait TG: Is there a superior occipitotemporal fasciculus? A microsurgical anatomic study, *Neurosurg* 40:1226, 1997. *Recent evidence that what has traditionally been thought to be a long association bundle is in fact fibers fanning out from the posterior limb of the internal capsule to interconnect the thalamus with frontal and parietal cortex.*

Villablanca J: Behavioral and polygraphic study of "sleep" and "wakefulness" in chronic decerebrate cats, *Electroencephalogr Clin Neurophysiol* 21: 562, 1966. *In the chronic state after a rostral mesencephalic transection, the portions of the CNS both rostral and caudal to the transection are capable of some manifestations of sleep and wakefulness; amazingly enough, they do so with completely independent rhythms.*

Wada JA, Davis AE: Fundamental nature of human infant's brain asymmetry, *Can J Neurol Sci* 4:203, 1977. *We are born not only with built-in anatomical asymmetries but apparently also with built-in physiological asymmetries.*

Wada J, Rasmussen T: Intracarotid injection of sodium amytal for the lateralization of cerebral speech dominance: experimental and clinical observations, *J Neurosurg* 17:266, 1960.

Watanabe M: Reward expectancy in primate prefrontal neurons, *Nature* 382:629, 1996.

Watson RT et al: Normal tactile threshold in monkeys with neglect, *Neurol* 34:917, 1984.

Woolsey TA, van der Loos H: The structural organization of layer IV in the somatosensory region (SI) of mouse cerebral cortex: the description of a cortical field composed of discrete cytoarchitectonic units, *Brain Res* 17:205, 1970. *A special kind of columnar organization described in a delightful paper.*

Yamadori A et al: Preservation of singing in Broca's aphasia, *J Neurol Neurosurg Psychiatry* 40:221, 1977.

Young AW: *Functions of the right cerebral hemisphere,* New York, 1983, Academic Press.

Zhang HQ et al: Parallel processing in cerebral cortex of the marmoset monkey: effect of reversible SI inactivation on tactile responses, *J Neurophysiol* 76:3633, 1996.

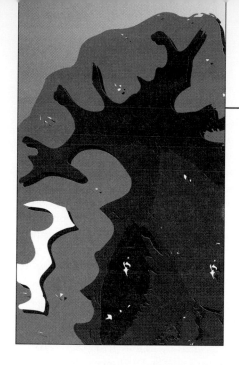

DRIVES, EMOTIONS, AND MEMORIES: THE HYPOTHALAMUS AND LIMBIC SYSTEM

We seldom perceive things in a completely neutral fashion. Various sights and sounds make us happy, sad, or angry; certain odors can make some individuals positively ecstatic. There is also a two-way connection between these emotional aspects of perception on the one hand and thoughts and memories on the other: appropriate aromas can conjure up images of meals and wines consumed in the past; in addition, the remembrance of something in the past can stir the same emotions that accompanied the original event, and even thinking about something that has not happened can arouse emotions. Assuming that "thinking" depends heavily on the neocortex, it would seem likely that the anatomical substrate for feelings and emotions would at least be closely connected with the neocortex. The same system would also need to be heavily interconnected with the hypothalamus because sensory inputs that arouse an emotion also initiate autonomic responses such as salivating and gearing up the alimentary tract, or pumping adrenalin and diverting blood to skeletal muscles. Finally, the types of stimuli that elicit emotion-laden responses in us—and the responses themselves—are, in a more general sense, crucial to all animals, for these are the drive-related activities central to the preservation of individuals and their species, activities such as feeding, defense, and sexual behavior.

The **limbic system** is the name given to the portions of the brain primarily concerned with such responses and behavior. As discussed in some detail later in the chapter, it includes the **cingulate** and **parahippocampal gyri** (see Figure 3-11), the **amygdala,** and the **hippocampus.** In view of the preceding discussion, it is not surprising that the components of the limbic system appeared early in vertebrate phylogeny and that in its connections the limbic system is interposed between the hypothalamus and the neocortex. That is, limbic structures serve as bridges between autonomic and voluntary responses to

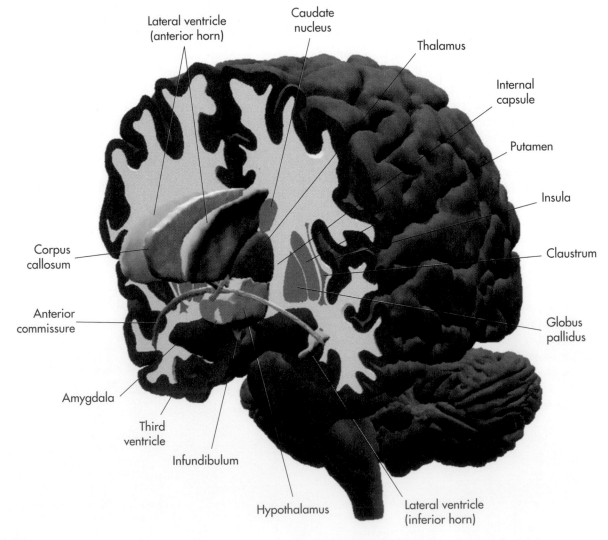

FIGURE 23-1

Three-dimensional reconstruction of the hypothalamus and surrounding cerebral structures. The hypothalamus has been rendered with a flat anterior surface because the preoptic area (Figure 23-4), which envelops the anterior end of the third ventricle but is not formally part of the diencephalon, was not included.

changes in the environment. Our response to a chilly room provides a simple example. There are autonomic responses to the chill, coordinated by the hypothalamus, such as cutaneous vasoconstriction and shivering. We also become consciously aware of the chill, and may choose to put on more clothes or turn up the heat.

THE HYPOTHALAMUS COORDINATES DRIVE-RELATED BEHAVIORS

The hypothalamus (Figure 23-1) is a small portion of the diencephalon (weighing only about 4 g) but is important as a nodal point in pathways concerned with autonomic, endocrine, emotional, and somatic functions (Figure 23-2) generally designed to maintain our internal environment in a physiological range (i.e., to promote homeostasis). For example, stimulation of appropriate hypothalamic areas in experimental animals can cause vasodilation, rage, feeding behavior, or alterations of pituitary function. Accordingly the connections of the hypothalamus are widespread and complex, but they fall into three principal categories: (1)

interconnections with various components of the limbic system, (2) outputs that influence the pituitary gland, and (3) interconnections with various visceral and somatic nuclei, both motor and sensory, of the brainstem and spinal cord. The hypothalamus is divided into a number of nuclei and areas, as described shortly. Each of these different nuclei and areas has more or less distinctive connections, but for the sake of simplicity most of these connections are discussed here as though the hypothalamus were by and large a uniform structure.

The Hypothalamus Can Be Subdivided in Both Longitudinal and Medial-Lateral Directions

The inferior surface of the hypothalamus (see Figures 3-14 and 3-15), exposed directly to subarachnoid space, is bounded by the optic chiasm, the optic tracts, and the posterior edge of the mammillary bodies. This area, exclusive of the mammillary bodies, is called the **tuber cinereum** (Figure 23-3, *A*). The **median eminence,** a swelling on the surface of the tuber cinereum, is continuous with the

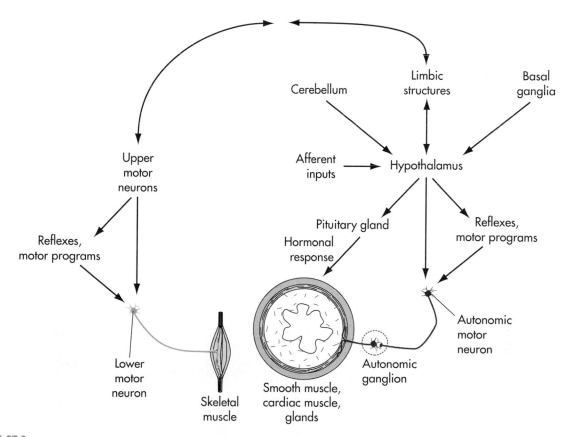

FIGURE 23-2

Overview of the pivotal role of the hypothalamus in drive-related activities. The hypothalamus can affect autonomic motor neurons both directly and through visceral motor programs in the brainstem and spinal cord, and can also influence visceral structures through its control over the pituitary gland (Figure 23-9). It can also stimulate somatic responses through connections with limbic structures that interconnect the hypothalamus and neocortex. The latter are two-way connections, providing us a degree of voluntary control over responses that may be physiologically desirable but do not fit the current circumstances in some other way (e.g., "grin and bear it"). The cerebellum and basal ganglia also have connections with the hypothalamus, but their role in the planning and coordination of drive-related activities are still poorly understood and are not discussed in this chapter.

infundibular stalk, which in turn is continuous with the **posterior lobe of the pituitary.** The median eminence, infundibular stalk, and posterior lobe together constitute the **neurohypophysis.**

The medial surface of the hypothalamus (Figure 23-3, *B*) extends anteriorly to the lamina terminalis, superiorly to the hypothalamic sulcus, and posteriorly to the caudal edge of the diencephalon. As in other parts of the diencephalon, these longitudinal boundaries are semiarbitrary; functionally related neural tissue continues through both the anterior and posterior boundaries. For example, the anterior border of the hypothalamus technically is the plane through the anterior edge of the optic chiasm and the posterior edge of the anterior commissure. However, the neural tissue immediately in front of this formal boundary is structurally and functionally continuous with the hypothalamus. Therefore this region (the **preoptic area**), traditionally considered to be part of the telencephalon, is usually treated instead as part of the anterior hypothalamus.

The hypothalamus can be subdivided longitudinally into **anterior, tuberal,** and **posterior** regions. The anterior region is the part above the optic chiasm, the tuberal region is the part above and including the tuber cinereum, and the posterior region is the part above and including the mammillary bodies. In addition, the entire hypothalamus of each side is divided into medial and lateral zones* by a parasagittal plane through the fornix as this fiber bundle traverses the hypothalamus (Figures 23-4 and 23-13, *C*). Thus the hypothalamus consists of six parts on each side: the medial and lateral zones of the anterior, tuberal, and posterior regions. The principal nuclei of these areas are indicated in Table 23-1 and Figure 23-4.

The lateral zone consists mainly of scattered cells interspersed among the longitudinally running fibers of the **medial forebrain bundle.** Anteriorly it is continuous with the lateral preoptic nucleus, and caudally it is continuous with the midbrain tegmentum. Part of the supraoptic nucleus intrudes into it, as do clumps of cells called **lateral tuberal nuclei.** It also contains the small **tuberomammillary nucleus,** the source of histaminergic fibers that project widely to the cerebral cortex and thalamus

---

*The part of the medial hypothalamus immediately adjacent to the wall of the third ventricle is often considered separately as a **periventricular** zone.

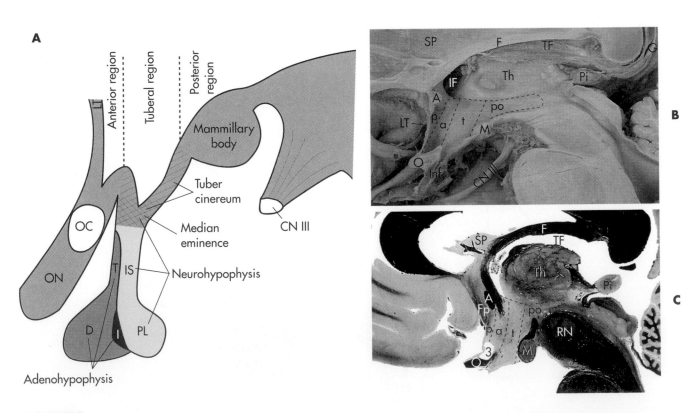

FIGURE 23-3

A, Regions of the hypothalamus and pituitary in midsagittal view. The entire area filled with diagonal lines is the tuber cinereum. The crosshatched portion of the tuber cinereum is the median eminence. **B,** The medial surface of the hypothalamus. **C,** Myelin-stained parasagittal section of the diencephalon, near the midline. *a, p, po, t,* Anterior, preoptic, posterior, and tuberal regions of the hypothalamus; *3,* third ventricle (optic recess); *A,* anterior commissure; *D,* distal part of the adenohypophysis; *F,* fornix; *Fp,* precommissural part of the fornix (Figure 23-13); *G,* great cerebral vein (of Galen); *IF,* interventricular foramen; *Inf,* infundibulum; *I,* intermediate part of the adenohypophysis; *IS,* infundibular stalk; *LT,* lamina terminalis; *M,* mammillary body (part of the posterior hypothalamus); *O* or *OC,* optic chiasm; *ON,* optic nerve; *Pi,* pineal gland; *PL,* posterior lobe of the pituitary; *RN,* red nucleus; *SP,* septum pellucidum; *Th,* thalamus; *T,* tuberal part of the adenohypophysis; *TF,* transverse fissure.

and participate in the sleep-wake cycle (see Figure 22-26). Otherwise it is undivided.

The medial zone, on the other hand, contains a number of nuclei. These include two distinctive nuclei containing large neurosecretory cells, the **supraoptic** and **paraventricular nuclei.** The supraoptic nucleus sits astride the optic tract, extending into the lateral hypothalamic zone; the paraventricular nucleus is higher up in the wall of the third ventricle, near the anterior commissure. Most cells of the supraoptic nucleus and many cells of the paraventricular nucleus secrete hormones that travel down the axons of these cells and are released in the neurohypophysis. The hormones involved and the pathway traversed by them are discussed later in this chapter (Figure 23-9). The supraoptic region also contains a small **suprachiasmatic nucleus** and a larger **anterior nucleus.** The anterior nucleus is continuous anteriorly with the medial preoptic nucleus. The suprachiasmatic nucleus, although tiny, is the "master clock" for most of our circadian rhythms (Figure 23-5, *A*). The free-running period of cells in the suprachiasmatic nucleus is typically about 25 hours (Figure 23-5, *B*), but it receives direct projections from the retina that entrain it to the actual day length.

Table 23-1 Hypothalamic Nuclei

Region	Medial area	Lateral area
Anterior	Medial preoptic nucleus	Lateral preoptic nucleus
	Supraoptic nucleus	Lateral nucleus
	Paraventricular nucleus	Part of the supraoptic nucleus
	Anterior nucleus	
	Suprachiasmatic nucleus	
Tuberal	Dorsomedial nucleus	Lateral nucleus
	Ventromedial nucleus	Lateral tuberal nuclei
	Arcuate (infundibular) nucleus	Tuberomammillary nucleus
Posterior	Mammillary body	Lateral nucleus
	Posterior nucleus	

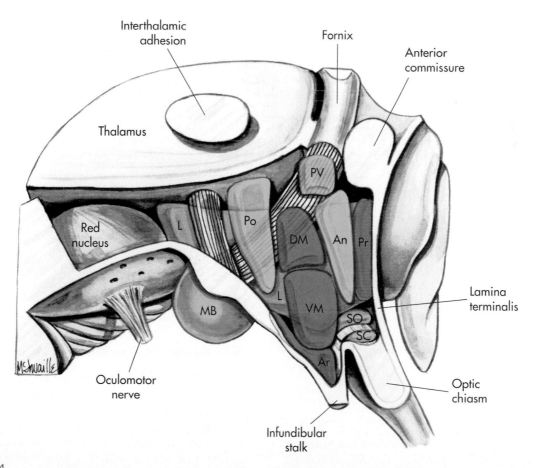

FIGURE 23-4

Principal nuclei of the hypothalamus. *An,* Anterior nucleus; *Ar,* arcuate (infundibular) nucleus; *DM,* dorsomedial nucleus; *L,* lateral nucleus; *MB,* mammillary body; *Po,* posterior nucleus; *Pr,* medial preoptic nucleus; *PV,* paraventricular nucleus; *SC,* suprachiasmatic nucleus; *SO,* supraoptic nucleus; *VM,* ventromedial nucleus. [Modified from Nauta WJH, Haymaker W: *The hypothalamus,* Springfield, Ill, 1969, Charles C Thomas, Publisher.]

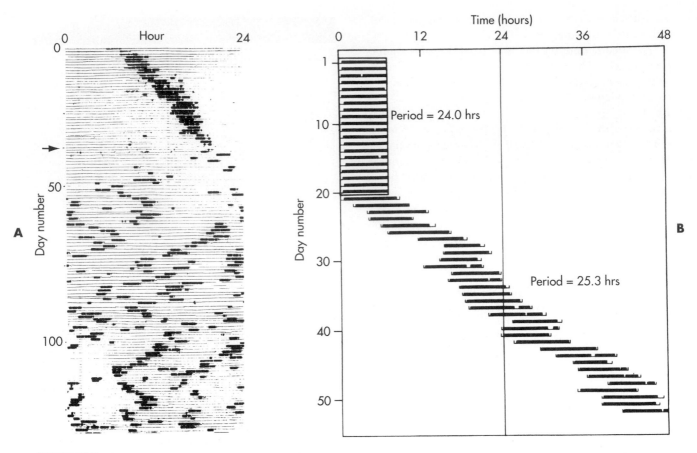

FIGURE 23-5

Dependence of circadian rhythms on the suprachiasmatic nucleus. **A,** Wheel-running behavior of a hamster over a period of several months while living in constant light. Each horizontal line represents a single day, and each thickening represents a period of wheel running. Wheel running starts out clearly rhythmic, with a prominent episode approximately every 25 hours. On day 37 *(arrow)* the suprachiasmatic nucleus was destroyed bilaterally, and the wheel running subsequently became almost random. **B,** Entrainment of circadian rhythms by environmental cues. These are sleep records of a 22-year-old man living in a laboratory situation with no cues about the time of day. Thick bars represent time asleep, and thin lines indicate time in bed but awake. For the first 20 days, the subject was awakened every 24 hours and chose to go to bed at about the same time every day (without knowing what time it was). After day 20 he self-selected his own sleep time (i.e., his circadian rhythms were allowed to run freely with no entraining cues). As a result, he went to bed about an hour later on each successive day; the free-running period was 25.3 hours. (**A** from Turek FW: Are the suprachiasmatic nuclei the location of the biological clock in mammals? *Nature* 292:289, 1981. **B** from Czeisler CA et al: Chronotherapy: resetting the circadian clocks of patients with delayed sleep phase insomnia, *Sleep* 4:1, 1981.)

The medial tuberal region is subdivided into dorsal and ventral portions called the **dorsomedial** and **ventromedial nuclei,** respectively. In addition, cells in the floor of the infundibular recess of the third ventricle constitute the **arcuate** (or **infundibular**) **nucleus.**

The medial mammillary region contains the **mammillary body** (actually a complex of several nuclei) and the **posterior hypothalamic nucleus,** which is continuous with the periaqueductal gray matter of the midbrain.

Hypothalamic Inputs Arise in Widespread Neural Sites

Neural inputs to the hypothalamus arise in two general areas (Figure 23-6): (1) various parts of the forebrain, particularly components of the limbic system, and (2) the brainstem and spinal cord. Afferents from the brainstem and spinal cord convey visceral and somatic sensory infor-

mation, whereas those from limbic structures convey information relevant to the role of the hypothalamus in mediating many of the autonomic and somatic aspects of affective states. The connections of limbic components with each other and with the hypothalamus are discussed later in this chapter and are only mentioned briefly here.

Most inputs from the forebrain arise in limbic structures

Major forebrain afferents to the hypothalamus arise in the (1) **septal nuclei** and nearby parts of the basal forebrain, including the ventral striatum, (2) hippocampus, (3) amygdala, (4) orbital cortex of the frontal lobe and some other cortical areas, and (5) retina. The septal nuclei (see Figure 24-2), prominent components of the limbic system located adjacent to the septum pellucidum, project fibers to the hypothalamus through the medial forebrain bundle.

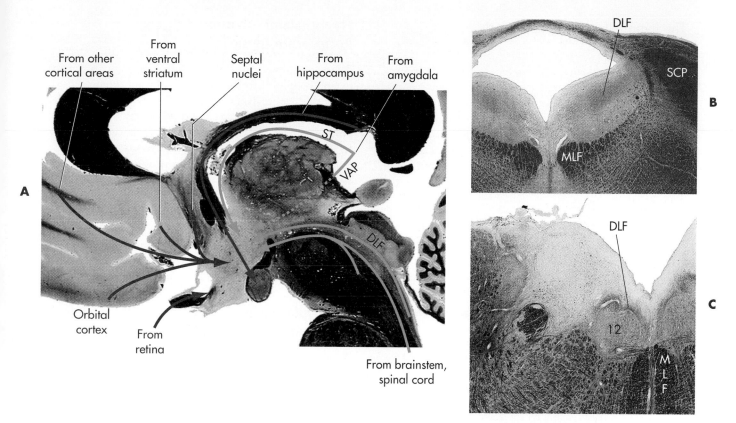

FIGURE 23-6

A, Major inputs to the hypothalamus. *DLF,* Dorsal longitudinal fasciculus; *ST,* stria terminalis; *VAP,* ventral amygdalofugal pathway (Figure 23-21). **B** and **C,** Location of the dorsal longitudinal fasciculus *(DLF)* in the rostral pons and rostral medulla. *12,* Hypoglossal nucleus; *MLF,* medial longitudinal fasciculus; *SCP,* superior cerebellar peduncle.

The medial forebrain bundle is built like a frayed rope, with fibers entering and leaving it at many levels as it traverses the lateral hypothalamic zone and extends into the brainstem tegmentum. This is a bidirectional bundle that also contains afferents from the brainstem to the hypothalamus as well as hypothalamic efferents passing both rostrally and caudally and fibers interconnecting different hypothalamic levels.

The major output from the hippocampus is contained in the fornix. This fiber bundle arches around under the corpus callosum and through the hypothalamus, where most of its fibers reach the mammillary body (Figure 23-15).

The amygdala projects fibers to the hypothalamus by two different routes. Some travel through the **stria terminalis,** a long, curved fiber bundle that accompanies the caudate nucleus. Others take a shorter course and pass under the lenticular nucleus directly to the hypothalamus (Figures 23-20 and 23-21).

Finally, there are direct projections from the cerebral cortex to the hypothalamus. These arise mainly in the orbital cortex of the frontal lobe and in the insula and join the medial forebrain bundle. There are also contributions from the cingulate gyrus and some other cortical areas.

Inputs from the brainstem and spinal cord traverse the medial forebrain bundle and dorsal longitudinal fasciculus

An assortment of sensory inputs reaches the hypothalamus by several routes. Some involve synapses in various portions of the reticular formation and periaqueductal gray; others arrive directly from sites such as the solitary and parabrachial nuclei. Some of these afferents travel in the medial forebrain bundle; others are contained in the **dorsal longitudinal fasciculus** (Figure 23-6, *B* and *C*), a collection of thinly myelinated fibers that pass through the periventricular and periaqueductal gray of the brainstem and then fan out in the hypothalamic wall of the third ventricle. Still other afferents enter the hypothalamus as collaterals of fibers in other pathways such as the spinothalamic tract. Finally, there is a small but functionally important projection (Figure 23-5) from a subset of retinal ganglion cells directly to the suprachiasmatic nucleus.

Ascending axons from brainstem monoamine-containing neuronal groups—locus ceruleus, raphe nuclei, ventral tegmental area—also traverse the medial forebrain bundle on their way to innervate the cerebral cortex (see Figures 11-20, 11-22, and 11-23). Along the way, some terminate in the hypothalamus.

The hypothalamus contains intrinsic sensory neurons

In addition to receiving various types of visceral and somatic information through the brainstem pathways just mentioned, the hypothalamus contains cells that are directly responsive to physical stimuli. Some of these cells are sensitive to the temperature of the hypothalamus itself, whereas the activity of others is sensitive to such things as blood osmolality (Figure 23-7) or the concentration of glucose or certain hormones in blood passing through the hypothalamus.

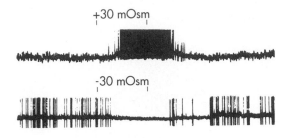

+30 mOsm

-30 mOsm

FIGURE 23-7
Patch-clamp recordings from a rat supraoptic neuron as it was exposed to hypertonic and hypotonic solutions. Hypertonic solutions cause the neuron to shrink, mechanosensitive ion channels to open, and a burst of action potentials. Hypotonic solutions cause the reverse. (From Oliet SHR, Bourque CW: Mechanosensitive channels transduce osmosensitivity in supraoptic neurons, *Nature* 364:341, 1993.)

Hypothalamic Outputs Largely Reciprocate Inputs

Efferent pathways from the hypothalamus are, to a great extent, reciprocal to the afferent pathways (Figure 23-8). Thus the hypothalamus projects to the septal nuclei, the hippocampus, the amygdala, and the brainstem and spinal cord by way of the same fiber bundles that carry afferents to the hypothalamus. In addition, a few pathways are totally or predominantly efferent in nature. The prominent **mammillothalamic tract** passes from the mammillary body to the anterior nucleus of the thalamus, and a considerably smaller number travel in the opposite direction as well (that is, from the anterior nucleus to the mammillary body). The **mammillotegmental tract** branches from the mammillothalamic tract near the latter's origin and projects to the midbrain reticular formation.

The hypothalamus controls both lobes of the pituitary gland

The final efferent pathways from the hypothalamus are of great functional importance because they control the **pituitary gland** (or **hypophysis**). This control is accomplished by two means: a neural projection to the neurohypophysis and a vascular link with the adenohypophysis.

The supraoptic and paraventricular nuclei, as mentioned previously, contain large neurosecretory cells. (The paraventricular nucleus also contains numerous smaller cells, many of which project as hypothalamic efferents to

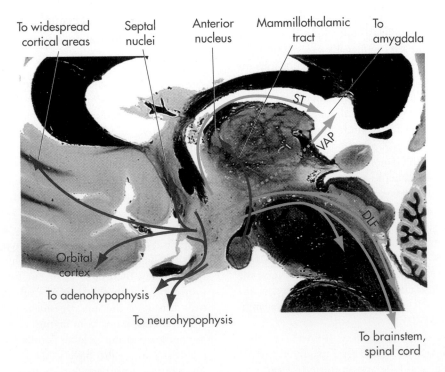

To widespread cortical areas   Septal nuclei   Anterior nucleus   Mammillothalamic tract   To amygdala

ST

VAP

DLF

Orbital cortex

To adenohypophysis

To neurohypophysis

To brainstem, spinal cord

FIGURE 23-8
Major outputs from the hypothalamus. *DLF*, Dorsal longitudinal fasciculus; *ST*, stria terminalis; *VAP*, ventral amygdalofugal pathway (Figure 23-21).

the dorsal motor nucleus of the vagus nerve, the intermediolateral cell column of the spinal cord, and other sites.) The larger neurosecretory cells of the supraoptic and paraventricular nuclei produce two peptide hormones, each nine amino acids in length; a given cell produces only one of the two hormones. The first is **antidiuretic hormone** (**ADH,** or **vasopressin**), whose principal physiological function as a hormone is to increase the reabsorption of water in the kidney and thereby decrease the production of urine.★ The second is **oxytocin** (from the Greek words meaning "rapid birth"), a similar peptide that causes contraction of uterine and mammary smooth muscle and is important in parturition and milk ejection. Both hor-

---

★Both vasopressin and oxytocin, like the hypothalamic releasing factors, also serve as neurotransmitters or neuromodulators, so their total physiological roles extend beyond their functions as hormones.

mones travel down the axons of their parent cell bodies by axoplasmic flow, bound to a carrier protein (**neurophysin**). These neurosecretory cells are electrically excitable, and the passage of action potentials down their axons causes release of their hormones from bulbous endings adjacent to capillaries in the median eminence, infundibular stalk, and posterior lobe of the pituitary (Figure 23-9, A). Most of the axons arise in the supraoptic nucleus, so this pathway is called the **supraopticohypophyseal tract.**

The adenohypophysis secretes a multitude of hormones whose discussion is beyond the scope of this book. It has been known for some time that electrical stimulation of certain areas of the hypothalamus can modulate the rates of secretion of these hormones, but no neural connections are known that could explain this modulation. This drew attention to the **hypophyseal**

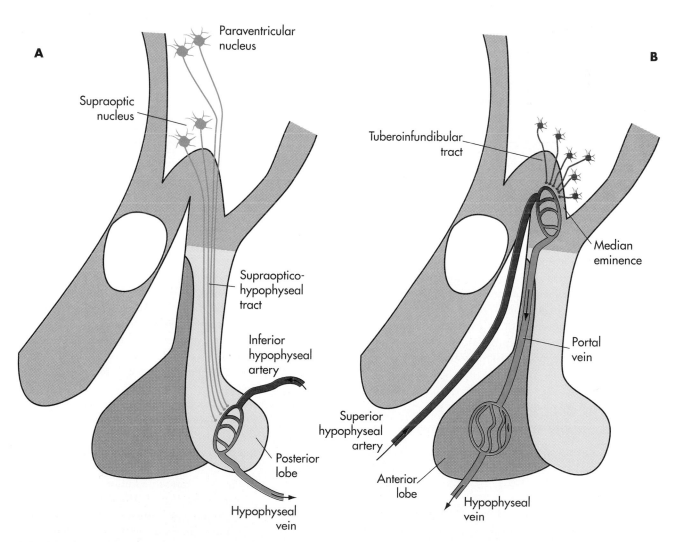

FIGURE 23-9
Routes by which the hypothalamus influences the pituitary gland. **A,** Oxytocin and vasopressin are transported down the axons of magnocellular neurons of the supraoptic and paraventricular nuclei, reaching capillaries of the posterior lobe. **B,** Parvocellular neurons in the arcuate nucleus and nearby regions of the walls of the third ventricle secrete releasing and inhibiting hormones in the median eminence, where they gain access to the hypophyseal portal system and through it reach the anterior lobe. The inferior hypophyseal artery (not shown) also participates in the hypophyseal portal system, giving rise to capillary sinusoids in the lower part of the infundibulum.

portal system as a vascular connection between the hypothalamus and the adenohypophysis (Figure 23-9, *B*). The **superior hypophyseal artery,** a branch of the internal carotid, breaks up into a capillary bed in the median eminence and proximal part of the infundibular stalk. Blood in these capillaries then re-collects into **hypophyseal portal vessels,** which travel down the infundibular stalk and break up into a second capillary bed in the adenohypophysis. Small peptides,★ called **hypothalamic releasing hormones** and **inhibiting hormones,** are secreted by cells of the arcuate nucleus and nearby sites in the wall of the third ventricle,† travel down the axons of these cells, and are released into the bloodstream in the first capillary bed (recall that the median eminence is one of the circumventricular organs (see Figure 6-26), and its capillaries are fenestrated (see Figure 6-27). From there the releasing and inhibiting hormones travel down the hypophyseal portal vessels to the adenohypophysis, where they act. As their names imply, releasing hormones promote the release of particular hormones, whereas inhibiting hormones prevent this release. The entire collection of axons carrying these releasing and inhibiting factors is called the **tuberoinfundibular** or **tuberohypophyseal tract.**

The relatively small cells that secrete releasing and inhibiting factors are commonly referred to as the **parvocellular neurosecretory system,** as distinguished from the **magnocellular neurosecretory system** of larger neurons in the supraoptic and paraventricular nuclei that secrete oxytocin and vasopressin.

The same small hypothalamic peptides are also found in other neurons in widespread areas of the CNS and in other cells of the body as well. This is reminiscent of the situation with enkephalins and endorphins, briefly discussed in Chapter 11. A slowly emerging picture is that in some respects the brain is a much more "distributed" organ than it is normally considered to be—that is, it may use the same chemical both as a neurotransmitter acting locally on a postsynaptic neuron and as a hormone acting at a distance, both actions working toward the same physiological goal.

Perforating Branches From the Circle of Willis Supply the Hypothalamus

Inspection of Figure 6-3 reveals that the infundibular stalk is located just about in the middle of the circle of Willis, and the inferior surface of the entire hypothala-

mus is more or less surrounded by the circle. The arterial supply of the hypothalamus is derived from a series of small ganglionic or perforating arteries arising from arteries in and adjacent to the circle of Willis (see Figure 6-8). Specifically the **anteromedial** group of ganglionic arteries, arising from the anterior cerebral and anterior communicating arteries, supplies the preoptic and supraoptic regions; the **posteromedial** group, arising from the posterior communicating arteries and the proximal portions of the posterior cerebral arteries, supplies the tuberal and mammillary regions; the **anterolateral** group (or lateral striate arteries), arising from proximal portions of the middle cerebral arteries, helps supply the lateral hypothalamus.

Hypothalamic Damage Disrupts Homeostasis

The connections of the hypothalamus with the limbic system, pituitary, and brainstem make it eminently suitable for controlling various visceral functions and activities involved in drives and emotional states. Consistent with this, many hypothalamic "centers" have been described that are concerned with feeding and drinking behavior, temperature regulation, gut motility, sexual activity, and numerous other functions. In most cases, however, fragments of a behavior pattern elicited by stimulating a hypothalamic location can be elicited by stimulating appropriate sites in the brainstem. Thus many of the hypothalamic sites associated with particular behaviors may really be trigger points that, when stimulated, initiate neural activity in other parts of the CNS, which in turn causes the behavior pattern (Figure 23-2). Furthermore, many parts of the hypothalamus are organized loosely enough that electrical stimulation of only a certain part of a certain nucleus is impossible. For example, the medial forebrain bundle runs through the lateral hypothalamus, so if a particular behavior were elicited by stimulating a particular site in the lateral hypothalamus, it could be the result of stimulating either a portion of the lateral hypothalamic nucleus or some fibers of the medial forebrain bundle that originated and will terminate outside the hypothalamus.

Given these caveats, it has nevertheless been found that certain types of changes consistently follow stimulation of or damage to particular hypothalamic areas in experimental animals. Because the hypothalamus is so small, discrete lesions affecting individual functional areas of the human hypothalamus are quite rare; in addition, lesions must be bilateral to disrupt most hypothalamic functions. However, the clinical findings in humans with hypothalamic damage are generally consistent with what would be expected from work on experimental animals. Only a few examples are cited here.

The hypothalamus is in overall control of the autonomic nervous system in the sense that practically any

---

★The major exception is dopamine, which inhibits the release of prolactin.

†Some of these are located in the paraventricular nucleus, which therefore contains three distinct cell types—large neurons that secrete oxytocin or vasopressin, smaller neurons that secrete releasing or inhibiting hormones, and neurons that project to the brainstem and spinal cord.

type of autonomic response can be elicited by stimulating some hypothalamic site. Although the sites overlap to a considerable degree, those associated with parasympathetic responses tend to be located anteriorly, and those associated with sympathetic responses tend to be located posteriorly. Appropriate somatic motor activity accompanies these autonomic responses, as the example of hypothalamic control of temperature regulation demonstrates. Stimulation of the anterior hypothalamus and preoptic area induces sweating (or panting in animals with fewer sweat glands than we have) and cutaneous vasodilatation, which in turn causes body temperature to fall. In contrast, stimulation of the posterior hypothalamus causes cutaneous vasoconstriction and shivering, which in turn causes an increase in body temperature. The hypothalamus thus acts as a thermostat: temperature-sensitive neurons in the anterior hypothalamus monitor the temperature of blood passing by them and activate anterior heat-dissipation or posterior heat-production mechanisms as necessary to maintain the desired value. Bilateral lesions of the anterior hypothalamus make an animal unable to dissipate heat in a warm environment. (Such lesions may also cause diabetes insipidus, in which large amounts of dilute urine are produced as a result of destruction of the supraoptic nuclei.) Bilateral lesions of the posterior hypothalamus may make an animal unable to regulate its body temperature in either a warm or a cold environment because the destruction involves not only the area concerned with the production and conservation of heat, but also the fibers descending from the more anterior heat-dissipation areas.

The role of the hypothalamus in more complex activities is demonstrated by its involvement in feeding behavior. Here again, two areas with opposing influences have been found. Bilateral destruction of the ventromedial nucleus ("satiety center") produces animals that overeat and get fat, whereas destruction of the lateral hypothalamus in the tuberal region ("feeding center") produces animals that do not eat and may actually starve to death unless force-fed during the postoperative weeks. The complete mechanism of these effects is not known, but they are not as simple as they sound. The obesity following ventromedial lesions, for example, results not only from overeating but also from decreased physical activity and from metabolic changes favoring the accumulation of fat.

One should not get the impression that discrete lesions in the hypothalamus cause single changes such as hypothermia or obesity. The case of bilateral lesions of the ventromedial nucleus provides an instructive example not only of multiple effects from discrete lesions but also of the involvement of the hypothalamus in emotional behavior. Cats with bilateral ventromedial lesions overeat and get fat and are also extremely

nasty.★ They respond with full-blown, hissing rages to the most innocuous of stimuli. Similar rage responses can be elicited by stimulation of the lateral hypothalamus adjacent to the ventromedial nucleus of an intact cat. The attacks are coordinated and well directed but cease the moment the stimulus does. The ways in which such emotional responses are related, under normal circumstances, to activity in the limbic system are discussed later in this chapter.

LIMBIC STRUCTURES ARE INTERPOSED BETWEEN THE HYPOTHALAMUS AND NEOCORTEX

In 1878 Broca pointed out that a general feature of mammalian brains is a great horseshoe-shaped rim of cortex surrounding the junction between the diencephalon and each cerebral hemisphere (see Figure 3-11). The ends of the arc are joined by olfactory areas at the base of the brain so that a complete loop is formed, with the olfactory tract and bulb extending anteriorly like the handle of a tennis racket. He referred to this ring of cortex at the margin of the hemisphere as the **limbic lobe** (from the Latin *limbus* meaning "border") and suggested that the entire lobe might be concerned with the sense of smell. However, the limbic lobe includes the cingulate and parahippocampal gyri and the hippocampus, and it soon became apparent that olfaction is not the primary responsibility of these areas. For example, although dolphins have no olfactory bulbs and are thought to be completely anosmatic, they nevertheless have well-developed hippocampi. A few cases have been reported of humans with congenital absence of the olfactory bulb and tracts but with apparently normal limbic lobes. Finally, subsequent anatomical and physiological experiments showed that, aside from the already mentioned olfactory areas at the base of the brain, the limbic lobe does not receive a particularly large amount of olfactory input.

The limbic lobe does, however, fit many of the previously described criteria for an anatomical substrate for drive-related and emotional behavior. As is shown in the remainder of this chapter, the limbic cortex is connected in one direction with widespread neocortical areas and in another direction with the hypothalamus. Physiological evidence has supported this view, and the conglomerate of the limbic lobe, its connections, and a few additional structures has come to be referred to as the **limbic system.** There is, unfortunately, no universal agreement on

---

★"One of my own most striking memories is of huge, fat, and extremely hostile cats with ventromedial hypothalamic lesions. When they observed laboratory visitors through the bars, thankfully strong bars, of their cages, they appeared to have a singular interest in attack. They gave every sign of dedication to the goal of destroying the visitor. Their great size made the threat something not to be taken lightly." (From Isaacson RL: *The limbic system*, New York, 1974, Plenum Press, p. 85)

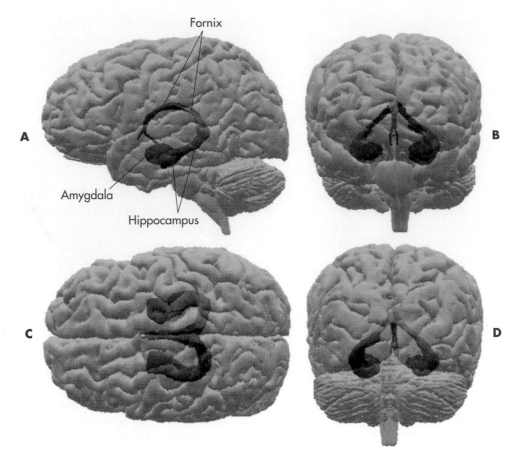

Fornix

Amygdala

Hippocampus

A

B

C

D

FIGURE 23-10
Three-dimensional reconstruction of the hippocampus, fornix, and amygdala inside a translucent CNS, seen from the left (**A**), front (**B**), above (**C**), and behind (**D**).

the total list of structures that should be included in the term "limbic system," but the concept should be clear by the end of this chapter. All authors would include the cingulate and parahippocampal gyri,* the hippocampus, the amygdala, and the sepal nuclei; most would include the hypothalamus, parts of the midbrain reticular formation, and the olfactory areas. Beyond that, the boundaries get fuzzy; some authors include various of the thalamic and neocortical regions interconnected with undisputed limbic components, whereas others do not.

The Hippocampus and Amygdala Are the Central Components of the Two Major Limbic Subsystems

The interconnections of limbic components are numerous and complex, but the overall concept of the system is not. The output end (in terms of programming or triggering behavioral outputs) is a continuous core of neural tissue

*Parts of the cingulate and parahippocampal gyri are intermediate in structure between the archicortex and paleocortex on the one hand and the neocortex on the other; they are therefore sometimes referred to as **mesocortex** or **juxtallocortex**.

extending from the septal area through the hypothalamus and into the midbrain reticular formation. The medial forebrain bundle is its principal longitudinal fiber pathway.* Two major limbic subsystems feed into this common output (Figure 23-10). The first (Figure 23-11, *A*) is centered around the hippocampus, utilizes the cingulate and parahippocampal gyri as its liaison with the neocortex gen-

*Activation of these output structures is also apparently responsible for triggering some of the feelings that are one object of drive-related behavior. Animals with electrodes implanted in certain CNS locations, if given control of the button that turns on stimulation through these electrodes, will push the button with great zest. Electrode locations that elicit self-stimulation are widespread in the limbic system, but the most effective sites are in the septal area and along the medial forebrain bundle; animals with electrodes there will stimulate themselves at great rates for long periods and may be willing to forego food or sleep or to endure painful stimuli to press the button. Sites with the opposite effect (i.e., sites at which animals will try hard to avoid being stimulated) are fewer and are principally located in the vicinity of the periaqueductal gray matter of the midbrain. These results have been generally confirmed for humans. Direct stimulation of the septal area, as an experimental treatment for certain psychiatric disorders, often yields a feeling of well-being, which is diffuse and hard to define but definitely pleasant. Stimulation near the periaqueductal gray matter sometimes causes unbearable feelings of horror and pain—an indication of the complexity of this region, as stimulation at very nearby sites can cause analgesia (see Chapter 11).

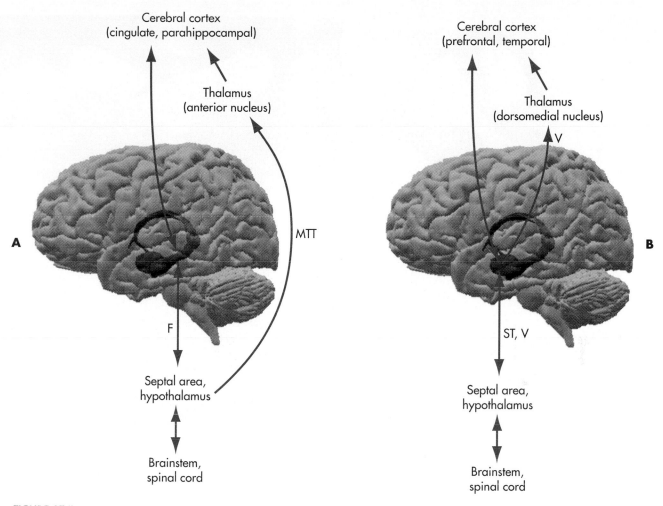

FIGURE 23-11
Schematic outline of hippocampal **(A)** and amygdalar **(B)** participation in the limbic system. The hippocampus is interposed between neocortex generally (through connections with the cingulate and parahippocampal gyri) and the septal-hypothalamic output core of the limbic system. Because the anterior thalamic nucleus is closely related to the cingulate gyrus, it plays a prominent role in hippocampal circuits, as does the mammillary body. The major fiber bundles interconnecting some of these structures are indicated by abbreviations. The fornix *(F)* is the major output pathway from the hippocampus but carries some afferents as well. The mammillary bodies (part of the hypothalamus) project to the anterior thalamic nucleus through the mammillothalamic tract *(MTT)*. The amygdala is interposed between neocortex generally (partly through connections with orbital and other prefrontal cortex, partly through widespread direct connections) and the septal-hypothalamic output core of the limbic system. Because the dorsomedial thalamic nucleus is closely related to the prefrontal cortex, this nucleus plays a prominent role in circuits formed by the amygdala. Some fibers passing to and from the amygdala travel in the stria terminalis *(ST)*. Others take a more diffuse ventral course *(V)*, passing underneath the lenticular nucleus (Figure 23-13)

erally, and has a close relationship with the anterior thalamic nucleus and the mammillary body. The second (Figure 23-11, *B*) is centered around the amygdala, utilizes prefrontal (especially orbital) and anterior temporal cortex as its liaison with the neocortex generally, and has a close relationship with the dorsomedial nucleus of the thalamus.

The Hippocampus Is a Cortical Structure That Borders the Inferior Horn of the Lateral Ventricle

Paleocortex and archicortex occupy most of the surface of each cerebral hemisphere in lower vertebrates. As the area devoted to neocortex expands through phylogeny, archicortex moves dorsally and then rolls around onto the

medial surface of the hemisphere, whereas the paleocortex moves ventrally onto the base of the brain (see Figure 2-12). With the continued expansion of the hemisphere in primates, the hippocampus becomes one more structure that is carried around in a great arc—in this case ending up in the temporal lobe as the floor of the inferior horn of the lateral ventricle (Figure 23-12). Traces of its heritage are revealed by a thin strand of rudimentary gray matter (the **hippocampal rudiment** or **indusium griseum**), continuous with the hippocampus, which is left behind on the dorsal surface of the corpus callosum and by the long, curved course of the fornix, the most prominent hippocampal output pathway (Figure 23-13).

The hippocampus is a curved and recurved sheet of cortex folded into the medial surface of the temporal lobe.

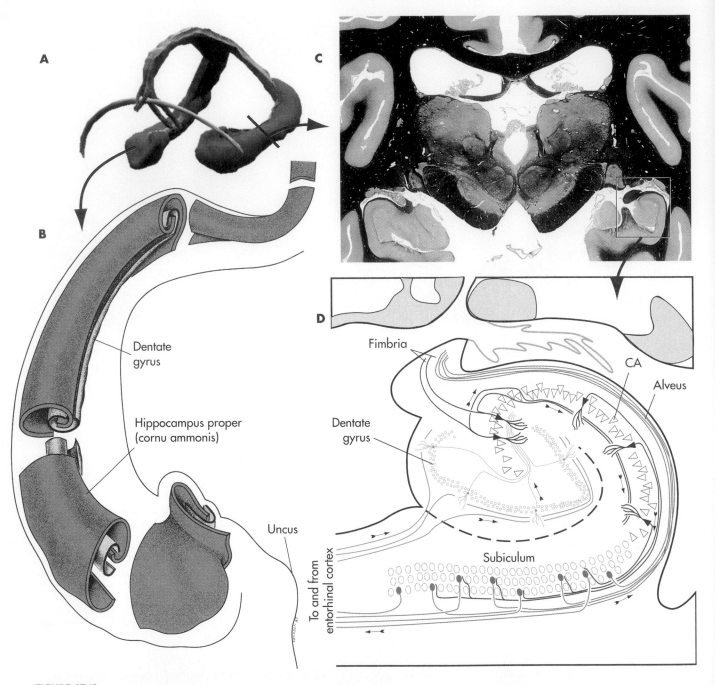

A

B

C

D

Dentate
gyrus

Hippocampus proper
(cornu ammonis)

Uncus

To and from
entorhinal cortex

Fimbria

Dentate
gyrus

CA

Alveus

Subiculum

FIGURE 23-12
Structure of the hippocampus. **A,** Three-dimensional reconstruction of the hippocampi and fornix. **B,** Arrangement of the dentate gyrus and hippocampus proper (cornu ammonis) as two interlocking C-shaped (in cross section) cortical structures. **C,** Coronal section through the dentate gyrus, hippocampus proper, and subiculum. **D,** Schematic diagram showing the general arrangements of cells and fibers in the hippocampus. A few hippocampal efferents arise from pyramidal cells of the hippocampus proper *(CA),* but most, as indicated, arise from the subiculum. Note that the major route of information flow through the hippocampal formation is a one-way circuit, starting with inputs from entorhinal cortex and then passing successively through the dentate gyrus, two sectors of hippocampal pyramidal cells, and the subiculum. Finally, subicular neurons project either through the fornix or directly back to cerebral cortex. (**B** modified from Duvernoy HM: *The human hippocampus: an atlas of applied anatomy,* Munich, 1988, JF Bergmann Verlag. **C** modified from Nolte J, Angevine JB Jr: *The human brain in photographs and diagrams,* St. Louis, 1995, Mosby.)

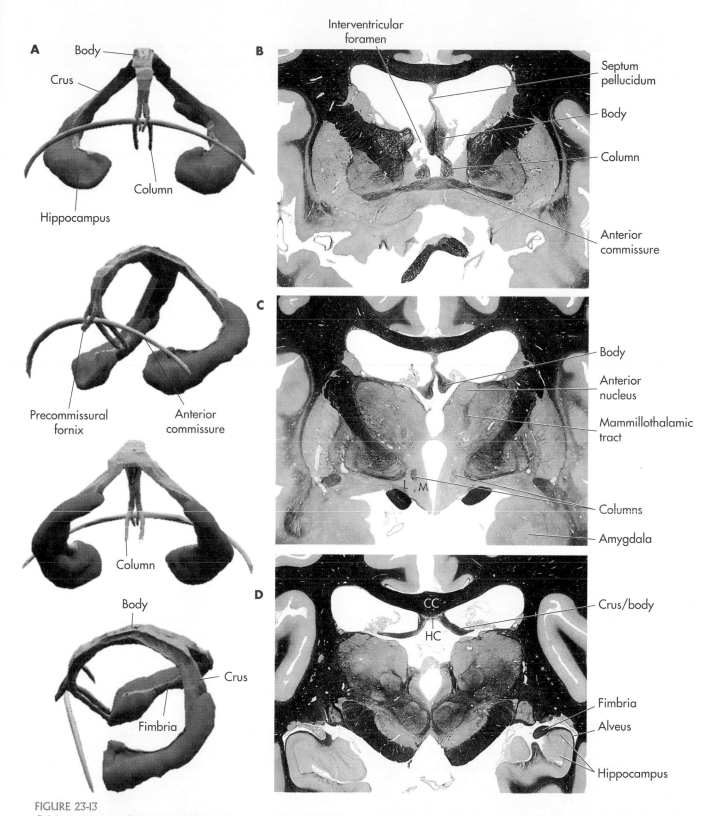

FIGURE 23-13

Origin and course of the fornix. This bundle, mostly efferent fibers from the hippocampus, begins as fibers that collect on the ventricular surface of the hippocampus proper as the alveus. The fibers move medially to form the fimbria of the hippocampus and then part company with the hippocampus near the splenium to become the crus of the fornix. The two crura converge on the midline, forming the body of the fornix; as they do so, a few fibers are exchanged between the two crura in the hippocampal commissure *(HC)*. The body of the fornix diverges again near the anterior commissure and interventricular foramen into the columns of the fornix. Most of these fibers continue on through the hypothalamus as the **postcommissural fornix**, ending primarily in the mammillary bodies. Some, however, split off in front of the anterior commissure as the **precommissural fornix**, ending primarily in the septal nuclei and ventral striatum. **A** shows three-dimensional reconstructions of this course. **B, C,** and **D** are coronal sections at the levels of the anterior commissure, anterior thalamus, and posterior thalamus. *CC,* Corpus callosum; *L, M,* lateral and medial zones of the tuberal hypothalamus. (**B-D** modified from Nolte J, Angevine JB Jr: *The human brain in photographs and diagrams,* St. Louis, 1995, Mosby.)

Transverse sections (Figure 23-12) reveal that it has three distinct zones: the **dentate gyrus,** the **hippocampus proper,**★ and the **subiculum.** In such sections, the dentate gyrus and the hippocampus proper have the form of two interlocking Cs. The subiculum is a transitional zone continuous with the hippocampus proper at one of its edges and the cortex of the parahippocampal gyrus at the other edge. The entire hippocampus has a length of about 5 cm in the inferior horn from its anterior end at the amygdala to its tapering posterior end near the splenium of the corpus callosum. Along this course numerous small blood vessels enter the hippocampus from the adjacent subarachnoid space by penetrating the dentate gyrus, thus giving this gyrus the beaded or toothed appearance for which it was named.

The fornix is a prominent output pathway from the hippocampus

The hippocampus and the dentate gyrus are three-layered, with a superficial **molecular layer** and a deep **polymorphic layer,** both similar to the layers of the same name in the neocortex. The intermediate stratum is a **granule cell layer** in the dentate gyrus and a **pyramidal cell layer** in the hippocampus proper. The molecular layer of the hippocampus proper faces the dentate gyrus, and the hippocampal equivalent of subcortical white matter is a layer of fibers called the **alveus** that lies just beneath the ependymal lining of the ventricle (Figure 23-12). The molecular layer of the dentate gyrus faces the subarachnoid space, and its output fibers, which do not leave the hippocampus, project directly into the hippocampus proper. The subiculum, as mentioned previously, is the zone of transition from the hippocampus proper to the parahippocampal gyrus and changes gradually from three-layered to six-layered cortex.

The alveus contains both afferents to and efferents from the hippocampus (primarily the latter). These fibers collect into a bundle called the **fimbria** (Latin for "fringe") **of the hippocampus** at the edge of the choroid fissure (Figure 23-12). When the hippocampus ends near the splenium of the corpus callosum, the fimbria becomes a detached bundle called the **crus** ("leg") **of the fornix.** The two crura converge and join in the midline to form the **body of the fornix,** which travels forward at the inferior edge of the septum pellucidum (Figure 23-13). At the interventricular foramen, the fornix turns inferiorly

and posteriorly, diverging into the **columns of the fornix,** which then pass through the middle of the hypothalamus toward the mammillary bodies (Figures 23-4 and 23-13, *C*).

The connections of the hippocampus have been mapped in ruthless detail and in three dimensions. Proceeding around its **C** shape (as seen in transverse sections), the hippocampus proper has been divided into several zones,★ all of whose connections differ somewhat from one another and from those of the subiculum and dentate gyrus. Along the course of the hippocampus through the temporal lobe, its connections change. Finally, afferents from different sources end at different levels on the apical dendrites of hippocampal pyramidal cells. The high degree of order has made the hippocampus very attractive for anatomical and physiological research, particularly in studies of neural plasticity and regeneration. However, to keep matters manageable the following account treats the hippocampus, by and large, as a uniform structure.

Entorhinal cortex is the principal source of inputs to the hippocampus

By far the most prominent source of afferents to the hippocampus is the adjacent entorhinal cortex (Figure 23-14). If the entorhinal cortex received only olfactory inputs, this would not be very impressive, but it also receives projections from the cingulate gyrus (via the cingulum), from the orbital cortex (via the uncinate fasciculus), and from the amygdala and other areas of the temporal lobe. Through these additional connections the hippocampus has access to virtually all types of sensory information. In addition, some septal and hypothalamic fibers reach the hippocampus through the fornix. Finally, a few fibers arrive from the contralateral hippocampus by passing from one crus of the fornix to the other beneath the splenium of the corpus callosum in the **hippocampal commissure** (Figure 23-13, *D*), a small commissure near the site where the two crura join to form the body of the fornix.

Hippocampal outputs reach entorhinal cortex, the mammillary body, and the septal area

Hippocampal output arises mainly in the subiculum, with some contribution from the hippocampus proper. Many fibers project directly back to the entorhinal cortex and also to other cortical areas, but the most anatomically prominent output pathway is the fornix (Figure 23-15). Fornix fibers arch forward under the corpus callosum

---

★Also called **Ammon's horn** (or **cornu ammonis,** after an Egyptian deity with ram's horns) because of the way the hippocampi curve downward and outward from the hippocampal rudiment into the temporal lobes. Hippocampal nomenclature has a long, colorful, and not entirely logical history, as discussed by F.T. Lewis in "The significance of the term hippocampus" (*J Comp Neurol* 35:213, 1923-1924). In this book I use the terms "hippocampus" and "hippocampal formation" interchangeably to refer to the combination of dentate gyrus, hippocampus proper, and subiculum.

★These zones, each a narrow longitudinal strip of the hippocampus proper, are commonly referred to as **CA fields** (derived from CA as an abbreviation for cornu ammonis). Hence neurons of the dentate gyrus project primarily to CA3 pyramidal cells, whose axon collaterals project to CA2 and CA1 pyramidal cells. CA1 in turn projects to the subiculum, where most of the output from the hippocampus arises (Figure 23-12).

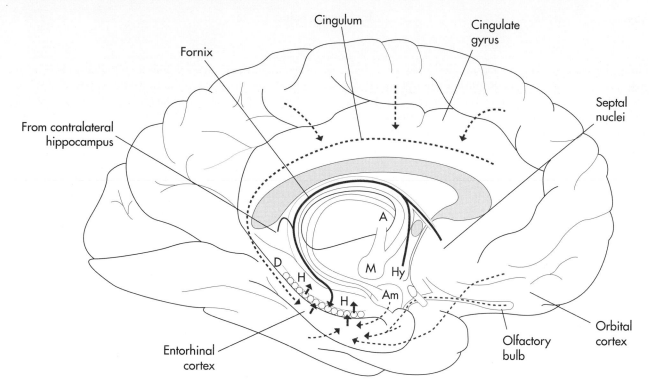

FIGURE 23-14

Afferents to the hippocampus *(H)*. The major source is the entorhinal cortex, which in turn collects inputs from cingulate, temporal, and orbital cortices and from the amygdala *(Am)* and olfactory cortex. Other hippocampal inputs arrive from the septal nuclei and hypothalamus *(Hy)* and from the contralateral hippocampal formation, all via the fornix. Indirect inputs are indicated by dashed pathways. This is a simplified diagram, and other connections, such as inputs from the locus ceruleus and direct inputs from the amygdala, are not indicated. *A*, Anterior thalamic nucleus; *D*, dentate gyrus; *M*, mammillary body. (The drawing of the brain in this and similar figures in this chapter was adapted from an illustration in Warwick R, Williams PL: *Gray's anatomy*, Br ed 35, Philadelphia, 1973, WB Saunders.)

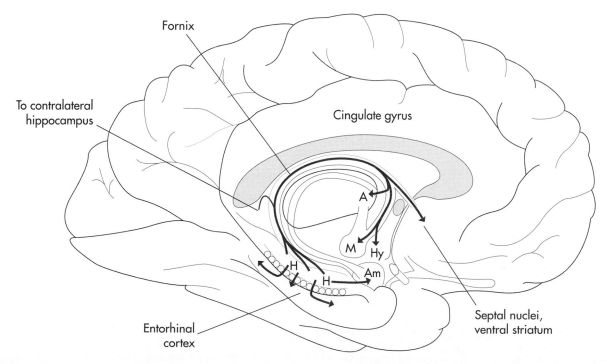

FIGURE 23-15

Efferents from the hippocampus *(H)*. One major efferent pathway is the fornix, through which fibers reach an assortment of anteriorly situated forebrain structures. In addition, many fibers pass directly from the subiculum to the entorhinal cortex, to the amygdala *(Am)*, or backward along the cingulum to the cingulate gyrus. Some fibers of the precommissural fornix spread beyond the septal nuclei and ventral striatum and reach orbital and anterior cingulate cortices. *A*, Anterior thalamic nucleus; *Hy*, nonmammillary regions of the hypothalamus; *M*, mammillary body.

along the path depicted in Figure 23-13 (except for the few that cross in the hippocampal commissure). At the level of the interventricular foramen, some fibers split off in front of the anterior commissure as the **precommissural fornix** (Figure 23-13, *A*). Most of these end nearby in the septal and preoptic nuclei and ventral striatum, but some continue on to reach orbital and anterior cingulate cortex. The remaining fibers of the fornix (the **postcommissural fornix**) do one of two things; some turn sharply posteriorly and end in the anterior thalamic nucleus, whereas the rest travel through the hypothalamus in the column of the fornix and end mainly in the mammillary body (although some end in other hypothalamic areas or in the midbrain reticular formation). Because the mammillothalamic tract ends in the anterior nucleus, the hippocampus can influence this part of the thalamus both directly and indirectly.

The anterior thalamic nucleus projects to the cingulate gyrus, thus completing a great loop through the diencephalon and telencephalon (Figure 23-16). Beginning in the hippocampus, the pathway proceeds through the fornix to the mammillary body, from there in sequence to the anterior thalamic nucleus, the cingulate gyrus and part of the parahippocampal gyrus (the entorhinal cortex), and finally back to the hippocampus. James Papez pointed out in 1937 that this loop provided for interactions among the neocortex, limbic structures, and the hypothalamus and proposed that it might be the anatomical substrate of emotional experience. Though undoubtedly a great oversimplification (for one thing, hippocampal connections are considerably more complex than this loop would indicate), this idea provided the impetus for a great deal of research into the structure and function of the limbic system; the loop is still known as the **Papez circuit.**

The hippocampus and nearby cortical regions are critical for some forms of memory

A variety of changes in autonomic and endocrine function have been described as resulting from hippocampal stimulation or damage in experimental animals, consistent with the connections between the hippocampus and the septal nuclei and hypothalamus; a number of behavioral changes have been described as well. Despite this, however, the most prominent role ascribed to the hippocampus in humans has to do with learning and memory. Neurosurgeons discovered (by accident) in the early 1950s that after bilateral removal of the medial parts of the temporal lobe* (or after unilateral removal from patients with preexisting damage on the other side), humans have a striking memory deficit. After such surgery, patients are unable to

*Even though the hippocampus underlies cortical areas usually described as parts of the limbic lobe, this area is also commonly referred to as the *medial temporal lobe* because of its continuity with the temporal lobe of gross anatomy.

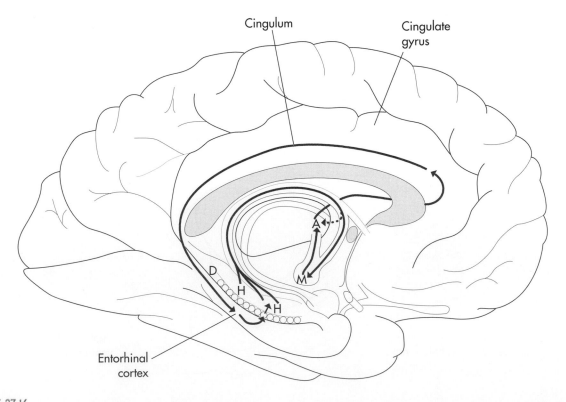

FIGURE 23-16
The Papez circuit. The shortcut from the hippocampus directly to the anterior thalamic nucleus, not part of the circuit as originally proposed, is indicated by a dashed line. *A*, Anterior thalamic nucleus; *D*, dentate gyrus; *H*, hippocampus; *M*, mammillary body.

form new memories of facts and events. There is typically some retrograde amnesia for events that occurred before the surgery, but beyond some point in the past, early memories are intact. However, a new item such as a list of numbers or a dictated phrase disappears at the first distraction, although it can be retained for a little while if the patient has nothing else to do but concentrate on that item. Intelligence is more or less undisturbed, but nevertheless, this is an enormously debilitating problem. Imagine being perpetually unable to remember new acquaintances; unable to keep track of events in the lives of relatives and old friends; unable to complete simple tasks because of the inability to remember why they were begun; unable to read a story because there is no memory of sentences preceding the current one.

Interestingly, the amnesia that occurs after bilateral hippocampal damage applies only to specific facts and events and not to the learning of new skills and procedures. Such a patient could, for example, learn in repeated attempts how to assemble a jigsaw puzzle more and more skillfully, at the same rate as a normal individual, despite never remembering having seen the puzzle before. Although we tend to think of memory as a unitary function and to associate it with remembering facts and events, there are in fact multiple kinds of memory, each depending on different sets of CNS structures (Figure 23-17). Memory of events and facts—remembering what you had for dinner last night or remembering that Yankee Stadium is in the Bronx—is called **declarative** memory, meaning that these items are accessible to consciousness and can be declared as facts. Memory of skills and procedures—how to play

handball or pinochle—is called **procedural** memory. Just as we normally combine the activities of multiple eye-movement control systems in real-life situations, so do we combine different kinds of memory in most learning tasks. The knowledge of how to get to school or work, for example, is a mixture of learned habits and procedures and remembered facts.

Because the hippocampus is a major part of the medial temporal lobe and a memory deficit occurs in cases in which little appears to be damaged other than the two hippocampi, the function of laying down or consolidating new memories has been attributed to this portion of the limbic system. (Memories themselves must reside elsewhere in the CNS—presumably as distributed sets of neocortical connections—because old memories can still be retrieved after medial temporal damage.)

Damage to the mammillary bodies (which occurs in the course of widespread damage to the periaqueductal and periventricular gray matter as a result of chronic alcoholism) is correlated with a similar memory deficit. The condition is called **Korsakoff's psychosis.** Patients so afflicted may have relatively intact intelligence but an inability to form new memories. They typically make up answers as they go along, concealing to some extent the memory loss (hence a wonderful alternate name for Korsakoff's psychosis: the **amnestic confabulatory syndrome**). This led to the appealing notion that the entire Papez circuit is involved in learning and memory. Unfortunately, things are rarely as simple as they seem, and acceptance of the hippocampal role in memory has developed slowly. For example, bilateral destruction of the

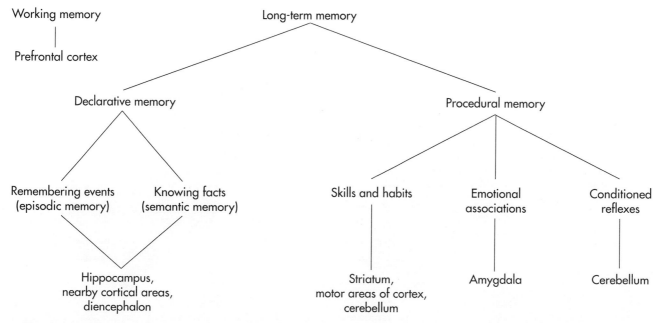

FIGURE 23-17
Different types of learning and memory and their probable anatomical correlates. Other types of memory have been described, and there is no universally accepted nomenclature. In addition, some of the anatomical correlates are speculative (e.g., the relative roles of the striatum, neocortex, and cerebellum in the learning of skills and habits are not known).

cingulum causes no particular memory loss,* and destruction of the fornix does not cause a memory deficit comparable in magnitude to that seen after medial temporal damage. In addition, there have been cases in which reported destruction of the mammillary bodies was not accompanied by memory loss. Some investigators claim that the only common factor in all cases of Korsakoff's psychosis is bilateral damage to the medial thalamus (i.e., the dorsomedial nuclei). Finally, it seemed for a long time that careful, selective damage to the hippocampi of experimental animals paradoxically did not produce the same severe memory deficit found in humans.

Explanations for these apparent discrepancies have come from the realization that there are multiple kinds of memory systems working in parallel with each other (Figure 23-17), and from increased knowledge of hippocampal anatomy. As mentioned previously, humans with amnesia can still learn new motor skills, indicating that this form of learning does not require an intact hippocampus. In general, it now appears that some varieties of learning and memory, such as pattern recognition, habits, conditioned autonomic reactions to stimuli, and motor skills (i.e., memories not built around the conscious recall of specific items) do not depend on the hippocampus. Rather, the hippocampus and nearby cortical areas (such as entorhinal cortex) play a crucial role, one that slowly di-

minishes over months or even years, in consolidating explicit memories of facts and events. Because the hippocampus has substantial outputs that do not travel through the fornix (Figure 23-15), damage to the fornix does not cause a major impairment of memory. Similarly, damage restricted to the hippocampus and sparing entorhinal and nearby cortices causes only partial amnesia. The critical structure whose damage causes Korsakoff's psychosis has still not been determined with certainty.

The Amygdala Is Centrally Involved in Emotional Responses

The amygdala is a collection of nuclei lying beneath the uncus of the temporal lobe at the anterior end of the hippocampus and the inferior horn of the lateral ventricle (Figure 23-18). It merges with the periamygdaloid cortex, which forms part of the surface of the uncus. The amygdala also abuts the putamen and the tail of the caudate nucleus as the latter ends in the temporal lobe (Figures 23-18, *B* and 23-21, *D*) and was considered at one time to be one of the basal ganglia, which by definition comprised all subcortical gray masses of the telencephalon. The amygdala does have some connections with the striatum (Figure 23-22), but the overall pattern of its connections is typical of the limbic system.

The amygdala receives a wide variety of sensory inputs

The amygdala receives a great deal of sensory input in a highly processed form. Single amygdalar cells may be se-

---

*Interestingly, bilateral section of the cingulum causes emotional changes similar to those seen after prefrontal leukotomy, a type of change that might be expected after damage to the limbic system. This operation has been used on an experimental basis as a treatment for intractable pain and for certain psychiatric disorders.

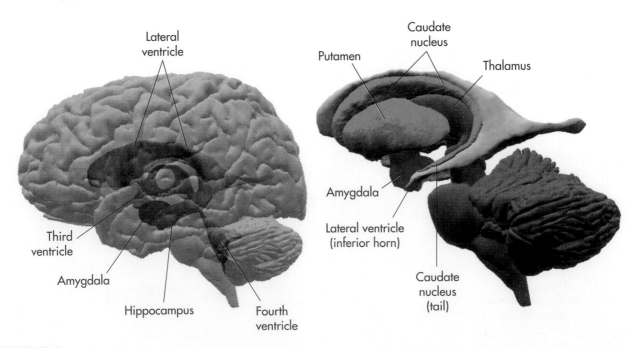

FIGURE 23-18
Three-dimensional reconstructions showing the spatial relationships between the amygdala, hippocampus, putamen, and caudate nucleus. (Modified from Nolte J, Angevine JB Jr: *The human brain in photographs and diagrams*, St. Louis, 1995, Mosby.)

lective or may respond to various combinations of many different sensory modalities, including somatosensory, visual, auditory, and all types of visceral inputs. The afferents carrying this information arise in several locations (Figure 23-19) and reach the amygdala by traveling in the reverse direction along the paths followed by amygdalar efferents (described in the next section).

Visceral inputs, particularly olfactory inputs, are especially prominent. Some olfactory tract fibers end in part of the amygdala, and this part in turn projects to the rest of the amygdala; olfactory inputs also arise in the piriform cortex. Additional visceral information reaches the amygdala indirectly from the hypothalamus, septal area, and orbital and insular cortex, and also by more direct routes; for example, the parabrachial nucleus projects to the amygdala, and it seems likely that the same may be true of other visceral nuclei in the brainstem. The temporal and anterior cingulate cortices also project to the amygdala and are probably responsible for most of the auditory, visual, and somatosensory information that reaches this structure.

The amygdala projects to the cerebral cortex and hypothalamus

Fibers leave the amygdala through two major pathways to reach many of the same areas that send afferents to it (Figure 23-20). The first pathway is the **stria terminalis,** which arches around from the temporal lobe toward the interventricular foramen in company with the caudate nucleus and the thalamostriate (or terminal) vein. In the body of the lateral ventricle, the stria terminalis lies in the groove between the caudate nucleus and the thalamus (Figure 23-21). Fibers of the stria terminalis distribute mainly to the septal nuclei and the hypothalamus.

The second efferent route goes by the awkward name of the **ventral amygdalofugal pathway** (particularly awkward as it also contains many afferents to the amygdala). These fibers pass underneath the lenticular nucleus (Figure 23-21) and spread out to blanket the base of the brain, ending in the septal nuclei and the hypothalamus, in olfactory regions such as the anterior olfactory nucleus, the anterior perforated substance, the piriform cortex, and in the orbital and anterior cingulate cortices. Some reach the **ventral striatum,** which includes the area of fusion of the putamen and the head of the caudate nucleus (the nucleus accumbens [see Figures 19-2 and 19-5]) as well as adjacent portions of the striatum. The ventral striatum in turn projects to an extension of the globus pallidus, the **ventral pallidum,** beneath the anterior commissure (Figure 23-22). The ventral striatum and pallidum are links in a basal ganglia circuit similar to that involved in motor functions. In this case, however, the inputs to the basal ganglia are from limbic structures such as the amygdala and hippocampus; the outputs relay in the dorsomedial

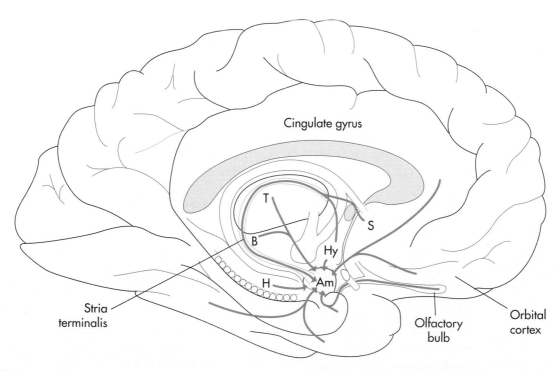

FIGURE 23-19

Afferents to the amygdala *(Am)*. These arrive via four routes: (1) from the hypothalamus *(Hy)* and septal nuclei *(S)* through the stria terminalis; (2) from the thalamus *(T)* and hypothalamus *(Hy)*, and from orbital and anterior cingulate cortex, through the ventral pathway; (3) from the olfactory bulb and olfactory cortex through the lateral olfactory stria; and (4) directly from temporal lobe structures such as neocortical areas and the hippocampus *(H)*. Additional inputs reach the amygdala from brainstem sites *(B)* such as the parabrachial nucleus.

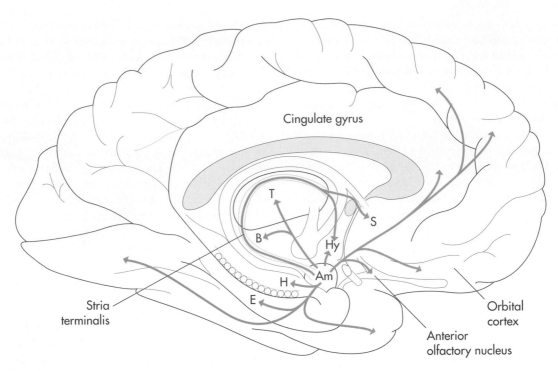

FIGURE 23-20
Efferents from the amygdala. These take three routes: (1) the stria terminalis, which reaches the septal nuclei *(S)* and hypothalamus *(Hy)*; (2) the ventral amygdalofugal pathway (Figure 23-21, *C*) to the hypothalamus *(Hy)*, thalamus *(T)*, widespread areas of frontal and insular cortex, olfactory structures, and various brainstem sites *(B)*; and (3) direct projections to the hippocampus *(H)*, entorhinal cortex *(E)*, and temporal and other neocortical areas.

nucleus of the thalamus rather than the VA/VL complex and influence prefrontal and orbital frontal cortex. This limbic connection with the basal ganglia is presumably a route through which drive-related information can influence decisions about movement, and apparently functions more generally in the neural circuitry that makes associations between stimuli and rewards (Figure 23-23). Many ventral amygdalofugal fibers turn dorsally in the diencephalon and reach the dorsomedial nucleus of the thalamus. Finally, some amygdalar efferents enter neither the stria terminalis nor the ventral pathway but rather pass directly to entorhinal cortex and other cortical areas in the temporal lobe and beyond.

The amygdala is involved in emotional learning

As complex as the connections of the amygdala appear, they are dominated by extensive interconnections with the septal area and hypothalamus on the one hand and with prefrontal cortex, both directly and indirectly (via the dorsomedial nucleus), on the other. This puts it in a position to influence both drive-related behavior patterns and the subjective feelings that accompany these activities. In the first of these two roles, the amygdala can be considered a sort of higher order modulating influence on the hypothalamus. Almost any visceral or somatic activity that can

be elicited by stimulating the hypothalamus (including such things as feeding or cardiovascular and respiratory changes) can also be elicited by stimulating some point in the amygdala. The responses to amygdalar stimulation tend to be more "natural" than those to hypothalamic stimulation, building up gradually and then decaying slowly at the end of the stimulus. Conversely, syndromes such as the aphagia or hyperphagia that follow selective lesions of parts of the hypothalamus can also be caused by amygdalar lesions, although in this case the syndromes are less severe.

The role of the amygdala in subjective feelings (presumably involving interactions with both the prefrontal cortex and the hypothalamus) has also been indicated in electrical studies. When an animal's amygdala is stimulated, it most often stops whatever it was doing and becomes very attentive. This may be followed by responses of defense, raging aggression, or fleeing. Amygdalar stimulation in humans can cause a variety of emotions, but the most common is fear accompanied by all its normal autonomic manifestations (for instance, dilation of the pupils, release of adrenalin, and increased heart rate). Conversely, bilateral destruction of the amygdala causes a great decrease in aggression, and as a result the animals are tame and placid. This is part of a different kind of memory deficit, one that impairs the ability to learn or remember the appropriate emotional and autonomic responses to stimuli. We all learn to have automatic sympathetic responses to danger-

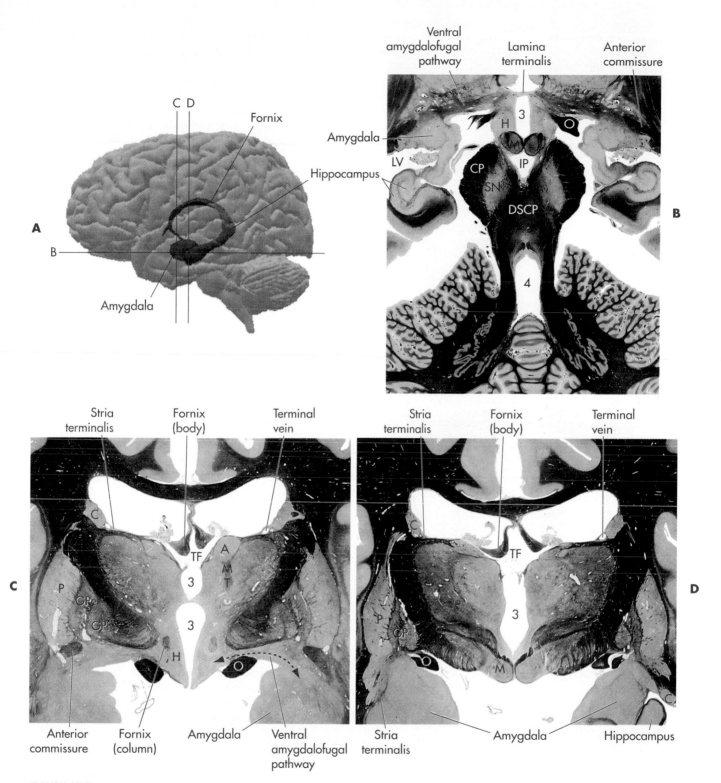

FIGURE 23-21

Location of the amygdala and related fiber bundles. **A,** Three-dimensional reconstruction with the planes of section shown in **B, C,** and **D** indicated. *3,* Third ventricle; *4,* fourth ventricle; *A,* anterior thalamic nucleus; *C,* caudate nucleus; *CP,* cerebral peduncle; *DSCP,* decussation of the superior cerebellar peduncles; *GP,* globus pallidus; *GPe,* globus pallidus (external segment); *GPi,* globus pallidus (internal segment); *H,* tuberal hypothalamus; *IP,* interpeduncular cistern; *LV,* lateral ventricle (inferior horn); *M,* mammillary body; *MT,* mammillothalamic tract; *O,* optic tract; *P,* putamen; *SN,* substantia nigra; *TF,* transverse fissure. [**B-D** modified from Nolte J, Angevine JB Jr: *The human brain in photographs and diagrams,* St. Louis, 1995, Mosby.]

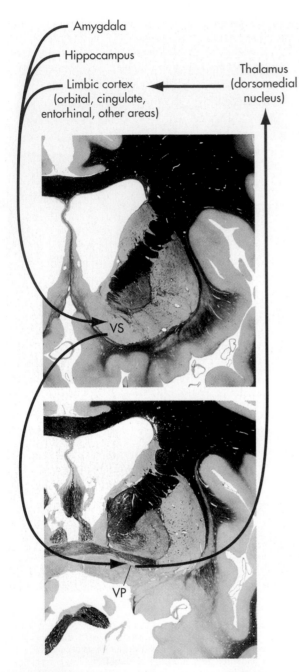

Amygdala

Hippocampus

Limbic cortex
(orbital, cingulate,
entorhinal, other areas)

Thalamus
(dorsomedial
nucleus)

VS

VP

FIGURE 23-22
Overview of the limbic loop through the basal ganglia. Only major connections are indicated, although others are known. For example, there are direct projections from the ventral striatum to the hypothalamus and amygdala. *VP*, Ventral pallidum; *VS*, ventral striatum.

Bilateral Temporal Lobe Damage Causes a Complex, Devastating Syndrome

The classic technique for studying the function of a structure is to remove it or destroy it and then see what happens. Removing the temporal lobe back to the level of the primary auditory cortex should certainly incapacitate the limbic system to a great extent because the amygdala and most of the hippocampus and parahippocampal gyrus would be lost. When this is done to animals bilaterally, a constellation of deficits results called the **Klüver-Bucy syndrome** for the investigators who first described it.

1. The animals are fearless and placid, showing an absence of emotional reactions. They do not respond to threats, to social gestures by other animals, or to objects they would normally flee from or attack.
2. Male animals become hypersexual and are impressively indiscriminate in their choice of sex partners. They are likely to mount other animals of the same sex, animals of whatever species may be available, or inanimate objects.
3. They show an inordinate degree of attention to all sensory stimuli, as though ceaselessly curious. They respond to every object within sight or reach by sniffing it and examining it orally. If the object can in any sense be considered edible, they eat it. Partly because of this, they eat much more than normal animals.
4. Although they incessantly examine all objects in sight, these animals recognize nothing and may pick up the same thing over and over. This was called "psychic blindness" by Klüver and Bucy and would now be called *visual agnosia*.

The Klüver-Bucy syndrome has been fractionated to some extent, and different parts of it can be attributed to the loss of different structures. Thus the placidity results from destruction of the amygdala, the hypersexuality from loss of the piriform cortex, and the visual agnosia from damage to visual association areas on the inferior surface of the temporal lobe. The composite syndrome is tremendously detrimental.* Leaving aside the visual agnosia, it is as though the animal still has intact all the behavior patterns central to satisfying basic drives but can no longer tell when and in what context to use them.

ous stimuli (here in the Southwest, for example, the sight of a scorpion or snake); amygdalar damage prevents the acquisition of these response patterns. In a simplified view, the hippocampus is involved in learning that an event happened or that something is a fact, and the amygdala is involved in learning whether to consider something "good" or "bad."

---

*"A monkey which approaches every enemy to examine it orally will conceivably not survive longer than a few hours if turned loose in a region with a plentiful supply of enemies. We doubt that a monkey would be seriously hampered under natural conditions, in the wild, by a loss of its prefrontal region, its parietal lobes or its occipital lobes, as long as small portions of the striate cortex remained intact." (Klüver H, Bucy PC: Preliminary analysis of functions of the temporal lobes in monkeys, *Arch Neurol Psychiatry* 42:979, 1939.)

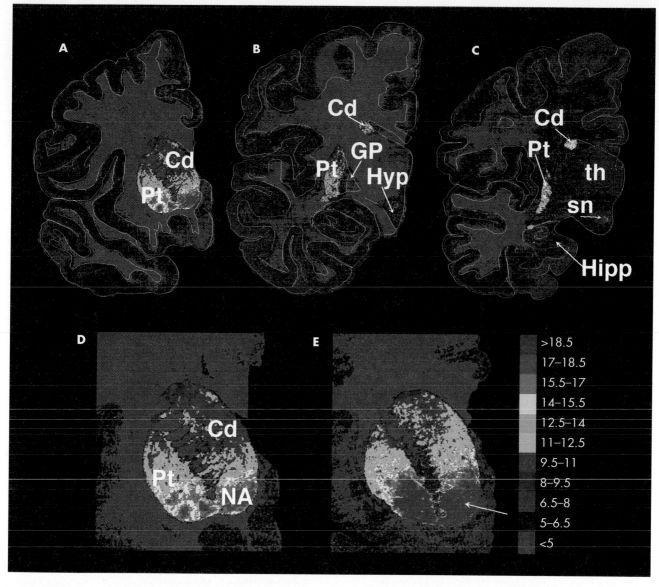

FIGURE 23-23

Mapping the distribution of a particular type of dopamine receptor (D$_3$ receptor) that has been implicated in reward circuitry, using a radioactive ligand. In coronal sections of normal brain (**A-D**) the receptor is preferentially localized in the ventral striatum, particularly nucleus accumbens *(NA)*. In the brain of a chronic cocaine user who died of a cocaine overdose (**E**), this preferential distribution is even more pronounced. The color bar at the lower right shows the color coding of receptor density, measured as radioligand binding (fmol/mg). (From Staley JK, Mash DC: Adaptive increase in D$_3$ dopamine receptors in the brain reward circuits of human cocaine fatalities, *J Neurosci* 16:6100, 1996.)

SUGGESTED READINGS

Adams JH, Daniel PM, Prichard MML: Observations on the portal circulation of the pituitary gland, *Neuroendocrinology* 1:193, 1965-66.

Aggleton JP, editor: *The amygdala: neurobiological aspects of emotion, memory, and mental dysfunction,* New York, 1992, Wiley-Liss.

Allen LS et al: Two sexually dimorphic cell groups in the human brain, *J Neurosci* 9:497, 1989. *Both are contained in the preoptic/anterior hypothalamus, a region known to be involved in the production of gonadotropin-releasing factor.*

Amaral DG, Insausti R: Hippocampal formation. In Paxinos G, editor: *The human nervous system,* San Diego, 1990, Academic Press.

Andy OJ, Stephan H: The septum in the human brain, *J Comp Neurol* 133:383, 1968. *There is a tendency to think of the septal area as small and rudimentary in humans, but this paper argues that in fact it reaches its highest development in us.*

Bandler R, Shipley MT: Columnar organization in the midbrain periaqueductal gray: modules for emotional expression? *Trends Neurosci* 17:379, 1994.

Bergland RM, Page RB: Pituitary-brain vascular relations: a new paradigm, *Sci* 204:18, 1979. *Results that indicate that the pituitary portal system may not be so straightforward; for example, it may at times function in reverse, transporting adenohypophyseal hormones to the brain.*

Blessing WW: *The lower brainstem and bodily homeostasis,* New York, 1997, Oxford University Press.

Braak H, Braak E: The hypothalamus of the human adult: chiasmatic region, *Anat Embryol* 175:315, 1987.

Buijs RM et al, editors: *Hypothalamic integration of circadian rhythms* (Prog Brain Res vol 111), Amsterdam, 1996, Elsevier.

Devinsky O, Morrell MJ, Vogt BA: Contributions of anterior cingulate cortex to behavior, *Brain* 118:279, 1995.

Dierickx K: Immunocytochemical localization of the vertebrate cyclic nonapeptide neurohypophyseal hormones and neurophysins, *Int Rev Cytol* 62:120, 1980.

Dietrichs E, Haines DE: Interconnections between hypothalamus and cerebellum, *Anat Embryol* 179:207, 1989.

Duggan JP, Booth DA: Obesity, overeating, and rapid gastric emptying in rats with ventromedial hypothalamic lesions, *Science* 231:609, 1986. *A satisfyingly simple partial explanation for why rats with ventromedial hypothalamic lesions eat too much. These authors propose that autonomic regulation of stomach emptying is disturbed, that the stomach empties too quickly, and that the rat doesn't feel full for long. Consequently it eats again sooner than a normal rat.*

Duvernoy HM: *The human hippocampus: functional anatomy, vascularization and serial sections with MRI,* ed 2, Berlin, 1998, Springer-Verlag. *A meticulously detailed and beautifully illustrated book.*

Gaffan D, Murray EA: Amygdalar interaction with the mediodorsal nucleus of the thalamus and the ventromedial prefrontal cortex in stimulus-reward associative learning in the monkey, *J Neurosci* 10:3479, 1990.

Guillemin R: Peptides in the brain: the new endocrinology of the neuron, *Science* 202:390, 1978.

Hardy JD, Hellon RF, Sutherland K: Temperature-sensitive neurones in the dog's hypothalamus, *J Physiol* 175:242, 1964.

Hayward JN: Functional and morphological aspects of hypothalamic neurons, *Physiol Rev* 57:574, 1977.

Heller HC, Crawshaw LI, Hammel HT: The thermostat of vertebrate animals, *Sci Am* 239(2):102, 1978.

Holmes EJ et al: Ablations of the mammillary nuclei in monkeys: effects on postoperative memory, *Exp Neurol* 81:97, 1983.

Holstege G, Bandler R, Saper CB, editors: *The emotional motor system* (Prog Brain Res vol 107), Amsterdam, 1996, Elsevier.

Isaacson RL: *The limbic system,* ed 2, New York, 1982, Plenum Press.

Johnston D, Amaral DG: Hippocampus. In Shepherd GM, editor: *The synaptic organization of the brain,* ed 4, New York, 1998, Oxford University Press.

Kaada BR: Stimulation and regional ablation of the amygdaloid complex with reference to functional representations. In Eleftheriou BE, editor: *The neurobiology of the amygdala,* New York, 1972, Plenum Press.

Katter JT, Burstein R, Giesler GJ Jr: The cells of origin of the spinohypothalamic tract in cats, *J Comp Neurol* 303:101, 1991.

Klüver H, Bucy PC: Preliminary analysis of functions of the temporal lobes in monkeys, *Arch Neurol Psychiatry* 42:979, 1939. *Still interesting reading.*

Knowlton BJ, Mangels JA, Squire LR: A neostriatal learning system in humans, *Science* 273:1399, 1996.

LeDoux JE, Romanski L, Xagoraris A: Indelibility of subcortical emotional memories, *J Cog Neurosci* 1:238, 1989. *Recent work on the role of the amygdala in learning the emotional significance of stimuli.*

Levin BE, Routh VH: Role of the brain in energy balance and obesity, *Am J Physiol* 271:R491, 1996.

Lewis FT: The significance of the term hippocampus, *J Comp Neurol* 35:213, 1923-24. *A caustic but interesting paper concerning "the flight of fancy which led Arantius, in 1587, to introduce the term 'hippocampus'...recorded in what is perhaps the worst anatomical description extant. It has left its readers in doubt whether the elevations of cerebral substance were being compared with fish or beast, and no one could be sure which end was the head."*

Lilly R et al: The human Klüver-Bucy syndrome, *Neurol* 33:1141, 1983.

Loewy AD, Spyer KM: *Central regulation of autonomic function,* New York, 1990, Oxford University Press.

Machne X, Segundo JP: Unitary responses to afferent volleys in amygdaloid complex, *J Neurophysiol* 19:232, 1956. *Single cells that respond equally well to a brief shock to the sciatic nerve and to a whiff of something.*

Malamud N: Psychiatric disorder with intracranial tumors of limbic system, *Arch Neurol* 17:113, 1967.

Morgane PJ, Panksepp J: *Handbook of the hypothalamus, vol 1, Anatomy of the hypothalamus,* New York, 1979, Marcel Dekker.

Mosko SS, Moore RY: Neonatal suprachiasmatic nucleus lesions: effects on the development of circadian rhythms in the rat, *Brain Res* 164:17, 1979.

Nathan PW, Smith MC: The location of descending fibres to sympathetic neurons supplying the eye and sudomotor neurons supplying the head and neck, *J Neurol Neurosurg Psychiatry* 49:187, 1986.

Papez JW: A proposed mechanism of emotion, *Arch Neurol Psychiatry* 38:725, 1937. *The evidence wasn't very strong by today's standards, but the idea has been extremely influential anyway.*

Penfield W, Mathieson G: Memory: autopsy findings and comments on the role of hippocampus in experiential recall, *Arch Neurol* 31:145, 1974. *The hippocampus-memory story in a well-written account by one of the neurosurgeons who made the unfortunate discovery.*

Raisman G, Brown-Grant K: The "suprachiasmatic syndrome": endocrine and behavioural abnormalities following lesions of the suprachiasmatic nucleus in the female rat, *Proc R Soc Lond* B198:297, 1977.

Reeves AG, Plum F: Hyperphagia, rage, and dementia accompanying a ventromedial hypothalamic neoplasm, *Arch Neurol* 20:616, 1969.

Reiman EM et al: Neuroanatomical correlates of anticipatory anxiety, *Science* 243:1071, 1989. *PET scanning studies implicating the anterior ends of the temporal lobes in the neural circuitry underlying feelings of fear and anxiety.*

Rosene DL, van Hoesen GW: Hippocampal efferents reach widespread areas of cerebral cortex and amygdala in the rhesus monkey, *Science* 198:315, 1977.

Salloway S, Malloy P, Cummings JL, editors: *The neuropsychiatry of limbic and subcortical disorders,* Washington, 1997, American Psychiatric Press, Inc.

Schwartz J-C et al: Histaminergic transmission in the mammalian brain, *Physiol Rev* 71:1, 1991.

Schwartz WJ: Understanding circadian clocks: from c-Fos to fly balls, *Ann Neurol* 41:289, 1997.

Sims KS, Williams RS: The human amygdaloid complex: a cytologic and histochemical atlas using Nissl, myelin, acetylcholinesterase and nicotinamide adenine dinucleotide phosphate diaphorase staining, *Neurosci* 36:449, 1990.

Solodkin A, Van Hoesen GW: Entorhinal cortex modules of the human brain, *J Comp Neurol* 365:610, 1996.

Swaab DF et al: Functional neuroanatomy and neuropathology of the human hypothalamus, *Anat Embryol* 187:317, 1993.

Swanson LW, Cowan WM: Hippocampo-hypothalamic connections: origin in subicular cortex, not Ammon's horn, *Science* 189:303, 1975.

Swanson LW, Sawchenko PE: Hypothalamic integration: organization of the paraventricular and supraoptic nuclei, *Ann Rev Neurosci* 6:269, 1983.

Victor M, Adams RD, Collins GH: *The Wernicke-Korsakoff syndrome: a clinical and pathological study of 245 patients, 82 with post-mortem examination*, Philadelphia, 1971, FA Davis Co.

Wasman M, Flynn JP: Directed attack elicited from hypothalamus, *Arch Neurol* 6:220, 1962.

Willingham DB: Systems of memory in the human brain, *Neuron* 18:5, 1997.

Young JK, Stanton GB: A three-dimensional reconstruction of the human hypothalamus, *Brain Res Bull* 35:323, 1994.

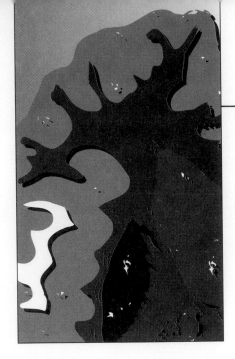

ATLAS OF THE HUMAN FOREBRAIN*

When the nervous system is discussed in terms of functional subsystems, as in the preceding chapters, it is sometimes difficult to envision how the various parts are related to the whole. Therefore an abbreviated atlas is provided here in the same philosophy as that in Chapter 15, with a wide variety of forebrain structures and a few brainstem structures labeled.

Only major structures that were mentioned prominently in this book are indicated. In addition, to keep the number of labels manageable, cerebral sulci and gyri were in general left unlabeled, and a number of structures that appear repeatedly were not labeled every time they appeared. Very abbreviated descriptions of labeled structures are provided; additional details can be found elsewhere in the text.

*All figures except 24–2 and 24–10 were modified from Nolte J, Angevine JB Jr: *The human brain in photographs and diagrams,* St. Louis, 1995, Mosby.

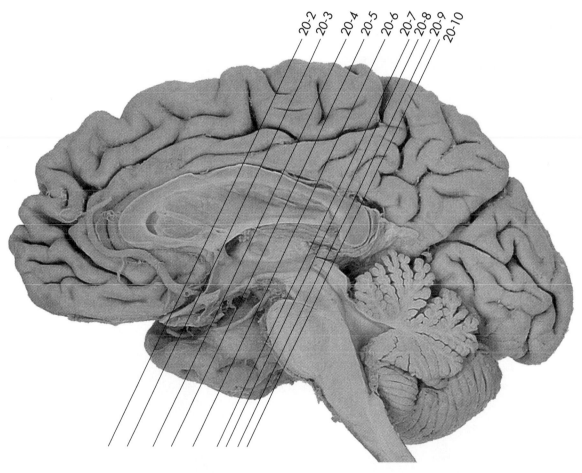

FIGURE 24-1
Planes of the sections shown in Figures 24-2 to 24-10.

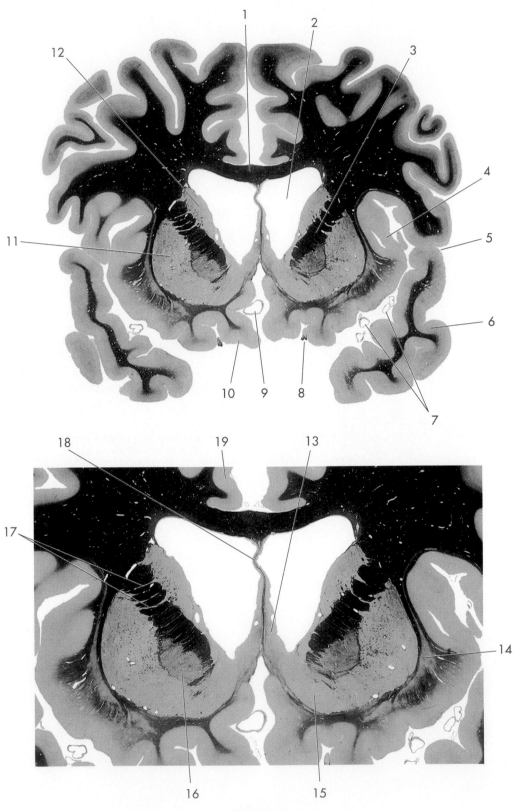

FIGURE 24-2

FIGURE 24-2

Anterior horn of the lateral ventricle.

1. Corpus callosum (body). Commissural fibers interconnecting most cortical areas.
2. Anterior horn of the lateral ventricle.
3. Anterior limb of the internal capsule. Contains projections to and from prefrontal and anterior cingulate cortex, including those from the dorsomedial and anterior nuclei.
4. Insula. Includes gustatory and autonomic areas.
5. Lateral sulcus.
6. Anterior end of the temporal lobe (temporal pole). Limbic cortex.
7. Branches of the middle cerebral artery. Will emerge from the lateral sulcus and supply the lateral surface of the cerebral hemisphere.
8. Olfactory tract. Projections from the olfactory bulb to the piriform cortex and amygala.
9. Anterior cerebral artery. Branches parallel the corpus callosum and supply the medial surface of the frontal and parietal lobes.
10. Gyrus rectus. Part of orbital frontal cortex; extensive limbic connections, particularly in circuits involving the amygdala.

11. Putamen. The part of the striatum with predominantly motor connections.
12. Head of the caudate nucleus, the part of the striatum predominantly connected with association cortex.
13. Septal nuclei. Reciprocally connected with the amygdala, hippocampus, hypothalamus, and other limbic structures.
14. Claustrum. Reciprocal connections with cerebral cortex, poorly understood function.
15. Nucleus accumbens. The part of the striatum with predominantly limbic connections.
16. Globus pallidus (lateral or external segment). Afferents from the striatum, efferents to the subthalamic nucleus.
17. Gray bridges between putamen and caudate nucleus; part of the reason the striatum got its name.
18. Septum pellucidum. Paired membrane separating the two lateral ventricles.
19. Cingulate gyrus. Extensive limbic connections, particularly in circuits involving the hippocampus.

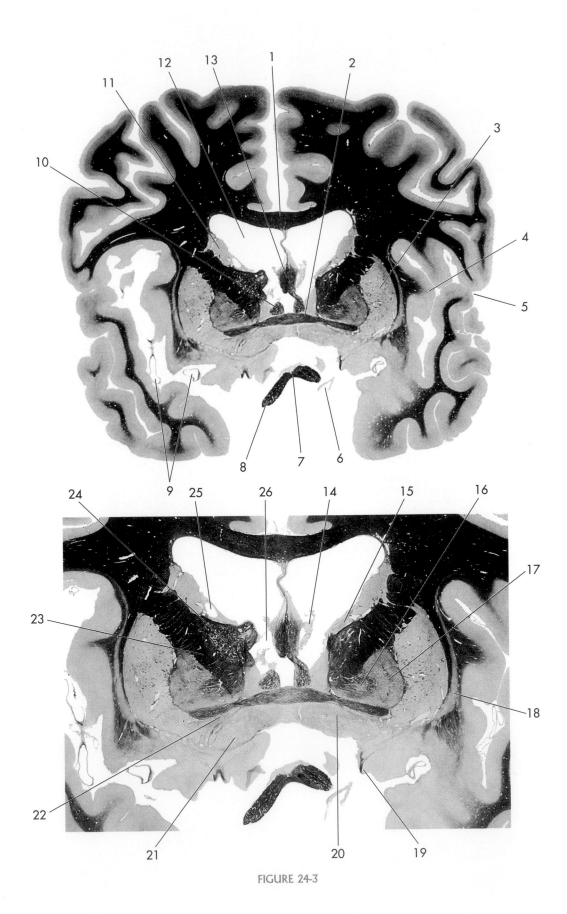

FIGURE 24-3

FIGURE 24-3

Anterior commissure.

1. Corpus callosum (body). Commissural fibers interconnecting most cortical areas.
2. Anterior commissure. Commissural fibers interconnecting the temporal lobes, together with a few crossing olfactory fibers.
3. Putamen. The part of the striatum with predominantly motor connections.
4. Insula. Includes gustatory and autonomic areas.
5. Lateral sulcus.
6. Internal carotid artery, just before it bifurcates into the anterior and middle cerebral arteries.
7. Optic chiasm, where optic nerve fibers from the nasal half of each retina decussate.
8. Optic nerve. Axons of retinal ganglion cells on their way to the lateral geniculate nucleus, superior colliculus, and a few other sites.
9. Branches of the middle cerebral artery. Will emerge from the lateral sulcus and supply the lateral surface of the cerebral hemisphere.
10. Column of the fornix. Efferents from the hippocampus to the septal area and mammillary bodies.
11. Junction between the head and body of the caudate nucleus, the part of the striatum predominantly connected with association cortex.
12. Junction between the anterior horn and body of the lateral ventricle.
13. Body of the fornix. Efferents from the hippocampus to the septal area and mammillary bodies.
14. Choroid plexus adjacent to the interventricular foramen.
15. Stria terminalis. Efferents from the amygdala to the septal area and hypothalamus.
16. Globus pallidus (medial or internal segment). Afferents from the striatum and subthalamic nucleus, efferents to the thalamus.
17. Globus pallidus (lateral or external segment). Afferents from the striatum, efferents to the subthalamic nucleus.
18. Claustrum. Reciprocal connections with cerebral cortex, poorly understood function.
19. Olfactory tract. Projections from the olfactory bulb to the piriform cortex and amygdala.
20. Location of the basal nucleus (of Meynert). Groups of large cholinergic neurons, situated in the substantia innominata, that innervate most forebrain areas.
21. Nucleus accumbens. The part of the striatum with predominantly limbic connections.
22. Ventral pallidum. Limbic extension of the globus pallidus, with inputs from the nucleus accumbens.
23. Genu of the internal capsule. Contains projections to and from frontal cortex.
24. Reticular nucleus, covering the anterior (and lateral) surface of the thalamus. Afferents from the thalamus and cerebral cortex, GABAergic efferents to the thalamus.
25. Terminal (thalamostriate) vein, adjacent to the stria terminalis.
26. Interventricular foramen.

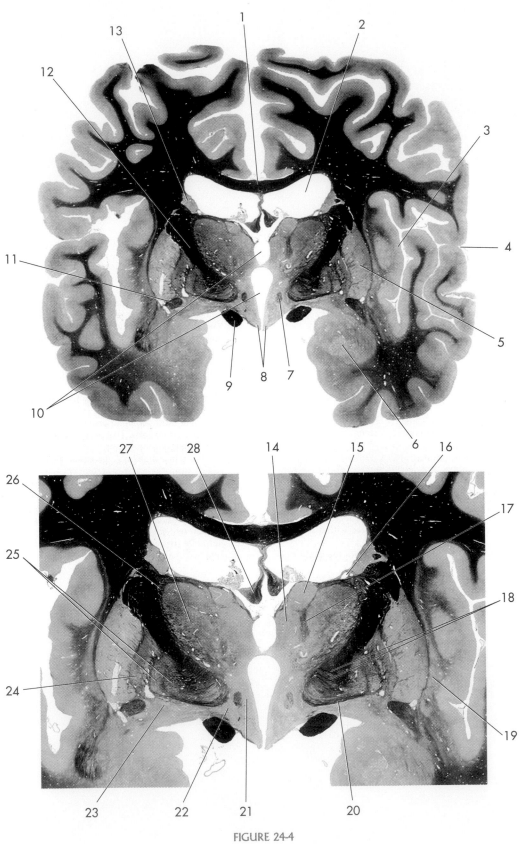

FIGURE 24-4

FIGURE 24-4

Anterior thalamus.

1. Corpus callosum (body). Commissural fibers interconnecting most cortical areas.
2. Body of the lateral ventricle.
3. Insula. Includes gustatory and autonomic areas.
4. Lateral sulcus.
5. Putamen. The part of the striatum with predominantly motor connections.
6. Amygdala. A collection of nuclei forming the core of one of the two major limbic circuits.
7. Column of the fornix. Efferents from the hippocampus to the mammillary bodies.
8. Median eminence of the hypothalamus. Former attachment point of the infundibular stalk.
9. Optic tract. Axons of ganglion cells from half of each retina, on their way to the lateral geniculate nucleus, superior colliculus, and a few other sites.
10. Third ventricle. The two portions indicated are separated by the interthalamic adhesion (massa intermedia).
11. Fibers that will cross in the anterior commissure, interconnecting the temporal lobes.
12. Posterior limb of the internal capsule. Contains projections to and from sensorimotor and parietal cortex, including corticospinal fibers and the somatosensory radiation.
13. Body of the caudate nucleus, the part of the striatum predominantly connected with association cortex.
14. Dorsomedial nucleus. Connections with prefrontal association cortex.
15. Anterior nucleus. Afferents from the mammillary body (via the mammillothalamic tract), efferents to the cingulate gyrus.
16. Terminal (thalamostriate) vein, adjacent to the stria terminalis.
17. Mammillothalamic tract. Projection from the mammillary body to the anterior nucleus of the thalamus. Part of the Papez circuit.
18. Lenticular fasciculus (passing through the internal capsule). Part of the projection from the globus pallidus to the thalamus.
19. Claustrum. Reciprocal connections with cerebral cortex, poorly understood function.
20. Ansa lenticularis. Part of the projection from the globus pallidus to the thalamus.
21. Medial zone of the hypothalamus. At this level, includes the ventromedial and dorsomedial nuclei.
22. Lateral hypothalamic nucleus.
23. Location of the basal nucleus (of Meynert). Groups of large cholinergic neurons, situated in the substantia innominata, that innervate most forebrain areas.
24. Globus pallidus (lateral or external segment). Afferents from the striatum, efferents to the subthalamic nucleus.
25. Globus pallidus (medial or internal segment). Afferents from the striatum and subthalamic nucleus, efferents to the thalamus.
26. Reticular nucleus of the thalamus. Afferents from the thalamus and cerebral cortex, GABAergic efferents to the thalamus.
27. Ventral anterior and ventral lateral nuclei (VA/VL). Afferents from the cerebellum and basal ganglia, efferents to motor areas of cortex.
28. Body of the fornix. Efferents from the hippocampus to the septal area and mammillary bodies.

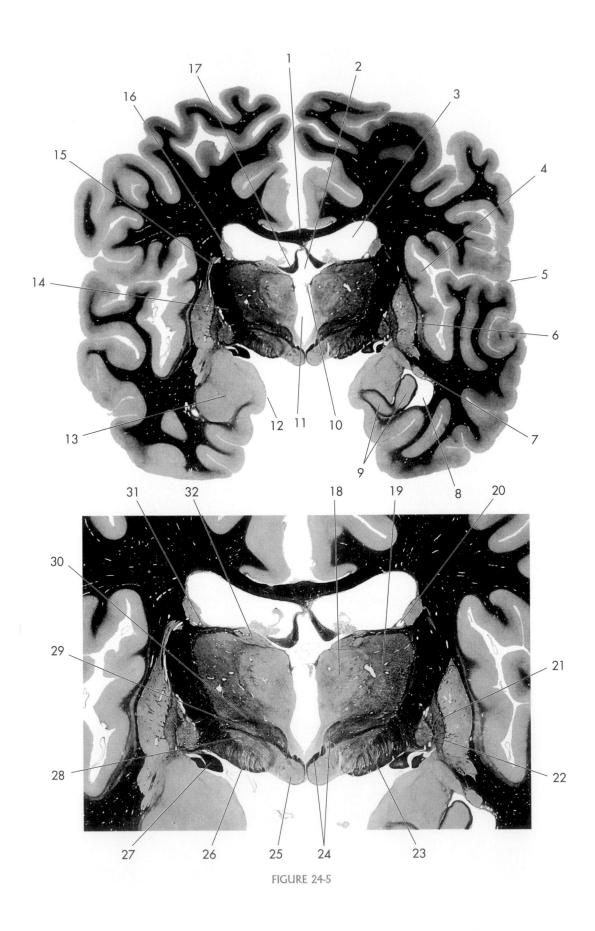

FIGURE 24-5

FIGURE 24-5

Midthalamus; mammillary bodies.

1. Corpus callosum (body). Commissural fibers interconnecting most cortical areas.
2. Transverse cerebral fissure. An extension of subarachnoid space, situated above the roof of the third ventricle and containing the internal cerebral veins.
3. Body of the lateral ventricle.
4. Insula. Includes gustatory and autonomic areas.
5. Lateral sulcus.
6. Putamen. The part of the striatum with predominantly motor connections.
7. Tail of the caudate nucleus, the part of the striatum predominantly connected with association cortex.
8. Inferior horn of the lateral ventricle.
9. Anterior end of the hippocampus, the core of one of the two major limbic circuits.
10. Choroid plexus in the roof of the third ventricle.
11. Third ventricle, the slit-shaped cavity of the diencephalon.
12. Uncus. The proximity of the surface of the uncus to the cerebral peduncle can cause clinical problems.
13. Amygdala. A collection of nuclei forming the core of one of the two major limbic circuits.
14. Posterior limb of the internal capsule. Contains projections to and from sensorimotor and parietal cortex, including corticospinal fibers and the somatosensory radiation.
15. Gray bridge between putamen and caudate nucleus; part of the reason the striatum got its name.
16. Body of the caudate nucleus, the part of the striatum predominantly connected with association cortex.
17. Body of the fornix. Efferents from the hippocampus to the septal area and mammillary bodies.
18. Dorsomedial nucleus. Connections with prefrontal association cortex.
19. Ventral lateral nucleus (VL). Afferents from the cerebellum and basal ganglia (primarily the former), efferents to motor areas of cortex.
20. Terminal (thalamostriate) vein, adjacent to the stria terminalis.
21. Globus pallidus (lateral or external segment). Afferents from the caudate nucleus and putamen, efferents to the subthalamic nucleus.
22. Globus pallidus (medial or internal segment). Afferents from the caudate nucleus, putamen, and subthalamic nucleus, efferents to the thalamus.
23. Lenticular fasciculus. Part of the projection from the globus pallidus to the thalamus.
24. Mammillothalamic tract. Projection from the mammillary body to the anterior nucleus of the thalamus. Part of the Papez circuit.
25. Mammillary body. Afferents from the hippocampus, efferents to the anterior nucleus of the thalamus. Part of the Papez circuit.
26. Substantia nigra. The reticular part receives inputs from the striatum and projects to the thalamus; the compact part contains pigmented, dopaminergic neurons that project to the striatum.
27. Optic tract. Axons of ganglion cells from half of each retina, on their way to the lateral geniculate nucleus, superior colliculus, and a few other sites.
28. Subthalamic nucleus. Afferents from motor cortex and the external segment of the globus pallidus, excitatory efferents to the internal segment of the globus pallidus.
29. Zona incerta. One more source of direct inputs to the cerebral cortex; function unknown.
30. Thalamic fasciculus. Projections from the cerebellum and basal ganglia to the ventral anterior and ventral lateral nuclei (VA/VL).
31. Stria terminalis. Efferents from the amygdala to the septal area and hypothalamus.
32. Lateral dorsal nucleus. Efferents to the cingulate gyrus.

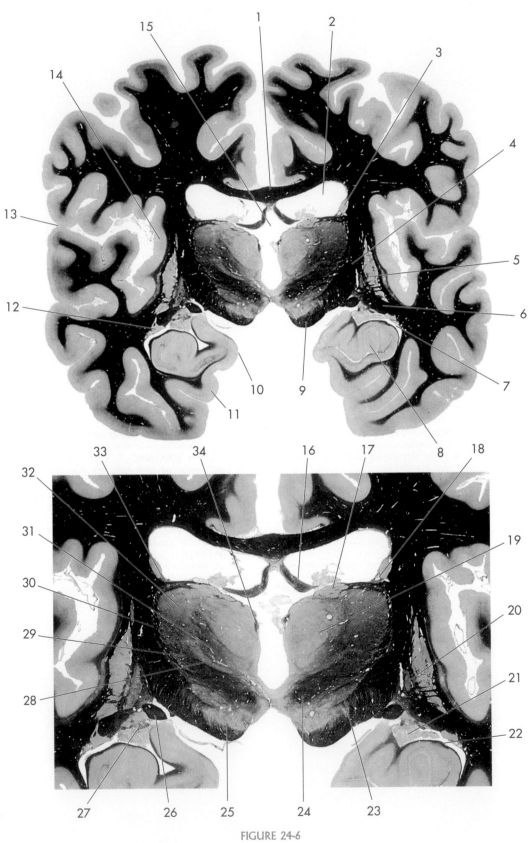

FIGURE 24-6

FIGURE 24-6

Midthalamus.

1. Corpus callosum (body). Commissural fibers interconnecting most cortical areas.
2. Body of the lateral ventricle.
3. Body of the caudate nucleus, the part of the striatum predominantly connected with association cortex.
4. Posterior limb of the internal capsule. Contains projections to and from sensorimotor and parietal cortex, including corticospinal fibers and the somatosensory radiation.
5. Putamen. The part of the striatum with predominantly motor connections.
6. Sublenticular part of the internal capsule. Contains projections to and from temporal and some other cortical areas, including the auditory radiation and part of the optic radiation.
7. Inferior horn of the lateral ventricle.
8. Hippocampus, the core of one of the two major limbic circuits.
9. Basis pedunculi (of the cerebral peduncle). Corticospinal, corticobulbar, and corticopontine fibers.
10. Uncus. The proximity of the surface of the uncus to the cerebral peduncle can cause clinical problems.
11. Parahippocampal gyrus. This anterior level is entorhinal cortex, source of most afferents to the hippocampus.
12. Tail of the caudate nucleus, the part of the striatum predominantly connected with association cortex.
13. Lateral sulcus.
14. Insula. Includes gustatory and autonomic areas.
15. Transverse cerebral fissure. An extension of subarachnoid space, situated above the roof of the third ventricle and containing the internal cerebral veins.
16. Body of the fornix. Efferents from the hippocampus to the septal area and mammillary bodies.
17. Lateral dorsal nucleus. Efferents to the cingulate gyrus.
18. Terminal (thalamostriate) vein, with adjacent stria terminalis.
19. Dorsomedial nucleus. Connections with prefrontal association cortex.
20. Globus pallidus (lateral or external segment). Afferents from the striatum, efferents to the subthalamic nucleus.

21. Choroid plexus in the inferior horn of the lateral ventricle.
22. Alveus. Hippocampal efferents on the ventricular surface of the hippocampus.
23. Subthalamic nucleus. Afferents from motor cortex and the external segment of the globus pallidus, excitatory efferents to the internal segment of the globus pallidus.
24. Rostral end of the red nucleus, surrounded by cerebellar efferents on their way to the thalamus.
25. Substantia nigra. The reticular part receives inputs from the striatum and projects to the thalamus; the compact part contains pigmented, dopaminergic neurons that project to the striatum.
26. Optic tract. Axons of ganglion cells from half of each retina, on their way to the lateral geniculate nucleus, superior colliculus, and a few other sites.
27. Stria terminalis, which has now emerged from the posterior surface of the amygdala. Efferents from the amygdala to the septal area and hypothalamus.
28. Ventral posteromedial nucleus (VPM). Afferents from trigeminal and solitary nuclei, efferents to somatosensory and gustatory cortex.
29. Ventral posterolateral nucleus (VPL). Afferents from the spinal cord (spinothalamic tract) and posterior column nuclei, efferents to somatosensory cortex.
30. Reticular nucleus of the thalamus. Afferents from the thalamus and cerebral cortex, GABAergic efferents to the thalamus.
31. Centromedian nucleus, the largest of the intralaminar nuclei. Afferents from the globus pallidus, efferents to the striatum.
32. Ventral lateral nucleus (VL). Afferents from the cerebellum and basal ganglia (primarily the former), efferents to motor areas of cortex.
33. Stria terminalis. Efferents from the amygdala to the septal area and hypothalamus.
34. Stria medullaris of the thalamus. Site of attachment of the roof of the third ventricle, and a route through which septal efferents reach the habenula.

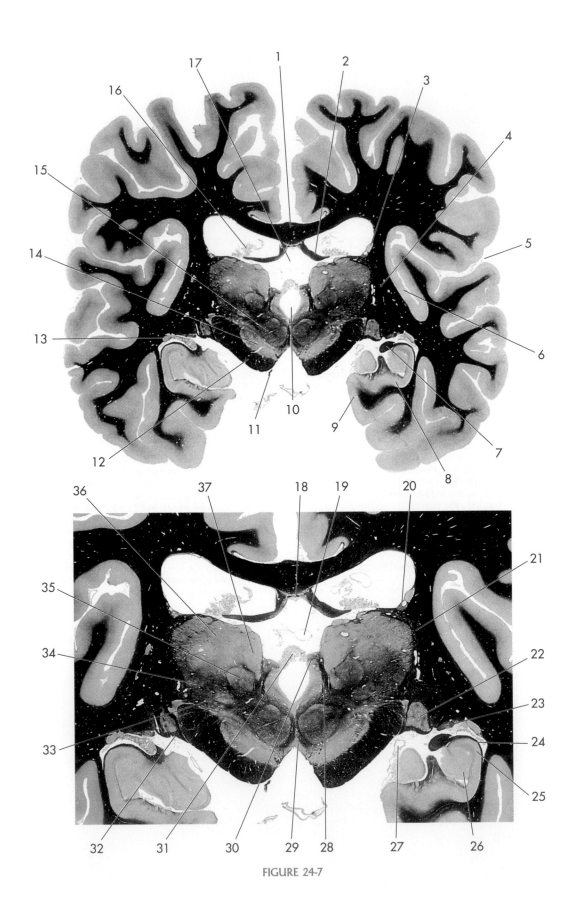

FIGURE 24-7

FIGURE 24-7

Posterior thalamus; habenula.

1. Corpus callosum (body). Commissural fibers interconnecting most cortical areas.
2. Body of the fornix. Efferents from the hippocampus to the septal area and mammillary bodies.
3. Body of the caudate nucleus, the part of the striatum predominantly connected with association cortex.
4. Retrolenticular part of the internal capsule. Contains projections to and from the parietal and occipital lobes, including part of the optic radiation.
5. Lateral sulcus.
6. Insula. Includes gustatory and autonomic areas.
7. Fimbria of the hippocampus. Hippocampal efferents that have assembled from the alveus, on their way into the fornix.
8. Subiculum, a subdivision of the hippocampus and its principal source of efferents. Afferents from the hippocampus proper.
9. Parahippocampal gyrus. This anterior level is entorhinal cortex, source of most afferents to the hippocampus.
10. Third ventricle, near the aqueduct.
11. Oculomotor nerve, just emerging from the midbrain.
12. Basis pedunculi (of the cerebral peduncle). Corticospinal, corticobulbar, and corticopontine fibers.
13. Tail of the caudate nucleus, the part of the striatum predominantly connected with association cortex.
14. Substantia nigra. The reticular part receives inputs from the striatum and projects to the thalamus; the compact part contains pigmented, dopaminergic neurons that project to the striatum.
15. Red nucleus. Afferents from the cerebellum, efferents to the inferior olivary nucleus and spinal cord.
16. Choroid plexus in the body of the lateral ventricle.
17. Transverse cerebral fissure. An extension of subarachnoid space, situated above the roof of the third ventricle and containing the internal cerebral veins.
18. Hippocampal commissure. Fibers interconnecting the two hippocampi.
19. Internal cerebral vein, on its way to the great cerebral vein (of Galen).
20. Stria terminalis (adjacent to terminal vein). Efferents from the amygdala to the septal area and hypothalamus.
21. Reticular nucleus of the thalamus. Afferents from the thalamus and cerebral cortex, GABAergic efferents to the thalamus.
22. Lateral geniculate nucleus. Afferents from the retina, efferents to visual cortex.
23. Stria terminalis. Efferents from the amygdala to the septal area and hypothalamus.
24. Alveus. Hippocampal efferents on the ventricular surface of the hippocampus.
25. Hippocampus proper (cornu ammonis), a subdivision of the hippocampus. Afferents from the dentate gyrus, efferents to the subiculum and septal area.
26. Dentate gyrus, a subdivision of the hippocampus. Afferents from entorhinal cortex, efferents to hippocampal pyramidal cells.
27. Posterior cerebral artery.
28. Fasciculus retroflexus (= habenulointerpeduncular tract!). Conveys limbic output from the habenula to the midbrain reticular formation.
29. Ventral tegmental area. Contains dopaminergic neurons that project to a variety of limbic and neocortical areas.
30. Habenula, a relay in caudally directed limbic projections. Afferents from the septal area, efferents to the midbrain reticular formation.
31. Choroid plexus in the roof of the third ventricle.
32. Optic tract entering the lateral geniculate nucleus.
33. Ventral posteromedial nucleus (VPM). Afferents from trigeminal and solitary nuclei, efferents to somatosensory and gustatory cortex.
34. Ventral posterolateral nucleus (VPL). Afferents from the spinal cord (spinothalamic tract) and posterior column nuclei, efferents to somatosensory cortex.
35. Centromedian nucleus, the largest of the intralaminar nuclei. Afferents from the globus pallidus, efferents to the striatum.
36. Lateral posterior nucleus. Connections, similar to those of the pulvinar, with parietal-occipital-temporal association cortex.
37. Dorsomedial nucleus. Connections with prefrontal association cortex.

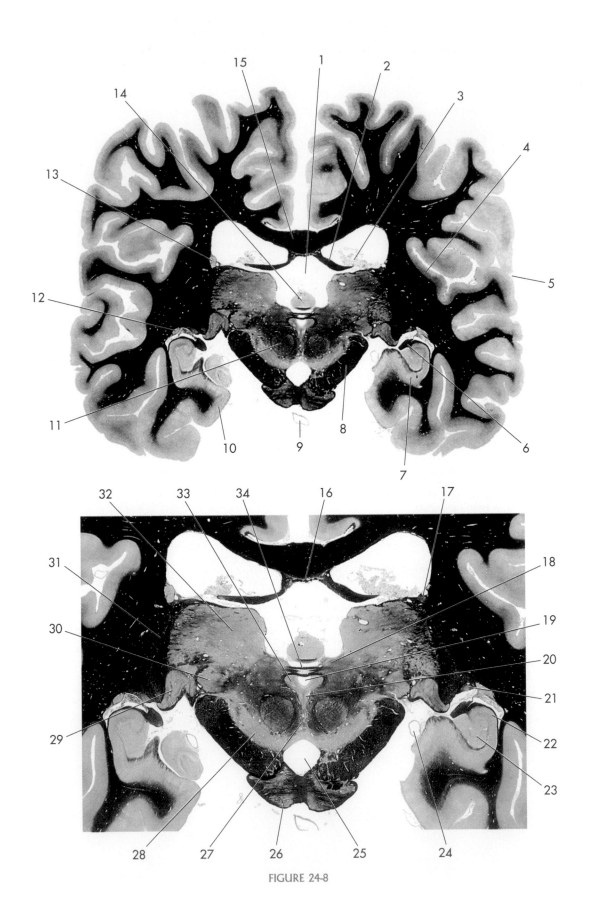

FIGURE 24-8

FIGURE 24-8

Posterior commissure.

1. Superior cistern, a subarachnoid cistern continuous anteriorly with the transverse fissure above the roof of the third ventricle.
2. Body of the fornix. Efferents from the hippocampus to the septal area and mammillary bodies.
3. Choroid plexus in the body of the lateral ventricle.
4. Insula. Includes gustatory and autonomic areas.
5. Lateral sulcus.
6. Fimbria of the hippocampus. Hippocampal efferents that have assembled from the alveus, on their way into the fornix.
7. Subiculum, a subdivision of the hippocampus and its principal source of efferents. Afferents from the hippocampus proper.
8. Basis pedunculi (of the cerebral peduncle). Corticospinal, corticobulbar, and corticopontine fibers.
9. Basilar artery.
10. Parahippocampal gyrus. This anterior level is entorhinal cortex, source of most afferents to the hippocampus.
11. Red nucleus. Afferents from the cerebellum, efferents to the inferior olivary nucleus and spinal cord.
12. Tail of the caudate nucleus, the part of the striatum predominantly connected with association cortex.
13. Body of the caudate nucleus, the part of the striatum predominantly connected with association cortex.
14. Pineal gland. An endocrine gland important in seasonal cycles of some animals; function unclear in humans.
15. Corpus callosum (body). Commissural fibers interconnecting most cortical areas.
16. Hippocampal commissure. Fibers interconnecting the two hippocampi.
17. Stria terminalis (adjacent to terminal vein). Efferents from the amygdala to the septal area and hypothalamus.
18. Pretectal area. Part of the pupillary light reflex pathway; afferents from retinal ganglion cells, efferents to the Edinger-Westphal nucleus.
19. Cerebral aqueduct, the connection between the third and fourth ventricles.

20. Oculomotor nucleus. Lower motor neurons for extraocular muscles and the levator palpebrae, preganglionic parasympathetic neurons for the ciliary muscle and pupillary sphincter.
21. Stria terminalis. Efferents from the amygdala to the septal area and hypothalamus.
22. Hippocampus proper (cornu ammonis), a subdivision of the hippocampus. Afferents from the dentate gyrus, efferents to the subiculum and septal area.
23. Dentate gyrus, a subdivision of the hippocampus. Afferents from entorhinal cortex, efferents to hippocampal pyramidal cells.
24. Posterior cerebral artery.
25. Interpeduncular cistern, the subarachnoid cistern between the cerebral peduncles.
26. Most rostral pontine nuclei. Afferents from cerebral cortex (via the cerebral peduncle), efferents to contralateral cerebellar cortex (via the middle cerebellar peduncle).
27. Ventral tegmental area. Contains dopaminergic neurons that project to a variety of limbic and neocortical areas.
28. Substantia nigra. The reticular part receives inputs from the striatum and projects to the thalamus; the compact part contains pigmented, dopaminergic neurons that project to the striatum.
29. Lateral geniculate nucleus. Afferents from the retina, efferents to visual cortex.
30. Medial geniculate nucleus. Auditory afferents via the inferior brachium, efferents to auditory cortex.
31. Reticular nucleus of the thalamus. Afferents from the thalamus and cerebral cortex, GABAergic efferents to the thalamus.
32. Pulvinar. Connections with parietal-occipital-temporal association cortex.
33. Periaqueductal gray. Part of a descending pain-control pathway.
34. Posterior commissure. Crossing fibers dealing with vertical eye movements and the pupillary light reflex.

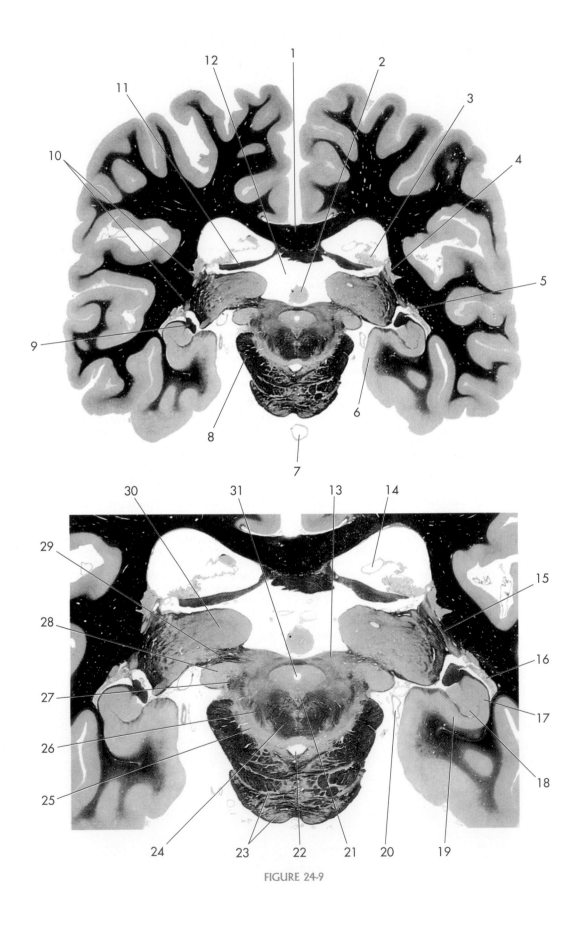

FIGURE 24-9

FIGURE 24-9

Posterior thalamus; midbrain.

1. Corpus callosum (splenium). Commissural fibers interconnecting most cortical areas.
2. Pineal gland. An endocrine gland important in seasonal cycles of some animals; function unclear in humans.
3. Choroid plexus in the body of the lateral ventricle.
4. Body of the caudate nucleus, the part of the striatum predominantly connected with association cortex.
5. Tail of the caudate nucleus, the part of the striatum predominantly connected with association cortex.
6. Parahippocampal gyrus, continuous with the cingulate gyrus near the splenium of the corpus callosum.
7. Basilar artery.
8. Basis pedunculi (of the cerebral peduncle). Corticospinal, corticobulbar, and corticopontine fibers.
9. Fimbria of the hippocampus. Hippocampal efferents that have assembled from the alveus, on their way into the fornix.
10. Stria terminalis. Efferents from the amygdala to the septal area and hypothalamus.
11. Crus of the fornix. Efferents from the hippocampus to the septal area and mammillary bodies.
12. Superior cistern, a subarachnoid cistern continuous anteriorly with the transverse fissure above the roof of the third ventricle.
13. Rostral end of the superior colliculus. Afferents from the retina and visual cortex, efferents to the pulvinar and other structures; functions in visual attention and eye movements.
14. Choroidal vein, draining the choroid plexus of the lateral ventricle.
15. Stria terminalis cut tangentially as it curves around with the lateral ventricle. Efferents from the amygdala to the septal area and hypothalamus.
16. Choroid plexus in the inferior horn of the lateral ventricle.
17. Hippocampus proper (cornu ammonis), a subdivision of the hippocampus. Afferents from the dentate gyrus, efferents to the subiculum and septal area.
18. Dentate gyrus, a subdivision of the hippocampus. Afferents from entorhinal cortex, efferents to hippocampal pyramidal cells.
19. Subiculum, a subdivision of the hippocampus and its principal source of efferents. Afferents from the hippocampus proper.
20. Posterior cerebral artery.
21. Oculomotor nucleus. Lower motor neurons for extraocular muscles and the levator palpebrae, preganglionic parasympathetic neurons for the ciliary muscle and pupillary sphincter.
22. Interpeduncular cistern, the subarachnoid cistern between the cerebral peduncles.
23. Pontine nuclei. Afferents from cerebral cortex (via the cerebral peduncle), efferents to contralateral cerebellar cortex (via the middle cerebellar peduncle).
24. Crossed superior cerebellar peduncle. Efferents from contralateral deep cerebellar nuclei, on their way to the red nucleus and VL.
25. Substantia nigra. The reticular part receives inputs from the striatum and projects to the thalamus; the compact part contains pigmented, dopaminergic neurons that project to the striatum.
26. Medial lemniscus. Somatosensory afferents from the posterior column nuclei and trigeminal main sensory nucleus, on their way to VPL/VPM.
27. Inferior brachium (brachium of the inferior colliculus). Auditory afferents from the inferior colliculus entering the medial geniculate nucleus.
28. Medial geniculate nucleus. Auditory afferents via the inferior brachium, efferents to auditory cortex.
29. Superior brachium (brachium of the superior colliculus). Contains afferents from the retina and visual cortex to the superior colliculus and pretectal area.
30. Pulvinar. Connections with parietal-occipital-temporal association cortex.
31. Cerebral aqueduct, the connection between the third and fourth ventricles.

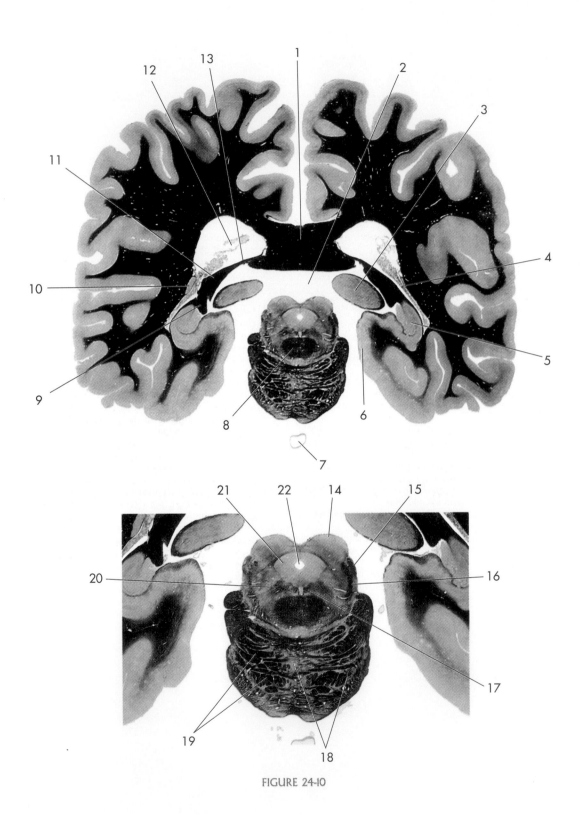

FIGURE 24-10

FIGURE 24-10

Atrium of the lateral ventricle.

1. Splenium of the corpus callosum. Commissural fibers interconnecting posterior cortical areas.
2. Superior cistern, a subarachnoid cistern continuous anteriorly with the transverse fissure above the roof of the third ventricle.
3. Pulvinar. Connections with parietal-occipital-temporal association cortex.
4. Choroid plexus, cut tangentially as it curves from the body into the inferior horn of the lateral ventricle.
5. Posterior end of the hippocampus, the core of one of the two major limbic circuits.
6. Parahippocampal gyrus, continuous with the cingulate gyrus near the splenium of the corpus callosum.
7. Basilar artery.
8. Decussation of the superior cerebellar peduncles. Efferents from the deep cerebellar nuclei, on their way to the red nucleus and VL.
9. Fimbria of the hippocampus. Hippocampal efferents that have assembled from the alveus, on their way into the fornix.
10. Caudate nucleus, cut tangentially as it curves around with the lateral ventricle.
11. Hippocampal efferent fibers passing from the fimbria of the hippocampus to the crus of the fornix.
12. Glomus, an expanded mass of choroid plexus in the atrium of the lateral ventricle.
13. Crus of the fornix. Efferents from the hippocampus to the septal area and mammillary bodies.
14. Superior colliculus. Afferents from the retina and visual cortex, efferents to the pulvinar and other structures; functions in visual attention and eye movements.
15. Inferior brachium (brachium of the inferior colliculus). Auditory afferents from the inferior colliculus on their way to the medial geniculate nucleus.
16. Medial lemniscus. Somatosensory afferents from the posterior column nuclei and trigeminal main sensory nucleus, on their way to the VPL/VPM.
17. Medial longitudinal fasciculus (MLF). Involved in coordinating horizontal eye movements; includes fibers from contralateral abducens interneurons on their way to medial rectus motor neurons.
18. Pontine nuclei. Afferents from cerebral cortex (via the cerebral peduncle), efferents to contralateral cerebellar cortex (via the middle cerebellar peduncle).
19. Corticospinal, corticopontine, and corticobulbar fibers.
20. Central tegmental tract. A complex bundle that contains fibers descending from the red nucleus to the inferior olivary nucleus, ascending gustatory fibers, and ascending and descending fibers of the reticular formation.
21. Periaqueductal gray. Part of a descending pain-control pathway.
22. Cerebral aqueduct, the connection between the third and fourth ventricles.

Page numbers in italics indicate illustrations; *t* indicates tables; *n* indicates notes.

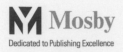
Mosby
Dedicated to Publishing Excellence

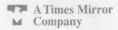
A Times Mirror
Company

WE WANT TO HEAR FROM YOU!

To help us publish the most useful materials for students, we would appreciate your comments on this book. Please take a few moments to complete the form below, then tear it out and mail it to us. Thank you for your input.

Nolte: The Human Brain 4e

1. What year and course of study are you in?

_____Medical school	_____1st year
_____Osteopathic school	_____2nd year
_____Dental school	_____3rd year
_____Pharmacy school	_____4th year
_____Physician assistant program	_____Other _____
_____Nursing school	
_____Other _____	

2. How are you using this book? Please be specific: as a textbook for a course, to refresh the material before a Board exam, etc. If you are using the book for a course, what is the name of the course?

3. Was this book useful to you? Why or why not?

4. What features of textbooks are important to you?

_____Color figures	_____Self-assessment questions
_____Summary tables and boxes	_____Price
_____Summaries	_____Concept-type headings
_____Other _____	

5. What influenced your decision to buy this text?
   _____Required/recommended by instructor
   _____Recommendation by student
   _____Bookstore display
   _____Other _____

6. What other instructional materials did/would you find useful in this course?
   _____Computer-assisted instruction
   _____Slides
   _____Other _____

Are you interested in doing in-depth reviews of our textbooks?   _____Yes   _____No

NAME: _____
ADDRESS: _____
_____
TELEPHONE: _____
FAX: _____
E-MAIL: _____

THANK YOU!